IMPACT OF EMERGING ZOONOTIC DISEASES ON ANIMAL HEALTH

8th Biennial Conference of the Society for Tropical Veterinary Medicine

ANNALS OF THE NEW YORK ACADEMY OF SCIENCES
Volume 1081

IMPACT OF EMERGING ZOONOTIC DISEASES ON ANIMAL HEALTH
8th Biennial Conference of the Society for Tropical Veterinary Medicine

Edited by Edmour F. Blouin and Jean-Charles Maillard

Published by Blackwell Publishing on behalf of the New York Academy of Sciences
Boston, Massachusetts
2006

Library of Congress Cataloging-in-Publication Data

Society for Tropical Veterinary Medicine. Meeting (8th : 2005 :
Hanoi, Vietnam)
    Impact of emerging zoonotic diseases on animal health / 8th
Biennial Conference of the Society for Tropical Veterinary
Medicine ; edited by Edmour F. Blouin and Jean-Charles Maillard.
        p. ; cm. – (Annals of the New York Academy of Sciences, ISSN
0077-8923 ; v. 1373)
    ISBN-13: 978-1-57331-637-8 (alk. paper)
    ISBN-10: 1-57331-637-7 (alk. paper)
    1. Zoonoses–Congresses. I. Blouin, Edmour Francis, 1954- II.
Maillard, Jean-Charles. III. New York Academy of Sciences. IV. Title.
V. Series.
    [DNLM: 1. Zoonoses–transmission–Congresses. 2. Bird
Diseases–prevention & control–Congresses. 3. Disease Transmission,
Horizontal–prevention & control–Congresses. 4. Swine
Diseases–prevention & control–Congresses. 5. Tropical
Medicine–Congresses. 6. Zoonoses–etiology–Congresses.
W1 AN626YL v. 1373 2006 / WC 950 S678i 2006]

    SF740.S63 2005
    636.089'6959–dc22

                                                    2006019684

The *Annals of the New York Academy of Sciences* (ISSN: 0077-8923 [print]; ISSN: 1749-6632 [online]) is published 28 times a year on behalf of the New York Academy of Sciences by Blackwell Publishing, with offices located at 350 Main Street, Malden, Massachusetts 02148 USA, PO Box 1354, Garsington Road, Oxford OX4 2DQ UK, and PO Box 378 Carlton South, 3053 Victoria Australia.

Information for subscribers: Subscription prices for 2006 are: Premium Institutional: $3850.00 (US) and £2139.00 (Europe and Rest of World).
Customers in the UK should add VAT at 5%. Customers in the EU should also add VAT at 5% or provide a VAT registration number or evidence of entitlement to exemption. Customers in Canada should add 7% GST or provide evidence of entitlement to exemption. The Premium Institutional price also includes online access to full-text articles from 1997 to present, where available. For other pricing options or more information about online access to Blackwell Publishing journals, including access information and terms and conditions, please visit www.blackwellpublishing.com/nyas.

Membership information: Members may order copies of the *Annals* volumes directly from the Academy by visiting www.nyas.org/annals, emailing membership@nyas.org, faxing 212-888-2894, or calling 800-843-6927 (US only), or +1 212 838 0230, ext. 345 (International). For more information on becoming a member of the New York Academy of Sciences, please visit www.nyas.org/membership.

Journal Customer Services: For ordering information, claims, and any inquiry concerning your institutional subscription, please contact your nearest office:
UK: Email: customerservices@blackwellpublishing.com; Tel: +44 (0) 1865 778315; Fax +44 (0) 1865 471775
US: Email: customerservices@blackwellpublishing.com; Tel: +1 781 388 8599 or 1 800 835 6770 (Toll free in the USA); Fax: +1 781 388 8232
Asia: Email: customerservices@blackwellpublishing.com; Tel: +65 6511 8000; Fax: +61 3 8359 1120
Members: Claims and inquiries on member orders should be directed to the Academy at email: membership@nyas.org or Tel: +1 212 838 0230 (International) or 800-843-6927 (US only).

Printed in the USA.
Printed on acid-free paper.

Mailing: The *Annals of the New York Academy of Sciences* are mailed Standard Rate.
Postmaster: Send all address changes to *Annals of the New York Academy of Sciences*,
Blackwell Publishing, Inc., Journals Subscription Department, 350 Main Street, Malden,
MA 01248-5020. Mailing to rest of world by DHL Smart and Global Mail.

Disclaimer: The Publisher, the New York Academy of Sciences, and the Editors cannot
be held responsible for errors or any consequences arising from the use of information
contained in this publication; the views and opinions expressed do not necessarily reflect
those of the Publisher, the New York Academy of Sciences, or the Editors.

Annals are available to subscribers online at the New York Academy of Sciences and also at
Blackwell Synergy. Visit www.annalsnyas.org or www.blackwell-synergy.com to search the
articles and register for table of contents e-mail alerts. Access to full text and PDF downloads
of *Annals* articles are available to nonmembers and subscribers on a pay-per-view basis at
www.annalsnyas.org.

The paper used in this publication meets the minimum requirements of the National Standard for Information Sciences Permanence of Paper for Printed Library Materials, ANSI
Z39.48_1984.

ISSN: 0077-8923 (print); 1749-6632 (online)
ISBN-10: 1-57331-637-7 (paper); ISBN-13: 978-1-57331-637-8 (paper)

A catalogue record for this title is available from the British Library.

Digitization of the *Annals of the New York Academy of Sciences*

An agreement has recently been reached between Blackwell Publishing and the New York
Academy of Sciences to digitize the entire run of the *Annals of the New York Academy of
Sciences* back to volume one.

The back files, which have been defined as all of those issues published before 1997, will
be sold to libraries as part of Blackwell Publishing's Legacy Sales Program and hosted on
the Blackwell Synergy website.

Copyright of all material will remain with the rights holder. Contributors: Please contact
Blackwell Publishing if you do not wish an article or picture from the *Annals of the New
York Academy of Sciences* to be included in this digitization project.

ANNALS OF THE NEW YORK ACADEMY OF SCIENCES
Volume 1081
October 2006

IMPACT OF EMERGING ZOONOTIC DISEASES ON ANIMAL HEALTH
8th Biennial Conference of the Society for Tropical Veterinary Medicine

Editors
EDMOUR F. BLOUIN AND JEAN-CHARLES MAILLARD

This volume is the result of a conference entitled **Impact of Emerging Zoonotic Diseases and Animal Health: 8th Biennial Conference of the Society for Tropical Veterinary Medicine,** held on June 26 through July 1, 2005, in Hanoi, Vietnam.

CONTENTS

Part I. Trends in Emerging Zoonoses

Surveillance and Control of Zoonoses

Trends in Avian Zoonoses

Part II. Trends in the Study of Disease Agents

Virology and Bacteriology

Financial assistance was received from:

- French Agricultural Research Center for International Development (CIRAD),
  France
- Food and Agriculture Organisation, United Nations
- APHIS, United States Department of Agriculture
- ARS, United States Department of Agriculture
- Merial Ltd.
- Asian Development Bank

Introduction

This volume represents the program of the 8th Biennial Conference of the Society for Tropical Veterinary Medicine (STVM) held from June 26 through July 1, 2005 in Hanoi, Vietnam. The aim of the society is to promote the international advancement of veterinary medicine, hygiene, and related disciplines in tropical countries all around the world. The conferences promote international information exchange on timely issues affecting global animal health. This was the first STVM conference in Asia, and the theme was the "Impact of Emerging Zoonotic Diseases on Animal Health." The Indochina peninsula and particularly Vietnam are among the most important hot spots for biodiversity in the world. This region of Southeast Asia is also an area of intense demographic development. The need to protect the great biodiversity of the region places great constraints on the use of natural spaces, such as forests and preserves, and often conflicts with the need for sustainable intensification of agricultural and animal production. Human, domestic animal, and wildlife habitats have increasingly overlapped, and the intersection has resulted in modified patterns of interaction between wild and domestic animals and humans. In such an environmental context we can expect to see changes in disease transmission between animals and humans. We have already seen an increase in incidence of previously identified zoonoses, but the recent epidemic crises associated with the emergence of new zoonotic diseases, such as severe acute respiratory syndrome (SARS) and avian influenza, emphasize our need to understand and control disease emergence. The necessity for sustained development and growth of animals in the tropics requires that we identify and control factors that contribute to the emergence of these and other diseases. These factors have a direct effect on the animal health and our ability to maintain it. We need to evaluate the risks of emergence at different levels, including the optimization of diagnostic tools and organization of control and prevention programs. Maintaining animal health in tropical Asian regions has a profound impact on tropical veterinary medicine and during a time of increased international trade and human mobility has implications for animal health worldwide.

This conference format included 12 symposia and plenary sessions and was attended by some 130 participants from 32 countries, with 40% representing Asian countries. Oral communications, poster sessions, and workshops provided many opportunities for discussions between the international and national participants. The majority of these presentations are collected in this

Ann. N.Y. Acad. Sci. 1081: xv–xvi (2006). © 2006 New York Academy of Sciences.
doi: 10.1196/annals.1373.000

special issue. One specific workshop on Highly Pathogenic Avian Influenza was very fruitful, especially regarding the management of vaccination, and recommendations from this session are included.

On behalf of the board and all the members of the Society for Tropical Veterinary Medicine, we take great pleasure in thanking the Vietnamese authorities, for their strong support in making the STVM 2005 Conference such a success, and particularly Drs. Bui Ba Bong, Truong Van Dung, and To Long Thanh from the Ministry of Agriculture and Rural Development.

We hope you find the papers in this volume interesting. We are grateful to the Editorial Board of the *Annals of the New York Academy of Sciences* and Blackwell Publishing for providing editorial assistance and the opportunity to present these proceedings.

—EDMOUR F. BLOUIN
Department of Veterinary Pathobiology
Center for Veterinary Health Sciences
Oklahoma State University, Stillwater
Oklahoma 74078, USA

—JEAN-CHARLES MAILLARD
CIRAD-EMVT/PRISE–c/o
NIAH, Thuy Phuong, Tu Liem
Hanoi, Vietnam

Dedication

Jim C. Williams

Dr. Jim Williams served as president of the American Society for Tropical Veterinary Medicine from 1989 to 1993. The organization was originally established as an affiliated organization of the American Society for Tropical Medicine and Hygiene. Dr. Williams restructured ASTVM into an independent organization, which subsequently became the Society for Tropical Veterinary Medicine.

Dr. Williams received his M.S. and Ph.D. from Texas A & M University. He served as chief of the Rickettsial Diseases Laboratory, Airborne Diseases Division, U.S. Army Medical Research Institute of Infectious Diseases from 1983 to 1987, and then became chief of the Intracellular Pathogens Branch of the Bacteriology Division at USAMRIID until 1991. He then was named Director of Regulatory Affairs, Food and Drug Administration, Office of Vaccines.

Dr. Williams joined industry and served in various administrative positions and presently is Chief Operating Officer of PharmaFrontiers in Woodlands, TX. He is an expert in product approval, scientific and regulatory review of investigational new drug applications, and in the development of criteria and standards for vaccine development and approval. His memberships in professional societies are numerous, including the American Society for Microbiology, Commissioned Officers Association, Reserve Officers Association, and the Regulatory Affairs Professional Society. He was honored in 1991 with a Scroll of Appreciation by USAMRIID during Operation Desert Shield and Desert Storm; in 1991 with the Public Health Service Commendation Medal, Individual Honor Award; and in 1994 with the Public Health Service Outstanding Unit Commendation for Excellence in Scientific and Regulatory Management of the CBER International Combined Vaccines Workshop.

When Jim became president of ASTVM, he inherited an organization fraught with problems and minimal funds in the treasury. However, together with Dr. Vanessa Sanchez (the organizing committee of two) they persevered to plan the first STVM Biennial meeting that was held in Puerto Rico in February 1991. Desert Storm, which began in January, greatly limited the attendance at the

Address for correspondence: Katherine M. Kocan, Department of Veterinary Pathobiology, Center for Veterinary Health Sciences, Oklahoma State University, Stillwater, OK 74078. Voice: 405-744-7271; fax: 405-744-5275.

e-mail: katherine.kocan@okstate.edu

Ann. N.Y. Acad. Sci. 1081: xvii–xviii (2006). © 2006 New York Academy of Sciences.
doi: 10.1196/annals.1373.084

last minute because of government travel restrictions. Nonetheless, the meeting, attended by approximately 65 quality scientists, was highly successful. An excellent keynote address was presented by Dr. Yilma on development of rinderpest vaccines. This first meeting became the model for future ones, in which a relevant scientific venue and social activities are combined in a tropical/international venue. Jim created in a new logo for ASTVM, and the organization name was subsequently changed to STVM, which reflects the international nature of the organization. Dr. Williams was named an honorary member of STVM in 1996. Because of Jim Williams' efforts, STVM has evolved into an international organization with members representing approximately 40 countries worldwide. The organization has developed a keen interest in promoting students, with the establishment of the Norval-Young Award, a Career Development Award, and most recently, the Alain Provost Award, sponsored by CIRAD-EMVT. Herein we dedicate STVM-05 to Dr. Jim Williams. Thank you Jim from all of us at STVM!

—KATHERINE M. KOCAN
Department of Veterinary Pathobiology
Center for Veterinary Health Sciences
Oklahoma State University, Stillwater,
Oklahoma 74078, USA

Biodiversity and Emerging Diseases

JEAN-CHARLES MAILLARD[a] AND JEAN-PAUL GONZALEZ[b]

[a] Cirad-Emvt/PRISE, Hanoi, Vietnam

[b] IRD/UR178, RCEVD, IST, Mahidol University, Nakhonpathom, Thailand

ABSTRACT: First we remind general considerations concerning biodiversity on earth and particularly the loss of genetic biodiversity that seems irreversible whether its origin is directly or indirectly linked to human activities. Urgent and considerable efforts must be made from now on to cataloge, understand, preserve, and enhance the value of biodiversity while ensuring food safety and human and animal health. Ambitious integrated and multifield research programs must be implemented in order to understand the causes and anticipate the consequences of loss of biodiversity. Such losses are a serious threat to sustainable development and to the quality of life of future generations. They have an influence on the natural balance of global biodiversity in particularly in reducing the capability of species to adapt rapidly by genetic mutations to survive in modified ecosystems. Usually, the natural immune systems of mammals (both human and animal), are highly polymorphic and able to adapt rapidly to new situations. We more specifically discuss the fact that if the genetic diversity of the affected populations is low the invading microorganisms, will suddenly expand and create epidemic outbreaks with risks of pandemic. So biodiversity appears to function as an important barrier (buffer), especially against disease-causing organisms, which can function in different ways. Finally, we discuss the importance of preserving biodiversity mainly in the wildlife ecosystems as an integrated and sustainable approach among others in order to prevent and control the emergence or reemergence of diseases in animals and humans (zoonosis). Although plants are also part of this paradigm, they fall outside our field of study.

KEYWORDS: biodiversity; emerging diseases; immunogenetics; breeding intensification

"Human beings modify the environment and the environment modifies part of human beings directly dependent on environmental change."
(Jiddu Krishnamurti, 1934)

Address for correspondence: Dr. Maillard Jean-Charles, CIRAD-EMVT/PRISE –c/o NIAH, Thuy Phuong, Tu Liem, Hanoi, Vietnam. Voice: 84-4-838-8068; fax: 84-4-757-2177.
e-mail: maillard@fpt.vn

Ann. N.Y. Acad. Sci. 1081: 1–16 (2006). © 2006 New York Academy of Sciences.
doi: 10.1196/annals.1373.001

INTRODUCTION

The earth is host to a vast biological diversity that includes greater than the millions of known species, a wealth of genomes, physiological mechanisms, and behaviors. This biological diversity of plants, animals, and microbes creates a complex ecosystem comprising a diversity of individuals and populations. These various levels of diversity are the result of over 3 billion years of continuing evolution, and are an important chapter in the earth's geological timeline. Fewer than two million of the estimated 30 million species have been described, of which 75% are invertebrates. Although biodiversity changes over the long term, man is coming to the realization that many of his harmful actions on the environment have had unprecedented effects on the distribution and number of living species, the stability of ecosystems, and the genetic drift and natural evolution of organisms. The current loss of species rate is notably higher than the natural rate of extinction. Moreover, tens of thousands of other species are already condemned to extinction in a term on a human timescale, largely due to the destruction of habitat across the globe. This loss of biodiversity is caused mainly by economic and demographic factors, and especially by the increasing demand for space and biological resources needed to sustain global production and the growth of human population, its consumption, and its trade. Furthermore, we are currently witnessing the loss, fragmentation, and degradation of natural habitat through the overexploitation of biological resources, the introduction of exotic species, soil, water, and atmospheric pollution, and more recently through the first signs of global climate change. The loss of genetic biodiversity seems irreversible whether its origin is directly or indirectly caused by humans. Ambitious integrated and multifield research programs must be implemented in order to understand the causes and anticipate the consequences of loss of biodiversity; *in fine*, their purpose would be to put forward rational strategies for the preservation of biodiversity. On a more general level, such losses have an influence on the natural balance of global biodiversity: "nature hates a vacuum" and manifests itself by systematically replacing destroyed spaces and extinct species with new organisms, which in turn invade and change the environment, adapt rapidly in order to survive, and more often than not, transmit this in their genotype and thus perpetuate this transformation (e.g., genetic mutation). Such "forced" mutations can be silent and without major effects on individuals, ecosystems, or their inhabitants. These changes can have a strong effect on individuals, which may evolve to have increased pathogenicity or fertility, etc., . . . and affect the functioning of an ecosystem, with severe consequences for the other species living within the same ecosystem. For example, from a medical perspective the crossing of species barrier may inflict a new (emerging) parasitism on an unprecedented host, or escaping natural defense mechanisms. However, if the genetic diversity of the affected populations is low (e.g., inbreeding in small populations that are isolated or fragmented, monoclonal populations bred in industrial farms, etc.), the invading microorganisms, will suddenly expand and create epidemic outbreaks with risks of pandemic. Such conditions provide the opportunity for emerging and reemerging diseases, with often severe clinical syndromes and epidemic outbreaks that can be devastating for animals as well as for humans (zoonosis) living in shared ecosystems or in overlapping territories (sympatry). Many pathogens thus threaten humans and domesticated animals when their own natural habitats have been disturbed. In such a context, the interactions between pathogens, the hosts' immune system (human and animal), resistance to drugs, and the density of human and animal populations can cause exotic species to become invasive to hosts without previous exposure or immune response. Inversely, exotic (exogenous) species can introduce pathogens that threaten the local endemic species.

Biodiversity thus appears to function as an important barrier (buffer), especially against disease-causing organisms, which can function in different ways. For example, the polymorphic major histocompatibility complex (MHC) that protects a population or as a dilution effect on pathogens when populations are diversified. This is the case for pathogens transmitted through vectors, such as malaria, sleeping sickness, or West Nile fever, whose vectors turn feed on humans and domesticated animals when the biodiversity of wildlife is restricted.

WHAT EXACTLY IS MEANT BY THE TERM BIODIVERSITY?

Biodiversity involves the entire diversity of the living world, from the very large (natural landscapes) to the very small (genes), and extending from the diversity of ecosystems (oceans, forests, cultivated plains, or desert areas) to the diversity of genomes with their organizations and functions. Biodiversity encompasses the diversity of all living species, including microorganisms (virus, bacteria, prions, rickettsia, parasites, and fungi), algae, plants, and animals, and of their biology, which are all regulated by climates and environments. Biodiversity is therefore a reflection of the manifestation of the differences between living entities (species, populations, individuals. . .) and of the ecological interactions within which species evolve.

It is very difficult to give a precise estimate of the number of species living on the planet. The evaluation bracket is very wide and varies between 5 and 100 million depending on the author. Of the average figure most commonly used of 30 million species, less than 2 million have been described and 75% of these are insects! If one takes into account the fact that each species has at least one species-specific parasitic species (e.g., Wolbachia in insects), this estimate of undescribed species would probably exponentially outnumber "visible" species.

Biological diversity (biodiversity) is descriptive (static) as well as evolutive (dynamic), if one takes into account the totality of interactions and variability of living beings in a heterogeneous and changing world. By interactions, we mean such phenomena of global change, such as climate change, which has a multitude of causes and consequences on the environment.[1] The history of planet earth is made up of a succession of climatic changes, and we are currently going through the sixth great planetary extinction crisis, with a rate of extinction 100 times higher than the average natural rate. Every day, several living species, mostly unknown to us, disappear from the earth. IUCN (World Conservation Union) has published a "red list" of over 7000 known threatened species[2] within the animal kingdom alone, and 25% of the mere 4600 described are threatened with extinction in the relatively short term. (http://www.iucn.org/themes/ssc/red-lists.htm).

The *variability of biodiversity* is largely due to gene mutations (genetic variability), which are random, mostly adaptive and self-preserving, and which allow all organisms to adapt and survive in constraining environments. Without constant and necessary modifications these species would be doomed to extinction.

Genes of epigenetic origin may also play an important role in the evolution of living beings, especially in the transmission of acquired characters, as well as using other evolutionary mechanisms outside of classical Mendelian genetics. This natural (genetic) selection is the theory of the evolution of species as initially developed by Darwin in 1859. Population is the unit of evolutionary change from which diversity originates. Indeed, the evolutionary processes, which maintain organisms in the realm of the living, or the ecological processes, which precipitate them toward extinction, operate at this very level of organic integration.

Local populations and their wealth of genetic diversity must be the focus of our greatest attention, in particular through preservation action. Preservation of biodiversity through the interactions between species and their natural environment has a considerable potential for the evolution of the planet, and one, which must be sustainable so as to allow adaptation and survival in the face of planetary changes. The environment's space–time dynamics is the force, which causes the emergence of species, safeguards their existence, or suddenly causes them to die out forever. This driving power at the heart of biodiversity manifests itself through all sorts of changes, which may be violent, as in the case of accidents and disturbances (natural disasters, storms, fire outbreaks, floods. . .). Less brutal changes to their own environment may be caused by the organisms themselves, and especially humans.

Humans have been interacting with their environment since the Paleolithic era over 12,000 years ago.[3] At first humans evolved in small family groups in very open ecosystems and lived primarily from hunting and gathering. Populations progressively formed villages and domesticated several animal species, as depicted in cave paintings. Such cohabitation between humans, as well as between humans and animals, has influenced both social and health issues.[4] Between 70% and 80% of infectious diseases present in humans have been shown to be of animal origin.[5] Some of these were acquired in the Neolithic era when the first sedentary societies were organized and humans began to practice agriculture and farming using domesticated animals that were once wild. Throughout his history, *Homo sapiens sapiens* has successfully eliminated predators and competitors; however, the same cannot be said for his parasites and pathogens. It is impossible to make even a rough estimate of the number of micro- or macroorganism species that have the potential to be pathogenic for human or animal populations. In human or animal populations, those individuals most susceptible to diseases die, while only those resistant will survive.

Demographic changes have gradually altered living conditions on earth. Today man finds himself responsible for situations far less propitious than ever, which are evolving rapidly. Pollution and the destruction of ecosystems are escalating. Demographic explosion, especially in developing countries, causes increased demand on food supplies of both vegetable and animal origins. Large concentrations of human and domesticated animal populations in the form of megalopolis and breeding units are growing in density with far-reaching consequences for the environment, especially the management of natural (human and animal) and industrial wastes. Contact between human beings, as well as between humans and animals, is increasing both in duration and intensity.[6] Among other things, ongoing contact due to overpopulation and overcrowding causes stresses, which induce discomfort and biological dysfunctions, especially of a physiological nature. Immune defense systems are often disturbed; giving way to the emergence of new (emerging) diseases, or diseases that were thought to be under control or eradicated may reemerge.

Epidemics have increasingly severe consequences and result in greater morbidity and mortality. Industrial farming, with several thousand individuals from the same species and often from the same genetic strain (clone), causes considerable loss of genetic diversity. Epidemics that arise from this environment can then become destructive, as was evidenced by the avian influenza epidemic in Taiwan and more recently in southeast Asia. Pandemics therefore will likely become more frequent and will be enhanced by international trade, especially through air transport. The incubation period of all infectious agents (virus, bacteria, or parasite) is longer than the length of time needed for an individual carrying the germ (with no clinical signs) to fly anywhere on earth, and a pathogen could contaminate the entire planet in less than 24 h.

WHAT IS MEANT BY EMERGING OR REEMERGING DISEASES?

The lightning spread of severe acute respiratory syndrome (SARS), unprecedented in its speed and scope, was a reminder of man's vulnerability in the face of constantly evolving infectious diseases. The current avian influenza epizooty, which once again poses threat to world populations, highlights the magnitude of social damage, and economic loss. For the past few decades, health specialists worldwide have been confronted with emergence of viral fevers, identification of pathologies linked to previously no described germs as well as with the overwhelming worldwide spread of acquired immune deficiency syndrome (AIDS). The increasing numbers of epidemic phenomena, which appear in specific epidemiological contexts, and which imply previously no described human risk (dams and water-related diseases; deforestation and zoonosis acquired through contact with wild animals) have led the scientific community to assess these infections and to research and define the concept of new or emerging disease associated with risk factors.[7]

While emergence of new diseases appears to be linked with human behavior, natural changes in the environment must also be taken into account in this analysis (e.g., health issues caused by supraseasonal climate trends, El Nino, global warming, degradation of the ozone layer). The serious risks of emergence of infectious diseases in general, and zoonosis in particular, justify the need for integrated studies with multifield scientific approaches. Whether in the northern or southern hemispheres, identification of factors and areas of disease emergence need to be defined, along with the fundamental mechanisms that result from environmental changes previously not described of natural or human origin. A broader knowledge of emergence factors linked with human, animal hosts (mammals), or vectors/vector-borne pathogens, will allow for definition risk factors that will provide a basis for designing prevention and control strategies. Genetics (phylogenies) research on arthropod vectors and studies on bioecology of hosts and pathogens coevolution are also much needed.

The concept of pathocenosis[8] can be developed when the interaction of pathogens and the events that lead to epidemization are defined. Prediction of outbreaks could then be made by modeling the emergence and diffusion of diseases, in relation to the balance of biotopes, and emergence of invasive species that result from extinction or suppression of populations, pathogens, or hosts.[9] Evolutionary biology (of hosts and parasites) as much as human and social sciences concerned with the evolution of societies are the domains in which this research could be conducted and where emergence intervention/prevention system could then be applied.

Our ability to understand the dynamics of emergence is tied to the following essential questions. Where do pathogens come from? Is it possible to detect pathogens with the potential for emergence? What are the conditions (macro- and microecological) that pave the way for their emergence? Under which conditions do they spread and exactly what role do pathogens play in ecosystems? What are the tools and administrative and scientific strategies needed in order to detect the antecedent occurrences that precede an epidemic? What mechanisms could explain the increased virulence of pathogens and which genetic modifications could explain emergence of virulence in previously nonpathogenic organisms? Are specific elements of a pathogen's genome responsible for all or part of this virulence? Is increase in virulence always associated with change, or with a transfer of populations or host species?

Study of pathogens' influence on host populations has demonstrated that their effect is significant.[10,11] Many studies have been conducted on the regulatory role of parasites and pathogens in human and animal populations, primarily because they are directly related to public and veterinary health. However, the impact of pathogens and parasites on the functioning of ecosystems is an area of research that has been ignored, despite the fact that pathogens are everywhere and represent a large proportion of the living world.[12] Moreover, pathogens play a very important role in preserving the balance of ecosystems by acting as regulators or "deregulators" of the ecological balance that has been established over time. Some of the answers to numerous human and animal public health issues, for example, resistance to antibiotics, require a better understanding of the ecology of pathogenic organisms and both their populations and species community. In the future, understanding this multispecies dimension will be essential.[13]

IMMUNOGENETICS, LOSS OF DIVERSITY, AND RISK OF EMERGENCE OF DISEASES

As we have established, description of all the scientific approaches that each take into account a different facet of biodiversity would be tedious and exhausting. We will limit our discussion to the "immunogenetics" aspect that essentially controls the mammal host immune defense mechanisms. The overall question could be stated as follows: *In terms of health, what are the risks and what could be the consequences, particularly at the host–pathogen interface, of the loss of genetic diversity (biodiversity) in the emergence or reemergence of infectious diseases?* Defense mechanisms at the host–pathogen interface involve both the host (mammal or arthropod) and pathogen. Defense mechanisms could include physical (skin's natural tissue barrier, mucus, cilium. . .) or biochemical nature (enzymatic action, fever. . .) to prevent infection/infestation by pathogens. The pathogens could also activate biochemical neutralization mechanisms or physical or molecular mimesis that would allow them to escape/circumvent the host defense mechanisms. If the pathogen manages to escape those initial defenses and penetrates inside the host, the host may deploy several cellular and molecular biochemical mechanisms and activate several nonspecific and specific immune defense systems to destroying/suppressing the totality of pathogens. In turn, pathogens may activate escape mechanisms, including genetic mutations that bypass the host-specific pathogen recognition functions. A successful parasite does not kill its host, which would jeopardize its survival. Finally, arthropod vectors, such as hematophagous fleas, ticks, and mosquitoes, have defense systems against pathogens that effect regulation of the parasite's diffusion and multiplication and the host, who contributes to the survival of the vector population with the blood meal (physical avoidance, chemotaxin, "bite" strategy). A more detailed look from a genomic perspective at these mechanisms at the host–pathogen interface reveals that many of them interact so as to perpetually neutralize each other, and that this opposition is all the more balanced if the hosts' genetic diversity is high enough to respond to that of the pathogens. In fact, the higher the hosts' genetic diversity, the greater the probability of neutralization/equilibrium. If genetic diversity were to decrease, the hosts would no longer be able to control the pathogens' genetic diversity adequately or correctly. The pathogens would develop relentlessly in the host population with various consequences for the latter, which could reach total extinction in the short to long term. Preserving current biodiversity means safeguarding its future evolution potential, a future as yet unknown to us since, although some repetition of the past is possible through DNA's and paleontology's archives, future prediction is not. Most importantly, evolution never turns back the clock: this irreversibility is the very cause of the irrevocable mechanisms of the extinction of species.

HOST–PATHOGEN GENOMICS AND IMMUNOGENETICS

We know all species are part of the chain of living beings whose remarkable unity expresses itself through the biochemical and genetic medium of DNA. DNA is like a "software," a sort of "unbroken link," a memory of the living world from the time of the species emergence. DNA is the universal code common to all plants and animals, a stock of information, the foundation of biological diversity, and the primary material on which evolution relies to maintain the species in a state of adaptation allowing them to resist environmental change. The majority of pathogens (prokaryotes) possess genomes that are smaller (between 10^3 and 10^7 base pairs [bp]) than those of their eukaryotic hosts, whether mammal or bird (3.10^9 bp). Prokaryotic pathogens have a genome whose DNA is almost 100% encoding, but the same does not apply to the genomes of mammals, in which only 10% are functional protein-encoding genes. The other 90% consist of noncoding sequences, introns, regulatory sequences, pseudogenes, etc. Random mutations occur every 10^6 bp during each DNA replication (cell division). This statistically means that the majority of mutations in prokaryotic pathogens occurs in encoding areas and has direct functional consequences. Inversely, the frequency of mutation every 10^6 bp, in relation to the 10^9 bp size of eukaryotic genomes, will cause a majority of mutations to occur in noncoding zones (silent mutations) and will accordingly have no direct functional consequence. Having considered this, it is apparent that pathogens' genetic mutation and, therefore, adaptation potential are far superior to those of the hosts. Moreover, replications occur during cell division and reproductions, and pathogens' reproduction cycles are considerably shorter than those of higher mammals, including man. In brief, the rate of mutation and therefore of genetic variability is much greater in prokaryotes than in higher eukaryotes. It grants them a considerable ability to adapt to their environment rapidly, especially by escaping the hosts' immune defense mechanisms by masking or molecular mimesis. Mammal hosts respond to the pathogens' large variability potential with genetic systems that are more complex, highly polymorphic, and with a large number of genes whose rearrangements allow for a considerable number of molecular combinations. Consider the example of the MHC, and in particular its class I and class II molecules involved in immune recognition mechanisms at an extracellular and intracellular level respectively, and the five different types of immunoglobulin (antibodies) IgA, IgE, IgD, IgG and IgM (http://imgt.cines.fr). All these structurally close molecules are made up of proteins with constant and variable chains encoded by a very large number of genes. MHC molecules are encoded by several dozen loci distributed across one or several chromosomes, and each of these loci presents several dozen different alleles. Immunoglobulin molecules are encoded by several hundred genes whose recombinations can statistically produce over 10^8 possible rearrangements. Taking only into account these two immune defense systems—MHC molecules and immunoglobulin—we begin to get a grasp of the mammal hosts' incredible reactivity potential, both in terms of speed and specificity, to recognize both the exogenous and endogenous antigens of pathogens and to deploy control and suppression processes immediately. Suppression of the host's pathogens must be complete, otherwise the few "surviving" (i.e., unsuppressed) pathogens can adapt rapidly through mutation and once again escape the hosts' specific defense systems or chemical treatments, as in the case of bacterial antibiotic resistance or chemoresistance mechanisms of parasites. Moreover, as the genetic system of mammals is autosomal with codominant expression and possible gene duplications, heterozygoty further multiplies allelic variability, which allows for the increase of the hosts' immune reactivity potential. This particular benefit of heterozygoty allows the hosts to adapt to the mutational capacity of pathogens. Inversely, any decrease in the hosts' genetic variability, whether at individual or population level (homozygoty, consanguinity rate, bottleneck, etc.) considerably reduces immune reactivity and the hosts' ability to control and suppress pathogens. Similarly, considering monospecific populations rather than individuals, Apanius[14] developed the theory of frequency-dependent coevolution of cyclic and antagonist mechanisms between a given pathogen population and a host population (FIG. 1). Taking the case of an equilibrium situation in which a host population shows a high frequency of a specific MHC allele, which strongly correlates with a given character, such as for instance resistance to a given disease. If the pathogen responsible for this disease manages to rapidly circumvent the host's immune defenses through mutation, a number of individuals within the host population will perish and the frequency of the "circumvented" resistant allele will decrease in the host population. Its proportion will thus progressively decrease in the overall population until a genetic rearrangement occurs in an individual from the host population, allowing it to control the

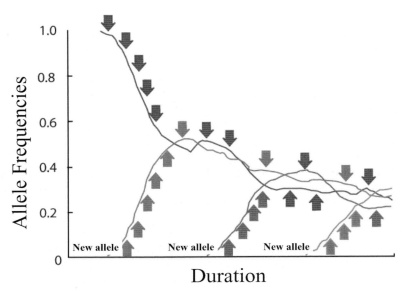

FIGURE 1. Frequence-dependence Apanius' theory on the cyclic and antagonist mechanisms of coevolution at the host–pathogen level populations.

pathogen's new variant. Natural selection eradicates sensitive hosts and only individuals having the new resistant allele survive. By reproducing, these individuals will cause the frequency of the new resistant allele to increase in the population, which will in turn see its numbers grow. Escape/circumvention by pathogens and genetic rearrangements in the hosts are constant and antagonist cyclical mechanisms at the host–pathogen interface, which occur over the time span of several generations of hosts. Each time the pathogen succeeds in circumventing the host population's defenses through mutation, the latter's probabilities of survival will be proportional to its genetic diversity. Indeed, the greater the gene diversity in a host population, the greater the possibilities of genetic rearrangements, the more the host population will be able to control pathogen infections/infestations cyclically and the greater the probability of survival over time. In the opposite case, it will eventually become extinct in the more or less short term as its reproduction cycles will not be sufficient to rebuild population equilibrium (i.e., population critical mass). The notion of population critical mass is essential for the understanding of relations between the host and the pathogen biological diversity (dilution effect, buffer effect), and of the probability of lateral transfers to other host species, including humans, by crossing of species barrier. In reality, mechanisms described for a given disease are much more complex, since pathogens' aggressions are manifold and often simultaneous and correlations are variable; one allele providing resistance to one specific disease can also be associated with greater sensitivity to another disease. One example would be hosts "tolerant" to a germ, which thus protects their population (i.e., the germ does not exert its pathogenicity on its natural host and its host does not recognize it as "immunologically" foreign). The germ, although potentially pathogenic for hosts other than its natural host, endures in the surrounding ecosystem without any visible damage to the community. Only emergence brought about by specific conditions will disturb this apparent equilibrium (pathocenosis).[8] This example is also played out as described above, according to constant interactions whereby natural selection through the rapid suppression of the most sensitive individuals will tend to reduce genetic diversity through the loss of sensitivity alleles on a population scale. Inversely, the hosts' gene rearrangements will preserve diversity. The rate of evolution of mutational frequencies is obviously highly variable in mammals and will depend on linkage disequilibrium in linked genes, on selective pressure on the various genetic systems taken into account, on the type of mutation (deletion, substitution, or insertion), their rate, and whether or not they are located in functional genomic areas. Human activity disturbs, interferes with, and often thwarts the cyclical mechanisms of natural equilibriums through breeding techniques, such as marker-assisted selection (MAS), or through chemical treatment (more or less adequately controlled use of antibiotics or antiparasitics). Hence, selection mechanisms can occur simultaneously within individuals, given groups or entire populations, with variable reactive time spans. The greater a population's genetic (gene) diversity, the greater the chances of survival of its individuals and the more sustainable will be the survival of its population.

BIODIVERSITY AND BREEDING SYSTEMS

Humans have developed a vast number of animal breeding methods that have varied greatly since the initial domestication of several animal species. We will only analyze the immunopathological risks associated with loss of biodiversity in modern industrial breeding farms, with regards, for example, to the latest great viral and bacterial epidemics, whether porcine or avian. The large concentration of animals farmed in overcrowded conditions in industrial batteries (several hundreds or even several thousands of individuals in a confined space), provides an extremely infectious context through contact with numerous pathogens, as opposed to natural extensive or semiextensive breeding conditions. This effect is enhanced when new species are added to an intensive monospecific breeding farm (e.g., poultry/porcine) whose overcrowded conditions will foster anomalous exchanges and cause a major risk of epidemic by crossing of species barrier. Where a small infectious dose would naturally be controlled by a normal immune system, there is no chance, even for an efficient immune system, of controlling huge infectious doses which "saturate" defense effector mechanisms and "overflow" the animals' immune mechanisms, all the more so when the animals are descended from consanguineous genetic strains (clones) with a high rate of homozygoty and therefore low genetic diversity, which reduces their immune reaction capacity. The "infectious dose effect" is an important factor for consideration, since the rapidity of emergence and magnitude of an epidemic, as well as relapse episodes (emergence) triggered by pathogens with high mutational potential, all depend on it. Important questions are: Where do the pathogens provoking epidemic outbreaks come from? Are they new (emerging) or do they reemerge (reemerging) through certain particular breeding or environmental conditions? Do they come from food? Do they originate in new and infected individuals, or from contact with wild animals, such as rodents? It is difficult to answer such questions. What we do know is that wild fauna is generally well adapted to its pathogenic environment through natural selection but that this is absolutely not the case for farmed individuals, whose contact with wild pathogenic strains always has severe pathological consequences. Many examples of pathogen transmission either direct or through vectors (West Nile Fever, blue tongue disease, malaria, trypanosomiasis, etc.), have demonstrated the real risks of such contact between wild and farmed environments, which should to a minimum. Domesticated hosts' genetic (bio)diversity is, however, an important factor, a type of protective barrier (buffer) against emerging and reemerging diseases. For example, the introduction of exotic genotypes in a specific environment, whether directly or by cross-breeding of exogenous genotypes, is a serious mistake. First, it presents a major risk of reducing the genetic diversity (with a weakening of immune defense capacities) of local populations often perfectly well adapted to their environment through natural selection (including resistance to endemic pathogenic strains); it also carries a major risk of introducing pathogenic strains unknown to the local population and which might provoke pathological outbreaks that can lead to the rapid extinction of endemic species. The extinction of endemic populations allows the exotic species to become invasive, which can induce huge environmental changes involving the emergence of ecosytemic disequilibrium. Will depleted ecosystems withstand the aggressiveness of invasive species whose worldwide threat is increasing as it becomes intensified by global trade? Will the extinction of certain species known as "key species" provoke the domino effect extinction of dependent species and cause a complex reorganization of ecosystems?[15] Will ecosystems be steered into new, detrimental directions, which would remain stable once certain irreversibility thresholds have been reached? Will we witness breakages of interactions between species in such diverse areas as competition, predation, and parasitism as well as all types of symbiosis? Will we observe new power relations in the never-ending "arms race" between pathogens and hosts, which could provoke the emergence of new pathologies or the reemergence of old ones we hoped had been suppressed. Indeed, if certain natural habitats disappear, especially wild ones, the absence of their usual wild hosts may cause pathogens to leave their ecosystem, and colonize and threaten domesticated environments or populations sensitive to them. The risks of emergence of new epidemic outbreaks are thus increased and threaten animals and humans alike (zoonosis) in the case of transmission by crossing of species barrier.

CONCLUSIONS AND RECOMMENDATIONS

Returning to a veterinary context that takes into account the various elements in this article, we can suggest what should be avoided in terms of breeding techniques, especially within sustainable and rational intensification; we can also make some concrete recommendations in order to avoid, or at least control, the emergence or reemergence of diseases including zoonosis. Human demographic evolution is evidently at the heart of the problems we are currently experiencing. Human penetration into new territories for the purposes of establishing new species, agriculture, farming, and for the tourist exploration of still untouched natural ecosystems, increase the probabilities of contact and therefore transmission of pathogens from unsuspected reservoirs or vectors.[16] Two interactive configurations must be taken into account: on the one hand, the worldwide growth of human population, and on the other hand biodiversity, a great part of which is the source of past, present, and probably future diseases. The central problem concerns demographic relations between human and other species. The more human population will grow, the more this population will compete with other animal species, increasing the risk of contacts with potentially dangerous agents it had not been previously confronted with.

Another aspect is one of relations between geographical areas. Countries in the intertropical zone are host to 30 to 35 times more infectious and parasitic agents currently responsible for diseases in human populations than temperate countries.[17] Yet to this day, huge numbers of microorganisms remain unknown in tropical regions where it is estimated that hardly 10% of biological diversity has been cataloged. We can only predict the number of pro- or eukaryotic organisms, which could be pathogenic to their new hosts when transmitted to human, animal, or vegetal populations. Modern societies could be incurring great risks by allowing the scourge of poverty to spread over the populations of the south.[18] As for the intensification of farming systems, which in the south even more than in the north, responds to the increasing demand for animal food products associated with human demographic growth, it should be sustainable and rational, and take into account a whole set of environmental (medical measures, effluent management. . .), sociological, and economical as well as genetic factors, as previously seen. We must avoid noncontrolled farming, as well as large, highly populated industrial breeding farms that generally use animals from the same species, the same origin, or even from monoclonal strains, which lead to a detrimental loss of genetic diversity. The numbers and density in which animals are bred result in overcrowded conditions, which, among other things, stress the animals, modify their metabolic performances, weaken their immune system, and above all maintain a high risk of hyperinfection by massive infectious loads. We should also avoid multispecies breeding (chicken, ducks, or pigs for example) within the same industrial farm or the same geographical zone: if a disease breaks out, there is a high risk of mutation/recombination/reassortment of pathogens and thus of crossing the species barrier. This is also the reason why contact with humans and especially breeding farm employees should be avoided as much as possible when a disease breaks out on an industrial farm; this can be achieved by applying strict rules on movement restriction and on the use of mechanical (masks, protective suits) and chemical protection (various disinfections, preventive vaccination). Such measures are generally already recommended by public services (OIE, WHO, relevant ministries), but are not always correctly implemented. In case of epidemic, stringent controls are required at all stages of the production pipeline. Possible alternatives that would reduce the risks of contact could for instance include replacing large industrial units with several smaller-scale production units containing lower densities of animals.[19] In other words, this means favoring product quality over industrial yield. There are many advantages to this: animals would be less stressed and thus more resistant to infectious aggressions; contact between individuals would be less intense, which would reduce infection rates since infectious doses would be lower. It would thus be possible to diversify the races bred in farms containing several mid-sized breeding units by using different animal strains for one species. Genetic diversity would be maintained and allow for a variable immune behavior in the face of infection/infestation by pathogens. In case of epidemic, this would reduce the risks of high mortality and their disastrous economic consequences for farmers, since not all the animals would die (as is the case on large industrial farms). The surviving animals would thus be selected *de facto* to recreate a population resistant to the given pathogen. All players involved in the farming production pipeline, whether political, economical, or professional, should be aware of the importance of valorizing biodiversity through the diversification of animal strains used for breeding. Strains with different potentials and qualities would in turn diversify economic markets and offer a wider choice of products to the consumer.

Last but not least, we suggest the development of an increased number of research projects specifically aimed at wild environments and species. The evaluation and characterization of wild genetic diversity will provide a wealth of information and thus allow correct modeling and valorization of biodiversity on the basis of the natural adaptation and survival potential of wild populations.[11] Obviously, we should avoid contact between wild fauna, which is an important pathogen reservoir, and domesticated animals, which are not adapted and so are for the most part sensitive to those pathogens. Inversely, biological diversity acquired by wild fauna through natural selection should be valorized as having considerable potential for the future, especially from a genetic perspective. Species with amazing properties have been sorted through natural selection. Many are still unknown to us and need to be discovered in order to be valorized. Although wild species act as pathogen reservoirs, they are also reservoirs of pathogen-resistant genes, more commonly of adaptation genes for various difficult or constraining environments (saline or desert habitat). Identifying such genes of interest would allow their introgression in domestic species with the use of various reproductive biotechnologies. We are convinced that the results of such research will in future contribute strongly to controlling the emergence of new diseases, or to the reemergence or spread of known diseases, by rational and sustainable farming of genetically resistant species.

ACKNOWLEDGMENT

We greatly appreciate and thank Dr. Kathy Kocan, from the Department of Veterinary Pathobiology, Center for Veterinary Health Sciences, Oklahoma State University, Stillwater, for her comments and correction of this manuscript.

REFERENCES

1. MARTENS, P. & A.J. MCMICHAEL. 2002. Environmental Change, Climate and Health. Issues and Research Methods. Cambridge University Press. Cambridge. ISBN 0–521782-36-8.
2. UICN. 2001. Catégories et critères de l'UICN pour la liste rouge; Version 3.1. Commission De La Sauvegarde Des Espèces De l'UICN. UICN, Gland, Suisse & Cambridge. UK. ii+30 pp.
3. MCMICHAEL, A.J. 2001. Human Frontiers, Environments and Disease. Past Patterns, Uncertain Futures. Cambridge University Press. Cambridge. ISBN 0-521004-94-2.
4. ARON, J.-L. & J.A. PATZ, 2001. Ecosystem Change and Public Health. 480. Johns Hopkins University Press. Baltimore, USA. ISBN 0-801886582-4.
5. ASHFORD, R.W. & W. CREWE. 1998. The parasites of homo sapiens: an annotated checklist of the protozoa, helminths and arthropods for which we are home.142. Liverpool School of Tropical Medicine, Liverpool. ISBN o-4152-7688-8.
6. DICKINSON, G. & K. MURPHY. 1998. Ecosystems. A functional approach,. Routledge Introductions to Environment Series —Environmental Science. 190. Routledge. Coll. New York. ISBN 0-415145-12-0/0-415145-13-9
7. HUGOT, J.P. & J.P. GONZALEZ. 2005. Maladies émergentes: un problème sociétal d'avenir. 121-125, In "Biodiversité et changements globaux." ADPF/MAE. Paris. ISBN 2-914935-27-7.
8. GRMEK, M. 1993. The concept of emerging disease. Hist. Philos. Life Sci. **15:** 281–296.
9. OSTFELD, R.S. & F. KEESING. 2000. The function of biodiversity in the ecology of vector-borne zoonotic diseases. Canadian J. Zool., no 78, Ottawa, p. 2061–2078.
10. GRENFELL, B.T. & A.P. DOBSON. 1995. Ecology of Infectious Diseases. In Natural Populations. 521p. Cambridge University Press, Cambridge. ISBN 0-521-46.502-8.

11. HUDSON, P., A. RIZZOLI, B.T. GRENFELL, *et al.* 2001. Ecology of Wildlife Diseases. 197. Oxford University Press, Oxford, UK. ISBN 0-19-850619-8.
12. DE MEEUS, T. & F. RENAUD. 2001. Parasites within the new phylogeny of eukaryotes. *In* Trends in Parasitology, no18, Londres, p. 247–251.
13. THOMAS, F., J.-F. GUEGAN & F. RENAUD. 2005. Parasitism and Ecosystems. Oxford University Press. Oxford.
14. APANIUS, V., D. PENN, P.R. SLEV, *et al.* 1997. The nature of selection on the major histocompatibility complex. Crit. Rev. Immunol. **17:** 179–224.
15. CHIVIAN, 2001. Species loss and ecosystem disruption: the implications for human health. Canadian Med. Assoc. J., no 164, Ottawa, p. 66–69.
16. SALUZZO, J.-F., P. VIDAL & J.-P. GONZALEZ. 2004. Les Virus émergents, Éd.: 192p. de l'IRD. Paris. ISBN 2-7099-1539-1.
17. GUERNIER, V., M. HOCHBERG & J.-F. GUEGAN. 2004. Ecology Drives the Worldwide Distribution of Human Diseases. 740–746. PloS (Biology). London. no 2.
18. FROMENT, A. 1997. Une approche écoanthropologique de la santé publique. Nature Sciences Sociétés. no 5, Paris, p. 5–11.
19. UN MILLENIUM PROJECT, 2005. Investing in Development: A Practical Plan to achieve the Millenium Development Goals. pp329. United Nations. New York. ISBN 1-84407-217-7.

Perspectives on Applied Spatial Analysis to Animal Health

A Case of Rodents in Thailand

VINCENT HERBRETEAU,[a,b] FLORENT DEMORAES,[a,b]
JEAN-PIERRE HUGOT,[b,c] PATTAMAPORN KITTAYAPONG,[a]
GÉRARD SALEM,[b,d] MARC SOURIS,[a,b] AND JEAN-PAUL GONZALEZ[b]

[a]*Center for Vectors and Vector-borne Diseases (CVVD), Faculty of Sciences, Mahidol University, Bangkok 10400, Thailand*

[b]*Institut de Recherche pour le Développement (IRD), Research Unit UT178, RCEVD/CVD, Mahidol University, Nakhon Pathom 73170, Thailand*

[c]*Muséum National d'Histoire Naturelle de Paris, Département Systématique et Évolution, UMR 5202 Origin, Structure and Evolution of Biodiversity, 75231 Paris Cedex 05, France*

[d]*Laboratoire Espace, Santé, Territoire, Université Paris-X, Nanterre, 92000 Nanterre, France*

ABSTRACT: Geographic information systems (GIS) and remote sensing have been increasingly used in ecology and epidemiology, providing a spatial approach for animal health issues. Recent development of earth environmental satellites—i.e., their growing number, improving sensor resolutions and capabilities—has offered new opportunities to delineate possible habitats and understand animals and associated parasites in their environment, by identifying the nature and structure of land use, hydrological network, soil hydromorphy, and human settlements. Integrated into GIS, remotely sensed and other geo-referenced data allow both spatial and temporal analyses of animal ecology and health. However, a review of their applications has showed the poor quality of data sources and processing used, revealing limitations between theory and practical implementations. As an example, the assessment of the expected distribution of Bandicoot rats, main agricultural pest and vector of zoonoses in Phrae province (North Thailand), illustrates a rational use of spatial analysis, with the choice of relevant data, scales, and processing. Vegetation indices are computed on a TERRA ASTER image and further classified using elevation data. The biotopes of *Bandicota indica* and *Bandicota savilei* are delimited, providing a major source of knowledge for rodent and human health analyses.

Address for correspondence: Vincent Herbreteau, PhD candidate in Health Geography, Master of Engineering in GIS and Remote Sensing, IRD-UT178, Center for Vectors and Vector-borne Diseases, Faculty of Sciences, Mahidol University, Thanon Rama VI, Phyathai, Bangkok 10400, Thailand. Voice: 66-24410227; fax: 66-24410227.
e-mail: Vincent.Herbreteau@ird.fr

Ann. N.Y. Acad. Sci. 1081: 17–29 (2006). © 2006 New York Academy of Sciences.
doi: 10.1196/annals.1373.002

KEYWORDS: geographic information systems; remote sensing; spatial analysis; rodents; biogeography; Bandicoot; *Bandicota indica*; *Bandicota savilei*; NDVI; SAVI; ASTER

INTRODUCTION

With an increasing access to a large variety of location-based data, including animal and animal health information, spatial analysis has emerged as a major method for describing and understanding diseases dynamics and risk of transmission.[1] The aims of spatial analysis are: (*a*) the epidemiological surveillance, with disease mapping of reported incidences, and further active surveillance, involving collection of animal health and animal population information; (*b*) the explanatory understanding of animal population and diseases dynamics, by identifying patterns in the spatio-temporal distribution of diseases and identifying risk factors or causes of the diseases (etiology), and (*c*) the disease prevention, by predicting outbreaks and assisting in decision making. Spatial analysis is conducted through a geographic information system (GIS), used as the central interface to integrate, manage, and process data.[2,3] A current trend is to combine other available tools, such as remote sensing (RS), with GIS software, in order to implement efficient computer-based systems for spatial analysis.

Most of the researches in health involving space technologies have been dedicated to human health. The few applications using RS in animal health were mainly studies of Blutetongue,[4–6] African horse sickness,[7] bovine tuberculosis,[8,9] Eastern equine encephalomyelitis virus,[10,11] and assessment of mosquitoes abundance.[12] Rare applications on rodent-borne diseases have been published.[13] The ecological approach of vectors has been the most direct contribution of RS to health studies, used in 96% of past researches.[14] Location-based data set usually gathers environmental variables, such as climate, topography, or land use, modeled as indicators of the animal ecology. Land use is extracted by RS from aerial pictures or satellite images, of which a large choice has been made available. However, an almost exhaustive review of the use of RS in health over the last 25 years has shown the gap between the theory and arguments of RS professionals and the limited use of these techniques in health, and especially epidemiology.[14] Most studies are based on the low-resolution images chosen, because they are free of charge or available at a low cost and not for their relevance regarding the objectives of the study. Considering that the choice of scales in health geography is a fundamental issue to understand diseases dynamics, being limited to the resolutions of the image is obviously a major weakness, though rarely mentioned. The second outcome of this article highlighted the limited processes performed on images; 49% of the studies used the normalized difference vegetation index (NDVI).[14] In addition, in most of these cases, authors rarely processed NDVI by themselves despite the simplicity of the calculation; they acquired already processed NDVI from National Oceanographic and Atmospheric Administration images that have been made available through the Internet. A conclusion of this review about RS in health is that the price of data has been the limiting factor to the relevance of such studies.

After reviewing the applications of spatial analysis to health and emphasizing their limits, this article aims to provide a descriptive and relevant example making use of RS for vector-borne diseases. It consists in assessing the potential distribution of a genus of common rodents in Thailand, *Bandicota*, which is a major vector of zoonoses. Three *Bandicota* species are described from India to South East Asia: *Bandicota indica* (Bechstein, 1800), the great bandicoot, *Bandicota savilei* (Thomas, 1916), the lesser bandicoot, and *Bandicota bengalensis* (Gray and Hardwicke, 1804), the Bengal bandicoot. Only the first two occur in Thailand, in different ecosystems. *B. indica* has been designated as the main vector of leptospirosis,[15,16] but both of them are suspected to be the vectors of other zoonoses, especially Scrub typhus and hantaviruses.

An explanatory approach of rodent distribution was used to identify potential indicators of presence, later compared with field sampling data and ecological observations (FIG. 1). *B. indica* is the largest murine rodent occurring in South East Asia, common in agricultural areas, particularly in rice fields, possibly close to houses and often wetlands.[17–19] Villagers regularly hunt *B. indica* for meat or to protect cultivations, and have always shown great knowledge of its ecology during interviews. *B. savilei* is a medium-sized rat, living in agricultural but dry areas, which is a major point of distinction between the two

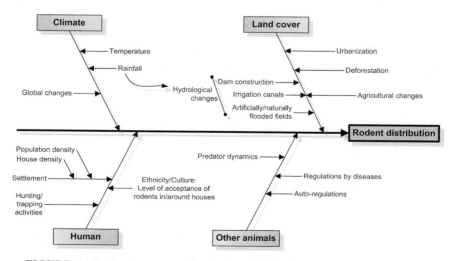

FIGURE 1. Explanatory approach of rodent distribution.

species.[19] Despite rare notifications of *B. savilei* during trapping in Thailand, it has shown great adaptation to agricultural changes, with populations rapidly colonizing and damaging corn fields.

MATERIALS AND METHODS

Since 1998, rodent surveys have been conducted in Phrae province and other Thai regions, in the frame of a research on rodent-borne zoonoses (IRD/UT178 in collaboration with Mahidol University/CVVD). Trappings were set up in different ecosystems to broadly sample murine rodents' diversity, invest their morphology and taxonomy, and identify ecological indicators of their distribution. In 2004, complementary interviews were conducted in Phrae province regarding Bandicoot rats' ecology, distribution, and dynamics.

The study area, centered on Phrae province, is located in the Central–Northern part of Thailand between longitude 99.5°E and 100.2°E and between latitude 17.5°N and 18.3°N. The topography comprises forested highland areas, with a North–South alignment, separated by large flood plains. Drastic changes in land use have occurred with the agricultural development, boosted by the construction of several reservoirs to irrigate lowland areas, and a continuous deforestation in the highland area that officials could slow down but have failed to stop. Phrae City, located by the side of Mae Yom River in the large flood plain, is one of the most frequently flooded localities in Thailand.

Regarding the price of data as a recurrent limiting factor in the choice of images, we carried out our research using only free data and tools, searching for the highest quality and relevance. We integrated, managed, and processed data using SavGIS, a GIS freeware under development by IRD (http://www.savgis.com), offering beyond GIS capabilities, integrated tools for RS. A TERRA EOS AM-1 (Earth Observing System) ASTER (Advanced Spaceborne Thermal Emission and Reflection Radiometer) image from the March 7, 2003 was acquired, for free, from the United States Geological Survey website (http://eros.usgs.gov/products/satellite.html). With a 15-m spatial resolution and 14 bands available, ASTER images are suitable for describing the land use on a large scale (small extent). Only three bands, in the green, red, and near-infrared electromagnetic spectrum portions were acquired, to use the specificities of high reflectance of vegetation in near-infrared wavelengths. They were merged and arranged in a false color composition, for an easier distinction of vegetation density and activity (FIG. 2).

Elevation data for Thailand were obtained from the international project Shuttle Radar Topography Mission (SRTM), providing a worldwide Digital Elevation Model (DEM), accessible via the Internet (http://srtm.usgs.gov/). Data points are located every 3-arc second (approximately 90 m) on a latitude/longitude grid. These data points were interpolated for the whole country, using SavGIS, and directly integrated into the GIS database (FIG. 3).

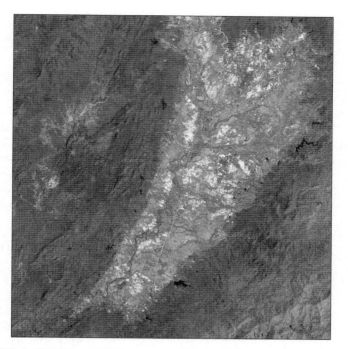

FIGURE 2. TERRA ASTER image. Phrae, Thailand 07/03/03 (False-color composition).

Vegetation indices (VIs) are calculations of reflectance values in different spectral portions helping to quantify the abundance and vigor of vegetation. While the NDVI is the most commonly used in health applications, there are nearly two dozen others. Most are ratios of a near-infrared and red bands, considering the proprieties of high reflectance for vigorous vegetation in near-infrared spectral portion.[20,21] In the present study, we used two different VIs (NDVI and SAVI) as described below. NDVI, introduced by Rouse *et al.*,[22] is a ratio-based index, ranging between −1.0 and +1.0, with vegetation having positive values:

$$NDVI = (NIR - R)/(NIR + R)$$

with NIR = value of pixel in near-infrared band,
R = value of pixel in Red band.

NDVI is a differential index for active vegetation, that is, forests or fields with a dense cover. Bare fields with some spontaneous vegetation or fields with little vegetation coverage are hardly separated. To minimize the effects of soil, Huete incorporated a soil adjustment factor (L) in the NDVI formula and proposed the soil-adjusted vegetation index (SAVI)[23,24]:

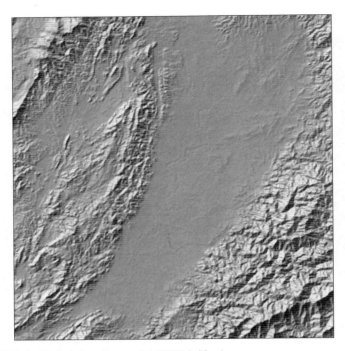

FIGURE 3. Digital elevation model (SRTM, 90 m).

$$SAVI = [(1 + L) \times (NIR - R)]/(NIR + R + L)$$

This correction factor is determined by the relative coverage of vegetation and color of soil. For this study, L was given a value of 1 for bare soils and emergent crops, 0.5 for an intermediate stage, and 0 to get the NDVI values for dense vegetation cover. Then, NDVI and SAVI are combined to separate the range of coverage, from sparse to dense, which can be found in a same area in tropical countries.

RESULTS

There were 1718 murine rodents, belonging to 30 different species, trapped between January 1998 and December 2004, in Northern, Northeastern, and Central Thailand, representative of the great biodiversity. *B. indica* constitutes 13.5% (232 specimens) of the total murine rodents trapped during this period. This ratio should not be interpreted in terms of abundance because of the multiple biases inherent in the trapping method. Of the species trapped, 55.9% were males, showing the active behavior of males going hunting while females protect the nest and litter after birth. *B. indica* was exclusively found during

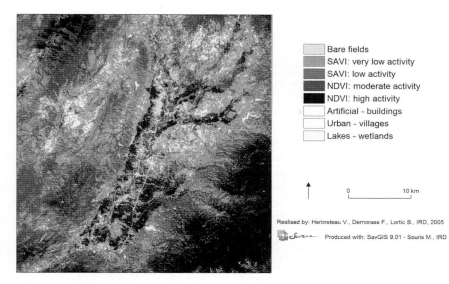

Bare fields
SAVI: very low activity
SAVI: low activity
NDVI: moderate activity
NDVI: high activity
Artificial - buildings
Urban - villages
Lakes - wetlands

0   10 km

Realised by: Herbreteau V., Demoraes F., Lortic B., IRD, 2005

Produced with: SavGIS 9.01 - Souris M., IRD

FIGURE 4. Classification (all classes).

sampling in the lowland rice fields, especially abundant after harvests, digging burrows on the edge of fields.

Sixty *B. savilei* (3.5% of total murine rodents) were trapped during the same period. Here again, the smaller number of *B. savilei* trapped, compared to *B. indica*, does not reflect any reality in the density of both species but the biases in trapping methods. Half of *B. savilei* specimens come from the mountains of Phrae province, where it has been a major agricultural pest since maize production has increased, replacing mung beans and other crops, in the foothills of the mountains. These fields provide dry habitats for *B. savilei*, with a seasonal but abundant source of food.

The supervised classification (FIG. 4) helps to separate what represent the human settlements, the city of Phrae, the villages, some large isolated buildings, and the main roads. Regarding the distribution of Bandicoot rats, the extent and structure of human settlements are a first indicator, considered as attractive for *B. indica*. Lakes and wetlands are also accurately extracted from optical satellite images. In the central flood plain, fields with no vegetation were classified as bare lands. Difficulties lie in distinguishing different vegetation covers, stages of cultivation, and agricultural practices, especially artificial flooding. The calculation of SAVI with an *L*-value equal to 0 (then SAVI = NDVI), first showed active vegetation. Two classes were isolated, based on ground proof: high activity: NDVI > 185, and moderate activity: 170 < NDVI < 185 (these values are stretched from 0 to 255 to use the full color range for the output map). These areas correspond to highland forests and rice fields in the lowland flood plain. With an *L*-value equal to 1, also two classes were identified: very low activity: $165 < SAVI < 195$ and low activity: $195 < SAVI < 215$, with the result that the first class corresponds to the previously described *B. savilei* habitat, that is, field areas, in the foothills of the mountains, in transition between lowland rice fields and highland forests, where corn fields have been replacing forests. The two classes group together, in lowland areas, agricultural fields, and sparse vegetations, where *B. indica* can occasionally be found.

VIs give similar values for lowland rice fields and highland forests, both characterized by a dense cover. This common limitation of RS, when only based on reflectance values, was solved by using the topography derived from the SRTM DEM. Rice field areas, only found in the large flood plain where *B. indica* occurs, correspond to fields with a very low slope. The slope was calculated from the DEM and almost flat areas (with slopes $<2°$) were delineated (FIGS. 5 and 6). In these lowland areas, high vegetation reflectance is classified as rice field instead of forests. Otherwise, high reflectance values with a slope greater than $2°$ were classified as forested areas.

The potential distribution of *B. indica*, present in the large flood plain, corresponds to both "NDVI high activity" and "SAVI very low activity" classes,

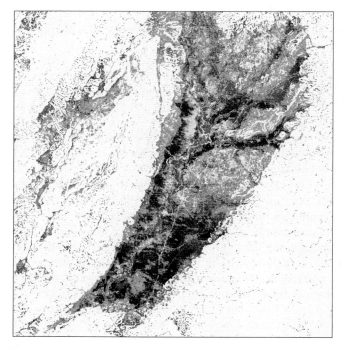

FIGURE 5. NDVI + SAVI in lowlands.

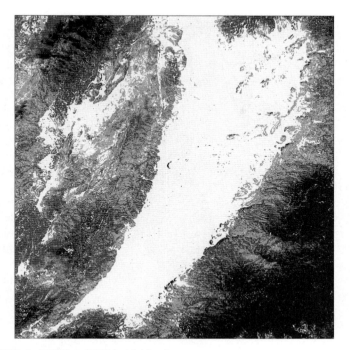

FIGURE 6. NDVI + SAVI in highlands.

within the lowland areas, while the potential distribution of *B. savilei* is de-limited by the "SAVI low activity" class. Maps of potential distribution were generated from these results (FIGS. 7 and 8).

DISCUSSION

Location-based data set integrated in a GIS are useful for RS analyses, illustrating with this example the need of GIS software directly integrating RS tools. VIs, based on reflectance values, show variations in the vegetation intensity but are not fully appropriate to differentiate the types of vegetation. Indeed, in the classified image, the same NDVI values can be attributed to both rice fields and forests. This is the reason why other RS techniques, such as texture or pattern discrimination processes, or other GIS queries, such as the merging of RS results with slopes or elevation as described above, should be used in complement.

The use of RS in tropical countries has a main restriction with the scarcity of exploitable satellite images during the rainy season when the widespread

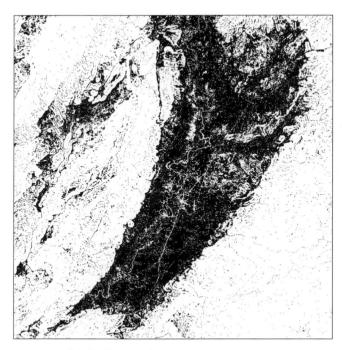

FIGURE 7. Potential distribution of *B. indica*.

cloud cover makes the ground not observable from the sky. As a result, observations are generally conducted during the dry season, limiting the analysis of
seasonal changes. However, radar sensors, emitting and recording radiations
with a longer wavelength (from 1 mm to 1 m), provide images that can be
used all through the year, with a particular interest for tropical diseases presenting a peak of incidence during the rainy season.[14] Access to low-cost but
high-resolution images should increase for higher relevance in health studies.
The emergence of web-based satellite images browser, after Google Earth®
initiative (http://earth.google.com/), which allows visualization for free, of
worldwide images at medium or even very high resolutions, is a new hope for
health geographers, seeking such an easy access to images but with different
bands for RS analysis.

Mapping the potential distribution of rats is a first step for pin-pointing
areas in which a risk of transmission of rodent-borne disease is likely to occur.
Future investigations should focus on the validation of these expected rodent
distribution maps through a higher number of trappings. Knowing the habitats
of murine transmitting pathogens is useful for both animal and human health
in order to define prevention and vector control campaigns.

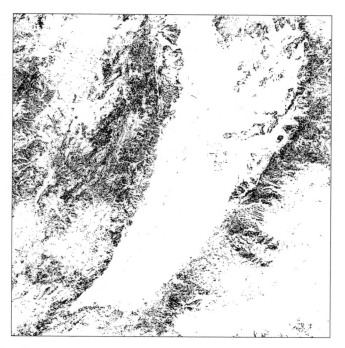

FIGURE 8. Potential distribution of *B. savilei*.

ACKNOWLEDGMENTS

We thank Bernard Lortic (IRD-UR029) for his precious help in image processing, Jean-Paul Cornet (IRD-UR178) and Jean-Louis Janeau (IRD-UR176/IWMI-SEA, Bangkok) for their continuous support all through this research. We also thank Arthorn Boonsaner (National Park, Wildlife and Plant Conservation Department, Thailand, Bangkok), Narissara Chatwatcharakul (IWMI-SEA, Bangkok), Wasana Khaungaew, and Primporn Moungthong (Ministry of Public Health, Phrae provincial office) for their assistance.

This research was supported by the Institut de Recherche pour le Développement (IRD) Research Unit UT178 "Fundamentals and Domains of Disease Emergence" and the program ≪Usages des Sols et Sédiments: Impacts Sanitaires≫ for field investigations.

REFERENCES

1. GATRELL, A. 1999. GIS and health: from spatial analysis to spatial decision support. *In* Geographic Information Research: Trans-Atlantic Perspectives. M. Craglia & H. Onsrud, Eds.: 143–158. Taylor and Francis. London.

2. ELLIOTT, P. & D. WARTENBERG. 2004. Spatial epidemiology: current approaches and future challenges. Environ. Health Perspect. **112:** 998–1006.
3. BAKER, R.D. 2004. Identifying space-time disease clusters. Acta Trop. **91:** 291–299.
4. TATEM, A.J., M. BAYLIS MELLOR, *et al.* 2003. Prediction of bluetongue vector distribution in Europe and north Africa using satellite imagery. Vet. Microbiol. **7:** 13–29.
5. CAPELA, R., B.V. PURSE, I. PENA, *et al.* 2003. Spatial distribution of Culicoides species in Portugal in relation to the transmission of African horse sickness and bluetongue viruses. Med. Vet. Entomol. **17:** 165–177.
6. PURSE, B.V., A.J. TATEM, *et al.* 2004. Modelling the distributions of Culicoides bluetongue virus vectors in Sicily in relation to satellite-derived climate variables. Med. Vet. Entomol. **18:** 90–101.
7. BAYLIS, M., H. BOUAYOUNE, *et al.* 1998. Use of climatic data and satellite imagery to model the abundance of *Culicoides imicola*, the vector of African horse sickness virus, in Morocco. Med. Vet. Entomol. **12:** 255–266.
8. WINT, G.R.W., T.P. ROBINSON, *et al.* 2002. Mapping bovine tuberculosis in Great Britain using environmental data. Trends Microbiol. **10:** 441–444.
9. MC KENZIE, J.S., R.S. MORRIS, *et al.* 2002. Application of remote sensing to enhance the control of wildlife associated *Mycobacterium bovis* infection. Photogrammetric Eng. Rem. **S68:** 153–159.
10. FREIER, J.W. 1993. Eastern equine encephalomyelitis. Lancet **342:** 1281–1283.
11. MONCAYO, A.C., J.D. EDMAN & J.T. FINN. 2000. Application of geographic information technology in determining risk of eastern equine encephalomyelitis virus transmission. J. Am. Mosq. Control **16:** 28–35.
12. GLEISER, R.M., G. SCHELOTTO & D.E. GORLA. 2002. Spatial pattern of abundance of the mosquito, *Ochlerotatus albifasciatus*, in relation to habitat characteristics. Med. Vet. Entomol. **16:** 364–371.
13. GLASS, G.E., J.E. CHEEK, J.A. PATZ, *et al.* 2000. Using remotely sensed data to identify areas at risk for hantavirus pulmonary syndrome. Emerging Infect. Dis. **6:** 238–247.
14. HERBRETEAU, V., G. SALEM, M. SOURIS, *et al.* 2005. Sizing up health through remote sensing: uses and misuses. Parassitologia **47:** 63–79.
15. PHULSUKSOMBATI, D., W. TANGKANAKUL, *et al.* 1999. Isolation of *leptospires* from wild rodents in Thailand, 1998. J. Health Sci. (Thai.) **8:** 360–369.
16. TANJATHAM, S., W. KHAUNGAEW & D. BOONYOD. 2003. Serological survey on Leptospira in animals and patients, Prae province. J. Health Sci. (Thai.) **12:** 265–272.
17. BOONSONG, L., J.A. MCNEELY & J.T. MARSHALL. 1988. Mammals of Thailand. Association for the Conservation of Wildlife. Bangkok.
18. CHAIMANEE, Y. 1998. Plio-Pleistocene Rodents of Thailand. Biodiversity Research and Training Program, National Center for Genetic Engineering and Biotechnology. Bangkok.
19. APLIN, K.P., P.R. BROWN, J. JACOB, *et al.* 2003. Field methods for rodent studies in Asia and the Indo-Pacific. ACIAR Monograph No. 100, ACIAR, Canberra.
20. JACKSON, R.D. & A.R. HUETE. 1991. Interpreting vegetation indices. Prev. Vet. Med. **11:** 185–200.
21. TUCKER, C.J. 1979. Red and photographic infrared linear combinations for monitoring vegetation. Remote Sens. Environ. **8:** 127–150.

22. ROUSE, J.W., R.H. HAAS, *et al.* 1973. Monitoring vegetation systems in the great plains with ERTS. Third ERTS Symposium, NASA SP-351. **1:** 309–317.
23. HUETE, A.R., R.D. JACKSON & D.F. POST. 1985. Spectral response of a plant canopy with different soil backgrounds. Remote Sens. Environ. **17:** 37–53.
24. HUETE, A.R. 1988. A soil-adjusted vegetation index (SAVI). Remote Sens. Environ. **25:** 295–309.

Epidemics of Emerging Animal Diseases and Food-Borne Infection Problems Over the Last 5 Years in Japan

ITSURO YAMANE

National Institute of Animal Health, Tsukuba-shi, Ibaraki, Japan 305-0856

ABSTRACT: There have been several emerging animal diseases and food-borne infection problems occurring in Japan over the last 5 years. We describe brief pictures of these epidemics and our control activities. As acute contagious and/or emerging animal diseases, the foot and mouth disease (FMD) outbreak caused by the Pan-Asian topotype of the type O virus occurred in March 2000 after 92 years of FMD-free status. In 2004, four cases of the highly pathogenic avian influenza (HPAI), which was the first outbreak after 79 years, and caused by the H5N1 subtype, were identified. As part of the responses against these outbreaks, all the animals in the affected farms were destroyed, and movement control areas were established around the infected premises, and a nation-wide intensive survey for FMD and HPAI was performed. As for food-borne or feed-borne infections, the first bovine spongiform encephalopathy (BSE) was identified in September 2001 and 19 more cases have been reported until June 2005. A large outbreak of food-borne infection caused by low-fat milk contaminated with enterotoxin A produced by *Staphylococcus aureus*, involving more than 13,000 patients, occurred in 2000. In 2003, people who consumed uncooked liver and meat from wild boar and deer developed clinical signs of hepatitis caused by the hepatitis E virus. Pork is also suspected as natural source of virus transmission. Early detection of the first cases and rapid action in preventing and controlling the spread of infections are very important combined with proper risk communication about correct information of the diseases.

KEYWORDS: foot and mouth disease; highly pathogenic avian influenza; bovine spongiform encephalopathy; hepatitis E virus

INTRODUCTION

Over the last 5 years, many emerging animal and human diseases have occurred in Japan, which resulted in social problems. Some of them were animal health issues, such as the foot and mouth disease (FMD) outbreak in 2000 and

Address for correspondence: Itsuro Yamane, 3-1-5, Kannondai, Tsukuba-shi, Ibaraki, Japan 305-0856. Voice: 81-29-838-7770; fax: 81-29-838-7880.
e-mail: iyamane@affrc.go.jp

Ann. N.Y. Acad. Sci. 1081: 30–38 (2006). © 2006 New York Academy of Sciences.
doi: 10.1196/annals.1373.003

the highly pathogenic avian influenza (HPAI) outbreak in 2004. Others were associated with food-borne or feed-borne infections, such as bovine spongiform encephalopathy (BSE) first detected in 2001, a food-borne infection caused by enterotoxin A produced by *Staphylococcus aureus* in 2000 and hepatitis E virus (HEV) infection that has been a concern since 2003. Since some of these diseases may have also occurred in other Asian countries, such as HPAI outbreaks, the lessons learned from the experiences in Japan may be shared with people in other countries. Therefore, overall pictures of all these emerging diseases that occurred in Japan in the last 5 years will be described and some of the actions taken are discussed in this article.

FMD OUTBREAKS

Livestock in Japan had been free from FMD since 1908, mainly because of strict border management and the preferable geographical condition for preventing FMD entries. On March 12, 2000, some beef cattle in the southern island of Japan (FIG. 1) showed clinical signs, such as pyrexia, anorexia, coughing, and erosions in the nasal and oral regions, and a field veterinarian reported

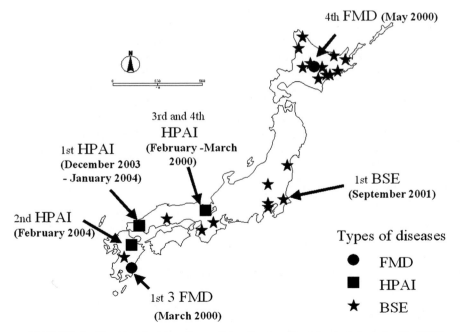

FIGURE 1. Geographical locations of the farms with animals infected with FMD, HPAI, and BSE.

the case to the local livestock hygiene center (LLHC). Sera and epithelial tissues were taken from animals and sent to the National Institute of Animal Health (NIAH) and all 10 animals in this farm were confirmed to be infected with FMD.[1]

The government ordered a state of emergency and a special committee was organized to tackle this problem. As the first action, animal movements within a radius of 20 km from the first farm with FMD infection were strictly restricted. All the cattle in this area were clinically examined and 1–5 animals from each of the farms were serologically tested, using liquid-phase blocking enzyme-linked immunosorbent assay (ELISA). Farms with introduced cattle from the prefecture of the initial case or those that imported hay or straw from FMD endemic countries were also investigated by the same method. For animals that reacted to the ELISA testing, a second ELISA testing, virus isolation attempts, and reverse transcript polymerase chain reaction (RT-PCR) using a probang sample were performed for confirmation. Within 1.5 months after the first case, approximately 52,000 serum samples from approximately 28,000 farms were obtained from all over Japan and were tested by ELISA resulting in two more infected farms in the same prefecture and one infected farm in Hokkaido being detected (FIG. 1).[2] All the animals raised in the farms ($n = 4$) with FMD confirmation were slaughtered, buried properly, and the premises were disinfected. The isolated FMD virus was designated as O/JPN/2000, a typical Asian strain. The epidemiological monitoring of the entire country was carefully continued, and the FMD-free status was declared by OIE at the end of September 2000, 6 months after the initial outbreak.

One of the reasons for the successful early eradication was early detection of the first case. This was done by a well-trained field veterinarian who first suspected FMD by the observed clinical signs. The second reason was early detection of the second group of three infected farms using mass serological testing. Since the clinical signs of the present FMD infection were not typical, mass serological testing was the key component combined with normal clinical examinations. Another important reason was strict animal movement control combined with the disinfection of vehicles and other materials. All these prevention and control measures were conducted properly with good collaboration among people in different sectors, such as the Ministry of Agriculture, Forestry and Fishery (MAFF), the LLHCs, and the NIAH.

HPAI OUTBREAKS

At the end of December 2003, the number of dying chickens increased rapidly in one layer chicken farm located in the western part of Japan (FIG. 1). The LLHC investigated this farm and the virus isolated from the dead chickens was suspected to be the avian influenza virus. Thereafter, isolated virus was submitted to the NIAH and the outbreak was confirmed to be caused by avian influenza virus H5N1 subtype, a causative agent of HPAI.

The movement of people, chickens, eggs, and premises of this farm were strictly restricted. All the chicken flocks were slaughtered, buried properly, and the premises were disinfected by January 21, 2004. The chickens and premises in farms located within a 30-km radius from the first case were also strictly restricted under the Domestic Animal Infectious Disease Control Law. And surveillance for clinical signs, serological testing, and virus isolation attempts for the chickens in this restricted area continued to confirm it to be free from infection until February 19, 2004.

On February 14, 2004, three pet birds, Japanese bantam, owned by a family in the southern island died suddenly (FIG. 1). The owner reported the evidence to the LLHC. The virus isolation attempts combined with pathological examination were initiated by the LLHC. The isolated virus was confirmed to be avian influenza H5N1 subtype. Similar actions were taken as in the first case, and the area has been confirmed to be free from infection on March 11, 2004.

On February 27, an anonymous person made a telephone call, which informed of evidence of a large number of chickens dying in one commercial layer chicken farm which owns more than 250,000 chickens in the central part of Japan (FIG. 1). Veterinarians from the LLHC started investigation on the above farm, and the virus isolated from the dead chicken was confirmed to be avian influenza H5N1 subtype. Because the size of the farm was bigger than in previous cases, the slaughtering, disinfection, and burying process also became bigger, which required the support of the members in the Japan Self Defense Forces. Only 4 km away from this farm, an outbreak of HPAI was also confirmed in a broiler chicken farm with 15,000 animals on March 8. Since the molecular characteristics of the virus isolated from the third and fourth cases were identical, combined with evidence of the close distance between these two farms, the fourth case was considered to be transmitted from the third case. Similar actions were taken as in the third case and the area was confirmed to be free from infection by April 1.

An epidemiological investigation team was established under the MAFF[3] to clarify the source of these HPAI outbreaks. This team investigated the potential source of virus entries, such as travel histories of the people working on the farms, source of the feeds and chickens, and other information. However, no specific factors were confirmative as a source of virus entries. Since Japanese and Korean isolates of avian influenza virus were closely related to each other by genetic analysis,[4] the investigation team hypothesized that the virus was brought from the Korean peninsula by some of the migratory birds. The virus might also have been brought onto domestic chicken farms by Japanese wild birds, which shared the water with the migratory birds or contaminated the water that was fed to the domestic chickens.

CASES OF BSE

The first case of BSE was reported on September 10, 2001,[5] which resulted in a social panic. The trading price of beef declined sharply and many barbecue restaurants closed because the number of customers decreased. Many people stopped purchasing beef, simply because they were afraid of being infected with variant Creutzfeldt–Jakob disease (vCJD). The beef cattle producers were not able to sell their products at proper prices and many cattle suitable for slaughter needed to be held on the farms because demand for beef declined drastically. Many media sources, including newspapers and TV, repeatedly reported the issues related to BSE every day.

In order to secure the safety of beef and investigate the source of the infection, surveillance systems for BSE have been initiated at both slaughterhouses and the farm level since October 2001.[5] At slaughterhouses, an ELISA test is used for all slaughtered cattle, and animals with positive ELISA results have been subjected to Western blotting and immunohistochemistry at several designated laboratories.[5] At the farm level, all the dead animals over 24 months old are requested to be tested for BSE since April 2002, using the same methods as for slaughterhouses.

Through all the surveillance systems, 20 heads of cattle were confirmed to be positive for BSE until June 20, 2005.[6] More than half of these were reported from Hokkaido, a northern island in which dairy production is the main industry (FIG. 1). From the preliminary survey, the positive rate of BSE among healthy, slaughtered animals in Japan was very low, in the order of 1.6×10^{-6}, which was lower than that reported in EU countries.[5] Combined with the mandatory testing of all slaughtered cattle, removing specific risk materials from all slaughtered animals and a ban on feeding meat bone meal to ruminants, the beef circulating in Japan can be considered to be extremely safe with regard to acquiring vCJD.

FOOD-BORNE INFECTION CAUSED BY ENTEROTOXIN TYPE A PRODUCED BY *STAPHYLOCOCCUS AUREUS*

The first report came from one hospital in Osaka City (FIG. 2) on June 27, 2000, which indicated a suspicion of food-borne infection in one family who consumed low-fat milk, resulting in clinical signs of vomiting, stomach ache, and diarrhea.[7] On June 28, more cases of patients with similar clinical signs were reported from the same prefecture and food hygiene inspectors started an investigation into one factory that produced low-fat milk, which was suspected as the cause of the outbreak. After Osaka City disclosed this outbreak on June 29, the number of reported cases increased until more than 14,000 people with similar clinical signs were identified. The outbreak pattern was a typical

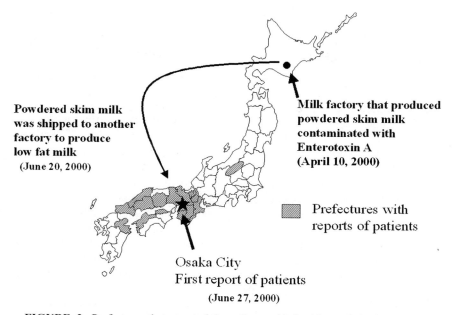

**Powdered skim milk
was shipped to another
factory to produce
low fat milk**
(June 20, 2000)

**Milk factory that produced
powdered skim milk
contaminated with
Enterotoxin A
(April 10, 2000)**

Prefectures with
reports of patients

Osaka City
First report of patients
(June 27, 2000)

FIGURE 2. Prefectures that reported the patients with food-borne infection caused by enterotoxin produced by *Staphylococcus aureus*.

point epidemic type with the highest number of patients greater than 2000 per day at the peak period of June 27–29 (FIG. 3). The patients were widely distributed throughout 15 prefectures, mainly located in the western part of Japan (FIG. 2).

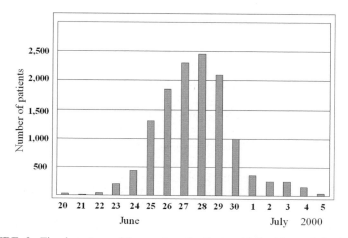

FIGURE 3. Timely pattern of the number of patients with food-borne infection caused by enterotoxin produced by *Staphylococcus aureus*.

Enterotoxin type A produced by *S. aureus* was identified from left-over milk of the patients; therefore, this toxin was suspected as the causative agent of this food-borne outbreak. The operation of the factory that produced the suspected low-fat milk was forced to stop. The police headquarters of Osaka City started an investigation of the corresponding milk company as a suspect of injury through professional negligence. Through the investigation, enterotoxin type A was identified from powdered skim milk produced in one factory located in the northern island. There was an accident of power failure for 3 h on April 1 at this factory and growth of *S. aureus* was suspected to have occurred. Thereafter, enterotoxin A produced from *S. aureus* contaminated powdered skim milk. Although some batches of the powdered skim milk produced during this period had higher bacteria counts than the required levels, some of them were resolved in water, mixed with other powdered skim milk, and re-used for producing other batches of powdered skim milk. This contaminated powdered skim milk was shipped from the factory in the northern island to a factory located in Osaka City on June 20, and the low-fat milk produced from this powdered skim milk contaminated with enterotoxin A became the source of the outbreak. Since enterotoxin is heat resistant, powdered skim milk remained toxic after the series of pasteurization processes.

In respect to the number of people infected, this outbreak became one of the biggest food-borne infection outbreaks in Japan after World War II. This outbreak was also a shocking event for food manufacturers, food hygiene officers, and researchers because a Hazard Analysis of Critical Control Point (HACCP) system has been authorized to the milk factory that produced powdered skim milk contaminated with enterotoxin A. The milk company, which was one of the biggest milk companies in Japan, was accused of negligence and received serious damage by social sanctions.

HEV INFECTION
AS A ZOONOTIC PROBLEM

HEV infections, which are endemic and frequently epidemic in developing countries, are also observed in developed countries in a sporadic form.[8] On March 2003, two hunters who repeatedly consumed uncooked liver from wild boars developed severe clinical signs of hepatitis and one of them died. Serum samples obtained from these patients revealed that the hepatitis was caused by HEV.[8] Similarly, 8 of 12 people who ate meat from wild boar were infected with HEV and five of them developed clinical signs.[9] In April 2003, four people who consumed uncooked meat from wild deer developed clinical signs of hepatitis and were diagnosed as being infected with HEV.[10] The HEV RNA was identified in the left-over portion of the deer meat by PCR. All the evidence indicated that HEV is transmissible from wild animals to human beings. Because Japanese are notorious for peculiar eating habits, such as uncooked fish and less frequently raw meat, this may at least partially explain the HEV infection in Japan.[10]

In August 2004, six people who consumed liver and intestine of pigs at a barbeque restaurant were infected with HEV and one of them died of acute hepatitis.[11] Thereafter, one of these infected people donated his blood without knowing of his infection and a blood transfusion infection also occurred. This evidence indicated that normal eating habits, such as consumption of pork, could be a potential risk for HEV infection. Researchers now suspect pork as a natural source of HEV infection because of the following reasons: (*a*) genetic similarity between isolates obtained from humans and pigs,[12] (*b*) virus is transmissible between pigs and monkeys,[13] and (*c*) seroprevalence of marketing pigs is high (90%).[12] Therefore, general cautions such as proper cooking of pork before consumption, in addition to avoiding contaminating of other food items with raw meats, needs to be carefully reminded to distributors and consumers.

CONCLUSIONS

All these emerging animal and human diseases, including food-borne infections, caused confusion for both producers and consumers. As general prevention and control practices for these diseases, early detection of the first case and rapid action for preventing and controlling the spread of infections are very important. Proper risk communication about correct information of the diseases to consumers as well as producers is also important in order to avoid unnecessary social confusion due to rumor or false information.

In addition, collaborations and understanding between producers and consumers, between veterinary medicine and human medicine, and between MAFF and Ministry of Health, Labour and Welfare (MHLW) have been emphasized after a series of these outbreaks. A new organization entitled the Food Safety Commission was established in July 2003 under the cabinet; therefore, this organization is considered to be neutral between MAFF and MHLW. The commission's main purposes are to undertake scientific risk assessment of food items, implement risk communication, and respond to food-borne accidents and emergencies.[14] By creating good collaboration among people in different sectors, we expect to prevent and control animal and human diseases more efficiently in the future.

REFERENCES

1. SUGIURA, K. *et al.* 2001. Eradication of foot and mouth disease in Japan. Rev. Sci. Tech. Off. Int. Epiz. **20:** 701–713.

2. YAMANE, I. *et al.* 2003. A foot and mouth disease outbreak (2000) in Japan and a trial of a geographic information system application for monitoring an eradication program. Proc. 10th Int. Sym. Vet. Epidemiol. Economics, Vol. 1, 891–893.

3. AN INVESTIGATION TEAM FOR THE INFECTION SOURCE OF HIGHLY PATHOGENIC AVIAN INFLUENZA, Ministry of Agriculture, Forestry and Fishery. 2004. Infection route of Highly Pathogenic Avian Influenza (in Japanese).

4. MASE, M. *et al.* 2005. Genetic comparison of H5N1 influenza A viruses isolated from chickens in Japan and Korea. Microbiol. Immunol. **49:** 871–874.

5. TSUTSUI, T. *et al.* 2004. Preliminary evaluation of the prevalence of BSE in Japan. Vet. Rec. **154:** 113–114.

6. NONAKA, T. *et al.* 2005. Geographical analysis of risk factors of bovine spongiform encephalopathy (In Japanese). J. Vet. Epidemiol. **9:** 15–20.

7. YAMAMOTO, S. 2001. Case of the toxin type food poisoning and hygienic control of the food (in Japanese). J. Vet. Epidemiol **5:** 41–44.

8. TEI, S. *et al.* 2003. Zoonotic transmission of hepatitis E virus from deer to human beings. Lancet **362:** 371–373.

9. TAMADA, Y. *et al.* 2004. Consumption of wild boar linked to cases of hepatitis E. J. Hepatol. **40:** 869–870.

10. MATSUDA, H. *et al.* 2003. Severe Hepatitis E virus infection after ingestion of uncooked liver from a wild boar. J. Infect. Dis. **188:** 944.

11. YOMIURI NEWSPAPER WEB VERSION. TOKYO, November 28 (in Japanese). Available at: http://www.geocities.jp/ewadai/wadai`0050.html (accessed June 20, 2005).

12. TAKAHASHI, M. *et al.* 2003. Swine hepatitis E virus strains in Japan form four phylogenetic clusters comparable with those of Japanese isolates of human hepatitis E virus. J. Gen. Virol. **84:** 851–862.

13. MENG, X.J. *et al.* 1998. Genetic and experimental evidence for cross-species infection by swine hepatitis E virus. J. Virol. **72:** 9714–9721.

14. FOOD SAFETY COMMISSION, TOKYO. http:/www.fsc.go.jp/english/index.html (accessed June 20, 2005).

Implication of Phylogenetic Systematics of Rodent-Borne Hantaviruses Allows Understanding of Their Distribution

VINCENT HERBRETEAU,[a] JEAN-PAUL GONZALEZ,[b] AND JEAN-PIERRE HUGOT[b]

[a]*Institut de Recherche pour le Développement (IRD), 75231 Paris Cedex 05, France*

[b]*Muséum National d'Histoire Naturelle, Département Systématique et Évolution, UMR Origin, Structure and Evolution of Biodiversity, 75231, Paris cedex 05, France*

ABSTRACT: Hantaviruses' distribution is reassessed after performing a cladistic analysis on 93 strains isolated from rodents, and one used as outgroup: *Thottapalayam* isolated from a shrew. While most hantaviruses found in wild animals were collected in northern Asia, Europe, North America, and South America, only *Thottapalayam* and *Thailand* were found in South and Southeastern Asia. *Thottapalayam* is highly divergent from the other known hantaviruses and may represent the emerging tip of a different lineage. Serological surveys carried out to detect evidence of Hantavirus in human populations revealed positive samples not only in West and Central Africa but also in Thailand, with a first case recently confirmed. This suggests that Hantaan-related viruses may infect humans out of their well-documented range. Thus, if rodents are probably the primary reservoir, other mammals may be involved in the cycle of hantaviruses. Additional work is needed out of the traditional areas where hantaviruses have been recorded. New viruses, different hosts, and different human syndromes may be discovered in the future mainly in Southeastern Asia and in Africa where Muridae rodents are present and highly diversified.

KEYWORDS: rodent-borne hantaviruses; *Thottapalayam*; S gene; phylogeny; Bayesian analysis; biogeography; co-evolution

INTRODUCTION

Wild rodents are the usual reservoirs of the zoonotically important hantaviruses (genus *Hantavirus*, family *Bunyaviridae*). Several serologically

Address for correspondence: Dr. Jean-Pierre Hugot, IRD, RCEVD-CVD, UT178, Mahidol University, 25/25 Phuttamonthon 4, Nakhon Pathom 73170, Thailand. Voice and fax: 66-2-441-01-89.
e-mail: hugot@mnhn.fr

Ann. N.Y. Acad. Sci. 1081: 39–56 (2006). © 2006 New York Academy of Sciences.
doi: 10.1196/annals.1373.004

distinct groups have been associated with different syndromes. In the Old World, *Hantaan, Dobrava, Seoul,* and *Puumala* cause the clinical forms of hemorrhagic fever with renal syndrome.[1] In the New World, *Sin Nombre* and *Andes* are responsible for hantavirus pulmonary syndrome.[2] A last group, *Tula,* widely distributed in Russia and Eastern Europe, has never been associated with a human disease.

The hantavirus genome has three segments—large (L 6.5 kb), medium (M 3.7 kb), and small (S 1.8 kb) encoding: viral transcriptase-replicase, surface glycoprotein precursor (G1 and G2), and nucleocapsid protein, respectively.[3,4] Different analyses based on the alignment of the M or S sequences[1,5–14] have been performed and used to discuss the distribution of these viruses, relative to the biogeography and evolutionary history of their hosts. Muridae rodents are the primary hosts, and because each virus group seems to be associated with a particular rodent group, the hypothesis of co-evolution has been suggested.[1,3,5,6] Since the methodology[15] to establish such co-evolution has been questioned and no firm conclusions have been reached, this article revisits the co-evolution of the virus by examining the evolutionary relationship of the S genes of various hantaviruses with their respective Muridae hosts.

MATERIALS AND METHODS

Sequences and Alignment

The data set includes *Hantavirus* S sequences, from 94 taxa, found in GenBank (TABLE 1): 92 isolated from different rodent hosts, one isolated in Korea from a bat (Kim, direct submission, 1995), and *Thottapalayam* detected in India from a shrew (*Suncus murinus*) by Carey *et al.*,[16] identified by Xiao *et al.*,[17] and recently introduced (complete S sequence) in GenBank by Schmaljohn and Toney (direct submission, 2004). Only complete coding part, whose wild host was certainly identified, were considered. The S sequence of Dugbe virus, previously used as outgroup by Hughes and Friedman,[11] was first considered but finally excluded as explained in the outgroup paragraph. A virus described in Thailand from a *Bandicota indica*[1] could not be included in the data set because the S sequence of this virus remains unknown. Selected sequences range between 1130 and 2082 nucleotides from which: first 42 correspond to the primer and nucleotides; 1342–2082 to the codon stop and noncoding region. Alignment of the coding part (nucleotides 43–1341) was performed using CLUSTAL-X automatic procedure,[18] then improved manually using SE-AL v2.0a11,[19] and validated using the amino acid translation. When applied to the noncoding part, the same procedure made visible the impossibility to detect real homologies between most of the sequences. Thus, only the coding part of the gene was used for phylogenetic analyses. Sequences were analyzed at nucleotide level.

Aligning and Coding Indels

Sequence alignment made it necessary to postulate several gaps, particularly between nucleotides 766 and 813. Various approaches have been employed to deal with insertions–deletions (indels), ranging from their total exclusion to their treatment as missing data or as a fifth character state. Gaps are considered reliable characters by many systematists; and the first approach means the loss of potential phylogenetic information.[20] In addition, in our data set, indels are observed within the hypervariable (HV) region where the percentage of parsimony informative characters is superior to 90% (<60% for the rest of the matrix). Therefore, we kept this region for analysis. Standard procedures for coding gaps suffer from several weaknesses: either the different sites are analyzed independently (gap = new state) and each gap is artificially over-weighted relatively to the number of sites, or each site is coded "?" (gap = missing data), and optimization procedure makes the whole zone devoid of phylogenetic information. To express the potential phylogenetic information contained in zones with internested insertions/deletions and substitutions, eight characters coding the presence/absence of deletions between nucleotides 766 and 813 were added. Finally, the matrix includes 1323 RNA characters and 8 presence/absence characters.

Outgroup Rooting

An outgroup sequence must be closely related to the rest of the sequences, but comparatively more different than the others are between themselves.[15] The introduction of the *Thottapalayam* sequence within the previously aligned rodent-borne sequences makes necessary the addition of several deletions and shows that *Thottapalayam* possesses several conservative parts of the rodent-borne sequences. Thus, if *Thottapalayam* may certainly be considered a Hantavirus, it is highly divergent from other members of the genus. This is confirmed by the values of the total character distances calculated using PAUP : within the rodent-borne group, distances vary from 2 to 516; between *Thottapalayam* and the others, distances range between 765 and 859. Thus, *Thottapalayam* may be considered a valuable outgroup and was included in the data set.

Sequence Analyses

Two methods likely to give results interpretable in an evolutionary context were used: maximum parsimony (MP) analysis and maximum Bayesian (MB) analysis. MACCLADE 4.0[21] and TREEVIEW 1.3[22] were used for data and tree handling and for computation of statistics. MP analysis was computed using PAUP*

TABLE 1. List of Hantavirus strains included in the present study

	Virus species and strain	Abbreviation	Host species	Family	Accession no.	Nucl	Region	Distribution
1	*Dobrava–Estonia*	DOBV-Estonia1	*Apodemus agrarius*	Murinae	AJ009773	1,671	PAL	Estonia (Saaremaa)
2	*Dobrava–Estonia*	DOBV-Estonia2	*Apodemus agrarius*	Murinae	AJ009775	1,671	PAL	Estonia (Saaremaa)
3	*Dobrava–Slovakia*	DOBV-Slovakia1	*Apodemus agrarius*	Murinae	AJ269549	1,704	PAL	Slovakia (Kosice)
4	*Dobrava–Bosnia*	DOBV-Bosnia	*Apodemus flavicollis*	Murinae	L41916	1,670	PAL	Bosnia
5	*Dobrava–Greece*	DOBV-Greece1	*Apodemus flavicollis*	Murinae	AJ410615	1,290	PAL	Greece (Northeast)
6	*Dobrava–Greece*	DOBV-Greece2	*Apodemus flavicollis*	Murinae	AJ410619	1,290	PAL	Greece (Northeast)
7	*Dobrava–Russia*	DOBV-Russia1	*Apodemus sylvaticus*	Murinae	AF442623	1,637	PAL	Russia (Krasnodar)
8	*Dobrava–Russia*	DOBV-Russia2	*Apodemus sylvaticus*	Murinae	AF442622	1,196	PAL	Russia (Goryachiy)
9	*Dobrava–Slovakia*	DOBV-Slovakia2	*Apodemus sylvaticus*	Murinae	AJ269550	1,704	PAL	Slovakia (Kosice)
10	*Hantaan–76118*	HTNV-76118	*Apodemus sylvaticus*	Murinae	M14626	1,696	PAL	South Korea
11	*Hantaan–Maaji*	HTNV-Maaji	*Apodemus sylvaticus*	Murinae	AF321094	1,700	PAL	Korea (Maaji)
12	*Hantaan–Amur AP61*	AMRV.AP61	*Apodemus peninsulae*	Murinae	AB071183	1,290	PAL	Russia FE (Solovey)
13	*Hantaan–Amur AP63*	AMRV.AP63	*Apodemus peninsulae*	Murinae	AB071184	1,696	PAL	Russia FE (Solovey)
14	*Hantaan–Guizhou*	HTNV-Guizhou	*Apodemus sylvaticus*	Murinae	AB027097	1,635	PAL	China (Guizhou)
15	*Hantaan–Anhui*	HTNV-Anhui	*Niviventer confucianus*	Murinae	AB027523	1,654	PAL	China (Anhui)
16	***Hantaan–Bat***	**HTNV-Bat**	***Rhinolophus ferrumequinum***	**Rinolophidae**	**U37768**	**1,696**	**PAL**	**Korea**
17	*Seoul–L99*	SEOV-L99	*Rattus losea*	Murinae	AF288299	1,764	PAL	China (Jiangxi)
18	*Seoul–Sapporo*	SEOV-Sapporo	*Rattus norvegicus*	Murinae	M34881	1,769	PAL	Japan (Sapporo)
19	*Seoul–Shanxi*	SEOV-Shanxi	*Rattus rattus*	Murinae	AF288643	1,772	PAL	China (Shanxi)
20	*Seoul–Tchoupitoulas*	SEOV-Tchoupi	*Rattus rattus*	Murinae	AF329389	1,785	NEA	USA (Louisiana)
21	*Seoul–Zhejiang*	SEOV-Zhejiang1	*Rattus rattus*	Murinae	AB027522	1,692	PAL	China (Zhejiang)
22	*Seoul–Zhejiang*	SEOV-Zhejiang2	*Rattus rattus*	Murinae	AF288653	1,772	PAL	China (Zhejiang)
23	*Sin Nombre*	SNV	*Peromyscus maniculatus*	Neotominae	L25784	2,059	NEA	USA (S-West & Central)
24	*SinNombre–Convict Creek*	SNV-Conv.74	*Peromyscus maniculatus*	Neotominae	L33683	1,287	NEA	USA (California)
25	*SinNombre–Convict Creek*	SNV-Conv.107	*Peromyscus maniculatus*	Neotominae	L33816	1,287	NEA	USA (California)
26	*SinNombre–Monongahela*	MGLV	*Peromyscus maniculatus*	Neotominae	U32591	2,082	NEA	USA (Appalachian)
27	*NewYork–RI1*	NYork-RI1	*Peromyscus leucopus*	Neotominae	U09488	2,078	NEA	USA (North East)
28	*Limestone Canyon*	Limestone Canyon	*Peromyscus boylii*	Neotominae	AF307322	1,209	NEA	USA (Arizona)
29	*El Moro Canyon*	El Moro Canyon	*Reithrodontomys megalotis*	Neotominae	U11427	1,896	NEA	USA (New Mexico)
30	*Rio Segundo*	RioSegundo	*Reithrodontomys mexicanus*	Neotominae	U18100	1,749	NEO	Costa Rica

Continued.

TABLE 1. Continued

	Virus species and strain	Abbreviation	Host species	Family	Accession no.	Nucl	Region	Distribution
31	Andes–AH1	ANDV-AH1	*Oligoryzomys longicaudatus*	Sigmodontinae	AF004660	1,876	NEO	Argentina
32	Andes–Bermejo	BMJV	*Oligoryzomys chacoensis*	Sigmodontinae	AF482713	1,933	NEO	Argentina (Oran)
33	Andes–Chile	ANDV-Chile1	*Oligoryzomys longicaudatus*	Sigmodontinae	AF291702	1,871	NEO	Chile (Aysen)
34	Andes–Chile	ANDV-Chile2	*Oligoryzomys longicaudatus*	Sigmodontinae	NC003466	1,871	NEO	Chile (Aysen)
35	Andes–Lechiguanas	LECV	*Oligoryzomys flavescens*	Sigmodontinae	AF482714	1,938	NEO	Argentina (Lechiguana)
36	Andes–Norte	ANDV-Norte	*Oligoryzomys chacoensis*	Sigmodontinae	AF325966	1,921	NEO	Argentina Norte
37	Andes–Oran	ORNV	*Oligoryzomys longicaudatus*	Sigmodontinae	AF482715	1,919	NEO	Argentina (Oran)
38	Andes–Pergamino	PRGV	*Akodon azarae*	Sigmodontinae	AF482717	1,860	NEO	Argentina
39	Maciel	Maciel	*Bolomys benefactus*	Sigmodontinae	AF482716	1,869	NEO	Argentina (Maciel)
40	Laguna Negra	Laguna Negra	*Calomys laucha*	Sigmodontinae	AF005727	1,904	NEO	Paraguay, Bolivia
41	Rio Mamore	RioMamore	*Oryzomys microtis*	Sigmodontinae	U52136	1,975	NEO	Bolivia
42	Bayou	Bayou	*Oryzomys palustris*	Sigmodontinae	L36929	1,958	NEA	USA (Louisiana)
43	Black Creek Canal	Black Creek	*Sigmodon hispidus*	Sigmodontinae	L39949	1,989	NEA	USA (Florida)
44	Muleshoe	Muleshoe	*Sigmodon hispidus*	Sigmodontinae	U54575	1,989	NEA	USA (Texas)
45	Caño Delgadito	CanoDelgadito	*Sigmodon alstoni*	Sigmodontinae	AF000140	1,130	NEO	Venezuela (Portuguesa)
46	Isla Vista	Isla Vista 1	*Microtus californicus*	Arvicolinae	U19302	1,720	NEA	USA (California)
47	Isla Vista	Isla Vista 2	*Microtus californicus*	Arvicolinae	U31534	1,720	NEA	USA (California)
48	Isla Vista	Isla Vista 3	*Microtus californicus*	Arvicolinae	U31535	1,302	NEA	USA (California)
49	Prospect Hill	ProspectHill1	*Microtus montanus*	Arvicolinae	M34011	1,675	NEA	USA
50	Prospect Hill	ProspectHill2	*Microtus montanus*	Arvicolinae	Z49098	1,675	NEA	USA
51	Prairie Vole	PrairieVole	*Microtus ochrogaster*	Arvicolinae	U19303	1,722	NEA	USA (?)
52	Topografov	Topografov	*Lemmus sibiricus*	Arvicolinae	AJ011646	1,951	PAL	Russia FE (Taymyr)
53	Khabarovsk	Khabarovsk	*Microtus fortis*	Arvicolinae	U35255	1,845	PAL	Russia FE (Khabarovsk)
54	Vladivostock	Vladivostock	*Microtus fortis*	Arvicolinae	AB011630	1,228	PAL	Russia FE (Vladivostok)
55	Tula–Germany1	TULV-Germany1	*Microtus arvalis*	Arvicolinae	AF164093	1,832	PAL	Germany
56	Tula–Germany2	TULV-Germany2	*Microtus arvalis*	Arvicolinae	AF289821	1,828	PAL	Germany
57	Tula–Lodz	TULV-Lodz1	*Microtus arvalis*	Arvicolinae	AF063892	1,852	PAL	Poland
58	Tula–Lodz	TULV Lodz2	*Microtus arvalis*	Arvicolinae	AF063897	1,852	PAL	Poland
59	Tula–Moravia	TULV-Moravia	*Microtus arvalis*	Arvicolinae	Z69991	1,831	PAL	Moravia
60	Tula–Slovakia	TULV-Slovakia1	*Microtus arvalis*	Arvicolinae	AJ223601	1,831	PAL	Slovakia (Koziky)

Continued.

TABLE 1. *Continued*

	Virus species and strain	Abbreviation	Host species	Family	Accession no.	Nucl	Region	Distribution
61	*Tula*–Slovakia	TULV-Slovakia2	*Microtus arvalis*	Arvicolinae	AJ223600	1,831	PAL	Slovakia (Koziky)
62	*Tula*–Slovakia	TULV-Slovakia3	*Microtus arvalis*	Arvicolinae	Z48235	1,831	PAL	Slovakia (Malacky)
63	*Tula*–Slovakia	TULV-Slovakia4	*Microtus arvalis*	Arvicolinae	Y13979	1,833	PAL	Slovakia (Kosice)
64	*Tula*–Slovakia	TULV-Slovakia5	*Microtus arvalis*	Arvicolinae	Y13980	1,832	PAL	Slovakia (Kosice)
65	*Tula*–Slovakia	TULV-Slovakia6	*Microtus arvalis*	Arvicolinae	Z68191	1,831	PAL	Slovakia (Malacky)
66	*Tula*–Russia	TULV-Russia	*Microtus gregalis*	Arvicolinae	Z30941	1,847	PAL	Russia (Tula)
67	*Tula*–Serbia	TULV-Serbia	*Microtus subterraneus*	Arvicolinae	AF017659	1,834	PAL	Serbia (Cacac)
68	*Puumala*–Bashkortostan	PUUV-Bashkor	*Clethrionomys glareolus*	Arvicolinae	AF442613	1,733	PAL	Russia (Bashkortostan)
69	*Puumala*–Belgium	PUUV-Belgium	*Clethrionomys glareolus*	Arvicolinae	AJ277030	1,837	PAL	Belgium (Thuin)
70	*Puumala*–CG1820	PUUV-CG1820	*Clethrionomys glareolus*	Arvicolinae	M32750	1,784	PAL	?
71	*Puumala*–Denmark	PUUV-Denmark	*Clethrionomys glareolus*	Arvicolinae	AJ238791	1,831	PAL	Denmark
72	*Puumala*–Evo	PUUV-Evo	*Clethrionomys glareolus*	Arvicolinae	Z30703	1,832	PAL	Finland
73	*Puumala*–Kamiiso	HOKV-Kamiiso	*Clethrionomys rufocanus*	Arvicolinae	AB010730	1,833	PAL	Japan (Hokkaido)
74	*Puumala*–Japan	HOKV-Japan	*Clethrionomys rufocanus*	Arvicolinae	AB010731	1,833	PAL	Japan (Tobetsu)
75	*Puumala*–Karelia	PUUV-Karelia1	*Clethrionomys glareolus*	Arvicolinae	AJ238790	1,832	PAL	Russia (Karelia, Gomselga)

Continued.

TABLE 1. *Continued*

	Virus species and strain	Abbreviation	Host species	Family	Accession no.	Nucl	Region	Distribution
76	*Puumala*–Karelia	PUUV-Karelia2	*Clethrionomys glareolus*	Arvicolinae	AJ238788	1,828	PAL	Russia (Karelia, Karhumaki)
77	*Puumala*–Karelia	PUUV-Karelia3	*Clethrionomys glareolus*	Arvicolinae	AJ238789	1,830	PAL	Russia (Karelia, Kolodozero)
78	*Puumala*–Kazan	PUUV-Kazan	*Clethrionomys glareolus*	Arvicolinae	Z84204	1,826	PAL	Sweden?
79	*Puumala*–Norway	PUUV-Norway1	*Clethrionomys glareolus*	Arvicolinae	AJ223369	1,849	PAL	Norway (Eidsvoll)
80	*Puumala*–Norway	PUUV-Norway3	*Clethrionomys glareolus*	Arvicolinae	AJ223374	1,828	PAL	Norway (Mellansel)
81	*Puumala*–Norway	PUUV-Norway4	*Clethrionomys glareolus*	Arvicolinae	AJ223375	1,829	PAL	Norway (Mellansel)
82	*Puumala*–Norway	PUUV-Norway5	*Clethrionomys glareolus*	Arvicolinae	AJ223376	1,871	PAL	Norway (Solleftea)
83	*Puumala*–Norway	PUUV-Norway6	*Clethrionomys glareolus*	Arvicolinae	AJ223377	1,882	PAL	Norway (Solleftea)
84	*Puumala*–Norway	PUUV-Norway7	*Clethrionomys glareolus*	Arvicolinae	AJ223380	1,827	PAL	Norway (Tavelsjo)
85	*Puumala*–Omsk	PUUV-Omsk1	*Clethrionomys glareolus*	Arvicolinae	AF367067	1,732	PAL	Omsk, Russia (W Siberia)
86	*Puumala*–Omsk	PUUV-Omsk2	*Clethrionomys glareolus*	Arvicolinae	AF367068	1,732	PAL	Omsk, Russia (W Siberia)
87	*Puumala*–Omsk	PUUV-Omsk3	*Clethrionomys glareolus*	Arvicolinae	AF367069	1,732	PAL	Omsk, Russia (W Siberia)
88	*Puumala*–Omsk	PUUV-Omsk4	*Clethrionomys glareolus*	Arvicolinae	AF367070	1,732	PAL	Omsk, Russia (W Siberia)
89	*Puumala*–Slovakia	PUUV-Slovakia	*Clethrionomys glareolus*	Arvicolinae	AF294652	1,809	PAL	Slovakia
90	*Puumala*–Sotkamo	PUUV-Sotkamo	*Clethrionomys glareolus*	Arvicolinae	X61035	1,830	PAL	Finland (Sotkamo)
91	*Puumala*–Udmurtia	PUUV-Udmurtia	*Clethrionomys glareolus*	Arvicolinae	Z21497	1,827	PAL	Finland (Udmurtia)
92	*Puumala*–Vranica	PUUV-Vranica	*Clethrionomys glareolus*	Arvicolinae	U14137	1,828	PAL	Bosnia (Vranica)
93	*Thottapalayam*	Thottalayam	*Suncus murinus*	Soricidae	AY526097	1,530	ORIENT	India (Thottalayam)

NOTE: First two columns: name of strain and acronym used in text and figures. Columns 3 and 4: scientific and family names of principal host. Columns 5 and 6: accession number of sequence and number of nucleotides given in GenBank. Region refers to biogeographic areas: Palearctic (PAL), Nearctic (NEA), Neotropical (NEO), Oriental (ORIENT). Column 7: in which country, and when possible in which province or locality, the virus strain has been collected.

4.0b10.[23] Robustness of nodes was assessed using bootstrap method[24] computed after 10,000 replicates of heuristic search, with closest stepwise addition of taxa. MODELTEST 3.0[25] was used to determine the best fitting likelihood settings: the general time-reversible model[26] with among-site substitution rate heterogeneity described by a gamma distribution with eight categories[27] and a fraction of sites (INV) constrained to be invariable (GTR+I+G, selected by AIC). MB analysis using these settings was performed using MRBAYES v3.0B4.[28] A Bayesian approach allows defining an explicit probability model of character evolution and obtaining a rapid approximation of posterior probabilities of trees, through the use of the Markov Chain Monte Carlo (MCMC) approach. MRBAYES also allows performing phylogenetic analyses of data sets combining information from different subsets, evolving under different evolutionary models. Two partitions were distinguished in our original data set: partition 1 = nucleotide (characters 1–1323) for which the likelihood model chosen was the GTR+I+G; partition 2 = indels (characters 1324–1331) treated as presence/absence. Analysis was conducted with four independent Markov chains, run for 2,000,000 metropolis-coupled MCMC generations, with tree sampling every 10 generations, and burn-in after 3300 trees. Consensus tree was computed using the "halfcompat" option, equivalent to the 50% majority rule. Proportion values of posterior probability of bipartition, considered equivalent to bootstrap values,[29,30] were used for evaluation of robustness of the nodes.

Virus Taxonomy

In the following and in the figures:

– Virus species listed in the Eighth Report of the International Committee on Taxonomy of Viruses[31] are in italic script.
– Strain names are in roman script, or are represented using their abbreviations in caps when an abbreviation has been proposed.
– When different strains of the same virus species are included, a number or an adjective (generally dealing with the geographic origin) is added.

The correspondence between the virus species, strain names, and abbreviations is given in TABLE 1.

RESULTS

General

MP or MB analyses yield consistent results. All bipartitions found by MP analysis with a bootstrap value superior or equal to 95% were also found by MB analysis with a posterior probability equal or superior to 95%. In addition,

MB analysis gave a resolution and a support superior or equal to 50% for several nodes, which were unresolved, or resolved with a bootstrap inferior to 50%, in the MP analysis. Even if MB analysis is likely to favor higher values when compared to bootstrap analysis,[28–30] the results are fully congruent and are represented in FIGURE 1. FIGURES 2 and 3 detail the composition of the three main clades.

The cladogram is rooted between a basal branch corresponding with *Thottapalayam* and a monophyletic group including all the rodent-borne parasites, distributed following the three main clades: CLADE-*1* includes "*Seoul, Hantaan, Dobrava*;" CLADE-*2* and CLADE-*3* are sister clades including: "*Bayou, Sinnombre, Andes*," and "*Islavista, Tula, Puumala*," respectively. Each clade and the sister-grouping of CLADE-*2* and CLADE-*3*, have a support superior or equal to 78%. CLADE-*1* groups 22 taxa: all the viruses hosted by Murinae rodents, and the single strain found on a bat; CLADE-*2* groups 23 taxa: all the viruses hosted by Sigmodontinae rodents; CLADE-*3* groups 48 taxa: all the viruses hosted by Arvicolinae rodents. Regarding the geographic distribution: CLADE-*1* is exclusively Palearctic, except Tchoupitoulas collected in the Nearctic (Louisiana); CLADE-*2* is found exclusively in the New World and associates strains from the Nearctic and the Neotropics; CLADE-*3* may be divided into one Nearctic subclade (*Islavista*) and the sister grouping of two Palearctic subclades (*Tula + Puumala*).

CLADE-*1*: "*Seoul, Hantaan, Dobrava*"

Viruses hosted by *Rattus* spp. are distinguished from those hosted by *Niviventer confucianus* and *Apodemus* spp. With the exception of the parasite of *Niviventer* (considered by taxonomists closer from *Rattus*), this distribution matches the taxonomy of the rodents at genus level. However, different virus strains hosted by the same rodent species are not grouped together. The bat virus is included in *Hantaan*; its closer relative is HT.76118. Regarding the geographic distribution: *Seoul* is found in eastern China, with the exception of Sapporo (Japan) and Tchoupitoulas (Louisiana), which are sister taxa. *Hantaan* is also restricted to the eastern part of the Palearctic region, but with a wider distribution, including several provinces in China, Korea, and the Amur area (northeastern Siberia). *Dobrava* has a European distribution extending from Estonia toward Greece, through western Russia, Slovakia, and Bosnia. The arrangement of *Dobrava* viruses on the cladogram generally fits with a North-to-South distribution (FIG. 2).

CLADE-*2*: "*Bayou, Sinnombre, Andes*"

From the three subclades, two are hosted by Sigmondontini rodents (*Bayou, Andes*), while Neotomini rodents host *Sinnombre*. *Bayou*, found in three states

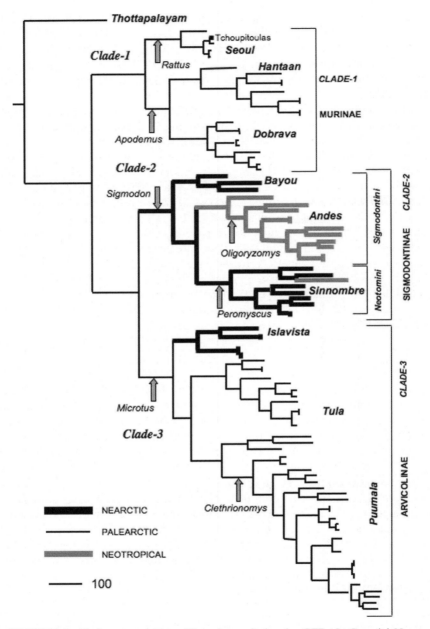

FIGURE 1. Cladogram resulting of Bayesian analysis using GTR+I+G model. Names given to the main groups according to previous publications, except "*Bayou*" and "*Islavista*," which are proposed as new names. Different color patterns are attributed to different geographic areas. Arrows point out optimization of the host genera on the cladogram.

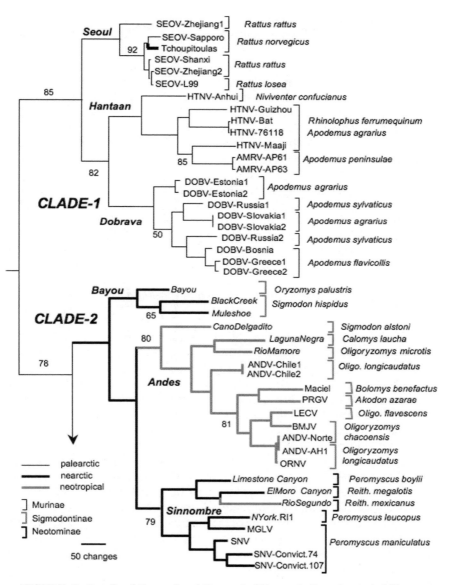

FIGURE 2. Details of CLADE-*1* and CLADE-*2* of FIGURE 1. Posterior probability numbered when inferior to 95% (probability of no-numbered nodes between 95 and 100). For each virus strain, the scientific name of the host is given; different color patterns are attributed to different host groups and to different biogeographic areas. *Reith. = Reithrodontomys*; *Oligo. = Oligoryzomys*.

of southeastern North America (Florida, Louisiana, and Texas) is hosted by two different genera, *Oryzomys* and *Sigmodon*. *Sinnombre* is subdivided into: a group of three taxa found in Arizona, New Mexico, and Costa Rica and hosted by *Peromyscus* sp. and *Reithrodontomys* spp.; a group hosted by *Peromyscus* spp. ranging from northeastern to southwestern and central United States. *Andes* is entirely found in the Neotropics and hosted by Sigmodontini rodents: *Oligoryzomys* is the most frequent, together with several other genera (*Akodon, Bolomys, Calomys, Sigmodon*). The most divergent species in this group is *Caño Delgadito* from Venezuela; the other species are arranged following their geographic origin: Laguna Negra and Rio Marmore (Bolivia and Paraguay); *Andes*-Chile 1 and 2 (Chile); the last seven from northern Argentina. Distribution of virus taxa within CLADE-2 generally fits with the taxonomy of rodents at host-tribe level and a dominant genus may be recognized for each of the main subgroups. However: the Sigmodontini parasites are not monophyletic; as in CLADE-*1*, no congruence is observed at host-species level (closely related viruses hosted by different host species, viruses hosted by the same host species not closely related on the cladogram) (FIG. 2).

CLADE-*3*: *"Prairie, Tula, Puumala"*

CLADE-*3* is the sister group of CLADE-2 and is hosted by Arvicolinae rodents. *Tula* and *Puumala* are strictly Palearctic, *Islavista* is strictly Nearctic. *Microtus* spp. is the dominant host for *Islavista* and *Tula*. *Islavista* may be subdivided into two groups: Isla Vista 1, 2, 3 are Californian, Prairie Vole and Prospect Hill 1 and 2 are from South Central United States. *Tula* has a European distribution extending from North to South, from Poland, Germany, Moravia, western Russia, and Slovakia. In *Puumala*: *Microtus*, associated with *Lemmus*, is present in a small basal group including three virus species found in the extreme East of Russian Siberia (Vladivostok, *Khabarovsk*, and *Topografov*), the other species are hosted by *Clethrionomys rufocanus* or *Clethrionomys glareolus*. Parasites of *C. rufocanus* are Japanese. Parasites of *C. glareolus* have a distribution extending from Northwestern Europe (Denmark, Belgium) to Scandinavia, Finland, and South Central Russia. In *Puumala*, a dominant host species may be recognized for each of the main subgroups. But, in *Islavista* and *Tula*, there is no general congruence between the virus and host classifications at the species level: closely related viruses hosted by different host species; viruses hosted by the same host species, not closely related on the cladogram (FIG. 3).

DISCUSSION

Clades, Groups, Robustness of the Nodes, and Molecular Data

Our analysis confirms the three main clades previously described within the hantaviruses[6,11] and supports the subdivision of each clade into three

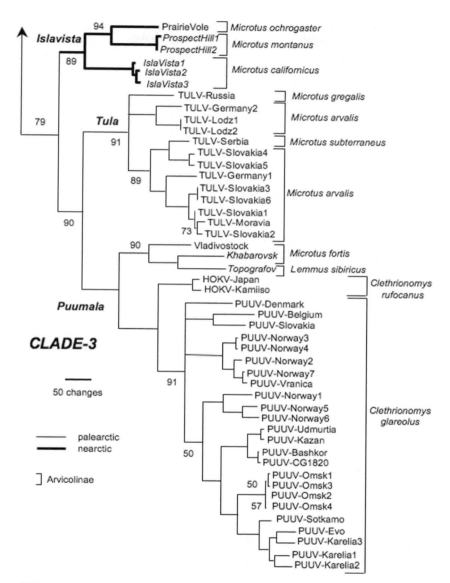

FIGURE 3. Detail of CLADE-*3* of FIGURE 1. See legend of FIGURE 2.

subclades. *"Seoul," "Hantaan," "Dobrava," "Andes," "Tula," "Puumala,"* already have been named. We propose new names for several new groups: *"Bayou,"* including *Bayou, Black Creek, Muleshoe*; *"Sinnombre,"* including: *Sin Nombre*, Convict, *Monongahela, New York*, and *Limestone, El Moro, Rio Segundo*; *"IslaVista,"* including: Prairie Vole, *Prospect Hill, Isla Vista*. The support for corresponding nodes of the cladogram is generally between 80 and 100. The alignment shows that main clades and subclades are supported by amino acid changes caused by synonymous or nonsynonymous nucleotide differences. Most changes occur in an HV region identified by several previous studies.[32,33] Hughes and Friedman[11] defined the HV region as residues 242–281. In our alignment, HV region corresponds to amino acid residues 249–317 and includes 92% of informative sites (62% in whole matrix). This region also includes several regular indels corresponding with the main subdivisions of the cladogram.

Host Specificity and Correspondence with Host Taxonomy

The topology of the three main clades matches the phylogeny of the three host subfamilies to which they are, respectively, devolved. Dominant host genera (pointed by arrows on FIG. 1) may be recognized by mapping the host genus, as a character, on the cladogram of the virus. Within CLADE-*1*, *Rattus* is dominant for *Seoul, Apodemus* for the association *Hantaan-Dobrava*. Within CLADE-*2,* each subclade is linked to a particular host tribe (Neotomini or Sigmodontini); *Sigmodon* appears as a potential primitive host; *Peromyscus* and *Oligoryzomys* are the dominant host genera for *Sinnombre* and *Andes*, respectively. Within CLADE-3, *Microtus* appears as a primitive host genus, and *Clethrionomys* is the dominant host genus for the *Puumala* subclade. The good correspondence of the phylogenies at their highest level is consistent with the hypothesis of co-evolution: the Hantavirus and the Muridae may have evolved and dispersed in parallel. But, whatever the clade considered, there is a mismatch of the host and parasite distributions at species level. This looks as if host specificity had disappeared somewhere between the species and/or the genus level. Depending on which clade is considered, this limit is variable: host switching at genus level appears difficult and unlikely within CLADE-*1* and CLADE-*3*, and easier in CLADE-*2*; within CLADE-*2*, the highest diversity, and thus the weakest specificity at genus level, are observed in *Andes*.

Biogeography of Rodent-Borne Hantaviruses

CLADE-*1* is Palearctic except *Tchoupitoulas*, reported from a wild *Rattus norvegicus* in New Orleans. *R. norvegicus* is a cosmopolitan species, whose dependence for human quarters is well known, and the presence of this Hantavirus in the New World may probably be interpreted as a case of dispersion by humans. CLADE-*2* is exclusively found in the New World: FIGURE 2 shows that, unexpectedly following the hypothesis of co-evolution, the parasites of the Nearctic Sigmodontini (*Bayou*) are not closely related to the parasites of Neotropical Sigmodontini (*Andes*). Most of the Sigmodontini biodiversity is found in the Neotropics, while their sister group, the Neotomini, is dominant in North America. *Bayou* seems limited to southeastern United States, and may perhaps be interpreted as resulting from an ancient isolation of its hosts in a remote part of their range. CLADE-*3* has a mixed distribution with one small Nearctic subclade (*Isla Vista*) and two Palearctic subclades (*Tula, Puumala*). *Prairie* and *Tula* are hosted by different species of genus *Microtus*, as are *Vladivostok* and *Khabarovsk*, which are the sister group of *Puumala* (hosted by *Clethrionomys* spp.). This distribution is consistent with a Palearctic origin, a passage into the New World probably transported by the Arvicolinae (*Microtus* looks a good candidate), a later dispersion in North and South America following the migrations of the Sigmodontinae. This scenario mimics the scenario generally accepted for the radiation of the Muridae, starting from their South Asian center of origin, and is compatible with the hypothesis of a parallel evolution. Within the subclades, a different pattern is suggested, because transmission between different rodent species in the same genus (and between different genera in the Neotropics) looks possible.

CONCLUSION

Two different patterns of dispersion explain the evolution of the hantaviruses: the first one, characterized by a strong specificity for a particular group of hosts, explains the ancient history of this group and its co-evolution with the Muridae; the second one, characterized by a slack specificity, is corresponding with the recent and current history of the viruses and their opportunistic circulation by using contacts between closely related rodent genera, species, and/or populations. This second pattern explains why, when the distribution of the hosts and parasites is sufficiently documented (*Dobrava, Tula, Puumala, Andes*), a geographic gradient becomes visible. Different patterns, following different specificities are in agreement with what is known about Hantavirus survival outside their hosts. Sauvage *et al.*,[34] considering the role of indirect transmission on virus persistence, suggest that viruses remain active outside the host, which could permit transmission without physical contact with the infectious rodents. This explains how hantaviruses may switch when the specific barrier is low and when different hosts have overlapping territories.

While most Bunyaviridae are hosted by arthropods, hantaviruses have rodents as principal hosts. However, two strains have been isolated from non-rodent mammals: *Thottapalayam,* isolated from a shrew; the *Hantaan* virus isolated from a bat. Considering its strong differences with the other hantaviruses, *Thottapalayam* cannot be interpreted as resulting from a recent host switching between a rodent and a shrew. Further investigations are needed to decide if this adaptation to a different group of mammals is an exception, or may represent the emerging tip of a different lineage.

The bat virus is included in *Hantaan*; its closer relative is HT.7611. No significant difference of branch length is observed between the two strains and their total-character distance equals 4; this suggests that the two sequences are almost identical: thus, the presence of a Hantavirus in *Rhinolophus ferrumequinum* must probably be interpreted as the result of an horizontal transfer.

Most of the hantaviruses found in wild animals were collected in the Holarctic, or the Neotropics (northern Asia, Europe, North America, and South America). But, *Thottapalayam* comes from South Asia, where is also found *Thailand*, hosted by *B. indica*, a Muridae rodent. Serological surveys carried out to detect the evidence of Hantavirus infection in human populations revealed that: in Thailand, in different provinces and/or in different environments, 1.2%–31.4% of the individuals tested had Hantavirus antibody[35–37]; the recent publication of the first human case in Thailand[38] confirms the presence of Hantavirus in South Asia; also, screenings performed in West and Central Africa, where a human case has not yet been reported, show that humans may have been infected by Hantaan-related virus.[39] All these suggest that, if rodents are probably the primary reservoir, other mammals may be involved in the cycle of hantaviruses; new viruses, different hosts, and different human syndromes may be expected to be discovered in the future. Additional work is needed out of the traditional areas where Hantaviruses have been recorded, mainly in Southeast Asia and in Africa where Muridae rodents are present and highly diversified.

REFERENCES

1. SCHMALJOHN, C.A., A. SCHMALJOHN & J. DALRYMPLE. 1987. Hantaan virus M RNA: coding strategy, nucleotide sequence, and gene order. Virology **157:** 31–39.
2. CHILDS, J.E., T.G. KSIAZEK, C.F. SPIROPOULOU, *et al.* 1994. Serologic and genetic identification of *Peromyscus maniculatus* as the primary rodent reservoir for a new hantavirus in the southwestern United States. J. Infect. Dis. **169:** 1271–1280.
3. SCHMALJOHN, C., G. JENNINGS, J. HAY & J.M. DALRYMPLE. 1986. Coding strategy of the S-genome segment of Hantaan virus. Virology **155:** 633–643.
4. ELLIOT, R.M., C.S. SCHMALJOHN & M.S. COLLETT. 1991. Bunyaviridae genome structure and gene expression. Curr. Top. Microbiol. Immunol. **69:** 91–141.
5. DEKONENKO, A., V. YAKIMENKO, A. IVANOV, *et al.* 2003. Genetic similarity of Puumala viruses found in Finland and western Siberia and of the mitochondrial DNA of their rodent hosts suggests a common evolutionary origin. Infect. Genet. Evol. **3:** 245–257.
6. NICHOL, S.T. 1999. Genetic analysis of hantaviruses and their host relationships. *In* Factors in the Emergence and Control of Rodent-Borne Viral Diseases. J.F. Saluzzo & B. Dodet, Eds.: 99–109. Elsevier SAS. Paris, France.
7. MONROE, M.C., S.P. MORZUNOV, A.M. JOHNSON, *et al.* 1999. Genetic diversity and distribution of *Peromyscus*-borne hantaviruses in North America. Emerg. Infect. Dis. **5:** 75–86.

8. HEISKE, A., B. ANHEIER, J. PILASKI, *et al.* 1999. A new *Clethrionomys*-derived Hantavirus from Germany: evidence for distinct genetic sublineages of Puumala viruses in Western Europe. Virus Res. **61:** 101–112.

9. HJELLE, B., F. CHAVEZ-GILES, N. TORREZ-MARTINEZ, *et al.* 1994. Genetic identification of a novel Hantavirus of the harvest mouse *Reithrodontomys megalotis*. J. Virol. **68:** 6751–6754.

10. HORLING, J., V. CHIZHIKOV, A. LUNDKVIST, *et al.* 1996. Khabarovsk virus: a phylogenetically and serologically distinct Hantavirus isolated from *Microtus fortis* trapped in far-east Russia. J. Gen. Virol. **77:** 687–694.

11. HUGHES, A.L. & R. FRIEDMAN. 2000. Evolutionary diversification of protein-coding genes of Hantaviruses. Mol. Biol. Evol. **17:** 1558–1568.

12. KARIWA, H., K. YOSHIMATSU & J. SAWABE. 1999. Genetic diversities of Hantaviruses among rodents in Hokkaido, Japan and Far East Russia. Virus. Res. **59:** 219–228.

13. LEVIS, S., S.P. MORZUNOV, J.E. ROWE, *et al.* 1998. Genetic diversity and epidemiology of hantaviruses in Argentina. J. Infect. Dis. **177:** 529–538.

14. LOPEZ, N., P. PADULA, C. ROSSI, *et al.* 1997. Genetic characterization and phylogeny of Andes virus and variants from Argentina and Chile. Virus Res. **50:** 77–84.

15. LI, W.-H. 1997. Molecular Evolution. Sinauer Associates. Sunderland, MA.

16. CAREY, D., R. REUBEN, K. PANICKER, *et al.* 1971. Thottapalayam virus: a presumptive arbovirus isolated from a shrew in India. Indian J. Med. Res. **59:** 1758–1760.

17. XIAO, S.-Y., J.W. LEDUC, Y.K. CHU & C.S. SCHMALJOHN. 1994. Phylogenetic analyses of virus isolates in the genus Hantavirus, family Bunyaviridae. Virology **198:** 205–217.

18. THOMPSON, J.D., D.G. HIGGINS & T.J. GIBSON. 1994. CLUSTAL W: improving the sensitivity of progressive multiple sequence alignment through sequence weighting, position-specific gap penalties and weight matrix choice. Nucleic Acids Res. **22:** 4673–4680.

19. RAMBAUT, A. 1996. Se-Al. Sequence Alignment Editor. Ver. 1.0 Alpha 1. University of Oxford, Oxford, UK.

20. BARRIEL, V. 1994. Phylogénies moléculaires et insertions-délétions de nucléotides. C. R. Acad. Sci. III **317:** 693–701.

21. MADDISON, D.R.W. & P. MADDISON. 2000. MacClade 4: Analysis of Phylogeny and Character Evolution. Version 4.0. Sinauer Associates. Sunderland, Massachusetts.

22. PAGE, R.D.M. 1996. TreeView: an application to display phylogenetic trees on personal computers. Comput. Appl. Biosci. **12:** 357–358.

23. SWOFFORD, D.L. 2001. PAUP*: Phylogenetic Analysis Using Parsimony (and Other Methods). Version 4. 0b10. Sinauer Associates. Sunderland, Massachusetts.

24. FELSENSTEIN, J. 1985. Confidence limits on phylogenies: an approach using the bootstrap. Evolution **39:** 783–791.

25. POSADA, D. & K.A. CRANDALL. 1998. Modeltest: testing the model of DNA substitution. Bioinformatics **14:** 817–818.

26. YANG, Z. 1994. Estimating the pattern of nucleotide substitution. J. Mol. Evol. **39:** 105–111.

27. YANG, Z. 1996. Among-site rate variation and its impact on phylogenetic analyses. Trends Ecol. Evol. **11:** 367–372.

28. HUELSENBECK, J.P. & F. RONQUIST. 2001. MRBAYES: Bayesian inference of phylogeny. Bioinformatics **17:** 754–755.

29. CUMMINGS, M.P., S.A. HANDLEY, D.S. MYERS, *et al.* 2003. Comparing bootstrap and posterior probability values in the four-taxon case. Syst. Biol. **52:** 477–487.
30. ZHAXYBAYEVA, O. & J.P. GOGARTEN. 2002. Bootstrap, Bayesian probability and maximum likelihood mapping: exploring new tools for comparative genome analyses. BMC Genomics **3:** 1–15.
31. NICHOLS, S.T., B.J. BEATY, R.M. ELLIOTT, R. GOLDBACH, A. PLYUSNIN, C.S. SCHMALJOHN & R.B. TESH. 2006. Family Bunyaviridae. *In*: Eighth Report of the International Committee on Taxonomy of Viruses. C. Fauquet, M. Mayo, J. Maniloff, U. Desselberger & L.A. Ball, Eds.: 695–715. Academic Press. New York.
32. LUNDKVIST, A., H. KALLIO-KOKKO, K.B. SJÖLANDER, *et al.* 1996. Characterization of Puumala virus nucleocapsid protein: identification of B-cell epitopes. Virology **216:** 397–406.
33. PLYUSNIN, A., O. VAPALAHTI & A. VAHERI. 1996. Hantaviruses: genome structure, expression and evolution. J. Gen. Virol. **77:** 2677–2687.
34. SAUVAGE, F., M. LANGLAIS, N.G. YOCCOZ & D. PONTIER. 2003. Modelling Hantavirus in fluctuating populations of bank voles: the role of indirect transmission on virus persistence. J. Anim. Ecol. **72:** 1–13.
35. ELWELL, M.R., G.S. WARD, M. TINGPALAPONG & J.W. LEDUC. 1985. Serologic evidence of Hantaan-like virus in rodents and man in Thailand. Southeast Asian J. Trop. Med. Public Health **16:** 349–354.
36. NITATPATTANA, N., G. CHAUVENCY, J. DARDAINE, *et al.* 2000. Serological study of Hantavirus in the rodent population of Nakhon Pathom and Nakhon Ratchasima provinces in Thailand. Southeast Asian J. Trop. Med. Public Health **31:** 277–282.
37. SAWASDIKOL, S., M. TAMURA & P. JAMJIT. 1989. Antibody to hemoragic fever with renal syndrome in man and rat in Thailand. Bull. Dept. Med. Sci. **31:** 125–130.
38. SUPUTTAMONGKOL, Y., N. NITATPATTANA, M. CHYAKULKEREE, *et al.* 2005. Hantavirus infection in Thailand: first clinical case report. Southern Asian J Trop. Med. Pub. Health **36:** 217–220.
39. GONZALEZ, J.-P., J.B. MCCORMICK, D. BAUDON, *et al.* 1984. Serological evidence for Hantaan-related virus in Africa. Lancet **324:** 1036–1037.

Epizootics of Yellow Fever in Venezuela (2004–2005)

An Emerging Zoonotic Disease

PEDRO M. RIFAKIS,[a*] JESUS A. BENITEZ,[b] JOSE DE-LA-PAZ-PINEDA,[c] AND ALFONSO J. RODRIGUEZ-MORALES[c]

[a]*Pérez de León Hospital, 1073 Caracas, Venezuela*

[b]*Environmental Health, Ministry of Health, Maracay, 2102 Aragua,Venezuela*

[c]*Center for Research Jose Witremundo Torrealba, Universidad de Los Andes, 3102 Trujillo, Venezuela*

ABSTRACT: Epidemics and epizootics of yellow fever (YF) have been occurring in the border area of eastern Colombia and western Venezuela since 2003; for this reason many epidemiological control measures were adopted by the Ministry of Health (MOH) trying to prevent their spreading. These activities included monkey deaths surveillance as well as immunization of susceptible individuals with YF vaccine. In this setting, we analyzed epidemiological and epizootical issues related to YF in Venezuela during 2004–2005. In this period, YF epizootics occurred initially without geographical links to the 2003 outbreaks (which occurred at the Southern Maracaibo lake epizootic wave), but in relation with the Guayana epizootic wave; beginning in Monagas state and then affecting Anzoátegui, Guárico, and Sucre states. Just months later, Apure was also affected. Mérida and Táchira also report epizootics for the end of 2004. This year concluded with 15 human deaths due to YF and more than 100 howler monkey deaths. In the same year, 715 suspected cases were investigated confirming YF in 0.7% of them. For these reasons, between 2002 and 2004, Venezuela's MOH has vaccinated approximately 1.9 million people in areas considered to be enzootic. The country's goal for 2006 is to have 7 million people residing in high-risk cities and towns vaccinated, and in this way, preventing and controlling this emerging zoonotic disease.

KEYWORDS: yellow fever; epizootics; epidemiology; Venezuela; South America

*In Memorian.

Address for correspondence: Jesus A. Benitez, C. R. Los Angeles, T-2, 10-2, Sec. Pque., Cigarral, Urb. La Boyera, Caracas 1083, Venezuela. Voice: 58-416-8269482; fax: 58-212-4429790.
e-mail: drjesusbenitez@yahoo.es

Ann. N.Y. Acad. Sci. 1081: 57–60 (2006). © 2006 New York Academy of Sciences.
doi: 10.1196/annals.1373.005

INTRODUCTION

Yellow fever (YF) virus is transmitted by the bite of infected mosquitoes and produces a severe hemorrhagic fever in humans. Despite a safe and effective vaccine (17D), YF continues to be a public health problem in tropical areas of Africa and South America.[1–3] In this region, the disease has been recently occurring in many tropical countries, such as Bolivia, Brazil, Colombia, Ecuador, French Guiana, Peru, and Venezuela.

The sylvatic cycle involves nonhuman primates and mosquitoes that breed in tree holes.[4] Persons living or working in proximity to such jungle or forest habitats who are bitten by infected mosquitoes (in Venezuela, *Haemagogus* and *Sabethes* species) can develop "jungle YF." Another cycle exists between humans and *Aedes aegypti* mosquitoes. *A. aegypti* mosquitoes are present in most urban centers of South and Central America,[5] the Caribbean, and parts of the southern United States[6]; persons in these areas are at risk for urban YF infection.

Recent epidemics and epizootics of YF have been occurring since 2003 in the area of the border of eastern Colombia with western Venezuela.[7] After these outbreaks begun, many epidemiological control measures were adopted and some of them reinforced by the Venezuela's Ministry of Health trying to prevent these situations. These activities included surveillance of monkey deaths as well as immunization of susceptible individuals with YF vaccine.[8] Although immunization rate and other medical factors have been considered critical, some studies have indicated a possible relation or influence on this YF emergence by the climatic variation and global climate change.[9]

In this setting, we analyzed epidemiological and epizootical issues related to YF in Venezuela during 2004–2005.

MATERIALS AND METHODS

Human and animal epidemiological data for this study were retrieved from the records of the Ministry of Health from Venezuela. With these data, a temporal–spatial analysis of the YF situation in Venezuela during 2004–2005 was done.

RESULTS

During 2004–2005, YF epizootics occurred initially without geographical relation to the 2003 outbreaks (occurred at the Southern Maracaibo lake epizootic wave) (FIG. 1), but in relation with the Guayana epizootic wave; beginning in Monagas state, then affecting Anzoátegui, Guárico, and Sucre states (FIG. 1).

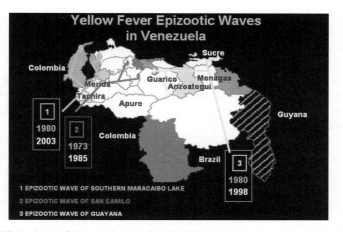

FIGURE 1. Map of Venezuela showing the YF epizootic waves, chronology of recent YF outbreaks, and affected states during 2004–2005 (gray colors).

During the middle of the year 2004, although it is not located directly in that epizootic wave, Apure state was also affected. Mérida and Táchira also report epizootics for the ending of the year 2004, but it was difficult to establish its relation with previous epizootics or with epizootics from the Southern Maracaibo lake epizootic wave (FIG. 1).

For the year ending 2004, mortality figures related to YF reached 15 deaths in humans and more than 100 in howler monkeys (*Alouatta* spp).

In the same year, 715 suspected cases were clinically, epidemiologically investigated in the laboratory confirming YF in five patients (0.70%).

CONCLUSIONS

World Health Organization (WHO) data suggest that YF transmission is increasing.[6,10] In Venezuela, since a "highlighted" case of YF in a U.S. traveler returning from the Venezuelan amazonic jungle in which the patient died from fulminant YF hepatitis,[11,12] there has been an increasing interest in the risk of the reemergence of this disease. These epidemic and epizootic outbreaks represented a challenge for national public health that has been facing it with many preventive measures to avoid the risk of reemergence of urban YF, given the high abundance of *A. aegypti* in the main urban centers of Venezuela.[5] The last human case registered of urban YF happened in 1918 in the city of Coro, Falcon State (northwestern Venezuela).[7]

In addition to environmental factors,[9] other possible reasons for the reemergence of YF are related to the high mobilization of displaced populations in remote areas and of difficult access, high concentration of indigenous populations (Bari, Yucpa, and Wayúu), and border conflict,[7] among others.

Under the International Health Regulations, monkey deaths from suspected YF epizootics must be reported to WHO within 24 h, with confirmation to follow when available.

When the first epizootics occurred at Monagas, it was inferred that the disease in primates was following a northward course within the state heading toward Anzoátegui and Sucre states; which corresponds to the typical behavior of disease in Venezuela, especially considering the activity of the Guayana wave implicated in this case (FIG. 1).

In 1973, 1980, 1985, 1998, and 2003 important YF epidemics and/or epizootics occurred. Fortunately, between 2002 and 2004, Venezuela vaccinated approximately 1.9 million people in areas considered to be enzootic. The country's goal for 2006 is to have 7 million people residing in high-risk cities and towns vaccinated, in this way preventing and controlling this emerging zoonotic disease. Further epidemiological and ecoepidemiological research is expected.

REFERENCES

1. VASCONCELOS, P.F., J.E. BRYANT, T.P. DA ROSA, et al. 2004. Genetic divergence and dispersal of yellow fever virus. Brazil. Emerg. Infect. Dis. **10:** 1578–1584.
2. MONATH, T.P. 1997. Epidemiology of yellow fever: current status and speculations on future trends. In Factors in the Emergence of Arbovirus Diseases. J.F. Saluzzo & B. Dodet, Eds.: 143–165. Elsevier. Amsterdam.
3. VAINIO, J. & F. CUTTS. 1998. Yellow fever. Global programme for vaccines and immunization. World Health Organization. Geneva. (WHO/EPI/GEN/98.11).
4. MONATH, T.P. 1999. Yellow fever. In Vaccines. S.A. Plotkin & W.A. Orenstein, Eds.: 815–879. WB Saunders. Philadelphia, PA.
5. BARBELLA, R.A., A.J. RODRIGUEZ & J. VARGAS. 2003. Update on epidemiological situation of dengue in Venezuela, 2001–2002. J. Clin. Virol. **28:** S62.
6. ROBERTSON, S.E., B.P. HULL, O. TOMORI, et al. 1996. Yellow fever: a decade of reemergence. JAMA **276:** 1157–1162.
7. VALERO, N. 2003. A propósito de la fiebre amarilla en Venezuela. Invest. Clin. **44:** 269–271.
8. MINISTERIO DE SALUD Y DESARROLLO SOCIAL (MSDS). 2003. Situación Epidemiológica de la Fiebre Amarilla. Alerta Epidemiológico Semanal **9:** 1–12.
9. RODRÍGUEZ, A.J., R.A. BARBELLA, G. CABANIEL, et al. 2004. Influence of climatic variations on yellow fever outbreaks in Venezuela, 2002–2003. Presented at the 20th Clinical Virology Symposium and Annual Meeting Pan American Society for Clinical Virology. Clearwater Beach. Florida, USA, April 25–28.
10. WORLD HEALTH ORGANIZATION. 1998. Yellow fever, 1996–1997. Wkly. Epidemiol. Rec. **73:** 354–359.
11. CENTERS FOR DISEASE CONTROL. 2000. Fatal yellow fever in a traveler returning from Venezuela, 1999. MMWR Morb. Mortal. Wkly. Rep. **49:** 303–305.
12. CENTERS FOR DISEASE CONTROL AND PREVENTION. 2000. Fatal yellow fever in a traveler returning from Venezuela, 1999. JAMA **283:** 2230–2232.

Risk Analysis and Bovine Tuberculosis, a Re-emerging Zoonosis

ERIC ETTER,[a] PILAR DONADO,[b] FERRAN JORI,[a]
ALEXANDRE CARON,[c] FLAVIE GOUTARD,[a] AND FRANÇOIS ROGER[a]

[a] CIRAD, EMVT Department, Epidemiology and Ecology Unit,
34098 Montpellier, France

[b] University of California, Davis, California 95616, USA

[c] CIRAD, EMVT Department, Integrated Wildlife Management Unit,
34398 Montpellier, France

ABSTRACT: The widespread of immunodeficiency with AIDS, the consequence of poverty on sanitary protection and information at both individual and state levels lead control of tuberculosis (TB) to be one of the priorities of World Health Organization programs. The impact of bovine tuberculosis (BTB) on humans is poorly documented. However, BTB remains a major problem for livestock in developing countries particularly in Africa and wildlife is responsible for the failure of TB eradication programs. In Africa, the consumption of raw milk and raw meat, and the development of bushmeat consumption as a cheap source of proteins, represent one of the principal routes for human contaminations with BTB. The exploration of these different pathways using tools as participatory epidemiology allows the risk analysis of the impact of BTB on human health in Africa. This analysis represents a management support and decision tool in the study and the control of zoonotic BTB.

KEYWORDS: bovine tuberculosis; risk analysis; participatory epidemiology; zoonosis; bushmeat

INTRODUCTION

Human tuberculosis (TB) of animal origin (zoonotic TB) is an important public health concern in developing countries. African nations pose a particular challenge in TB control, because of deficiencies in public health control measures for cattle and animal products, coupled with a high prevalence and incidence of HIV in the human population. Risk analysis is an important tool in defining the public health danger posed by zoonotic TB in Africa. Using risk analysis, two potential pathways are proposed as comprehensive models

Address for correspondence: François Roger, CIRAD, EMVT Department, Epidemiology and Ecology Unit, 34098 Montpellier Cedex 5, France. Voice: +33 4 67 59 37 06; fax: +33 4 67 59 37 54.
e-mail: francois.roger@cirad.fr

Ann. N.Y. Acad. Sci. 1081: 61–73 (2006). © 2006 New York Academy of Sciences.
doi: 10.1196/annals.1373.006

when considering different routes of human infection: (*a*) from domestic and wild animals; and (*b*) from animal products including milk and bushmeat.

Globally, wildlife reservoirs threaten the success of TB eradication programs (e.g., badgers in the United Kingdom;[1] however, according to Donnelly *et al.*,[2] the presence of badgers seems actually to keep transmission of TB down in cattle, possums in New Zealand, white-tailed deer in Michigan, USA, wild boar and deer in Spain and France). In Africa, little is known about wildlife reservoir, but in southern Africa (mainly South Africa), in the Kruger National Park, 15 years of studies clearly indicate that the African buffalo (*Syncerus caffer*) is the main reservoir of the pathogen agent, with other species like the greater kudu (*Tragelaphus strepsiceros*) and common warthog (*Phacochoerus africanus*) having a potential role in the continued prevalence of the disease.[3] Depending on the specific ecosystem with respect to species abundance, diversity, and anthropic factors, such as habitat impact and wildlife management, wildlife species seem to be more or less susceptible to the *Mycobacterium* spp. and therefore, the disease dynamics and the role of species have been varying accordingly.

The purpose of this article is to examine the impact of bovine tuberculosis (BTB) on human health in Africa and to propose an approach for its study and its control using risk analysis.

ECOLOGY, EPIDEMIOLOGY, AND ZOONOTIC ASPECTS OF BTB IN AFRICA

In Africa, BTB primarily affects cattle.[4-9] However, infection in other farm and domestic animals are sometimes reported. *Mycobacterium bovis* has a broad host range as the principal cause of TB in free-living wildlife, captive wildlife, domestic livestock, and non-human primates.[10] Wild ruminants and carnivores, such as African buffalo, lion, cheetah, greater kudu, leopard, warthog, and eland, can be infected.[11-13] Scavengers (hyenas, genet) and Chacma baboons in Kenya became infected through the ingestion of abattoir wastes.[14] Most of the time, BTB transmission is considered as passing from livestock to wildlife. In wild ruminants, the disease has been documented worldwide, and lesions and symptoms are very similar to those of domestic ruminants.[15]

Depending on the susceptibility of a species to, and on the prevalence of BTB, these animals could act as reservoirs or spill-over hosts to other species.[13-16] In reservoir or maintenance hosts, infection can persist through horizontal transfer in the absence of any other source of *M. bovis* and may well be transmitted to other susceptible hosts. Only a limited number of species act as maintenance or reservoir hosts of TB, which include brush-tailed possum (*Trichosurus vulpecula*), European badgers (*Meles meles*), bison (*Bison bison*), African buffalo

TABLE 1. Worldwide TB Figures (WHO 2002)

World population		6 219 000 000
TB-infected people		2 073 000 000
Estimated incidence	Tuberculosis	8 797 000
	Pulmonary TB (Smear-positive cases)	3 887 000
Deaths due to TB		1 800 000
TB cases due to HIV		9%
Deaths of TB patients due to HIV		12%

(*Syncerus cafer*), and white-tailed deer (*Odocoileus virginianus*). In contrast, spill-over hosts become infected with *M. bovis*, but the infection only occurs sporadically, or persists within these populations if a true maintenance host is present in the ecosystem. In the case of high density populations, spill-over hosts can act as reservoir hosts of *M. bovis*.[17]

In Africa, TB infection in humans is principally caused by *Mycobacterium tuberculosis*. However, human TB of animal origin caused by *M. bovis* is becoming increasingly prevalent in developing countries[18] due to the lack of both control and diagnostic measures and pasteurization of milk.[19,20] Concomitantly, TB is a major opportunistic infection in HIV-infected persons, and the World Health Organization (WHO) estimated that 70% (6 million) of the people co-infected with TB and HIV live in Sub-Saharan Africa.[19] The prevalence, incidence, and deaths caused by TB, reported in 2002 by WHO, are given in TABLE 1. Every year, there are 8–10 million new cases of TB reported, and 2–3 million deaths attributed to TB,[21] but the exact percentage of TB that may be caused by *M. bovis* is not known. Global prevalence of human TB due to *M. bovis* is estimated at 3.1% of all human TB cases, of which 2.1% are pulmonary infections, and 9.4% extra pulmonary.[19] However, the proportion of *M. Bovis* in Africa and within the TB–HIV complex is unknown.

Information regarding human disease due to *M. bovis* is rare. In Africa, where *M. bovis* is present in animal species, there is substantial lack of knowledge about the distribution, epidemiological patterns, and transmission dynamics of this important zoonosis. The fact that 50% of total African cattle happen to be in countries without any control measures for BTB[22] is a matter of concern. Results from several studies conducted in different African countries have clearly established the importance of BTB as a major public health problem. In Malawi, a survey of human sputum cultures from human TB patients revealed that 42.8% of the culture-positive specimens were *M. bovis* (Ministry of Health, 1985, cited by Wedlock *et al.*[20]). In Egypt, a study reported that 9 out of 20 randomly selected patients with TB peritonitis were infected with *M. bovis*.[23] Jiwa *et al.*,[4] in Tanzania, suggested that the presence of BTB in cattle necessitates further investigation into the role of animal-derived BTB in human health. In Burkina Faso, the Ministry of Health reported 1,334 human cases of zoonotic TB.[24] Ameni et al.[25] reported high occurrences of BTB in cattle and cattle owners, respectively, in central Ethiopia, and pointed out the need to assess and evaluate the impact of zoonotic TB on human populations in order to design cost-effective control methods throughout the country. The risk of contracting TB is 20–50 times greater in Africa than in Europe.[18]

The importance of M. bovis in human TB cases is not mentioned in any of the national reports submitted to OIE (World Organization of Animal Health) and WHO by African member states. Cases of M. bovis infection in humans are underreported as a result of diagnostic limitations and non-adapting sampling for searching extra pulmonary TB.[19]

TB infection may occur via contaminated materials (fomites), aerosolization (human to human), and predation, or by vertical and/or horizontal transmission in humans.[15] Zoonotic TB caused by M. bovis could be acquired by humans through the inhalation of cough sprayed from infected cattle, or from handling or consumption of milk contaminated with the organism.[20] BTB in humans affects young individuals and causes cervical lymphadenopathy, intestinal lesions, chronic skin TB (Lupus vulgaris), and other non-pulmonary forms.[19] If M. bovis is acquired by inhalation, humans typically develop pulmonary TB.[19]

Another factor which increases the risk of acquiring zoonotic TB in Sub-Saharan Africa is the active competition in all Sub-Saharan African countries between large-scale commercial food enterprises and smaller, less-regulated farmers who frequently ignore safety standards for hygiene and product quality. These smaller farmers sell directly to final consumers and contribute to the spread of TB.[19] Furthermore, 90% of the total milk produced by these countries and consumed by people is either fresh or soured, and not pasteurized (Walshe et al., 1991, cited by Cosivi et al.[19]

Finally, we can underline that the recent development of wildlife activities, such as game tourism, farming, and hunting to develop the peripheral zones of protected areas contributes to the exposure of specific persons to Mycobacterium spp.

RESEARCH QUESTION, TOOLS, AND METHODOLOGIES

Efficient risk analysis could become an important tool in assessing and overcoming the public health danger posed by zoonotic TB. Risk analysis is a relatively new research tool that encompasses qualitative, deterministic, and probabilistic health assessment. This tool requires interdisciplinary collaborations to satisfy the demands for high quality characterization of risk. Risk could be defined as the likelihood of occurrence of an adverse event and the severity of the consequences if the result does occur.[26] MacDiarmid and Pharo[27] defined risk analysis as a tool intended to provide decision-makers with an objective, repeatable, and documented appraisal of the risk posed by a particular action.

Based on the OIE (World Organization for Animal Health) code, risk analysis constitutes four steps: (1) hazard identification; (2) risk assessment; (3) risk management; and (4) risk communication.[28] Risk assessment evaluates the probability of entry, the establishment or spread of a disease under existing conditions, predetermined control measures, and the associated potential biological and economic consequences of establishment of the disease. In the case of zoonotic TB, it consists of the identification, estimation of statistical probabilities, and evaluation of the consequences of all risks associated with the transmission of BTB from animals to humans. Release assessment is the probability of releasing viable *M. bovis* to bordering communities from (*a*) cattle; (*b*) contaminated carcasses and meat; (*c*) contaminated milk; and (*d*) bushmeat. Exposure assessment is the probability of being exposed to viable *M. bovis*. Factors involved in this assessment are: (*a*) rural and peri-urban populations; and (*b*) abattoir workers, farm workers, and people with a high degree of contact with animals (e.g., game farm workers, rangers, wildlife vets). Consumption of contaminated food and hunting habits are also exposure variables. Consequence assessment is the probability of becoming infected, diseased, or of dying. Consequences of human BTB are sickness, death, as well as the potential for one group to be the release source for human-to-human transmission. Risk analysis can be quantitative providing a numeric, or qualitative estimate, when a descriptive approach is used.[29] Both types of assessments are equally valid if they are based on good quality data and concentrate on all the defined stages of the infective process.[29] Some of the inputs and variables of this model are unknown, which requires that we incorporate uncertainty and variability into the model. These variations are modeled using Monte-Carlo simulation technique, a stochastic iterative approach.[30] Input parameters should be defined through the collection of existing data, expert opinions, and the use of field surveys including participatory epidemiology (PE).

PE is an emerging field based on epidemiological technique using participatory methods to collect epidemiological data by the widely accepted methods of Rapid Rural Appraisal and Participatory Rural Appraisal. PE relies on observation, existing veterinary knowledge of traditional livestock owners, and oral history from the local communities. PE is based on the principle of flexibility with the use of iterative analysis and on the principle of triangulation which is the cross-checking of information gained from several intentionally different perspectives. A wide range of PE tools are available and can be categorized into three main groups, complemented with secondary sources and direct observation in the field: informal interviews of key informants, visualization methods, and ranking or scoring methods. Information derived from all these sources is then combined and cross-checked to build a picture of the issues under investigation. Use of conventional veterinary diagnostic tools is an integral part of, and in some cases overlaps with PE methods. PE can make use of quantitative information coming from previous formal epidemiological surveys, and uses qualitative intelligence to fill the gaps between available data.[31] Examples of PE used in veterinary research include: basic research on the epidemiology of endemic and epizootic diseases, used with Orma communities in Kenya for the Bovine Trypanosomiasis,[32] participatory disease searching which is a widely applied method of assessing Rinderpest risk, verifying eradication, and substantiating disease-free herd status,[33] disease modeling done on the construction of a model of the contagious bovine pleuropneumonia (CBPP) transmission in transhuman production systems.[34] PE methods augment the capacities of conventional epidemiological methods to provide reliable and fast epidemiological information on complex disease concerns. For risk factor identification and assessment of the local epidemiological situation of BTB, qualitative and semi-qualitative data are needed. The use of PE methods could provide guidance on local attitudes and behavior with regard to: animal husbandry practices, social and cultural habits (e.g., milk processing, milk consumption, and hunting and consumption of bushmeat).[35]

Risk assessment for *M. bovis* human infection is exemplified using one scenario pathway model: the milk pathway. This pathway determines an orderly series of events which would ultimately lead to the acquisition of BTB by humans in Uganda. The pathway looks at the probability that an individual is infected with *M. bovis* at the source.

Proposals will be based on the milk and meat pathways in African countries.

FRAMEWORK PROPOSED FOR RISK ANALYSIS OF ZOONOTIC BTB IN AFRICA MILK PATHWAY

In Uganda, as in most Sub-Saharan countries, human TB has a high prevalence. The Ugandan Ministry of Health reported in 1995 a mean annual incidence rate of human TB of 1.34/1000 person-years, and the role of BTB is unknown.[9] The same authors, using intradermal TB-skin testing, reported a 74% prevalence of TB reactors among cattle herds, 6% of individual-animals, and a within-herd range of 1–50% that could be 100% if suspicious reactors were included.[9] A regular high prevalence of BTB in cattle can be correlated with the isolation of *M. bovis* in milk samples. Vekemans *et al*.[36] reported isolation of *Mycobacteria* in 26% of 60 retailed milk samples collected from markets in Burkina Faso.

The high prevalence of BTB in Ugandan cattle could have public health implications; however, there is no information about the risk of zoonotic infections of BTB to humans. Because of this unknown transmission potential, we are proposing a BTB risk analysis in order to make recommendations to public health agencies for prevention and control of the disease. During their 6 years of study in the region, CIRAD (*Centre de Coopération Internationale en Recherche Agronomique pour le Développement*) established a series of comprehensive social and political networks. The public health authorities are aware of CIRAD's study and wish to understand the risk presented by

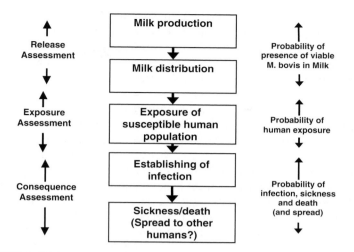

FIGURE 1. Risk assessment for the milk pathway.

zoonotic TB. CIRAD has proposed a basis for a comprehensive quantitative risk analysis (FIG. 1) with evidence of a potential risk, thorough knowledge of the structure of the culture, networks within the population and the dairy production industry, links to public health authorities and agencies, and organizing efficient field investigation capabilities. Risk hazard identification for zoonotic TB is currently based on a cross-sectional study with TB patients of the Mbarara Hospital in Uganda, in order to determine the risk factors for TB caused by *M. bovis*. A laboratory study component includes bacterial isolation of *Mycoplasma* spp. and characterization of *M. bovis* using molecular techniques. Risk factors are being categorized using a questionnaire that accounts for general information about the patients and their medical history, occupational information, household information, habits of milk consumption, habits of meat consumption, and knowledge of TB transmission routes (including the zoonotic aspects).

MEAT PATHWAYS WITH WILDLIFE AND DOMESTIC ANIMALS APPROACH

Eating raw or undercooked meat is one of the ways of contracting BTB. Because of local habits concomitant with a high prevalence of BTB in cattle, some countries present a real zoonotic risk of BTB transmission. Ameni *et al.* showed 99% of either raw meat or raw and cooked meat consumption versus 1% of only cooked meat consumption in Central Ethiopia.[25] The same study showed herd and individual animal prevalences of BTB of 42.6% and 7.9%, respectively. At the end, 24.5% of the interviewed households had experienced at least one human TB case in the family. In Ethiopia, BTB prevalence is a major concern for veterinary services ranging from 3.4% in smallholder production systems to 87% in intensive farms.[37,38] Because of the lack of sensibility of the routine post-mortem examination in the abattoirs and because of the high proportion of backyard slaughtering, this problem is in reality a public health problem.

The bushmeat trade and meat consumption have been increasing at an alarming rate in Sub-Saharan Africa, particularly in the forested areas of West and Central Africa.[39] Its relative importance as a source of proteins as compared to domestic animals and fish varies between 6% (southern Africa) and 55% (Central Africa) of total protein consumption.[40] This practice has demonstrated that in areas where bushmeat is important, hunters and persons involved in the bushmeat trade are exposed to the transmission of several wildlife diseases.[41,42] Despite the possibilities of human TB infection through bushmeat, these protein products have rarely been considered as a source of TB. In order to assess the risk of BTB infection from wildlife to humans, we need to investigate the problem at different levels. Data on BTB in wildlife in most of West and Central African countries are scarce or nonexistent. Proteins come from both wildlife hunted in the neighboring forests, and from cattle herds arriving from pastoral regions in several areas of Sub-Saharan Africa, such as the Central African Republic and Cameroon. Because prevalence of TB is important in transhuman herds,[43] there is a risk of transmission from cattle to wildlife as described in literature when wild and domesticated animals share the same territory.[11,17,19,44,45] A surveillance of BTB in bushmeat markets can be a method to monitor the presence of *M. bovis* in wildlife species. An advantage for sampling wildlife carcasses is that in bushmeat markets in West and Central Africa, a variety of species are available. The choice of species to be examined will depend on the likely prevalence of *M. bovis* within each species, their abundance, and the ease of sampling different hosts.[17] In some cases, spill-over species such as carnivores and other species at the top of the food chain have become useful sentinel species for the detection of BTB in other wildlife animals.[46] The level of detection of BTB in wildlife species will also depend on the kind of diagnosis used to test for the presence of the organism. In infected white-tailed deer in Michigan, it has been demonstrated that acid fast staining histopathology and PCR methods can underestimate the prevalence of BTB as compared to culture methods.[47] The chances of detecting *M. bovis* in a diseased carcass are also variable depending on the anatomical site used for screening the carcasses. The body parts harboring the most infectiveness will depend on the pathogenesis of *M. bovis* in the species being tested. Most wild ruminants present with gross lesions in the lymph nodes of the head,[48] while mesenteric lymph nodes lesions are more common in carnivores or scavengers.[17]

The risks of TB transmission from wildlife to humans have been insufficiently studied in Sub-Saharan areas where bushmeat consumption prevails. Indeed, in those areas, contact with wildlife carcasses from a wide variety of species is probably more widespread and common than in southern Africa. There, the most likely source of infection might be the cutaneous route, because slaughtering is performed in open areas. On the other hand, overcooking meat is a common measure used to prevent gastro-intestinal infections in African countries, and venison is seldom consumed insufficiently cooked. However, socioeconomic conditions, such as a lack of hygiene, informal trade, lack of veterinary inspection and food safety services, lack of disease awareness, and not using gloves, can be considered as risk factors for bushmeat traders, butchers, hunters, and middlemen to become infected via the cutaneous route, particularly when they cut themselves while dressing the carcass, or when they dress an unprotected, open wound or abrasion on their arms or forearms.[49]

Consequences for humans infected with *M. bovis* through bushmeat pathways are probably very similar to those assessed for milk consumers. The difference might be that the most exposed persons are adults, but with milk consumers, children are also exposed. Women are usually involved in the bushmeat trade and marketing, while men are more involved in hunting activities. Dressing carcasses is more commonly done in the field by men, who deal with heavy species (e.g., antelopes, bushpigs), while small species, such as primates, rodents, and reptiles are more likely to be dressed by women in the markets.

In addition, some molecular characterization techniques—for example, spacer oligonucleotide typing,[50] Single-step DNA-based assay[51] RFLP[52]—if tested specifically for *M. bovis* in multi-species model could permit, if successful, to introduce an idea of the historical contingency of disease strains in wildlife and domestic populations and at their interface. From these links, hypothetical pathways can be proposed and tested.

Last, the understanding of BTB dynamics in and between wildlife and domestic reservoirs is an important issue to be looked at. Pathogens' dynamics between the wildlife and domestic reservoirs in some areas will explain the incidence of the disease in cattle and therefore, will have an impact on the risk assessment in humans. Later in the analysis, risk management can take into account wildlife reservoir management options, inducing a change in prevalence in the domestic reservoir and changing the risk exposure of human population at a higher level.

CONCLUSION

Despite the lack of study coverage related to the impact of BTB in human TB cases, one can hypothesize that immunodepressed HIV patients would be more susceptible to BTB contamination when a specific threshold of risk factors is encountered. Contamination from human to human of *M. bovis* is usually considered as a rare event. But in the context of high HIV prevalence and the presence of many risk factors, the epidemiology of the disease in the human host could be changed and human-to-human transmission could be more common.[43]

The increase of population in Africa is leading to the use of more and more marginal lands by pastoral societies and agricultural "colons." These marginal lands correspond to areas where the remaining population of wildlife has been pushed by land-use pressure. Most of the national parks in Africa are based in these areas. Therefore, one can observe an increased contact between livestock production systems and wildlife ecosystems, leading to the potential for pathogen transmission in both ways. Another consequence linked to the political agenda trying to integrate development and conservation issues in the areas surrounding the national parks is the development sustainable activities, including game hunting and sustainable natural resources harvest. These activities also constitute new risk factors for the transmission of pathogens. Thus, contamination from buffalo and other wildlife species to humans has to be taken into account in terms of bushmeat consumption, as also including game hunting and traditional hunting. Other potential pathways should be studied and included as direct transmission from livestock. Modeling of the interface between wild and domestic animals will also help in building up comprehensive risk assessment models.

REFERENCES

1. GORMLEY, E. & J.D. COLLINS. 2000. The development of wildlife control strategies for eradication of tuberculosis in cattle in Ireland. Tuber. Lung Dis. **80:** 229–236.
2. DONNELLY, C.A. *et al.* 2003. Impact of localized badger culling on tuberculosis incidence in British cattle. Nature **426:** 834–837.
3. BENGIS, R.G. *et al.* 2004. The role of wildlife in emerging and re-emerging zoonoses. Rev. Sci. Tech. **23:** 497–511.
4. JIWA, S.F. *et al.* 1997. Bovine tuberculosis in the Lake Victoria zone of Tanzania and its possible consequences for human health in the HIV/AIDS era. Vet. Res. Commun. **21:** 533–539.
5. OMER, M.K. *et al.* 2001. A cross-sectional study of bovine tuberculosis in dairy farms in Asmara, Eritrea. Trop. Anim. Health Prod. **33:** 295–303.
6. BONSU, O.A., E. LAING & B.D. AKANMORI. 2000. Prevalence of tuberculosis in cattle in the Dangme-West district of Ghana, public health implications. Acta Trop. **76:** 9–14.
7. KAZWALA, R.R. *et al.* 1998. Isolation of Mycobacterium species from raw milk of pastoral cattle of the Southern Highlands of Tanzania. Trop. Anim. Health Prod. **30:** 233–239.
8. MARTRENCHAR, A. *et al.* 1993. Problems associated with tuberculosis and brucellosis skin-test methods in northern Cameroon. Prev. Vet. Med. **15:** 221–229.
9. BERNARD, F. *et al.* 2005. Tuberculosis and brucellosis prevalence survey on dairy cattle in Mbarara milk basin (Uganda). Prev. Vet. Med. **67:** 267–281.
10. O'REILLY, L.M. & C.J. DABORN. 1995. The epidemiology of *Mycobacterium bovis* infections in animals and man: a review. Tuber. Lung Dis. **76**(Suppl 1): 1–46.

11. WOODFORD, M.H. 1982. Tuberculosis in wildlife in the Ruwenzori National Park, Uganda (Part II). Trop. Anim. Health Prod. **14:** 155–160.
12. KEET, D.F. *et al.* 1996. Tuberculosis in buffaloes (*Syncerus caffer*) in the Kruger National Park: spread of the disease to other species. Onderstepoort J. Vet. Res. **63:** 239–244.
13. MICHEL, A.L. 2002. Implications of tuberculosis in African wildlife and livestock. Ann. N. Y. Acad. Sci. **969:** 251–255.
14. TARARA, R. *et al.* 1985. Tuberculosis in wild olive baboons, *Papio cynocephalus anubis* (Lesson), in Kenya. J. Wildl. Dis. **21:** 137–140.
15. BIET, F. *et al.* 2005. Zoonotic aspects of *Mycobacterium bovis* and *Mycobacterium avium*-intracellulare complex (MAC). Vet. Res. **36:** 411–436.
16. DELAHAY, R.J., C.L. CHEESEMAN & R.S. CLIFTON-HADLEY. 2001. Wildlife disease reservoirs: the epidemiology of *Mycobacterium bovis* infection in the European badger (*Meles meles*) and other British mammals. Tuberculosis (Edinb.) **81:** 43–49.
17. DE LISLE, G.W. *et al.* 2002. Tuberculosis in free-ranging wildlife: detection, diagnosis and management. Rev. Sci. Tech. **21:** 317–334.
18. BEDARD, B.G., S.W. MARTIN & D. CHINOMBO. 1993. A prevalence study of bovine tuberculosis and brucellosis in Malawi. Prev. Vet. Med. **16:** 193–205.
19. COSIVI, O. *et al.* 1998. Zoonotic tuberculosis due to *Mycobacterium bovis* in developing countries. Emerg. Infect. Dis. **4:** 59–70.
20. WEDLOCK, D.N. *et al.* 2002. Control of *Mycobacterium bovis* infections and the risk to human populations. Microbes Infect. **4:** 471–480.
21. DAVIES, P.D. & J.M. GRANGE. 2001. Factors affecting susceptibility and resistance to tuberculosis. Thorax **56**(Suppl 2): ii23–ii29.
22. WHO. 1994. TB: a Global Emergency, WHO Report on the TB Epidemic/WHO Global Tuberculosis Programme. World Health Organization. Geneva, Switzerland.
23. NAFEH, M.A. *et al.* 1992. Tuberculous peritonitis in Egypt: the value of laparoscopy in diagnosis. Am. J. Trop. Med. Hyg. **47:** 470–477.
24. COULIBALY, N.D. & K.R. YAMEOGO. 2000. Prevalence and control of zoonotic diseases: collaboration between public health workers and veterinarians in Burkina Faso. Acta Trop. **76:** 53–57.
25. AMENI, G., K. AMENU & M. TIBBO. 2003. Bovine tuberculosis: prevalence and risk factor assessment in cattle and cattle owners in Wuchale-Jida District, Central Ethiopia. Int. J. Appl. Res. Vet. Med. http://www.jarvm.com/articles/Vol1Iss1/AMENIJVM.htm
26. NORTH, D.W. 1995. Limitations, definitions, principles and methods of risk analysis. Rev. Sci. Tech. **14:** 913–923.
27. MACDIARMID, S.C. & H.J. PHARO. 2003. Risk analysis: assessment, management and communication. Rev. Sci. Tech. **22:** 397–408.
28. OIE. 2002. International Animal Health Code: Mammals, Birds and Bees. OIE. Paris.
29. ZEPEDA, C. 2004. Risk Communication. OIE Conference. Panama. http://www.oie.int/downld/Panama_riskcom_nov04.pdf
30. VOSE, D.J. 2000. Risk Analysis—A Quantitative Guide. John Willey & Sons, Ltd. New York.
31. CATLEY, A. & B. ADMASSU. 2003. Using participatory epidemiology to assess the impact of livestock diseases. FAO-OIE-AU/IBAR-IAEA Consultative Group Meeting on Contagious Bovine Pleuropneumonia in Africa.

32. CATLEY, A. & P. IRUNGU. 2000. Participatory research on bovine trypanosomosis in Tana river district, Kenya: preliminary findings and identification of best–best interventions. PAVE Project and Kenya Trypanosomiasis Research Institute, Nairobi, Kenya. http://www.participatoryepidemiology.info/Tana%zoRiver%zoresearch.pdf

33. AU/IBAR. 2001. Rinderpest eradication strategy in the West and East Nile ecosystems. Community-based Animal Health and Participatory. Epidemiology Unit, African Union/Interafrican Bureau for Animal Resources. Nairobi.

34. AU/IBAR. 2002. Contagious bovine pleuropneumonia in pastoralist areas of East Africa: disease dynamics and control options. African Union/Interafrican Bureau for Animal Resources. Nairobi.

35. ROBIN, R.A., A. CATLEY & D. HIRD. 2004. Significance of participatory epidemiology in veterinary public health community-based. Expert Consultation on Community-Based Veterinary Public Health Systems FAO **2:** 27–37.

36. VEKEMANS, M. *et al*. 1999. Potential source of human exposure to *Mycobacterium bovis* in Burkina Faso, in the context of the HIV epidemic. Clin. Microbiol. Infect. **5:** 617–621.

37. REDI, N. 2003. Prevalence of bovine tuberculosis and zoonotic implication in Asela Twon, South East, Ethiopia. Doctorate of Veterinary Medecine Thesis, Addis Ababa University, Debre-Zeit.

38. AMENI, G., P. BONNET & M. TIBBO. 2003. A cross-sectional study of bovine tuberculosis in selected dairy farms in Ethiopia. Int. J. Appl. Res. Vet. Med. http://www.jarvm.com/articles/Vol.Iss4/Tibbo.htm

39. ROBINSON, J.G. & E.L. BENNETT. 2000. Hunting for Sustainability in Tropical Forests. Columbia University. New York.

40. CHARDONNET, P. *et al*. 2002. The value of wildlife. Rev. Sci. Tech. **21:** 15–51.

41. KRUSE, H., A.M. KIRKEMO & K. HANDELAND. 2004. Wildlife as source of zoonotic infections. Emerg. Infect. Dis. **10:** 2067–2072.

42. LEROY, E.M. *et al*. 2004. Multiple Ebola virus transmission events and rapid decline of Central African wildlife. Science **303:** 387–390.

43. AYELE, W.Y. *et al*. 2004. Bovine tuberculosis: an old disease but a new threat to Africa. Int. J. Tuberc. Lung Dis. **8:** 924–937.

44. GALLAGHER, J. & R.S. CLIFTON-HADLEY. 2000. Tuberculosis in badgers: a review of the disease and its significance for other animals. Res. Vet. Sci. **69:** 203–217.

45. GORTAZAR, C. *et al*. 2005. Molecular characterization of *Mycobacterium tuberculosis* complex isolates from wild ungulates in south-central Spain. Vet. Res. **36:** 43–52.

46. CARON, A., P.C. CROSS & J.T. DU TOIT. 2003. Ecological implication of bovine tuberculosis in African buffalo herds. Ecol. Appl. **13:** 1338–1345.

47. O'BRIEN, D.J. *et al*. 2004. Estimating the true prevalence of *Mycobacterium bovis* in hunter-harvested white-tailed deer in Michigan. J. Wildl. Dis. **40:** 42–52.

48. SCHMITT, S.M. *et al*. 1997. Bovine tuberculosis in free-ranging white-tailed deer from Michigan. J. Wildl. Dis. **33:** 749–758.

49. WILKINS, M.J. *et al*. 2003. *Mycobacterium bovis* (bovine TB) exposure as a recreational risk for hunters: results of a Michigan Hunter Survey, 2001. Int. J. Tuberc. Lung Dis. **7:** 1001–1009.

50. ARANAZ, A. *et al*. 1996. Spacer oligonucleotide typing of *Mycobacterium bovis* strains from cattle and other animals: a tool for studying epidemiology of tuberculosis. J. Clin. Microbiol. **34:** 2734–2740.

51. COETSIER, C. *et al.* 2000. Duplex PCR for differential identification of *Mycobacterium bovis*, *M. avium*, and *M. avium* subsp. paratuberculosis in formalin-fixed paraffin-embedded tissues from cattle. J. Clin. Microbiol. **38:** 3048–3054.
52. BLAZQUEZ, J. *et al.* 1997. Genetic characterization of multidrug-resistant *Mycobacterium bovis* strains from a hospital outbreak involving human immunodeficiency virus-positive patients. J. Clin. Microbiol. **35:** 1390–1393.

Status of Mastitis as an Emerging Disease in Improved and Periurban Dairy Farms in India

SACHIN JOSHI AND SURESH GOKHALE

BAIF Development Research Foundation and Central Research Station, Uruli Kanchan, Pune, Maharashtra 412202, India

ABSTRACT: While reviewing present status of mastitis in India, results of investigations from periurban dairy farms on epidemiological, clinical manifestations, diagnosis, bacterial isolation, *in vitro* drug sensitivity, and treatment of subclinical mastitis have been presented. Mastitis, on account of its causing serious wastage and undesirable milk quality, is emerging as a major challenge among the others (like breeding improvement, nutrition management, control of infectious, tick-borne, blood, and internal parasitic diseases) in dairy development of tropics. Subclinical mastitis was found more important in India (varying from 10–50% in cows and 5–20% in buffaloes) than clinical mastitis (1–10%). The incidence was highest in Purebred Holsteins and Jerseys and lowest in local cattle and buffaloes. An investigation on 250 animals from periurban farms indicated that the monsoon season was more prone to subclinical mastitis than summer or winter, prevalence increased with higher lactation number and animals in 4th–5th month of lactation were found more susceptible (59.49%), hind quarters were found more affected (56.52%) than fore quarters (43.47%). The factors like herd size, agro climatic conditions of the region, variations in sociocultural practices, milk marketing, literacy level of the animal owner, system of feeding, and management were found important affecting the incidence of subclinical mastitis. Comparison of efficacy of different diagnostic techniques for subclinical mastitis, such as modified California mastitis test (MCMT), bromo thymol blue (BTB), modified whiteside test, trypsin inhibition test, milk pH, and electric conductivity indicated MCMT to be most sensitive (95.16%) and specific (98.02%) test. The antimicrobial susceptibility test revealed that most of the bacterial strains (gram positive, gram negative, and mixed) isolated from subclinical mastitis milk samples, were highly sensitive to enrofloxacin 53.91%, least sensitive to oxytetracycline 17.39% and ampicillin 7.83%, and resistant to streptomycin. The therapy with enrofloxacin and nimesulide was found more efficacious (92.30%) in treating subclinical mastitis cows. It was concluded that consideration of socioecological factors for mastitis control

Address for correspondence: Sachin Joshi, BAIF Development Research Foundation and Central Research Station, Uruli Kanchan, Pune, Maharashtra 412202, India. Voice: 91-020-26926248/448; fax: 91-020-26926347.

e-mail: crs@pn2.vsnl.net.in

Ann. N.Y. Acad. Sci. 1081: 74–83 (2006). © 2006 New York Academy of Sciences.
doi: 10.1196/annals.1373.007

in periurban area would help to reduce the cost of mastitis control in clean milk production.

KEYWORDS: clinical mastitis; subclinical mastitis; incidence; diagnostic methods; India

INTRODUCTION

While selection programs in buffaloes and successful attempts of crossing local low-milk-yielding cattle with Purebred Holstein and Jersey have been producing animals of high milk potential, the physiological stress and strain of heavy milk production, deep caudo-ventral placement of udder, large size and carriage of large volume of milk by the udder makes them more sensitive and prone to injury and subsequent udder infection and inflammation resulting into mastitis.

Mastitis is known to be an economically devastating disease hampering desired progress in dairy industry. The overall national economic loss in India due to mastitis was to the tune of Rs.16,072 million[1] (that due to clinical mastitis to be Rs.2,856.4 million and Rs.2,345.9 million and due to subclinical mastitis Rs.6,038.7 million and Rs.4,831 million in cattle and buffaloes, respectively). Average decrease in milk yield due to clinical and subclinical mastitis was estimated to be 50% and 17.5%, respectively.

Clinical mastitis is an individual problem and it is characterized by changes in the udder and milk drawn from it. Whereas subclinical mastitis is herd problem because it constituents a reservoir of infection which could be transmitted to other animals of herd.

INCIDENCE

The frequency, severity, and economic impact of mastitis are known to depend upon the preventive and management approaches. It has also been observed that the incidence and the patterns of causative agents markedly differ from place to place, herd to herd, and time to time. Studies conducted in different states within India reflect high incidence of the disease for past seven decades.

The incidence level of clinical and subclinical mastitis in various parts of the country ranged from 11.51%[2] to 23.55%,[3] 3.94%[4] to 17.25%,[2] and 1.99%[5] to 12.28%[6] in crossbred cows, local cows, and buffaloes, respectively. The figures for subclinical mastitis were from 18.40%[7] to 72.60%,[8] 15.78%[9] to 81.60%,[10] and 20.72%[4] to 61.73%,[11] respectively for the same classes of livestock.

EFFECT OF SEASON

The seasonality in the incidence of mastitis is well known. Incidence is recorded more both in cows (15.05%) and in buffaloes (8.89%) in rainy season

TABLE 1. Quarter number-wise prevalence of subclinical mastitis in HF crossbred cows

| Total no. of HF crossbreds examined | No. of animals of subclinical mastitis | Distribution of subclinical mastitis quarters | | | |
		One quarter	Two quarters	Three quarters	Four quarters
250	115 (46.00)	52 (45.21)	41 (35.65)	15 (13.04)	7 (6.08)

NOTE: Figures in parenthesis indicate percentage.

than in summer (13.97% and 7.04%, respectively). The seasonal prevalence of subclinical mastitis was recorded in monsoon, summer, and winter as 37.02%, 27.42%, and 26.04%, respectively.[12] Less hygienic farms favored higher incidence of mastitis than hygienic farms in both cows and buffaloes.

The periurban dairy farms are located 40 km radius from the main city. The production characteristics of dairying, such as use of crop residues, fodder crop rotation, and production of organic fertilizer, provide a strong synergy with other parts of farming system.

An investigation covering 250 animals from periurban bovine farms in Maharashtra state was carried out to study epidemiological, clinical manifestations, diagnosis, bacterial isolation, *in vitro* drug sensitivity, and treatment of subclinical mastitis.

The study indicated overall incidence of subclinical mastitis in Holstein-Friesian (HF) crossbred cows to be 46%.

QUARTER NUMBER-WISE PREVALENCE

Quarter number-wise prevalence was found varying (TABLE 1). Infection with one, two, three, and four quarters was 45.21%, 35.65%, 13.04%, and 6.08%, respectively.

The similar quarter infection rate (QIR) were recorded,[13,14] higher QIR of subclinical mastitis in dairy cattle is reported,[15] and lower incidence was observed in Uttar Pradesh.[16] The variation in the incidence could be due to variations in the managerial practices, cattle population, stage and number of lactations, environment, breed, nutritional status, size of herd, year of study, region, and zoogeography.[17] Predisposing factors like physical condition of teat, integrity of teat, tissue injury, defective sphincters, and variation from quarter to quarter could also contribute to variation.

QUARTER INFECTION RATE

The prevalence of QIR was studied (TABLE 2). The QIR was observed to be 20.7%; the lower QIR mentioned was 9.95%,[18] and higher 35.45% QIR was

TABLE 2. Quarter-wise prevalence of subclinical mastitis in HF crossbred cows

Total no. of quarter examined	No. of quarters positive for subclinical mastitis	Quarter infection rate (%)	Distribution among infected quarters			
			RF	RH	LF	LH
1000	207	20.7	49 (23.67)	60 (28.98)	41 (19.80)	57 (27.53)

NOTE: Figures in parenthesis indicate percentage. RF = right fore; RH = right hind; LF = left fore; LH = left hind.

also recorded.[19] The differences in QIR could be due to genetic resistance, variation in sample size, difference in teat length, teat shape, teat orifice morphology, breed, and management of houses.[17] As regard to distribution among infected quarters, the incidence was found more in hind quarters (56.52%) than fore quarters (43.47%). The reason for higher infection in hind quarters could be attributed to more exposure to the dung and urine, excessive forward and side way pulling, while walking undue stress, milking management, and other husbandry practices.[14]

EFFECT OF LACTATION RANK

The prevalence of subclinical mastitis increased with increasing lactation number. It was 45.16%, 50.00%, 55.55%, 63.15%, 47.22%, and 29.57% in first, second, third, fourth, fifth, and above fifth lactation, respectively (TABLE 3).

Lower resistance of animals, might be due to stress of peak milk yield in the 3rd to 5th lactations and improper contraction of teat sphincter could be some of the reasons.[14] The break down of streak canal barrier (harboring wax like material containing long chain fatty acids providing bacteriostatic effect) with advancing age leads to increased susceptibility to infection with successive increase in lactation number.[20]

TABLE 3. Lactation-wise prevalence of subclinical mastitis in HF crossbred cows

No. of lactation	No. of HF crossbreds examined	No. of cows positive for subclinical mastitis	Percentage of affected HF crossbreds
First	31	14	45.16
Second	38	19	50.00
Third	36	20	55.55
Fourth	38	24	63.15
Fifth	36	17	47.22
Above fifth	71	21	29.57
Total	250	115	

EFFECT OF LACTATION STAGE

The HF crossbreds during their 4th to 5th month of lactation stage were found more susceptible (59.49%) to subclinical mastitis, followed by 1st to 3rd month (42.22%), 6th to 7th month (40.29%), and 8th month of lactation stage and above (21.42%) (TABLE 4).

While similar findings in Nilliravi buffaloes and Sahiwal cows were reported,[21] the higher rate of incidence in early lactation phase could be due to physiological stress of high milk yield and alterations in homeostasis.

DIAGNOSIS OF SUBCLINICAL MASTITIS

Diagnosis is very essential for control and prevention of subclinical bovine mastitis, although various indirect tests have been described to detect subclinical mastitis,[20] each test has its own limitations to detect subclinical mastitis at all stages. Screening of individual milk samples or bulk milk by indirect method is necessary to detect subclinical mastitis and take effective control measures.

Leukocyte count was considered as standard reference test, to detect subclinical mastitis of 250 cows. The leukocyte count was more than 350 thousands/mL of milk, signifying subclinical mastitis. Average somatic cell count (SCC) of 207 quarters from 115 cows was 548,531 ± 11,900/mL of milk. Two hundred seven positive milk samples detected by SCC were also subjected to routine diagnostic test viz. modified California mastitis test (MCMT), chloride test, modified whiteside test (MWST), and trypsin inhibition (TI) test for their comparative efficacy. The results are presented in (TABLE 5). The overall efficacy of MCMT was found more efficacious (96.73%) followed by TI test (94.55%), chloride test (92.82%), and MWST (89.08%). The sensitivity and specificity of MCMT, chloride test, MWST, and TI test were 95.16% and 98.02%, 90.82% and 90.46%, 82.12% and 96.04%, and 92.27% and 96.83%, respectively.

The efficacy of MCMT was reported 90%[22] using CMT reagent with varied compositions.

TABLE 4. Lactation stage-wise prevalence of subclinical mastitis in HF crossbred cows

Months of lactation	No. of HF crossbreds examined	No. of cows positive for sub-clinical mastitis	Percentage of affected crossbreds
1 to 3	90	38	42.22
4 to 5	79	47	59.49
6 to 7	67	27	40.29
8 and above	14	3	21.42
Total	250	115	

TABLE 5. Efficacy of various indirect tests employed for diagnosis of subclinical mastitis in HF crossbred cows with reference to SCC

No.	Test	No. of samples examined	True +	True −	False +	False −	Sensitivity (%)	Specificity (%)	Overall percentage efficacy
1	Reference test (SCC)	460	207	253	−	−	−	−	−
2	MCMT	460	197	248	5	10	95.16	98.02	96.73
3	Chloride test	460	188	239	14	19	90.82	94.46	92.82
4	MWST	460	170	243	10	37	82.12	96.04	89.08
5	TI test	460	191	245	8	16	92.27	96.83	94.55

Hence, among all indirect test, MCMT is more immediate and efficient test and recommended in field condition. Similar observations were recorded for TI test.[23]

The average pH of infected milk was 6.82 ± 0.01 whereas in SCC less than 3.5 lacs/mL it was 6.55 ± 0.01. High rise in pH in mastitis milk has also been recorded.[17] The electrical conductivity of subclinical mastitis milk samples was 6.09 ± 0.7 mScm^{-1} while in below normal SCC it was 4.28 ± 0.06 mScm^{-1}. The increase in value of conductivity in infected quarter to increased concentration of sodium and chloride was also mentioned.[24]

BACTERIOLOGICAL EXAMINATION

The culturing of milk samples and Gram's staining revealed 41 (35.65%) gram positive, 31 (26.95%) gram negative, and 43 (37.39%) mixed infection. The culturing and antimicrobial sensitivity revealed that gram-positive isolates were highly sensitive to enrofloxacin 53.65%, followed by amoxicillin 48.78%, gentamicin 43.90%, ciprofloxacin 39.02%, cloxacillin 34.14%, chloramphenicol 29.26%, and least sensitive to oxytetracycline 21.95% and ampicillin 9.75%, respectively. Gram-negative strains were highly sensitive to enrofloxacin 58.06%, followed by ciprofloxacin 48.38%, gentamicin 45.16%, cloxacillin 41.93%, amoxicillin 32.25%, chloramphenicol 29.03%, and least sensitive to oxytetracycline 12.90% and ampicillin 9.67%, respectively.

Mixed strains were highly sensitive to enrofloxacin 51.16%, followed by gentamicin 37.20%, cloxacillin 34.88%, ciprofloxacin 32.55%, chloramphenicol 32.55%, amoxicillin 30.23%, and least sensitive to oxytetracycline 16.27% and ampicillin 4.65%, respectively. It is necessary to mention that the most of the bacterial strains (gram positive, gram negative, and mixed) isolated from subclinical mastitic milk samples during the course of investigation were resistant to streptomycin and least sensitive to oxytetracycline and ampicillin. Comparable antibiogram have been reported earlier from mastitis milk samples.[25]

Similar to present antibiogram resistant with streptomycin, oxytetracycline and ampicillin have also been reported.[26] Multiple resistance and cross resistance to these drugs probably attributes to the fact that, oxytetracycline, streptomycin, and penicillin drugs indiscriminately used for the treatment of bovine mastitis, over last 30 years, and the frequent and injudicious use of these antibiotics in animal practice have resulted in the development of resistance.

The subclinical mastitic cows were treated with enrofloxacin injection 250 mg (2.5 mL diluted in equal volume of water for injection) given intramammary per quarter and 1250 mg (12.5 mL) by intramuscular route. Along with antimicrobial therapy a recent but potent NSAID—Nimesulide, 500 mg (10 mL) was injected intramuscularly to all the affected cows. The therapy was repeated after 24 h for 5 days. After completion of therapy, 92.30% quarters recovered normally. Both the drugs were tolerated by the animals and no local or systemic untoward reactions were observed. Fluoroquinolones are potent DNA gyrase inhibitor causing powerful bacterial action at exceptionally low concentration.[27] Fluoroquinolones are active in alkaline pH and this explains reason of excellent efficacy of enrofloxacin. Excellent efficacy of new quinolones against mastitis has been reported.[17] The recovery and restoration of milk yield was faster due to concurrent therapy with Nimesulide. Nimesulide selectively inhibits inflammatory tissue enzyme—cyclooxygenase-2 (Cox-2) and thereby impairing production of prostaglandins by infected tissue.[28] Nimesulide, recent sulphonamilides exhibits significant selective inhibitory activity toward—Cox-2 without affective—cyclooxygenase-1 (Cox-1) and can be used in clinically in relieving the pain and inflammation.

FUTURE PROSPECTS FOR MASTITIS CONTROL

A thorough understanding of the epidemiology of pathogens in dairy herds is the key to the development of successful control schemes. Bacteria that most probably cause mastitis can be divided into two large groups based on the source: contagious pathogens and environmental pathogens. The primary contagious pathogens are *Staphylococcus aureus, Streptococcus agalactiae*, and *Mycoplasma spp.* Important environmental pathogens include *Coliform bacteria, Streptococcus dysgalactiae,* and *Streptococcus uberis.* The source of contagious and environmental pathogens in infected cows and the surroundings in which a cow lives. Therefore, methods of control adopted for contagious pathogens are not effective against environmental pathogens.

Post-milking teat dipping reduces the spread from cow to cow while dry cow therapy reduces the reservoir, which further augments the reduction in the teat exposure,[29] whereas, barrier teat dips generally containing a germicidal agent have been developed to aid in the control of the environmental pathogens.[30] Hygienic milking practice would also decrease exposure.

The streak canal is the primary defense mechanism of mammary gland as the portal of entry for almost microorganism that causes mastitis. During dry period, a keratin protein substance appears to protect streak canal.[31] The presence or absence of the keratin plug during dry period coincides with the period of known resistance and susceptibility to the environmental pathogens.

CYTOKINES

Nonspecific or innate responses are predominant during the early stage of infection. Central in the regulation of these responses, is the production of regulatory cytokines. Cytokines are naturally produced product that play important role in essentially all aspects of inflammation and immunity. One of the more existing potential applications of cytokines is for the control of mastitis.[32]

It has clearly demonstrated that diets of the dairy animals can influence the resistance to intramammary infection.[33] Specific components, like vitamins E, A, and B-carotene, and trace minerals, like selenium, copper, and zinc, are important from udder resistance point of view.

Strategies aimed at enhancing immune system of the mammary gland would greatly impact animal ability to resist mastitis. Vaccination is the method to develop specific resistance against potential pathogens. Vaccine efforts for bovine mastitis have concentrated mainly on common contagious and environmental pathogens. The efforts for assessing use and efficacy of such vaccines in developing countries are the urgent need to reduce the economic losses.

USE OF HERBAL EXTRACTS

Renewed interest has emerged for therapeutic use of nontoxic, economic traditional herbal preparations. Several products are released for alternate mastitis treatment, for example, uddermint,[34] golden udder,[35] mastilep,[36] and therapeutic use of oil extracts of *Ocimum sanctum* (tulsi) with *Azadirachta* (neem), and aqueous extract of *Tinospora cordifola* found good results for reducing bacterial load and enhancement of phagocytic capacity.[37] Efforts to the use of herbal products will reduce the treatment cost, adverse reactions of the drugs, and human being health hazards.

CONCLUSIONS

It was concluded that consideration of socioecological factors, like region, season, and cropping pattern, farming system, herd size, animal type, etc., for mastitis control in periurban area would help to reduce the cost of mastitis control in clean milk production.

With the advent of improved diagnostic tests, more understanding of the disease and availability of third generation antibiotics, and improved ways and means to upkeep the hygiene and management, the opportunities of clean milk production in periurban area are increasing.

REFERENCES

1. SINGH, P.J. & P.B. SINGH. 1994. A study of economic losses due to mastitis in India. Indian J. Dairy Sci. **47:** 265–272.
2. SETHI, R.K. & D.S. BALAINE. 1978. An approach to quantification of threshold traits in dairy cattle. Indian J. Dairy Sci. **31:** 311–315.
3. TANEJA, V.K., V.K. DWIVEDI, M.M. SAXENA, et al. 1989. Incidence of mastitis and production losses in crossbreds. Indian J. Ani. Sci. **59:** 1346–1348.
4. DHANDA, M.R. & M.S. SETHI. 1962. ICAR Series no.35, ICAR, N. D.
5. KUMAR, B. 1988. Studies on incidence, chemotherapy and control of mastitis in cattle and buffalo. M. V. Sc. thesis, Punjab agriculture University, Ludhiyana, India.
6. SHINDE, S.S., G.B. KULKARNI, G.R. GANGANE, et al. 2001. Incidence of mastitis in buffaloes in Parbhani District, Maharashtra. Indian Vet. Congress 22–23 Feb, 2001. **2:** 35–38.
7. SINGH, W., V.K. SHARMA, H.B. RAJANI, et al. 1982. Indian economy and test efficacy of subclinical mastitis in dairy animals. Indian Vet. J. **59:** 693–696.
8. ALI, S.L., P.G. SUPEKAR & P.C. SHUKLA. 1989. A study of the incidence of subclinical mastitis in cows in Mhow region. Guj. Vet. **16:** 16–28.
9. SWARUP, D. & K. PRABHUDAS. 1985. A note on occurrence and treatment of Streptococcus aureus sub-clinical mastitis in cows and goats. Indian J. Vet. Med. **5:** 35–38.
10. NARAYANAN, T. & K.K. IYA. 1953. Studies on bovine mastitis. 1. Incidence of mastitis in cows and buffaloes. Indian J. Dairy Sci. **6:** 169–173.
11. KARLA, D.S. & M.R. DHANDA. 1964. Vet. Rec. **76:** 219.
12. PATEL, P.R., S.K. RAWAL, et al. 2001. Status of mastitis in Gujarat state. Indian Vet. Congress **1:** 45–52.
13. VERMA, T.N., L.N. MANDAL & B.K. SINHA. 1978. Indian J. Pub. Health **22:** 249.
14. SINGH, K.B. & K.K. BAXI.1980. Studies on the incidence of diagnosis of subclinical mastitis in milk animals. Indian Vet. J. **57:** 723–729.
15. JOSHI, H.D., J. PRASAD & A. REKIB. 1976. Studies on field diagnosis of sub-clinical mastitis. Indian Vet. J. **53:** 752–756.
16. SHARMA, S.D. & P. ROY. 1977. Studies on the incidence of bovine sub-clinical mastitis in Uttar Pradesh. Indian Vet. J. **54:** 435–439.
17. RADOSTITS, O.M., D.C. BLOOD, C.C. GAY, et al. 2000. Veterinary Medicine, 9th ed.: 603–685. ELBS-Bailliere Tindal. London.
18. PARAI, J.P., N.N. PANDEY & S.B. LAL. 1992. Incidence of sub-clinical mastitis in crossbred and exotic cows. Indian Vet. Med. **12:** 16–20.
19. PRASAD, H., R.K. ROYCHAUDHARY & G. PATGIRI. 2001. Incidence of subclinical mastitis at drying-off. Indian Vet. J. **78:** 316–318.
20. SCHALM, O.W., E.J. COROLL & N.C. JAIN. 1971. Bovine Mastitis. Lea and Febiger. Philadelphia.

21. RASSOL, L.G., M.A. JABBAR, S.E. KAZMI, *et al.* 1985. Incidence of sub-clinical mastitis in Nilli-Ravi buffaloes and Sahiwal cows. Pakistan Vet. J. **5:** 76–78.

22. CHANDA, A.A., C.R. ROY, P.K. BANERJEE, *et al.* 1989. Studies on incidence of bovine mastitis. It's diagnosis, etiology and in vitro sensitivity of isolated pathogens. Indian Vet. J. **66:** 277–282.

23. AWAZ, K.B. & Abdul SAMAD. 1993. A rapid enzyme inhibition assay for detection and quantitation of trypsin inhibitors in biological materials. J. Bom. Vet . Coll. **4:** 25–31.

24. NAGRAJAN, B. 1999. Recent trends in the diagnosis of subclinical mastitis. Advanced diagnostic procedures in veterinary practice. Centre of advanced studies in clinical medicines and therapeutic. Manual of Madras Veterinary College. 189–194.

25. PARNJAPE, V.C. & A.M. DAS. 1986. Mastitis among buffalo population of Bombay—A bacteriological report. Indian Vet. J. **63:** 438–441.

26. ANJANEYULU, Y., N. SASIDHAR BABU & R.M. JAMES. 1998. Efficacy of commonly used antibiotics in bovine mastitis: A field study. Indian Vet. J. **75:** 460–461.

27. PRESSCOTT, J.G. & J.D. BAGGOT. 1985. JAMA **187:** 363–368.

28. XAVIR, R.1997. Safety profile of Nimesulide: ten years of clinical experience. Drugs Today **33:** 41–50.

29. SMITH, K.L. & J.S. HOGAN. 1995. Epidemiology of Mastitis. *In* Third IDF international mastitis seminar, Lachmann Printers Ltd. Haifa, Israel. pp. 82–83.

30. NICKERSON, S.C. & R.L. BODDIE. 1995. Efficacy studies on barrier teat dips. National mastitis council, Annual meeting proceeding, Fort Worth, Texas. pp. 38–47.

31. EBERTHART, R.J. 1986. Management of dry cows to reduce mastitis. J. Dairy Sci. **69:** 1721–1732.

32. VAN MIERT, A.S.J.P.A.M. 1990. Cytokines: modulation of host resistant against infection in: mastitis: physiology or pathology? Proceedings of international Congress Ghent, Belgium held during September 18–22, 1990, 69–91.

33. HOGAN, J.S.,W.P. WEISS & K.L. SMITH. 1996. Nutrition and mammary host defense against disease in dairy cattle *In* Progress in Dairy Science: 45–57. CAB International Wallinford. Oxon, UK.

34. OLDAKAR, G. 1990. Mastitis—One School of Thought. Dairy Farmer **86:** 4, 41,43.

35. ALLEN, J.1990. Good as gold. Dairy Farmer **37:** 48–49.

36. SAXENA, M.J. *et al.* 1995. Nonantibiotic herbal therapy for mastitis. Sem. Tel Aviv Israel S-**5:** 79–80.

37. DASH, P.K. 2001. Immunomodulatory therapy—A new approach in the management of sub-clinical mastitis. Indian Vet. Congress **2:** 87–91.

Role of Import and Export Regulatory Animal Health Officials in International Control and Surveillance for Animal Diseases

BOB H. BOKMA

United States Department of Agriculture, Animal and Plant Health Inspection Service, Veterinary Services, Riverdale, Maryland 20737, USA

ABSTRACT: The challenges to those who regulate the import and export of animals and animal products are escalating, due to the evolving nature of animal and human disease agents. The diseases and agents of interest may include low pathogenic avian influenza, bluetongue, bovine spongiform encephalopathy, and foot-and-mouth disease. Fear of an incursion of an unknown or incompletely understood threat can significantly limit risk tolerance. The fear may be that an incursion will affect export trade or tourism. An incomplete knowledge of the animal health situation in the exporting country, due to insufficient surveillance for the disease agent of concern, may limit the application of science in import decisions. In addition, the disease agent may be inappropriately considered exotic if it has not been described. As a result, excessive safeguards for disease agents that do not present any new threat may be employed. To confront these challenges, we are striving toward transparency in international reporting. Moreover, regulatory import decisions exceeding the recommendations of the Terrestrial Animal Health Code and the Aquatic Animal Health Code of the World Organization for Animal Health must be fair and science-based.

KEYWORDS: regulatory veterinary medicine; tropical veterinery medicine; import decisions; export certification; animals; animal genetics; animal products

INTRODUCTION

There are numerous bibliographic sources on the concept of public good, which in our view can be described as doing the right thing for the public's benefit. In our review of informal sources, public good is oftentimes described

Address for correspondence: Bob H. Bokma, United States Department of Agriculture, Animal and Plant Health Inspection Service, National Center for Import and Export, 4700 River Road, Unit 40, Riverdale, MD 20737. Voice: 301-734-8066; fax: 301-734-3222.
e-mail: Bob.H.Bokma@aphis.usda.gov

Ann. N.Y. Acad. Sci. 1081: 84–89 (2006). © 2006 New York Academy of Sciences.
doi: 10.1196/annals.1373.009

in economic terms, but it can equally be applied toward social benefits, such as prevention of human or animal disease or of an invasive species.[1] Related to this topic are numerous articles and discussions that contain a critical take-home message—the stakes are high.

In reviewing the proceedings and abstracts of the biennial meetings of the Society for Tropical Veterinary Medicine (STVM), several participants have discussed the obligations that countries have to implement appropriate importation safeguarding requirements with the exporting countries in the tropics for their animals and animal products. At the STVM 2003 meeting, Tom Walton reviewed important obligations of World Trade Organization (WTO) member countries and outlined animal health initiatives for enhancing a country's abilities to safeguard without being overly restrictive. WTO member countries are obliged to limit import restrictions to those recommended by the World Animal Health Organization, aka Organization International des Epizooties (OIE) or to demonstrate through risk assessments shared with trading partners when its requirements are more restrictive.[1] Leonardo Mascitelli gave a similar message from an Argentine perspective.[2] Previously, Dan Sheesley, Yoshihiro Ozawa, Tom Walton, and Bob Bokma have also discussed these obligations during the STVM 2001, 1999, 1997, and 1995 meetings, respectively.[3-6]

With regard to animal disease agent threats, there are risks and the perception of risk. In an April 2005 press release, the United Nations Food and Agriculture Organization pointed out that global livestock markets can increase national income and improve nutrition. However, they pose potential risks to livelihoods, human health, and the environment. And the list of potential human health threats is seemingly getting longer with the recent additions of avian influenza, West Nile virus (in the Americas), severe acute respiratory syndrome, bovine spongiform encephalopathy, and murine hantavirus. Public awareness of zoonotic diseases has increased to new levels and includes the zoonotic agents mentioned above as well as toxoplasmosis from cats; giardia from beavers; trichinella from swine, horses, and wildlife; rabies from various animal hosts; avian salmonella of public health impact; bovine *Escherichia coli* infections; and even Newcastle disease of poultry and wild birds.

During December 2004, Lonnie R. King, Dean, Michigan State University, College of Veterinary Medicine, discussed the ongoing convergence of veterinary and public health with some 60 public policy officials in the United States. According to King, in very recent times, this interrelationship has increased dramatically, following an earlier lull when vaccines and antibiotics slowed the previous trend. Many important examples of zoonoses have occurred in Southeast Asia during these last few years. King pointed out that infectious organisms cause some 1620 human diseases. Some 60% of these are zoonotic. Of the 35 major human outbreaks occurring over the last $2\frac{1}{2}$ years, 75% are zoonotic.[7]

At the STVM 2003 meeting, Peter Daszak discussed a new agenda for emerging diseases, relying heavily on team work and risk analyses to predict future emerging diseases.[8] He pointed out the increasing number of emerging disease agents such as Nipah and Hendra viruses, west Nile virus, which are zoonotic, as well as amphibian chytridiomycosis, which is decimating amphibian populations.

In addition to emerging diseases that may occur through traditional modes of transmission, potential agroterrorism or actual cases directed toward plant or animal health is another avenue for the spread of disease. When a dangerous animal or public health disease agent is introduced to a naïve animal population, low innate immunity may be an important factor affecting the severity of the disease that presents.

At the STVM 1999 meeting, Linda Logan-Henfrey discussed bio/ agroterrorism threats and what governmental veterinary regulators and researchers are doing to reduce the risk of animal and human disease agents.[9] She looked at this threat from the perspective of where potential agents are available and discussed the availability of weapons program agents. The real agroterrorism risk may not be from this grade of veterinary or public health disease agent, rather it may be from a disease agent that occurs in many countries but is not present at all in other regions. At the same meeting, John Williams and Dan Sheesley, as well as Frank Norn and Roger Breeze, focused on bio-terrorism threats and the responsibilities of government to protect the public and animal health.[10,11]

Roger Breeze examines the potential that exists for a terrorist to take action against a developed country such as the United States. He emphasizes that the prudent government should implement controls internally, such as vaccination, measures for rapid diagnosis, and inspection at border ports. He points out that the risk from agroterrorism due to the intentional introduction of an agent, such as foot-and-mouth disease, will have significant economic and social impact in a country with a highly susceptible non-vaccinated animal population. His thesis is that the implementation of appropriate safeguarding measures could easily be applied. One safeguard he recommends is detection of a terrorist threat at ports of entry, including screening of items that could harbor biological agents. Another safeguard is the registration and inspections of laboratories, which might have high impact disease agents that in the wrong hands could easily be applied in agroterrorism.[12] Clearly, this viewpoint, though pessimistic, is addressing the public good and merits significant consideration by governmental regulators.

IMPORT AND EXPORT DECISION-MAKING BY VETERINARY REGULATORY OFFICIALS

Through a veterinary infrastructure that is based on cooperation with State and Federal agencies and industry, U.S. import and export regulatory animal health officials carry out their functions for the public's benefit. As a result, many animal diseases have been eradicated in the United States, and many more are prevented from coming across the U.S. borders. Further, exporters in the United States have been able to send U.S. animals and animal products safely to a large number of trading partners, meeting important needs in those countries.

To prevent the introduction of foreign disease agents to a country or region, veterinarians accredited by the United States Department of Agriculture's Animal and Plant Health Inspection Service (APHIS) and official Federal and State veterinarians ensure that exported animals meet the requirements of the importing country as well as the minimum export requirements of the United States. Veterinarians in other countries also ensure that animals entering the United States can be safely imported. Ensuring that animals are free of foreign diseases promotes safe trade. The OIE's Terrestrial Animal Health Code and Aquatic Animal Health Code provide guidance for safe trade.

APHIS employs safeguards including taking steps to implement the provisions of the OIE animal health codes. APHIS' National Center for Import and Export (NCIE) provides the regulatory and procedural guidance to APHIS field forces and the Department of Homeland Security's Customs and Border Protection. NCIE regulates the trade of animals or animal products between the United State and other nations.

To protect animal health, APHIS enacts regulations. Our regulations are contained in Title 9, *Code of Federal Regulations*. When a need has been identified to reflect current science or import requirements, we must amend the regulations. In many cases, such as for regionalization requests, APHIS conducts a risk assessment before determining whether to proceed with rulemaking. Amending the regulations engenders a rulemaking process that consists of multiple steps specified by the Administrative Procedures Act, various executive orders, and other documents. While often a lengthy process, it provides the public and other interested parties an opportunity to comment and contribute to the decision-making process. The public is concerned about zoonotic threats to animal and public health.

The role of import and export regulatory animal health officials is to facilitate the safe trade of animals and animal products following international guidelines. However, the balance between the risk of disease and safe trade is sometimes difficult to achieve. Common overreactions to the potential threat of disease outbreaks include complete bans on trade of low-risk animal products and commodities. As an example, at the STVM 2003 meeting, Cheryl Hall described restrictions on poultry products from the United States due to low pathogenic avian influenza. She stated that concern over the potential for H5 and H7 virus to mutate into highly pathogenic avian influenza may result in overly restrictive import measures applied to other viruses that have not been observed to have this ability.[13]

However, a decision that causes a ban of all trade of live birds and poultry, swine, or ruminants and their products and is based on perceived threat of a significant animal or public disease agent fails to consider international guidelines. While the OIE's animal health codes allow for the implementation of emergency measures and the due notification and comment period may follow when a true emergency exists, the codes contain reasonable recommendations for response, including measures to allow safe trade of commodities that have been determined to be of low risk. A scientifically reasonable reaction would be to strive toward an efficient implementation of the safeguards recommended by the OIE animal health codes. By extension, the logical recourses might include announcements of emergency measures. However, the measures should be the full implementation of the OIE recommendations, rather than bans of all imports or trade in low-risk commodities.

CONCLUSIONS

In this conference, we are challenged to discuss and come to conclusions regarding the impact of emerging zoonotic diseases on animal health. Discussions among import and export officers in two countries can protect the public good, principally in the importing country. While an importing country needs to implement mitigation measures to protect animal health, mitigation measures should not hinder trade unnecessarily. Unsuccessful trade leads to mistrust and the potential to harm. Fair and safe trade leads to respect.

ACKNOWLEDGMENT

Acknowledgement goes to Mr. Alejandro Asin, for assistance related to this key concept.

REFERENCES

1. ACORD, B.A. & T.E. WALTON. 2004. Animal health organizations: roles to mitigate the impact of ecologic change on animal health in the tropics. Ann. N. Y. Acad. Sci. **1026:** 32–40.
2. CANÉ, B.G., LF LEANES & L.O. MASCITELLI. 2004. Emerging diseases and their impact on animal commerce: the Argentine lesson. Ann. N. Y. Acad. Sci. **1026:** 12–18.
3. SHEESLEY, D.J. & J.K. GREIFER. 1996. Implications of international trade agreements for global animal health. Ann. N. Y. Acad. Sci. **791:** 296–302.
4. OZAWA, Y. 2000. International trade: multinational aspects. Ann. N. Y. Acad. Sci. **916:** 31–35.
5. WALTON, T.E. 2000. The impact of diseases on the importation of animals and animal products.. Ann. N. Y. Acad. Sci. **916:** 36–40.

6. BOKMA, B.H. 2001. Balancing international animal movement restrictions with animal health status and veterinary infrastructure [abstract]. Biennial meeting of the Society for Tropical Veterinary Medicine, Pilanesberg, South Africa.
7. KING, L.R. 2005. Comments quoted in the Journal of the American Veterinary Medicine Association. J. Am. Vet. Med. Assoc. **226:** 500–502.
8. DASZAK, P., G.M. TABOR, A.M. KILPATRICK, *et al.* 2004. Conservation medicine and a new agenda for emerging diseases. Ann. N. Y. Acad. Sci. **1026:** 1–11.
9. LOGAN-HENFREY, L. 2000. Mitigation of bioterrorist threats in the 21st century. Ann. N. Y. Acad. Sci. **916:** 121–133.
10. WILLIAMS, J.L. & D. SHEESLEY. 2000. Response to bio-terrorism directed against animals. Ann. N. Y. Acad. Sci. **916:** 117–120.
11. HORN, F. & R.G. BREEZE. 1999. Agriculture and food security. Ann. N. Y. Acad. Sci. **894:** 9–17.
12. BREEZE, R. 2004. Agroterrorism: betting far more than the farm. Biosecur. Bioterror. **2(4):** 251–264.
13. HALL, C. 2004. Impact of avian influenza on U.S. poultry trade relations 2002: H5 or H7 low pathogenic avian influenza. Ann. N. Y. Acad. Sci. **1026:** 47–53.

Regional and International Approaches on Prevention and Control of Animal Transboundary and Emerging Diseases

J. DOMENECH,[a] J. LUBROTH,[a] C. EDDI,[a] V. MARTIN,[a] AND F. ROGER[b]

[a]*FAO, Rome, Italy*

[b]*CIRAD EMVT, Montpellier, France*

ABSTRACT: Transboundary animal diseases pose a serious risk to the world animal agriculture and food security and jeopardize international trade. The world has been facing devastating economic losses from major outbreaks of transboundary animal diseases (TADs) such as foot-and-mouth disease, classical swine fever, rinderpest, peste des petits ruminants (PPR), and Rift Valley fever. Lately the highly pathogenic avian influenza (HPAI) due to H5N1 virus, has become an international crisis as all regions around the world can be considered at risk. In the past decades, public health authorities within industrialized countries have been faced with an increasing number of food safety issues. The situation is equally serious in developing countries. The globalization of food (and feed) trade, facilitated by the liberalization of world trade, while offering many benefits and opportunities, also represents new risks. The GF-TADs Global Secretariat has carried out several regional consultations for the identification of priority diseases and best ways for their administration, prevention and control. In the questionnaires carried out and through the consultative process, it was noted that globally, FMD was ranked as the first and foremost priority. Rift Valley fever, and today highly pathogenic avian influenza, are defined as major animal diseases which also affect human health. PPR and CBPP, a disease which is particularly serious in Africa and finally, African swine fever (ASF) and classical swine fever (CSF) are also regionally recognised as top priorities on which the Framework is determined to work. The FAO philosophy— shared by the OIE—embraces the need to prevent and control TADs and emerging diseases at their source, which is most of the time in developing countries. Regional and international approaches have to be followed, and the FAO and OIE GF-TADs initiative provides the appropriate concepts and objectives as well as an organizational framework to link international and regional organizations at the service of their countries to better prevent and control the risks on animal and human health and the economic impact of TADs and emerging animal diseases.

Address for correspondence: Joseph Domenech.
e-mail: joseph.domenech@fao.org

Ann. N.Y. Acad. Sci. 1081: 90–107 (2006). © 2006 New York Academy of Sciences.
doi: 10.1196/annals.1373.010

KEYWORDS: transboundary animal diseases; emerging animal diseases; prevention; control; early warning

INTRODUCTION

With increasing globalization, the persistence of transboundary animal diseases (TADs) anywhere in the world poses a serious risk to the world animal agriculture and food security and jeopardizes international trade.[1]

In recent decades, the world has been facing devastating economic losses to livestock farmers from major outbreaks of TADs, such as foot and mouth disease (FMD), in Europe,[2] classical swine fever in the Caribbean and Europe (1996–2002),[3] rinderpest (RP) in Africa in the 1980s,[4] peste des petits ruminants in India and Bangladesh,[5] contagious bovine pleuropneumonia in Eastern and Southern Africa (late 1990s),[6] as well as Rift Valley fever in the Arabian Peninsula (2000).[7]

Amblyomma variegatum, the tropical bond tick that produce heavy economic loses in Africa, has infested several islands in the Caribbean region. It has been estimated that if the tick were to enter the American continent, the economic damage of the tick would be about 1 billion U.S. dollars.[8]

The avian influenza epidemic in Asia due to highly pathogenic H5N1 strain in poultry, which spread rapidly, and is characterized by mortality in chickens between 75% and 100%, resulted in the deaths and culling of some 40 million birds. The economic impact of the disease to the South East Asia was evaluated in more than 60 billion U.S. dollars.[9]

In the past two to three decades, public health authorities in industrialized countries have been faced with an increasing number of food safety problems. The situation is equally serious in developing countries. In addition to known food-borne diseases, public health communities are being challenged by the emergence of new or newly recognized types of food-borne illnesses, often with serious health and economic consequences.[10] For example, result of the BSE crises, the world suffered economic loses of more than 10 billion U.S. dollars[11,12] (FIG. 1).

The globalization of food (and feed) trade, facilitated by the liberalization of world trade, while offering many benefits and opportunities, also represents new risks. Food, a major trade commodity, is also an important vehicle for transmission of infectious diseases. Because food production, manufacturing, and marketing are now global, infectious agents can be disseminated from the original point of processing and packaging to locations thousands of kilometers away.

Currently, perhaps more than ever, sanitary and phytosanitary (SPS) measures play a role of high-priority in international trade and access to new export markets. SPS measures which conform to international standards, guidelines, or recommendations shall be deemed to be necessary to protect human, animal,

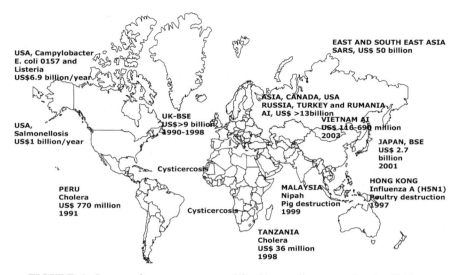

FIGURE 1. Impact of some zoonoses and food-borne diseases outbreaks, 2005.

or plant life or health, and presumed to be consistent with the relevant provisions of this Agreement and of GATT 1994. In assessing the risk to animal or plant life or health and determining the measure to be applied for achieving the appropriate level of SPS protection from such risk, states shall take into account the complexity of the context including socioeconomic factors and the share of responsibilities between many actors from the public and private sectors. A global vision encompassing animal and public health, food security, trade, development of developing countries, and environmental aspects must be followed. In the wake of the 2001 FMD epidemics in Europe, South America, Africa, and Asia, the OIE International Committee, through a Resolution of its 69th General Session, in 2001, and another Resolution of its 70th General Session, in 2002, called on both the OIE and FAO to pursue an international concerted effort against a certain number of diseases having significant effects on food security, poverty alleviation, food safety, public health, and access to formal markets. The report of the Temporary Committee on Foot and Mouth Disease of the European Union Parliament (October 3, 2002), concluded: "In view of the intensification of world trade and global warming, a thorough analysis of the existing and likely future threats arising from the introduction of animal diseases into the EU which could cause major economic damage is urgently needed at European level.... Lasting success can be achieved in efforts to control FMD worldwide only if it proves possible, through close international cooperation, to curb the disease decisively in areas where it is still endemic. The Commission should therefore do more to assist the countries concerned in their efforts to control or eradicate FMD and seek to improve cooperation with regard to information (early warning systems)."

The global nature of the problem of FMD and other TADs was also highlighted during the Ministerial Meeting on the occasion of the 31st Session of the FAO Conference in 2001. The Conference recognized the widespread and increasing impact of epidemic animal diseases, like FMD, on agricultural development, trade and food security; and stressed the need to continue the work at the national, regional and international level to combat the disease by involving all relevant stakeholders. The World Food Summit: 5 years later (WFS:*fyl*, 2002) reiterated the 1996 commitment and called for specific action and voluntary financial contribution to the FAO Global Trust Fund to facilitate food security programs and combat TADs.

The increasing importance of trade and expanded access to world markets by developing countries has also received high attention at the Doha Ministerial Meeting of WTO in November 2001, the UN Conference for Development in Monterrey in March 2002 and the World Summit on Sustainable Development in Johannesburg in September 2002. Enhanced trade in agricultural products in the south-to-north direction as well as among developing countries themselves is increasingly seen as a major factor in poverty reduction strategies. However, in order for developing countries to participate in formal trade in livestock products it is imperative that a concerted international effort be made for these countries to be able to fulfill the conditions and measures described in SPS.

SOCIOECONOMIC AND TRADE CONSIDERATIONS FOR THE CONTROL OF TADs

TADs impose major social and economic costs and risks to infected countries, their neighbors, and trading partners. The varying impact of TADs among stakeholders and the threat to existing and potential trade in wealthier countries complicates the question of appropriate control.

For all livestock producers, the threat of TADs increases the risk of lost production and impacts on livelihood, increasing vulnerability to poverty particularly for small-scale producers. The impact of TADs and of their control varies depending on the virulence of the disease, number of animals at risk, dependency on livestock for livelihood, and method of control.

On the consumption side, domestic consumers are concerned with the zoonotic potential of TADs and emerging infectious diseases, such as porcine Nipah virus, and the increased cost of livestock products resulting from disease outbreaks. In addition, when outbreaks of disease occur, there is inevitably an erosion of consumer confidence in the nation's food security. Particularly in the more developed countries, consumers demand guarantees for safer products, heightened government action (at no additional cost or taxation). In the aftermath of an outbreak, heightened border controls and inspections occur, and often there are stricter standards imposed for international trade. Apart from international commerce, investment in TADs control protects a vital and ready food resource—inexpensive animal protein on which consumers depend.

Certainly, the protection of trade interests is a major incentive for many countries to invest in prevention and control of TADs. Exporting countries are concerned with maintaining or expanding market shares and importing countries are concerned with protection of their domestic livestock populations. Those countries that have ability to meet and demonstrate adherence to international standards regarding TADs increases their competitiveness in the regional and international markets for livestock, commodities, and products of animal origin.

ROLE OF INTERNATIONAL AND REGIONAL ORGANIZATIONS

The two main international agencies, the Food and Agricultural Organisation (FAO) and the World Organisation for Animal Health (OIE, Office International des Epizooties) have developed their programs and activities to address the problem of controlling transboundary and emerging diseases.

The Emergency Prevention System for Transboundary Animal Diseases and Plant Pest and Diseases (EMPRES) is one of the major programs of FAO. EMPRES has four major precepts: early warning, early reaction, coordination, and enabling research. With regard to surveillance, FAO/EMPRES analyzes and disseminates warning messages, sets up surveillance networks, prepares prevention and prediction models, implements risk communication and develops systems for the management and analysis of the health information (TADinfo, EMPRES-i). The information and dissemination are done through an EMPRES discussion list (FIG. 2: 92 countries, 437 members) and discussion Forum. They also go through publications such as the *EMPRES Bulletin*, Early Warning Messages, Emergency Bulletins (FAO *Avian Influenza Disease Emergency News*), EMPRES watch and through its internet website[13,14] http://www.fao.org/ag/againfo/home/en/home.html; http://www.fao.org/ag/againfo/programmes/en/empres/home.asp. Manuals and thematic CDs are prepared (manuals on disease surveillance and recognition, contingency planning, information systems, and Good Emergency Management Practices) and distributed widely through the FAO representations in the country members. EMPRES has international and regional partners among them are OIE, WHO, Reference Laboratories and Collaborating Centers, Regional Organizations, Donors, and NGOs.

The World Organization for Animal Health (OIE) Website[15] www.oie.int. is an intergovernmental organization with 167 Member Countries, each represented by the country's senior veterinary health official. OIE has four main objectives—to guarantee the transparency of animal disease status worldwide;

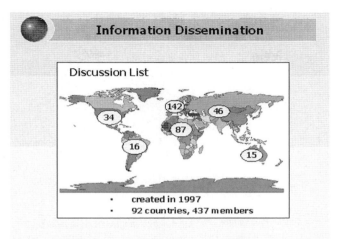

FIGURE 2. Worldwide distribution of EMPRES members.

to collect, analyze, and disseminate veterinary scientific information; to provide expertise and promote international solidarity for the control of animal diseases; and to guarantee the sanitary safety of world trade by developing sanitary rules for international trade in animals and animal products. OIE standards are recognized by the WTO as reference international sanitary rules. OIE has a network of reference laboratories and collaborating centers to provide scientific and technical assistance and expert advice on topics linked to disease surveillance and control. With regard to its specific mandate on disease information and early warning, OIE has a Global Information System (FIG. 3) which provides alert warning messages and weekly disease information electronic messages to its subscribers, based on official reports from OIE delegates in each country and from the OIE Reference Laboratories and from International Organizations among them FAO being the main partner.

The World Health Organization (www.who.org[16]) is the United Nations' specialized agency for health with a mission to attain the highest level of health for all people, particularly the poor and most vulnerable. The WHO established global influenza program which is the oldest disease control program at WHO with a major task to provide global influenza surveillance. The program has a network of laboratories commissioned to study circulating influenza viruses, collected from around the world, and document changes in the viruses' genetic make-up. Today, the WHO Global Influenza Surveillance Network consists of 113 national influenza centers located in 84 countries, and four WHO collaborating centers for influenza reference and research, located in London (England), Atlanta (USA), Melbourne (Australia), and Tokyo (Japan). A fifth collaborating center, located in Memphis, USA, performs specialized work on

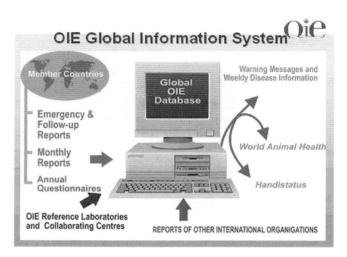

FIGURE 3. OIE global information system.

influenza viruses in animals. The WHO network has thus contributed greatly to the understanding of influenza epidemiology and assists vaccine manufacturers both by ensuring that influenza vaccines contain antigens of the most appropriate strains and by providing them with high-yielding "seed" virus for vaccine production. WHO is also an important partner in the GF-TADs initiative and will share and pool resources to develop common disease information system with FAO and OIE to keep the international community constantly alert to the threat of outbreaks of infectious diseases.

The Regional Organizations are equally important to the success of the implementation of programs on controlling epidemic diseases. They have the mandate and authority to facilitate and conduct regional and subregional activities related to trade and socioeconomic development and some of them have a focus or a specific mandate on animal production and health, such as the Inter African Bureau for Animal Resources (IBAR) or the Association for Southeast Asian Nations (ASEAN).

FAO/OIE GLOBAL FRAMEWORK FOR THE PROGRESSIVE CONTROL OF TRANSBOUNDARY ANIMAL DISEASES

The Global Framework for Transboundary Animal Diseases (GF-TADs)[17] is a joint FAO/OIE initiative which combines the strengths of both the organizations to achieve more than would be feasible by separate efforts. GF-TADs is a facilitating mechanism meant to empower countries and regional alliances in the fight against TADs, to provide capacity building, and to assist in the establishment of program strategies for the targeted control of certain TADs based on their regional priorities. The proposal presented here has been drawn up after extensive regional and expert consultations, with inputs from stakeholders throughout the world.

Goals and Objectives of GF-TADs

The goals and objectives of GF TADs are the following:

1. To safeguard the livestock industry of developed as well as developing countries from repeated incursions of infectious disease epidemics;
2. To improve food security and economic growth of developing countries through the reduction of the damaging effects of epidemic animal diseases;
3. To promote safe trade in livestock and animal products at national, regional, and international levels.

To obtain the necessary information for the promotion of early prevention and early reaction, close interaction among national animal health services for achieving a sound regional understanding of disease occurrence is required. GF-TADs will rely on the action of countries' veterinary service and those of the Regional Organizations and their specialized animal health bodies (FIG. 4). Since international animal health monitoring is able to single out geographical dynamics of disease occurrence only when countries report disease presence, GF-TADs intends to contribute to the strengthening of national structures and mechanisms to fulfill such reporting functions effectively.

The GF-TADs initiative is designed to initiate and support strategic regional cooperation for the control of TADs, such as avian influenza, FMD, RP, African

Regional Support Units

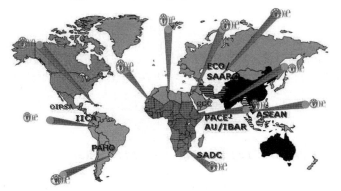

FIGURE 4. GF-TADs regional support units.

and classical swine fevers, peste des petits ruminants, caprine and bovine pleuropneumonia, Rift Valley fever, Newcastle disease of poultry, hemorrhagic septicemia, and sheep and goat pox, among others.

Specific Aims for GF-TADs

The specific aims of GF-TADs are the following:

1. Establish Regional Support Units (RSU), with a cadre of epidemiologists and initially funded through the GF-TADs, integrated in relevant Regional Organization specialized bodies (Fig. 4). Support of the development of regional strategies and their implementation. Support of a program for the deployment and upgrading of young professionals, integrated in the RSU.
2. Establishment of regional early warning nodes in RSU, to collect better quality epidemiological information and feed into the FAO/OIE/WHO Global Early Warning Systems.
3. Establishment of early response capacity at national, regional, and intercontinental levels for targeted disease control, based on prompt and authoritative disease investigation and diagnosis. Organize and manage a network of national and regional Epidemiology Units, with OIE-FAO Collaborative Centers alliances.
4. Strengthening of referral diagnostic and molecular biological capacity of OIE-FAO Reference Laboratories and follow-up technology transfer to National Agricultural Research Systems (NARS).
5. Securing the global status of internationally verified freedom from RP (declaration planned for 2010).
6. Definition of primary endemic areas (sources) for FMD and other selected TADs for focused efforts for the reduction of disease occurrence.
7. Provision of emergency contingency funds to countries that require immediate assistance in containment of an outbreak until other sources can be mobilized.
8. Identification of research programs in support of GF-TADs goals in collaboration with OIE-FAO Reference Laboratories and Collaborating Centers, other advanced research institutes, and national and regional laboratories and epidemiology units.
9. Promotion of north–south and south–south collaboration.

Development of Regional and Global Early Warning Systems

A Regional and Global Early Warning Systems (GLEWS) for major animal diseases co-managed by FAO and OIE (and WHO for zoonotic diseases)

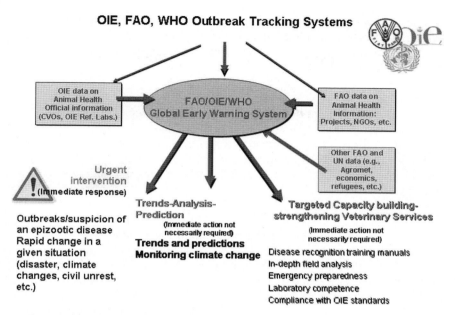

FIGURE 5. Global early warning systems.

has been developed in order to include tracking of rumor diseases occurrences. The RSU in charge of epidemiological data collection are linked with GLEWS. In these systems, the utilization of georeferenced information is promoted to better define primary endemic areas where focused action is required, risk factors are identified (e.g., refugee and other migration patterns, climatic changes that influence disease or disease-transmitting vectors, price differentials across borders), and information on marketing and trade routes is enabled down to the village level. The proposed systems will complement but not duplicate the existing OIE Animal Health Information System and will support the established obligations of member countries in international official disease reporting (FIG. 5).

Regional Support Units

Geographical areas, based on agroecological and traditional animal production practices, have been identified in conjunction with the importance of TADs for livestock production and trade, and of their significance for the maintenance of the most important infectious agents with potential for spread between countries and regions.

Through a process of regional consultation, countries sharing similar epidemiological and ecological status with respect to the major TADs were asked to evaluate their TAD status and prioritize situations they considered to be particularly pressing and needing attention.

The regional groupings tentatively identified with proposed RSU, with the priorities identified by constituent countries (TABLE 1).

Some Examples of Regional and International Approaches

The FAO/OIE GF-TADs agreement was signed in 2004 but its basic concept and objectives have been or are already applied to address the problems of several international crises such as RP, FMD, and highly pathogenic avian influenza (HPAI).

Global Rinderpest Eradication Programme

The Global Rinderpest Eradication Programme (GREP) is an international program which started in the mid 1990s as a unification mechanism that was a result of several regional efforts in RP eradication. RP was widely spread in Africa, Middle East, and Asia and a need for a Global Program was seen as an advantage to unify criteria and assist countries in gaining international recognition for RP freedom and their efforts. The organization of the control campaigns were based on a strong regional approach, with a global strategy which was jointly defined by the FAO, OIE, and the Regional Organizations involved. The GREP secretariat was established in FAO Rome and a time bound program was agreed. The OIE pathway for the declaration of freedom from the disease and then the infection was followed. The map (FIG. 6) shows the progress of the control of RP. The disease has disappeared from Asia, Middle East, Western, and Central Africa as well as from most of Eastern Africa. The Somali Pastoral ecosystem which includes parts of Somalia, Ethiopia, and Kenya is the only region of the world where there are still concerns of virus circulation. Intensive surveillance and disease search is implemented and no outbreak has been detected since 2003. The results of this GREP approach are such that RP could be the first animal disease to be eradicated from the entire world by 2010.

Foot and Mouth Disease

FMD is a widespread disease, and devastating crises occur regularly, as was the case in Europe four years ago.

A need for a global strategy with international surveillance and awareness are recognized and FAO and OIE are very active on that field. The European Commission for FMD (EU FMD) was established in 1954 as a statutory body

TABLE 1. Regional groupings *tentatively* identified with proposed RSU with the priorities identified by constituent countries

Clusters	Constituent countries (tentative)	Relevant regionalized specialized organizations (RSOs)
The Americas		
Andean cluster	Colombia, Bolivia, Peru, Venezuela, Ecuador	PAHO, IICA, Andean Pact (with Chile)
Southern Cone	Argentina, Brazil, Chile, Paraguay, Uruguay	PAHO (Panaftosa), IICA, Mercosur (Comité Veterinario Permanente)
Mesoamerica and Caribbean	Cuba, Dominican Republic, Haiti, Jamaica, Mexico, Costa Rica, Nicaragua, Guatemala, Panama, El Salvador, Belize, Honduras, Suriname, Guyana, French Guyana, other island countries and protectorates of the Caribbean	PAHO, IICA, OIRSA
Asia		
East Asia	Cambodia, Laos, Vietnam, Thailand, Myanmar, Indonesia, Malaysia Philippines, PR China, Taiwan Province of China, PDR Korea, DR Korea, Mongolia	ASEAN, (APHCA)
South Asia	India, Bangladesh, Sri Lanka, Nepal, Bhutan	SAARC, (APHCA)
Central Asia	Afghanistan, Kazakhstan, Kyrgyzstan, Turkmenistan, Uzbekistan, Tajikistan, Pakistan	ECO, (APHCA)
Middle East	Turkey, Iran, Syria, Iraq, Jordan, Lebanon, Palestine, Israel, Egypt	ECO, EU-FMD (APHCA, AHCNENA)
Arabian Peninsula	Saudi Arabia, Oman, Yemen, UAE, Qatar, Kuwait, Bahrain	GCC, AOAD (AHCNENA)
Africa		
North	Morocco, Algeria, Tunisia, Libya	AMU, AOAD, (AHCNENA)
West and Central	Senegal, Gambia, Mauritania, Côte d'Ivoire, Guinea Conakry, Guinea Bissau, Equatorial Guinea, Sierra Leone, Liberia, Mali, Togo, Benin, Burkina Faso, Ghana, Nigeria, Niger, Chad, CAR, Cameroon, Gabon,Congo Brazza	AU-IBAR,
Horn of Africa	Ethiopia, Eritrea, Sudan, Somalia, Djibouti, Kenya,Uganda	AU-IBAR,
Southern Africa and Indian Ocean	South Africa, Namibia, Zambia, Botswana, Mozambique, Swaziland, Lesotho, Angola, Rwanda, Burundi, Tanzania, Congo Kinshasa, Malawi, Madagascar, Island countries of the Indian Ocean	SADC, AU-IBAR
Eastern Europe	Russia, Belarus, Ukraine, Balkan Countries (Serbia-Montenegro, Kosovo, Moldova, Macedonia), Albania, Bulgaria, Armenia, Georgia, Azerbaijan	EU-FMD

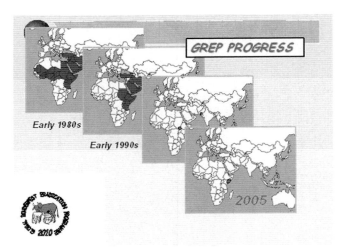

FIGURE 6. GREP progress.

of FAO, and European counties are members. The Secretariat is hosted by FAO in Rome, and the Executive Committee and the General Assembly are in charge of defining general policies and making sure that programs are following their guidance.

EU FMD has clear objectives with the initial goal to combat and eradicate FMD from Europe. The current thrusts are to prevent its reintroduction, to limit the risk from countries surrounding Europe and other countries (FIG. 7),

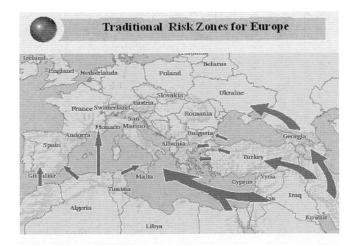

FIGURE 7. Risk map of FMD for Europe.

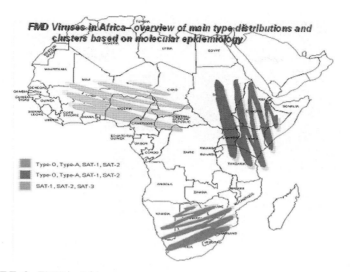

FIGURE 8. FMD in Africa.

and to elevate technical expertise. The approach is global and regional with the definition of the traditional immediate risk zones for Europe (Turkey, Middle East, North Africa, the Caucasus, and Central Asia). EU FMD also plays a role as global surveillance group for early detection of any changes in any region of the world which could suffer a new epidemic. The situation of Africa is considered to be of particular interest since five types (FIG. 8: O, A, SAT1, SAT2, and SAT3) of viruses are circulating (FIG. 8). The EU FMD sent warning messages a few months before the last epizootic in Europe.

A Technical Committee has been set up to regroup most of the internationally recognized experts and FAO OIE Reference Laboratories, including the World Reference Laboratory in the United Kingdom (Animal Health Laboratory, Pirbright). The partnership between FAO, EU FMD country members, reference laboratories, and OIE are developed. The support from the European Commission to develop and coordinate control programs in certain regions is important, and Tripartite meetings (FAO, OIE, and EC) are organized regularly according to the situation (in Thrace or the Caucasus, for example).

The EU FMD has an objective to become an international observatory of the FMD virus circulation "at source of risk."

Highly Pathogenic Avian Influenza

HPAI resulting from H5N1 virus has hit Asia since the end of 2003 and has had disastrous socioeconomic consequences on the poultry sector, on small farmers' livelihoods, on food security, and on rural development and

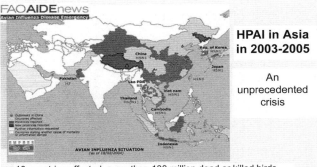

FIGURE 9. Avian influenza in Asia.

trade (FIG. 9). It has been devastating to several countries in Asia, where over 140 million chickens and ducks have died from the disease or have been culled. The impact on the economies of those countries, in terms of lost revenue, is estimated at much beyond $10 billion. The impact is greatest on millions of small farmers, i.e., the rural poor, whose livelihoods have been heavily affected by the disease.

It has become an international crisis since all regions in the World can be considered under risk due to the globalization of exchanges, with movements of animals, products, and humans and because of the possible spread of the virus through the migration of wild birds.

Avian influenza is also of concern because of its transmission from domestic poultry to humans in over 120 documented cases, causing the death of more than 60 people. If its mutation or reassortment events occur which allow the virus to become transmissible between human hosts, a serious human influenza pandemic is likely to ensue unless detection and containment efforts from those responsible for human health and welfare are stepped up. The veterinary community has a responsibility to ensure that cases of avian influenza in birds and other animals are properly controlled. To stop it in its tracks, avian influenza requires extraordinary political commitment, substantial investments, concerted international cooperation, and determinate actions at the country level, keeping in mind that the best way to prevent a human pandemic is to control the disease at source in animals.

Since the beginning of the crisis in early 2004, the concepts and approaches of GF-TADs have been applied, which basically means the development of a strong partnership with OIE, with the Regional Organizations and with the countries.

To combat avian influenza at its source, FAO has, from the outset, adopted a three-pronged approach.

First, and foremost, we are working with all affected and at risk countries to strengthen their veterinary services and to improve local capacity at the farm and market levels in order to: (*a*) improve the surveillance, detection, and reporting of the disease in both wildlife and domestic birds, (*b*) implement biosecurity measures aimed at preventing the spread of the disease; and (*c*) efficiently control the disease, once detected, and to limit its spread. There are known and proven practices for this operation, such as isolating poultry, good farm hygiene, use of effective vaccines, close monitoring, and quick culling when necessary, among others. These practices work, and there are success stories in several countries to report. FAO has been providing advice on how to apply these practices, offering capacity building workshops, developing guidelines and manuals, helping equip veterinary laboratories, provision of diagnostic reagents, assisting access to vaccines, facilitating sample transfer between countries and OIE/FAO Reference Laboratories, and assisting countries in the design of prevention and control strategies.

A second facet of FAO's work deals with the establishment of regional networks for improved information-sharing and collective efforts to confront a regional problem. The epidemiology of avian influenza is complex and requires understanding to search for the best intervention measures. Timely reporting of outbreaks and sharing of epidemiological data and of virus samples has been stressed by FAO. This is crucial to analyze the characteristics of the viruses in order to understand and control the disease and prevent human infection. FAO and OIE have repeatedly appealed to governments to improve the exchange of viral strains between veterinary and human health scientific communities.

A third dimension of FAO's work is to provide technical information globally and to advocate for an internationally coordinated effort against HPAI. FAO has, for example, collaborated jointly with OIE, WHO, and Ministries in the affected countries to organize several international and regional meetings to raise the profile of the avian influenza control program. FAO provides regular information updates through our websites[13,14] and through various publication instruments, such as the avian influenza Disease Emergency News Bulletin (e.g., *FAO AIDE News* and *EMPRES Watch*). We have also extensively communicated with multilateral and bilateral donors and government officials in a sustained effort to sound the alarm and mobilize action.

At this point, it is important to stress that FAO is not working in isolation. The world is up against a complex problem, with overwhelming human and economic consequences. Working alone, no organization will resolve it. Partnerships are needed. In particular, as it has already stated, FAO is in very close partnership with OIE. The two organizations have developed jointly a Global Strategy[18] and Guidelines[19] for the Progressive Control of Highly Pathogenic avian influenza. They have canvassed WHO support for that strategy and are working hand-in-glove to implement it.

FAO is also working in collaboration with other UN partners and with bilateral donors and several NGOs.

CONCLUSIONS

Transboundary and emerging diseases are becoming ever more important since they can spread throughout an entire region, impact trading partners and commerce, tourism, consumer confidence, and occur in distant countries, with devastating economic and livelihood consequences. With the globalization of trade and the increasing movements of people, these major crises will continue to menace the global animal and human populations; the FAO philosophy—shared by the OIE—is a need to prevent and control them at the *source*, which is most of the time in developing countries. Regional and international approaches have to be followed and the FAO OIE GF-TADs initiative provides the appropriate concepts and objectives as well as an organizational framework to link the international and regional organizations at the service of the countries to better prevent and control these diseases.

The GF-TADs Global Secretariat has carried out several regional consultations for the identification of priority diseases and best ways for their administration and prevention. This is an ambitious challenge, as there are wide range of serious diseases of concern, all of them transboundary and trade-limiting. In the questionnaires carried out and through the consultative process, it was noted that globally, FMD was ranked as the first and foremost priority. Rift Valley Fever, and today Highly Pathogenic Avian Influenza are defined as major animal diseases which also affect human health. PPR and CBPP, a disease which is particularly serious in Africa and finally, African swine fever (ASF) and classical swine fever (CSF) are also regionally recognized as top priorities on which the Framework is determined to work.

REFERENCES

1. SEIN ZEPEDA, C. 1998. Perspectives of Veterinary Services in Latin America in the face of globalization. Second FAO Electronic Conference on Veterinary Services. FAO.
2. THRUSFIELD, M., L. MANSLEY, P. DUNLOP, *et al*. 2005. The foot-and-mouth disease epidemic in Dumfries and Galloway, 2001. 2: Serosurveillance, and efficiency and effectiveness of control procedures after the national ban on animal movements. Vet. Rec. **156**: 269–278.
3. VARGAS TERAN, M., N. CALCAGNO FERRAT, J. LUBROTH. 2004. Situation of classical swine fever and the epidemiologic and ecologic aspects affecting its distribution in the American continent. Ann. N. Y. Acad. Sci. **1026**: 54–64.
4. RWEYEMAMU, M., R. PASKIN, A. BENKIRANE, *et al*. 2000. Emerging diseases of Africa and the Middle East. Ann. N. Y. Acad. Sci. **916**: 61–70.

5. ROEDER, P.L. & T.U. OBI. 1999. Recognizing peste des petits ruminants: a field manual. FAO Animal Health Manual (5) 28 p.
6. THIAUCOURT, F., L. DEDIEU, J.C. MAILLARD, *et al.* 2003. Contagious bovine pleuropneumonia vaccines, historic highlights, present situation and hopes. Dev. Biol. (Basel)**114:** 147–160.
7. BALKHY, H.H. & Z.A. MEMISH. 2003. Rift Valley fever: an uninvited zoonosis in the Arabian peninsula. Int. J. Antimicrob. Agents **21:** 153–157.
8. PEGRAM, R. & C. EDDI. 2002. Progress towards the eradication of *Amblyomma variegatum* from the Caribbean. Exp Appl. Acarol. **28:** 273–281.
9. LOKUGE, B., K. LOKUGE & T. FAUNCE. 2005. Avian influenza, agriculture trade and WTO rules: the economics of transboundary disease control in developing countries. Working Paper: Centre for Governance of Knowledge and Development.
10. ECONOMIC IMPACT OF FOOD BORNE ILLNESS. WHO. www.who.int//entity/foodsafety/publications/capacity/en/1.pdf.
11. VERBEKE, W. 2001. Consumer reactions and economic consequences of the BSE crisis. Verh. K. Acad. Geneeskd. Belg. **63:** 483–492.
12. SCOTT, A., M. CHRISTIE & P. MIDMORE. 2004. Impact of the 2001 foot-and-mouth disease outbreak in Britain: implications for rural studies. J. Rural. Studies **20:** 1–14.
13. FAO EMPRES SITE. http://www.fao.org/ag/againfo/home/en/home.html.
14. FAO AGS site.http://www.fao.org/ag/againfo/programmes/en/empres/home.asp.
15. OIE Web site. http://www.oie.int.
16. WHO Web site. www.who.org.
17. FAO OIE. 2004. The Global Framework for the Progressive Control of Transboundary Animal Diseases.
18. FAO OIE. 2005. A Global Strategy for the Progressive Control of Highly Pathogenic Avian Influenza (HPAI). http://www.fao.org/ag/againfo/subjects/documents/ai/HPAIGlobalStrategy31Oct05.pdf.
19. FAO POSITION PAPER. 2004. Recommendations on the prevention, control and eradication of Highly Pathogenic Avian Influenza (HPAI) in Asia.

Linking Human and Animal Health Surveillance for Emerging Diseases in the United States

Achievements and Challenges

TRACEY LYNN,[a] NINA MARANO,[b] TRACEE TREADWELL,[b] AND BOB BOKMA[c]

[a]USDA-APHIS, Veterinary Services, National Center for Animal Health Surveillance, Fort Collins, Colorado 80526, USA

[b]Centers for Disease Control and Prevention, National Center for Infectious Diseases, Atlanta, Georgia 30333, USA

[c]USDA-APHIS, Veterinary Services, National Center for Import and Export, Riverdale, Maryland 20737, USA

Recent events affecting public health, including SARS, Monkeypox, and Avian Influenza have highlighted the potential adverse health effects of human interaction with animals. Outbreaks of zoonotic diseases are occurring with increasing frequency, and it is apparent that the public health and agriculture sectors must seek new partnerships and new ways to detect these microbial threats. Both nationally and internationally, there has been an increasing recognition of a critical need to develop these partnerships. In May 2004, 70 veterinary and public health representatives from 29 countries met in Geneva for a WHO/FAO/OIE Consultation on Emerging Zoonoses.[1] The Regional Americas Surveillance Working Group identified diseases of concern in North, Latin, and South America, including West Nile fever, bat and wildlife rabies, equine encephalitis, hantavirus, monkeypox, and others. The concerns and issues documented in that report are mirrored in other documents and directives, such as the Animal Health Safeguarding Review,[2] the WHO Technical Report "Future Trends in Veterinary Public Health,"[3] the article "Converging Issues in Veterinary and Public Health,"[4] the 2002 Public Health Security and Bioterrorism Act,[5] and Homeland Security Presidential Directives 5-10.[6] These documents and associated agencies call for an integration of agriculture, public health,

Address for correspondence: Tracey Lynn, DVM, MS, DACVPM, United States Department of Agriculture (USDA), Animal and Plant Health Inspection Service (APHIS), National Center for Animal Health Surveillance, Natural Resources Research Center, 2150 Centre Ave, Bldg B, MS 2E7, Fort Collins, CO 80526-8117. Voice: 970-494-7597; fax: 970-494-7174.

e-mail: Tracey.V.Lynn@aphis.usda.gov

Ann. N.Y. Acad. Sci. 1081: 108–111 (2006). © 2006 New York Academy of Sciences.
doi: 10.1196/annals.1373.011

and food safety surveillance to most effectively protect both human and animal health.

The use of early warning systems, such as sentinel surveillance in vectors, wildlife, companion animals, and zoological parks, has been identified as one method for improving surveillance for emerging diseases.[1] Beginning in 2001 and 2003, the Centers for Disease Control and Prevention (CDC) sponsored two projects in zoo animal[7] and companion animal[8] surveillance. Innovative surveillance and reporting systems have also been developed, such as ArboNet for West Nile Virus surveillance.[9] ArboNet, a collaborative effort between CDC and the state health and agriculture departments, is unique in its ability to collate and report surveillance data from humans, mosquitoes, birds, mammals, and sentinel chicken flocks, marking one of the first times that such data have been integrated into a single reporting system. United States Department of Agriculture (USDA) and CDC are currently working together to improve completeness and timeliness of reporting.

In addition, USDA's National Surveillance Unit is developing the National Animal Health Surveillance System (NAHSS), a comprehensive, coordinated, integrated surveillance system.[10] The goal of the NAHSS is to establish and maintain the expertise and infrastructure for early detection and global risk surveillance for foreign and emerging diseases; evaluation and enhancement of surveillance for current disease control and eradication programs; monitoring of disease trends and threats to animal and veterinary public health in the United States and other countries; assessment of risks and timely dissemination of animal health information, especially to those partners obligated to respond.[11]

Various laboratory networks—the National Animal Health Laboratory Network (NAHLN), the Laboratory Response Network (LRN), and the Food Emergency Response Network (FERN)—represent a very promising potential for coordinating zoonotic disease surveillance. A USDA-coordinated network of Federal and State veterinary diagnostic laboratories, NAHLN is being developed to conduct targeted surveillance for early detection of disease outbreaks and to ensure rapid and sufficient laboratory capacity in response to animal health emergencies.[12] The LRN is a CDC-coordinated network of Federal and State laboratories, which is working to expand its membership to include one animal disease diagnostic laboratory in each state for bioterrorism preparedness and integrated response capacity to other public health emergencies.[13] The FERN, coordinated jointly by FDA and the Food Safety Inspection Service, is a national network of food-testing laboratories designed to integrate the detection of threat agents in the food supply.[14] The NAHLN, LRN, and FERN are working to maximize efficiencies between the three networks, and together represent a cornerstone in the development of comprehensive agriculture, public health, and food safety monitoring systems.

During 2002, a CDC–FDA–USDA Working Group was tasked to address coordination of human and animal disease surveillance. This group was reinvigorated in 2004 with the addition of dedicated staff at CDC and USDA, and is working to (1) identify needed elements and essential partners, (2) develop a system of communication and triggers for action, (3) divide the workload to maximize efficiency and identify roles and responsibilities, and (4) incorporate animal health surveillance into existing systems. In collaboration with the U.S. Animal Health Association, the Working Group has developed a survey, to be administered, beginning July 1, 2005, to all designated state animal and public health veterinarians, as a tool to generate data to partially inform the objectives 1 and 2 above. The data generated from the survey will help identify the needed elements and formulate possible solutions for improved networking and effective communication between state public health and state animal agriculture officials, and other potential partners.

Another of the Working Group's first projects was to bring the laboratory networks together to begin discussions on how to coordinate laboratory surveillance activities to mutual benefit. An initial meeting was held in December 2004, consisting of representaives from LRN, NAHLN, and FERN, using Avian Influenza as the model. At the end of that meeting, three focus groups were formed: an Epidemiology and Laboratory Notification and Response Group, a Laboratory Technology/Management Group, and a Reservoir Surveillance Group. The focus group for Epidemiology and Laboratory Notification and Response is working to document current communications between USDA and CDC epidemiology and laboratory groups. Currently, these communications primarily occur on an *ad hoc* basis through the established liaison positions, and the focus group is trying to identify methods to make communications more routine and less person-dependent, as well as identify and remove any roadblocks to good communication. To that end, the focus group is developing a memorandum of understanding to formalize how USDA and CDC will work together if a new pathogenic influenza strain, be it human or animal, is introduced into the United States.

Professionals within public health and agriculture face many challenges as they begin integrating agriculture, public health, and food safety surveillance. However, improved coordination of human and animal health surveillance at the state, national, and global levels is possible by utilizing the current infrastructure as well as developing new strategies. Our vision for successful partnering is to operate with mutual understanding and respect, using clearly defined communication strategies, coordinated surveillance and response strategies, a standardized system for sharing information, and a strategy for deployment of multisectoral and interdisciplinary response teams, when needed to face threats to human and animal health posed by emerging microbial threats.

REFERENCES

1. REPORT OF THE WHO/FAO/OIE JOINT CONSULTATION ON EMERGING ZOONOTIC DISEASES. Available from http://whqlibdoc.who.int/hq/2004/WHO_CDS_CPE_ZFK_2004.9.pdf. Accessed June 23, 2005.

2. ANIMAL HEALTH SAFEGUARDING REVIEW. 2001. Available from http://www.nasda-hq.org/ASGRwebsite/Index.pdf. Accessed May 3, 2005.
3. WHO TECHNICAL REPORT "FUTURE TRENDS IN VETERINARY PUBLIC HEALTH". Available from http://whqlibdoc.who.int/trs/WHO_TRS_907.pdf. Accessed May 3, 2005.
4. KING, L. & R. KHABBAZ. 2003. Converging issues in veterinary and public health. Emerg. Infect. Dis. [serial online] Apr [*May 3, 2005*]. Available from: URL: http://www.cdc.gov/ncidod/EID/vol9no4/03-0037.htm.
5. 2002 Public Health Security and Bioterrorism Act. Available from http://www.fda.gov/oc/bioterrorism/bioact.html. Accessed May 3, 2005.
6. HOMELAND SECURITY PRESIDENTIAL DIRECTIVES 5-10. Available from http://www.fas.org/irp/offdocs/nspd/. Accessed May 3, 2005.
7. Additional information available from http://www.aza.org/ConScience/GroupPop Mgt/Documents/ZIMS.pdf. Accessed June 23, 2005.
8. Additional information available from http://www.vet.purdue.edu/epi/index.htm. Accessed June 23, 2005.
9. Additional information available from http://www.cdc.gov/ncidod/dvbid/westnile/index.htm. Accessed June 23, 2005.
10. Additional information available from http://www.aphis.usda.gov/vs/ceah/ncahs/nsu/index.htm. Accessed June 23, 2005.
11. Additional information available from http://www.aphis.usda.gov/vs/nahss. Accessed August 14, 2006.
12. Additional information available from http://www.aphis.usda.gov/vs/highlights/section6/section6-6.html. Accessed June 23, 2005.
13. Additional information available from http://www.bt.cdc.gov/lrn/. Accessed June 23, 2005.
14. Additional information available from http://www.crcpd.org/Homeland_Security/Food_Emergency_Response_Network.pdf. Accessed June 23, 2005.

Development of a Monoclonal Antibody-Based Immunohistochemistry Method for BSE Surveillance in China

XIAODONG WU, ZHILIANG WANG, YUTIAN LIU, YONGQIANG ZHANG, YIPIN CHEN, AND YANLI ZOU

National BSE Reference Laboratory, National Diagnostic Center for Exotic Animal Diseases, National Animal Quarantine Institute MOA, Qingdao, 266032, China

ABSTRACT: Five hybridoma cell lines secreting anti-PrP antibodies were established from the fusion between mouse myeloma Sp2/0 and spleen cells from mice immunized with recombinant Chinese Luxi yellow cattle (*Bos taurus*, Luxi) PrP (24–234) or recombinant Chinese small-tailed Han sheep PrP (94–227). According to their Western blot reactivity, five monoclonal antibodies (mAbs) could be divided into two groups. Group A, mAbs 1H2, 4C6, and 4C11 recognized re-PrP, PrP^C, and PrP^{Sc} from both bovine and sheep. Group B, mAbs 2H3 and 4H10 only recognized re-PrP and PrP^{Sc} of sheep, and especially, these two mAbs could not recognize PrP^C from both bovine and sheep. In immunohistochemistry (IHC) test, mAb 4C11 immunostained the PrP^{Sc} accumulation in tissue sections from BSE cattle and Scrapie sheep, and compared with mAb 6H4, it had the same immunohistochemical pattern. An IHC method based on mAb 4C11 for the detection of BSE was established and had been applied for the long-term surveillance of BSE in China. From 2001 to 2004, 12,692 samples from the whole country had been tested and all had negative results.

KEYWORDS: mAb; bovine spongiform encephalopathy (BSE); immunohistochemistry; surveillance

INTRODUCTION

Bovine spongiform encephalopathy (BSE), so-called mad cow disease, is one type of transmissible spongiform encephalopathies (TSEs). BSE is an invariably fatal disease of domestic cattle, cases of which were first recognized in Great Britain in November 1986.[1] BSE has an insidious onset and usually a

Address for correspondence: Professor Zhiliang Wang, National BSE Reference Laboratory, National Diagnostic Center for Exotic Animal Diseases, National Animal Quarantine Institute MOA, 266032, Qingdao, China. Voice: +86-532-87839188; fax: +86-532-87839922.
e-mail: zlwang111@yahoo.com.cn

Ann. N.Y. Acad. Sci. 1081: 112–123 (2006). © 2006 New York Academy of Sciences.
doi: 10.1196/annals.1373.012

slowly progressive course,[1–3] and the causative agent is thought to consist of an aberrant isoform (PrP^{Sc}) of the cellular prion protein (PrP^{C}), termed *prion*.[4] PrP^{Sc} is generated from a host-encoded PrP^{C} by certain conformational transformation. Although the two PrP isoforms share the same primary structure, PrP^{Sc} is distinguished from PrP^{C} by biochemical and biophysical properties, such as high β-sheet content, partial resistance to protease digestion.[5–7]

There is evidence of a causal link between the BSE agent and a new variant form of the human TSE, variant Creutzfeldt–Jakob disease (vCJD),[8–11] which has caused a panic in the world. Most countries have paid great attention to BSE, and in China BSE has also been listed as a type I animal disease. The BSE risk status, epidemic status, and surveillance systems of a country have been important markers of international trade of cattle product. Whether surveillance systems are effective depends on the dependability of detection technology. To confirm the diagnosis of BSE, histological examination of the brain is principal, but this method is influenced by many factors, such as sample preparation and result judgment. Detection of accumulations of abnormal PrP^{Sc} in the central nervous system (CNS) of affected cattle by immunological methods offers a disease-specific diagnostic approach. PrP^{Sc} can be detected in unfixed brain extracts by immunoblotting and other enzyme immunoassay methods, and also be detected in fixed brain by immunohistochemistry (IHC) method. Both approaches are now widely used as confirmatory diagnostic methods and are recommended as adjuncts to histological examination. IHC method can provide a BSE diagnosis in animals that appear clinically normal with minimal (or no) spongiform lesions in the brain. Moreover, IHC method is simple in operation and easy in judgment with a low cost (under the condition in China, the workforce being very cheap).

Showing higher reproducibility and specificity than normal anti-PrP serum, monoclonal antibody (mAb) was expected to improve PrP test in multiple ways. Also, anti-PrP mAbs are unique tools for structural and biochemical analysis of PrP. Many commercial anti-PrP mAbs have been marketed and their price is very high. In our study, several hybridoma cell lines secreting mAbs to PrP were derived from PrP null mice immunized with either recombinant Chinese Luxi yellow cattle (*Bos taurus*, Luxi) PrP (24–234) or Chinese small-tailed Han sheep PrP (94–227). An IHC method based on anti-PrP mAb for the detection of PrP^{Sc} was established and has been applied for the long-term active surveillance of BSE in China.

MATERIALS AND METHODS

Expression and Purification of Recombinant PrP (re-PrP)

The cDNAs coding for Chinese Luxi yellow cattle (*Bos taurus,* Luxi) PrP (24–234 codons, without the N-terminal signal sequence and the C-terminal

GPI sequence) and Chinese small-tailed Han sheep PrP27–30 (94–227 codons, protease-resistant part of PrP^{Sc}) were amplified by polymerase chain reaction (PCR) using the genosome DNA as template and cloned into the prokaryotic expression vector pET-32a(+) (Novagen; EMD Biosciences Inc., Darmstadt, Germany), respectively. After transformation into *E. coli* BL21(DE3) (Novagen), two kinds of re-PrP were expressed, fusing with His-tag and Trx-tag. After we optimized the expressing conditions, large-scale re-PrP in inclusion bodies were prepared and purified by His•Bind® Purification Kit (Novagen) and analyzed by sodium dodecyl sulfate-polyacrylamide gel electrophoresis (SDS-PAGE), Western blot test using mAbs 6H4 and F89 as probe.

Brain Tissues

Brain homogenates from Scrapie sheep, BSE cattle, normal controls, and formalin-fixed brain tissues (obex) from BSE cattle were provided by OIE Reference Laboratory for BSE and Scrapie (Veterinary Faculty University of Berne, Switzerland).

Normal brain homogenates from Chinese Luxi yellow cattle (*Bos taurus*, Luxi) and Chinese small-tailed Han sheep were made by us. Every 0.15 g brain sample was homogenized (HYBRAID Ribolyser; HYBRAID Limited, Ashford, Middlesex, UK) in 1.5 mL 320 mM sucrose solution. Homogenates were centrifuged for 10 min at 5000 g at 4°C, and supernatants were aliquoted quickly and stored at –80°C.

Preparation of Anti-PrP mAbs

Eight-week-old PrP-null mice were subcutaneously immunized with 10 μg re-PrP emulsified in Freund's complete adjuvant (Sigma-Aldrich Co., St. Louis, MO).[12] Two weeks later, they received the same antigen emulsified in Freund's incomplete adjuvant (Sigma). Four days before cell fusion, each mouse was boosted intravenously with 5 μg re-PrP. Mice were sacrificed and single cell spleen suspensions were fused with SP2/0. Hybridoma cell supernatant was screened by an indirect enzyme-linked immunosorbent assay (ELISA). Ninety-six-wells plates were coated for 2 h at 37°C with 50 μL re-PrP at a concentration of 5 μg/mL in carbonate-buffered saline (CBS) and blocked with 1% bovine serum albumin (BSA) for 2 h at room temperature. The hybridomas secreting anti-PrP mAbs were cloned by limiting dilution. The isotypes of the mAbs were determined by the mouse mAb isotyping reagents (Sigma). Large-scale mAbs ascites were produced by BALB/CA mice and purified by ImmunoPure (G) IgG Purification Kit (Pierce, Rockford, IL). All procedures involving the animals were performed under the authorization of China Ministry of Agriculture.

Western Blot Analysis of mAbs

Normal brain homogenates and re-PrP were separated by 15% SDS-PAGE gels, and then transferred onto polyvinylidene difluoride membrane (PVDF, Immobilon P; Millipore Co., Bedford, MA). Membranes were blocked with 2% BSA in TBST (10 mM Tris, 150 mM sodium chloride, 0.1% Tween-20, pH7.4) for 1.5 h at 37°C and incubated for 1 h at room temperature with different mAbs. After washing in TBST, membranes were incubated with peroxidase-conjugated rabbit anti-mouse IgG at a dilution of 1:20,000 (Sigma). PVDF of homogenates was developed with an LumiGLO® Chemiluminescent Substrate (KPL Inc., Gaithersburg, MD) and visualized on X-Omat BT film (Kodak; Eastman Kodak Co., Rochester, NY). PVDF of re-PrP was developed with substrate 3,3′-diaminoben (DAB).

For the analysis of whether mAbs could recognize the PrP27-30 of brain homogenates from BSE cattle and Scrapie sheep, we used a commercial BSE Test Kit (Prionics check Western; Prionics AG, Wagistrasse, Switzerland), and replaced the mAb 6H4 with our mAbs.

Development of mAb-Based IHC Method

Several protocols have been applied successfully to the IHC detection of PrP for the diagnosis of BSE.[13–16] The technical procedures described below come from OIE Reference Laboratory for BSE and Scrapie (Vetsuisse Faculty University of Berne, Switzerland) with minor modifications.

Sample Preparation

The whole brain should be removed as soon as possible after death, and placed in 4–6 L of 10% formol saline fixative, which should be changed twice weekly. After fixation for 2 weeks, the brain was cut into coronal slices, leaving intact the diagnostically important areas at the obex, the cerebellar peduncles, and the rostral colliculi. A single block cut at the obex of the medulla oblongata should be selected for histological processing by conventional paraffin wax embedding methods for neural tissue.

Detection of PrP^{Sc}

The sections were deparaffinized through descending alcohol concentrations down to distilled water. After 3 × 5 min washing with phosphate-buffered saline (PBS), the samples were treated with proteinase K at a concentration of 5 μg/mL for 15 min at 37°C. Sections were immersed in boiling distilled water and autoclaved at 121°C for 20 min, cooled at room temperature. Following

3 × 5 min washing with PBS, the slides were immersed in 3% hydrogen peroxide in methanol for 20 min for inactivation of endogenous peroxidase. After rinsing for 3 × 5 min with PBS, slides were blocked by 5% normal swine serum for 20 min at room temperature. The sections were incubated for 4 h at 37°C (or alternatively for 12–18 h at 4°C) with mAb ascite at a dilution of 1:10,000, and then washed 3 × 5 min with PBS, mAbs 6H4, and F89 as control. According to the manufacturer's instruction of ChemMate™ AEC/H_2O_2 substrate solution (DakoCytomation; Dako Denmark A/S, Glostrup, Denmark), sections were subsequently incubated with solution of bottle A for 10 min at room temperature, subsequently washed 3 × 5 min with PBS, and then with solution of bottle B for 10 min at room temperature. After rinsing for 3 × 5 min with PBS, and for 1–2 min with distilled water, sections were incubated with solution of bottle C for 5–10 min to visualize immunoreactivity. After rinsing for 1–2 min with distilled water, the slides were covered with Glycergel and cover slip.

Interpretation of Results

Under the microscope, on both sides of obex, positive samples exhibit reddish brown PrP^{Sc} accumulation in clusters or along the axons, while negative samples do not show.

BSE Surveillance in China

In accordance with the "Terrestrial Animal Health Code" of OIE, we conducted the surveillance in China and the quantity of sampling is five case per100,000 in the adult cattle population every year, which is five times that of type A surveillance stipulates. From 2001 to 2004, 12,692 samples from the whole country, that were all formalin fixed brain, had been detected by the mAb-based IHC method, formalin fixed brain tissues (obex) from BSE cattle, and Scrapie sheep as positive control. At the same time, all samples were stained with hematoxylin and eosin (H.E), and examined for characteristic spongiform change and neuronal vacuolation.

RESULTS

Re-PrP

Two kinds of re-PrP were highly expressed by *E. coli* BL21(DE3) transformed with recombinant prokaryotic expression vector pET-32a(+), when bacteria were grown up to an OD of 0.8 at 28°C, then stimulated with 0.1 mM isopropylthiogalactoside (IPTG) and further grown for 2 h at 28°C. SDS-PAGE

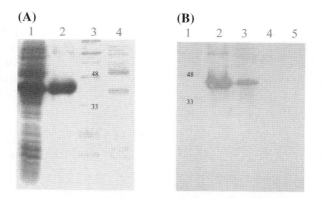

FIGURE 1. (A) The SDS-PAGE profile of purified recombinant Chinese yellow cattle (*Bos taurus*, Luxi) PrP fused with His-tag and Trx-tag, Coomassie blue staining. Purified re-PrP (lane 2). The inclusion bodies from *E. coli* BL21(DE3) transformed with pET-32a(+)/PrP (24–234) (lane 1) and pET-32a(+) (lane 4) induced with IPTG. Prestained protein marker, broad range in kilodaltons (kDa) (lane 3). **(B)** The purified re-PrP identified by mAb 6H4 in Western blot. Purified re-PrP (lane 2). The inclusion bodies form *E. coli* BL21(DE3) transformed with pET-32a(+)/PrP (24–234) (lane 3) and pET-32a(+) (lane 5′) induced with IPTG. The inclusion bodies from *E. coli* BL21(DE3) transformed with pET-32a(+)/PrP (24–234) (lane 4) not induced. Prestained protein marker, broad range in kDa (lane 1).

revealed that the molecular size of two kinds of fused re-PrP was identical to the expected value, and the purity of re-PrP is above 95%. Western blot test confirmed the successful expression of re-PrP (FIGS. 1 and 2).

mAb Specific for PrP

One mAb 4C11 against Chinese yellow cattle (*Bos taurus,* Luxi) PrP (24–234) and four mAbs 1H2, 2H3, 4C6, 4H10 against Chinese small-tailed Han sheep PrP (94–227) were screened by indirect ELISA and their immunoreactivity was characterized by Western blot analysis of normal and TSE brain tissues. According to the results of Western blot test, five mAbs could be divided into two groups. Group A, mAbs 1H2, 4C6, and 4C11 recognized re-PrP, PrP^C, and PrP^{Sc} from both bovine and sheep. Group B, mAbs 2H3 and 4H10 recognized re-PrP, and PrP^{Sc} only from sheep, and especially, these two mAbs could not recognize PrP^C from both bovine and sheep (FIG. 3). Antibody isotyping identified five mAbs as IgG1.

mAb-Based IHC Method

Among the five mAbs, 4C11 could immunostain the PrP^{Sc} accumulation in tissue sections from both BSE cattle and Scrapie sheep, and compared with

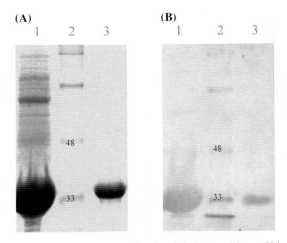

FIGURE 2. (A) The SDS-PAGE profile of purified recombinant Chinese small-tailed Han sheep PrP (94–227) fused with His-tag and Trx-tag, Coomassie blue staining. Purified re-PrP (lane 3). The inclusion bodies from *E. coli* BL21(DE3) transformed with pET-32a(+)/PrP (94–227) (lane 1). Prestained protein marker, broad range in kilodaltons (kDa) (lane 2). (B) The purified re-PrP identified by mAb F89 in Western blot. Purified re-PrP (lane 3). The inclusion bodies from *E. coli* BL21(DE3) transformed with pET-32a(+)/PrP (94–227) (lane 1). Prestained protein marker, broad range in kDa (lane 2).

mAb 6H4, it had an identical immunohistochemical pattern (FIG. 4). Using it as a key regent, we succeeded in establishing an mAb-based IHC method for BSE surveillance, which has been issued as national standard of China (BSE diagnostic technique, GB/T19180-2003).

BSE Surveillance in China

For BSE surveillance in China, we apply two kinds of mAbs, 4C11 and 6H4, respectively in the IHC test, and the detection coincidence rate of two kinds of mAbs is 100%. It was found that all 12,692 samples (2001–2004) from the whole country showed negative results in IHC test, as well as in H.E staining test, meanwhile positive control showed typical PrP^{Sc} accumulation pattern. All the test results (including reports, formalin fixed brain section, slides) were kept in the archives and supported a claimed BSE status that China poses a negligible BSE risk.

DISCUSSION

At present, PrP^{Sc} accumulation represents the only available marker of prion diseases and the immunological detection of its presence in brain is required for a definite diagnosis of TSEs. In China, some institutes have carried out a research on the detection technique of PrP^{Sc}. PrP peptide or

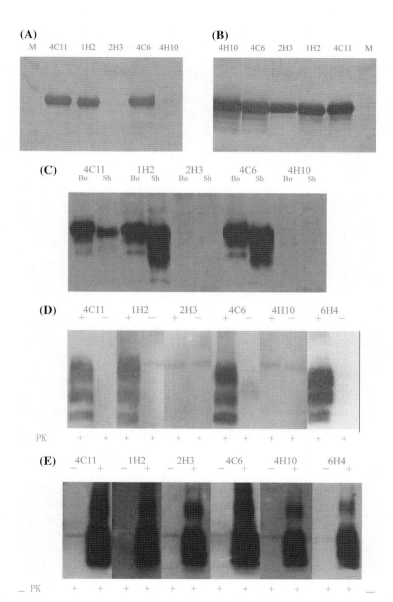

FIGURE 3. Immunoreactivities of five mAbs in Western blot analysis. (**A**) recombinant Chinese yellow cattle (*Bos taurus*, Luxi) PrP (24–234). (**B**) recombinant Chinese small-tailed Han sheep PrP (94–227). (**C**) Brain homogenates from normal bovine and sheep. (**D**) Brain homogenates from BSE cattle. (**E**) Brain homogenates from Scrapie sheep. In **D** and **E**, we used a commercial BSE Test Kit (Prionics check Western, Prionics), and replaced the mAb 6H4 with our mAbs; positive brain homogenates samples (+) from BSE cattle and Scrapie sheep, and negative samples (−) from normal cattle and sheep, were all treated by proteinase K.

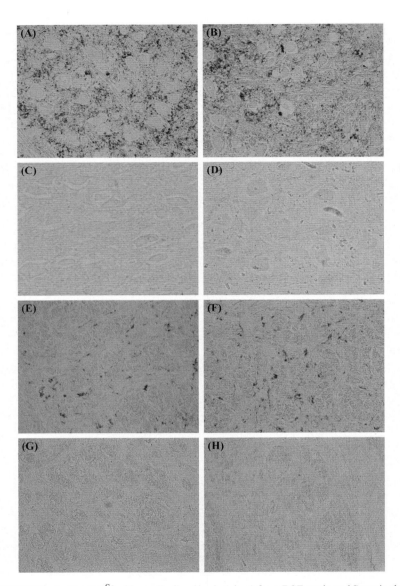

FIGURE 4. The PrP^{Sc} of formalin fixed brain (obex) from BSE cattle and Scrapie sheep identified by mAbs 4C11and 6H4. (**A**) PrP^{Sc} of formalin fixed brain (obex) from BSE cattle stained by 4C11. (**B**) PrP^{Sc} of formalin fixed brain (obex) from BSE cattle stained by 6H4. Reddish brown PrP^{Sc} accumulation in clusters in both **A** and **B**. (**C**) Negative control from normal cattle stained by 4C11. (**D**) Negative control from normal cattle stained by 6H4. (**E**) PrP^{Sc} of formalin fixed brain (obex) from Scrapie sheep stained by 4C11. (**F**) PrP^{Sc} of formalin fixed brain (obex) from Scrapie sheep stained by 6H4. Reddish brown PrP^{Sc} accumulation along the axons in both **E** and **F**. (**G**) Negative control from normal sheep stained by 4C11. (**H**) Negative control from normal sheep stained by 6H4.

re-PrP was used as antigen to prepare polyclonal antibody, for detection of PrP^{Sc} from mice brain infected by 263 K stain of scrapie.[17,18] In our study, we developed the five anti-PrP mAbs and established an mAb-based IHC method for the surveillance of BSE. Compared with rabbit anti-PrP polyclonal antibody, mAbs improved the sensitivity of IHC test, at the same time, reduced its nonspecificity (data not shown), making the detection level of the BSE of our country realize a great-leap-forward development. We have broken the international technological barrier of BSE completely.

Our laboratory, national BSE test center has undertaken active surveillance of BSE in China since 1999. The result showed that all samples were negative in both IHC and H.E test, accumulating the important test data for "international authentication of without BSE" of our country. According to the stipulations of the "Terrestrial Animal Health Code" of OIE, all countries should carry on BSE risk analysis and BSE long-term surveillance plan. According to the present test data, we have not detected BSE in our country, and will continue active surveillance of BSE, preventing BSE from invading our country, ensuring the safety of livestock produce, and promoting international trade of our country.

A lot of anti-PrP mAbs have been developed, using various antigens, such as PrP^{Sc}, PrP^{C}, re-PrP, PrP peptides.[19–31] Most of these mAbs recognize both PrP^{C} and PrP^{Sc} treated with denaturant, and are widely used for the immunodetection of PrP^{Sc} based on partial resistance to protease digestion, while few mAbs could distinguish the two PrP isoforms. The mAb 15B3 was reported to recognize a PrP^{Sc}-specific conformational epitope.[24] Recent report describes that mAb KG9 enables immunohistological detection of abnormal accumulation of PrP^{Sc} in the brain from BSE cattle but not from Scrapie sheep.[29] Remarkably, in our study, mAbs 2H3, 4H10 react only with PrP^{Sc} from Scrapie sheep in the Western blot test. We will carry out further research for understanding whether two mAbs could recognize sheep PrP^{Sc}-specific linear epitope.

ACKNOWLEDGMENTS

We thank Prof. Marc Vandevelde, Prof. Andreas Zurbriggen, and Dr. Torsten Seuberlich (Vetsuisse Faculty University of Berne, Switzerland) for the generous gift of formalin fixed brain tissues from BSE, for expert technical assistance in the development of mAb-based IHC method, and in the identification of mAbs by WB test. The financial support was provided by a grant from the National Natural Science Foundation of China (30270981) and a grant from the Ministry of Science and Technology of China (2004BA519A53).

REFERENCES

1. WELLS, G.A.H., A.C. SCOTT, C.T. JOHNSON, *et al.* 1987. A novel progressive spongiform encephalopathy in cattle. Vet. Rec. **121:** 419–420.

2. KIMBERLIN, R.H. 1992. Bovine spongiform encephalopathy. Rev. Sci. Tech. **11:** 347–390.
3. WILESMITH, J.W., G.A.H. WELLS, M.P. CRANWELL, *et al.* 1988. Bovine spongiform encephalopathy: epidemiological studies. Vet. Rec. **123:** 638–644.
4. PRUSINER, S.B. 1982. Novel proteinaceous infectious particles cause scrapie. Science **216:** 136–144.
5. HOPE, J., L.J. MORTON, C.F. FARQUHAR, *et al.* 1986. The major polypeptide of scrapie-associated fibrils (SAF) has the same size, charge distribution and N-terminal protein sequence as predicted for the normal brain protein (PrP). EMBO J. **5:** 2591–2597.
6. PAN, K.M., M. BALDWIN, J. NGUYEN, *et al.* 1993. Conversion of alpha-helices into beta-sheets features in the formation of the scrapie prion proteins. Proc. Natl. Acad. Sci. USA **90:** 10962–10966.
7. SAFAR, J., P.P. ROLLER, D.C. GAJDUSEK, *et al.* 1993. Conformational transitions, dissociation, and unfolding of scrapie amyloid (prion) protein. J. Biol. Chem. **268:** 20276–20284.
8. BRUCE, M.E., R.G. WILL, J.W. IRONSIDE, *et al.* 1997. Transmissions to mice indicate that 'new variant' CJD is caused by the BSE agent. Nature **389:** 498–501.
9. SCOTT, M.R., R. WILL, J. IRONSIDE, *et al.* 1999. Compelling transgenetic evidence for transmission of bovine spongiform encephalopathy prions to humans. Proc. Natl Acad. Sci. USA **96:** 15137–15142.
10. COLLINGE, J., K.C.L. SIDLE, J. MEADS, *et al.* 1996. Molecular analysis of prion strain variation and the aetiology of 'new variant' CJD. Nature **383:** 685–690.
11. HILL, A.F., M. DESBRUSLAIS, S. JOINER, *et al.* 1997. The same prion strain causes vCJD and BSE. Nature **389:** 448–450.
12. BÜELER, H., M. FISCHER, Y. LANG, *et al.* 1992. Normal development and behaviour of mice lacking the neuronal cell-surface PrP protein. Nature **356:** 577–582.
13. GRABER, H.U., R.K. MEYER, R. FATZER, *et al.* 1995. In situ hybridization and immunohistochemistry for prion protein (PrP) in bovine spongiform encephalopathy (BSE). J. Vet. Med. Assoc. **42:** 453–459.
14. HARITANI, M., Y.I. SPENCER & G.A.H. WELLS 1994. Hydrated autoclave pretreatment enhancement of prion protein immunoreactivity in formalin-fixed bovine spongiform encephalopathy-affected brain. Acta Neuropathol. (Berl.) **87:** 86–90.
15. KATZ, J.B., A.L. SHAFER & J.M. MILLER 1995. Production of antiserum for the diagnosis of scrapie and bovine spongiform encephalopathy using a baculovirus-expressed prion protein. J. Vet. Diagn. Invest. **7:** 245–247.
16. WELLS, G.A.H. & J.W. WILESMITH 1995. The neuropathology and epidemiology of bovine spongiform encephalopathy. Brain Pathol. **5:** 91–103.
17. SUN, X.F. *et al.* 2000. Generation and application of prion peptide antibody to human prion. Chin. J. Microbiol. Immunol. **20:** 70–73.
18. SUN, X.F. *et al.* 2000. PrP-res protein and neuropathological analysis of the brain tissues from hamsters infected with Scrapie 263K. Chin. J. Virol. **3:** 48–53.
19. BARRY, R.A. & S.B. PRUSINER 1986. Monoclonal antibodies to the cellular and scrapie prion proteins. J. Infect. Dis. **154:** 518–521.
20. KASCSAK, R.J., R. RUBENSTEIN, P.A. MERZ, *et al.* 1987. Mouse polyclonal and monoclonal antibody to scrapie-associated fibril proteins. J. Virol. **61:** 3688–3693.

21. HORIUCHI, M., N. YAMAZAKI, T. IKEDA, *et al.* 1995. A cellular form of prion protein (PrPC) exists in many non-neuronal tissues of sheep. J. Gen. Virol. **76:** 2583–2587.

22. WILLIAMSON, R.A., D. PERETZ, N. SMORODINSKY, *et al.* 1996. Circumventing tolerance to generate autologous monoclonal antibodies to the prion protein. Proc. Natl. Acad. Sci. USA **93:** 7279–7282.

23. KRASEMANN, S., M.H. GROSCHUP, S. HARMEYER, *et al.* 1996. Generation of monoclonal antibodies against human prion proteins in PrP0/0 mice. Mol. Med. **2:** 725–734.

24. KORTH, C., B. STIERLI, P. STREIT, *et al.* 1997. Prion (PrPSc)-specific epitope defined by a monoclonal antibody. Nature **390:** 74–77.

25. ZANUSSO, G., D. LIU, S. FERRARI, *et al.* 1998. Prion protein expression in different species: analysis with a panel of new mAbs. Proc. Natl. Acad. Sci. USA **95:** 8812–8816.

26. HARMEYER, S., E. PFAFF & M.H. GROSCHUP 1998. Synthetic peptide vaccines yield monoclonal antibodies to cellular and pathological prion proteins of ruminants. J. Gen. Virol. **79:** 937–945.

27. O'ROURKE, K.I., T.V. BASZLER, J.M. MILLER, *et al.* 1998. Monoclonal antibody F89/160.1.5 defines a conserved epitope on the ruminant prion protein. J. Clin. Microbiol. **36:** 1750–1755.

28. YOKOYAMA, T., K.M. KIMURA, Y. USHIKI, *et al.* 2001. *In vivo* conversion of cellular prion protein to pathogenic isoforms, as monitored by conformation specific antibodies. J. Biol. Chem. **276:** 11265–11271.

29. LAFFLING, A.J., A. BAIRD, C.R. BIRKETT, *et al.* 2001. A monoclonal antibody that enables specific immunohistological detection of prion protein in bovine spongiform encephalopathy cases. Neurosci. Lett. **300:** 99–102.

30. KIM, C.L., A. UMETANI, T. MATSUI, *et al.* 2004. Antigenic characterization of an abnormal isoform of prion protein using a new diverse panel of monoclonal antibodies. Virology **320:** 40–51.

31. MATUCCI, A., G. ZANUSSO, M. GELATI, *et al.* 2005. Analysis of mammalian scrapie protein by novel monoclonal antibodies recognizing distinct prion protein glycoforms: an immunoblot and immunohistochemical study at the light and electron microscopic levels. Brain Res. Bull. **65:** 155–162.

A Serological Survey of Pigs, Horses, and Ducks in Nepal for Evidence of Infection with Japanese Encephalitis Virus

GANESH R. PANT

Central Veterinary Laboratory, Tripureshwor, Kathmandu, Nepal

ABSTRACT: Japanese encephalitis (JE) is an emerging disease of animals and humans in Nepal. A serological study for antibody to JE virus was conducted in Nepal from September 2003 to August 2004 by collecting 280 sera from pigs, ducks, and horses covering 10 districts of the country. These sera were tested by performing competitive enzyme-linked immunosorbent assay for the detection of antibodies against JE virus. The total number of tested sera was 280, of which 43.92% were found positive for the presence of antibodies against JE virus infection in Nepal. Sero-prevalence of JE in pigs, ducks, and horses was 48.11%, 26.79%, and 50.0%, respectively.

KEYWORDS: Japanese encephalitis; emerging disease and competitive enzyme-linked immunosorbent assay

INTRODUCTION

Japanese encephalitis (JE) is a mosquito-borne viral disease and causes encephalitis in humans as well as in horses and abortion in pigs. JE is a disease of major public health importance in Nepal. Cases of JE were first reported in Nepal in 1978.[1] The Nepal Health Authority reported 26,666 cases and 5381 deaths, with an average of 20.2% fatality rate from 1978 to 2003. Epidemics of JE usually occur with the onset of the monsoon season in July and end in October. Annually, around 1000–3000 cases and 200–400 deaths have been reported due to JE in Nepal. JE is prevalent in 24 districts of the country; therefore, 12.5 million people living in these districts are considered at risk. The Culex mosquito (*Culex tritaeniorhynchus*) has been reported to be the principal vector for the transmission of JE in Nepal.[2] The total irrigated land for cultivation of rice is 771,759 hectares in Nepal, which acts as a favorable environment for the breeding of the vector.[3] The prevalence of JE infection in

Address for correspondence: Dr. Ganesh R. Pant, Central Veterinary Laboratory, Tripureshwor, Kathmandu, Nepal. Voice: +97714261938; fax: +97714261867.

e-mail: ganeshrajpant@yahoo.co.uk

Ann. N.Y. Acad. Sci. 1081: 124–129 (2006). © 2006 New York Academy of Sciences.
doi: 10.1196/annals.1373.013

children has been reported 62% in the 1 to 15 year age group.[4] The number of JE cases and deaths reported in Nepal in 2004 were 1545 and 133 respectively (personal communication with Mr. L.N. Shah of Epidemiology and Diseases Control Division).

The total number of pigs in Nepal is approximately 1 million, with the distribution 0.22 per household.[5] The population of pigs is around 400,000 in 24 JE-endemic districts. Abortion is one of the most common problems among the pigs. Total 286 outbreaks and 800 affected cases of abortion were reported in pigs from 2000 to 2004 in Nepal (personal communication with Veterinary Epidemiology Center). Pigs are considered the most important natural amplifying host for JE virus. However, only limited studies of JE infection in pigs and other susceptible animals are available for Nepal. The aim of this article was to investigate the status of JE virus infection in pigs, ducks, and horses in 10 districts of Nepal.

MATERIALS AND METHODS

A total of 280 serum samples was collected randomly from September 2003 to August 2004 from pigs, ducks, and horses in 10 districts. Out of 280 sera, 240 were inactivated for 30 min at 56°C and sent to the Australian Animal Health Laboratory Australia for laboratory investigation and only 40 were tested at Central Veterinary Laboratory in Nepal. All (280) samples were tested by performing competitive enzyme-linked immunosorbent assay (C-ELISA) test.[6] In brief, polyvinyl 96-well plates were coated first with JE antigen. The test sera were added at 1:10 dilution and JE-989 monoclonal antibody was added to serum in ELISA plate. Anti-mouse/horseradish peroxidase was added as a conjugate. Tetramethyl-benzidine was used as color detection. The reaction was stopped by adding 1 M sulphuric acid. The ELISA plates were read in a microplate photometer for absorption at wavelength 450 nm. Resultant optical densities were converted to percentage inhibition relative to a normal pig serum control. The sera resulting in less than 40% inhibition were considered negative, whereas those with greater than 40% inhibition were considered positive.

RESULTS AND DISCUSSION

The results of C-ELISA of different districts are described in TABLE 1. Out of 280 tested sera, 123 were positive for the presence of antibodies (IgG) against JE virus, whereas the rest were negative. In total, 43.92% of tested sera were found to be test-positive. This study has shown that the highest percentage of sero-positive cases was observed in Central region, which does not directly correlate with the incidence of JE in humans. For the first time, antibodies against JE virus in pigs were detected in the Kathmandu valley. According to the Health Authority of Nepal, the incidence of JE in humans was higher in

TABLE 1. Prevalence of Japanese encephalitis in different districts, Nepal, 2005

Region	District	Positive samples	Tested samples	Sero-positive %	Mean*
Far-Western					47.00
	Kailali	10	21	47.6	
Mid-Western					9.60
	Banke	5	52	9.6	
Western					35.30
	Kapilbastu	14	30	46.6	
	Rupendehi	6	25	24.0	
Central					69.50
	Kathmandu	13	31	42.0	
	Bhakatpur	3	4	75.0	
	Lalitpur	32	35	91.4	
Eastern					48.90
	Sunsari	16	40	40.0	
	Morang	19	31	61.3	
	Jhapa	5	11	45.4	
Total	10	123	280		43.92

*Mean sero-prevalence of each region of Nepal.

Dang, Kailali, Banke, Bardiya, Rupendehi, Kanchanpur, Morang, and Sunsari districts among the other endemic districts. The incidence of JE in humans in Lalitpur, Bhaktapur, and Kathmandu is very low, which may be due to the well-organized pig farming in these areas. Pig farms are located far from human inhabitation in urban areas. In contrast, the people living in the rural areas of highly endemic districts are compelled to live very close to their pig farming due to socioeconomic factors.

JE is principally considered as a disease of rural areas where the vector mosquitoes live and grow in a close association with pigs (main vector-amplifying host). In this study, the serum samples were collected and tested only from 10 districts; therefore, the result of this study does not necessarily reflect the whole situation of JE in the country (FIG. 1). However, the findings of this study indicate the prevalence of JE virus infection in pigs in seven JE-endemic districts and three districts of Kathmandu valley. The analysis of human cases indicates that only 8.6% were found to be test-positive when 1055 serum samples (collected from JE-infected patients) were tested in 2004 by performing IgM C-ELISA (personal communication with Epidemiology and Disease Control Division). The percentage of low positive result is not surprising because IgM antibodies do not persist in the patient's blood for a long time. However, this test is very useful to detect antibodies in the early and acute stages of JE infection in human beings.

The positive result in different species of animals like pigs, ducks, and horses were 48.11%, 26.79%, and 50.0%, respectively (TABLE 2). Out of 12 horse sera collected from Kailali district, only 50% were found positive. Joshi

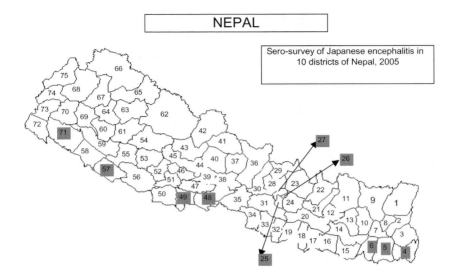

FIGURE 1. Sero-survey of Japanese encephalitis in 10 districts of Nepal, 2005.

S. No.	District	S.No.	District	S.No.	District
1	Taplejung	26	Bhaktapur	51	Argakhanchi
2	Panchthar	27	Kathmandu	52	Pyuthan
3	Ilam	28	Nuwakot	53	Rolpa
4	Jhapa	29	Rasuwa	54	Rukum
5	Morang	30	Dhading	55	Salyan
6	Sunsari	31	Makwanpur	56	Dang
7	Dhankuta	32	Rautahat	57	Banke
8	Terathum	33	Bara	58	Bardiya
9	Sankhushava	34	Parsa	59	Surkhet
10	Bhojpur	35	Chitwan	60	Dailekh
11	Solukhumbu	36	Gorkha	61	Jajarkot
12	Okhaldhunga	37	Lamjung	62	Dolpa
13	Khotang	38	Tanahun	63	Jumla
14	Udayapur	39	Syanga	64	Kalikot
15	Saptari	40	Kaski	65	Mugu
16	Siraha	41	Manang	66	Humla
17	Dhanusha	42	Mustang	67	Bajura
18	Mahottari	43	Myagdi	68	Bajhang
19	Sarlahi	44	Parbat	69	Achham
20	Sindhuli	45	Baglung	70	Doti
21	Ramechhap	46	Gulmi	71	Kailali
22	Dolakha	47	Palpa	72	Kanchanpur
23	Sindhupalchok	48	Nawalparasi	73	Dadeldhura
24	Kavre	49	Rupandehi	74	Baitadi
25	Lalitpur	50	Kapilbastu	75	Darchula

and Gaidamovisch[7] had reported that 28.1% of tested samples from domestic animals and birds were found positive for JE infection in Nepal. In that study, they also reported that the positive cases were 36.3% and 20% in pigs and ducks, respectively. Although clinical signs are not a feature of JE in adult

TABLE 2. Prevalence of Japanese encephalitis in various species of animals, Nepal, 2005

Species of animal	Total samples	Positive samples	Sero-prevalence
Pig	212	102	48.11%
Duck	56	15	26.79%
Horse	12	6	50.00%

pigs, abortion, stillbirth, abnormal fetuses, and infertility are closely associated with JE infection in pigs.[8] Piglet mortality and abortion are the most common problems reported by the field veterinarians in Nepal, which has not been fully investigated until now. The positive results of this study may be associated with the commonly observed pig abortion and infertility in the country. JE is a disease of zoonotic importance and therefore, further epidemiological studies are essential to design effective disease control measures in the JE-endemic areas in this country.

ACKNOWLEDGMENTS

The author would like to acknowledge AAHL and the Crawford Fund of Australia for providing technical and financial support to perform this study in Nepal. My sincere thanks go to Dr. Peter Daniels and Mr. Ross Lunt of AAHL for their technical guidance and moral support during the conduct of this study. I highly appreciate the financial support and help provided to me from the organizer of Eighth Biennial Conference of the Society for Tropical Veterinary Medicine in Hanoi, Vietnam, 2005.

REFERENCES

1. KHATRI, I.B., D.D. JOSHI & T.M.S. PRADHAN. 1981. Epidemiological study of viral encephalitis in Nepal. J. Inst. Med. **14:** 133–144.
2. EPIDEMIOLOGY AND DISEASE CONTROL DIVISION. 2005. Annual Report 2002 and 2003 pp 22–31. Epidemiology and Disease Control Division, Kathmandu, Nepal.
3. AGRIBUSINESS PROMOTION AND STATISTICAL DIVISION. 2003. Statistical Information on Nepalese Agriculture pp 5–7. Agribusiness Promotion and Statistical Division Ministry of Agriculture and Co-operatives, Singh Darbar, Kathmandu, Nepal.
4. BIST, M.B., M.K. BANERJEE, S.H. SINGH, et al. 2001. Efficacy of single dose SA 14-14-14-2 vaccine against Japanese encephalitis: a case control study. Lancet **358:** 791–795.
5. VETERINARY EPIDEMIOLOGY CENTER. 2004. Annual Epidemiological Bulletin January–December 2004, pp 128. Veterinary Epidemiology Center, Directorate of Animal Health, Kathmandu, Nepal.
6. WILLIAMS, D.T., P.W. DANIELS, R.A. LUNT, et al. 2001. Experimental infection of pigs with Japanese encephalitis virus and closely related Australian falvivirus. Am. J. Trop. Med. Hyg. **65:** 379–387.

7. JOSHI, D.D. & S. GAIDAMOVISCH. 1981–1982. Serological surveillance of virus encephalitis in Nepal. Bull. Vet. Sci. Anim. Husbandry Nepal **10:** 8–12.
8. JOO, H.S. & R.M. CHU. 1999. Japanese B Encephalitis. *In* Disease of Swine, 8th ed. B.E. Straw, S. D'Allaire, W.L. Mengeling & D.J. Tailor, Eds.: 173–178. Blackwell Science Limited. London.

Porcine Innate and Adaptative Immune Responses to Influenza and Coronavirus Infections

BERNARD CHARLEY,[a] SABINE RIFFAULT,[a] AND KRISTIEN VAN REETH,[b]

[a]INRA, 78350 Jouy-en-Josas, France

[b]Ghent University, 9820 Merelbeke, Belgium

ABSTRACT: Both innate and adaptive immune responses contribute to the control of infectious diseases, including by limiting the spreading of zoonotic diseases from animal reservoirs to humans. Pigs represent an important animal reservoir for influenza virus infection of human populations and are also naturally infected by coronaviruses, an important group of viruses, which includes the recently emerged severe acute respiratory syndrome (SARS) virus. Studies on both innate and adaptative immune responses of pigs to influenza virus and coronaviruses contribute, therefore, to a better control of these infections in their natural hosts and will be briefly reviewed in this article. Pro-inflammatory cytokines, including type I interferon (IFN), tumor necrosis factor-α (TNF-α), and interleukin-6 (IL-6), were found in lung secretions of influenza virus infected pigs, and correlated with the intensity of clinical signs, whereas prior vaccination against influenza strongly reduced the production of infectious virus and cytokines in the lungs upon challenge, which was associated with clinical protection. An early type I IFN production was also found in coronavirus infected pigs, including at mucosal sites. IFN induction by coronavirus is shown to involve interaction between a viral glycoprotein and a leukocyte subset, likely equivalent to plasmacytoid dendritic cells, present in the mucosae and associated lymphoid tissues. Given the IFN mediated antiviral and immunomodulatory effects, the use of IFN or IFN inducers may prove an efficient strategy for a better control of influenza virus and coronavirus infections in pigs. Because influenza and coronaviruses target mucosal surfaces, adaptative immune responses have to be characterized at mucosal sites. Thus, nasal and pulmonary antibody responses were analyzed in influenza virus infected or vaccinated pigs showing short-lived, but potentially protective local IgA and IgG antibody (Ab) responses. Interestingly, primary influenza virus infection induced long-lived increase of lung CD8+ T cells and local lymphoproliferative responses. Pigs infected by a respiratory coronavirus (PRCV) showed virus-specific IgG Ab-secreting cells

Address for correspondence: Bernard Charley, INRA, Virologie Immunologie moléculaires, 78350, Jouy-en-Josas, France. Voice: +331-34-65-26-00; fax: +331-35-65-26-21.
e-mail: bernard.charley@jouy.inra.fr

Ann. N.Y. Acad. Sci. 1081: 130–136 (2006). © 2006 New York Academy of Sciences.
doi: 10.1196/annals.1373.014

in the bronchial lymph nodes, whereas the transmissible gastroenteritis coronavirus (TGEV) induced more IgA Ab-secreting cells in gut tissues, which illustrates the importance of the route of antigen administration for inducing local immune effector mechanisms. Porcine viral infections provide, therefore, valuable models for evaluating the immune parameters that are important for controlling transmission of important viral zoonotic infections.

KEYWORDS: immunology; pigs; interferon; influenza; coronavirus

INTRODUCTION

Eleven of 18 emerging zoonotic infections listed over the last 5 years are caused by viruses, most of them being RNA viruses,[1] including major respiratory viral diseases, such as influenza or the recently emerged severe acute respiratory syndrome (SARS) virus. The easy and rapid airborne transmission of respiratory viruses between the natural host animals and the possibility for transmission from animals to humans point out the need for an efficient control of virus excretion at the site of replication, namely the respiratory tract mucosae. Such mechanisms for control involve therefore local, mucosa-associated, antiviral immune mechanisms.

Animals are both reservoirs and natural hosts of several important zoonotic respiratory viral infections, like influenza virus in birds, pigs, horses,[2] or SARS coronavirus in civets and other animals including pigs.[3–5] Pigs are also naturally infected by several coronaviruses, either respiratory (porcine respiratory coronavirus [PRCV]) or enteric (transmissible gastroenteritis virus, [TGEV]).[6] In addition, pigs show anatomical, physiological, and immunological similarities to humans. Pigs are, therefore, a relevant animal species for studying host responses and immune mechanisms to influenza and coronavirus infections.

The aim of this article is to briefly summarize our current knowledge about porcine immune responses, including innate and adaptive immunity, to both of these viral infections, with a special emphasis on effector mechanisms at mucosal sites.

Antiviral Innate Immune Mechanisms

The innate immune response to viral infections includes cell-mediated effector mechanisms such as natural killer (NK) activity, and soluble effectors among which type I interferons (IFN) play a major role. IFNs are a group of cytokines, initially identified by their ability to induce resistance to viral infection,[7] but also currently recognized as pro-inflammatory molecules and potent modulators of both innate and adaptive immune responses.[8,9] In the course of an experimental influenza infection of pigs, type I IFN is present in the bronchoalveolar secretions together with tumor necrosis factor-α (TNF-α), and interleukins (IL-1 and IL-6).[10] The IFN response starts within 12 h post inoculation (PI) and lasts for several days. Peak cytokine titers occur within 18–24 h PI and they are correlated with the peak of virus replication, clinical signs, and infiltration of neutrophils in the bronchoalveolar lavage fluids. In addition, the level of lung pro-inflammatory cytokines is correlated with the intensity of clinical signs. Thus, prior vaccination of pigs against influenza strongly reduced the production of infectious virus and cytokines in the lungs upon challenge, which was associated with clinical protection.[11] IFN-α producing leukocytes have been detected in the bronchiolar epithelium of infected pigs, at the peak of virus replication by immunohistochemistry. The IFN-producing cells were found at very low numbers, and in close contact with influenza virus infected cells.[12] An early type I IFN production was also characterized in coronavirus infected pigs, including at mucosal sites. Within 24 h after an experimental respiratory coronavirus infection (PRCV) in pigs, type I IFN started to be produced in the lung secretions, for more than 4 days, in the absence of significant levels of other pro-inflammatory cytokines (TNF-α and IL-1). At the same time, there were few if any clinical signs and lung neutrophil infiltration was much less prominent than during a swine influenza infection, which suggests that lung type I IFN in itself is not involved in pro-inflammatory and harmful effects.[13] The coronavirus TGEV experimental infection in newborn piglets is also characterized by a high and early IFN-α production, in intestinal secretions, and in several other organs.[14,15] This coronavirus experimental infection model has generated original data pertaining to mechanisms of IFN-α induction by viral glycoproteins: thus, only one viral external glycoprotein, gM, was shown to play a major IFN inducing role,[16,17] accordingly, virus-like particles, made of only two TGEV proteins (M and E) and devoid of viral genome, were as effective as native virus to induce IFN-α production by porcine leukocytes.[18] The IFN-α producing cells, referred to as natural interferon producing cells (NIPC)[19] were recently identified as plasmacytoid dendritic cells (PDC), in both humans/mice[20,21] and pigs.[22] PDC are low-density cells, negative for CD11c and lineage markers (CD3, CD19, CD56, and CD14), but positive for MHCII, CD4, and CD123.[23] In the course of coronavirus induced in vivo IFN-α production in pigs, NIPC were detected in spleen and secondary lymphoid organs and shared several phenotypic features with PDC.[14,24] Regarding mucosal innate responses, IFN-producing cells were investigated in situ by immunohistochemical staining of duodenum, jejunum, ileum, mesenteric lymph node, popliteal lymph node, and spleen cryosections collected from TGEV-infected piglets at the time of highest IFN production. This showed that the vast majority of IFN-α producing cells were located in the small intestine (inside lamina propria and surrounding Peyer's patches) and accumulated in the mesenteric lymph nodes.[14] It was, therefore, concluded that most if not all circulating IFN-α in TGEV-infected piglets originates from gut and mesenteric lymph node. These intestinal IFN-producing cells are in contact with but distinct from TGEV-antigen positive cells and express MHCII, therefore resembling potential intestinal porcine pDC. Nevertheless, the frequency of intestinal NIPC is very low compared to 'ordinary' DC that are extremely numerous, sometimes filling the whole lamina propria of a villus.[25] One can wonder about their function at such site: their small number makes them unlikely to be a major antigen-presenting DC subset. On the other hand, even a rare intestinal NIPC in mesenteric lymph node will flood the T cell area with IFN-α which is very likely to influence the outcome of the immune response. Contrary to their murine counterpart but in common with humans, porcine NIPC/pDC are the only DC subset able to bind bacterial/viral components via TLR9, TLR7 or yet unknown receptors.[26] Mucosal porcine NIPC/pDC could therefore be preferential targets for using natural ligands of TLR9 (bacterial and viral DNA or CpG-ODN[27]) as immunomodulators and IFN inducers. Given the potent IFN mediated antiviral and immunomodulatory effects,[7] the use of IFN or IFN inducers may prove an efficient strategy[28] for a better control of influenza virus and coronavirus infections in pigs. Besides type I IFN, other antiviral innate immune mechanisms include NK cell activity and both influenza virus and coronavirus were shown to activate porcine NK activity.[29]

Antiviral Adaptative Immune Mechanisms at Respiratory Surfaces

Antiviral adaptative immune mechanisms involve neutralizing antibody (Ab), including secretory IgA at mucosal surfaces, and cytotoxic T lymphocytes (CTL). Because influenza virus and coronaviruses target mucosal surfaces, adaptive immune responses have to be specifically characterized at mucosal sites. Thus, nasal and pulmonary antibody responses were analyzed in influenza virus infected or vaccinated pigs, showing short-lived IgG, but more durable IgA local Ab responses,[30,31] which resulted in protection to virus challenge.[32] Interestingly, primary influenza virus infection in pigs induced local antigen-specific lymphoproliferative responses[33] and a long-lived increase of lung CD8+ T cells which could play a role in the broad-spectrum immune protection to heterotypic virus strains.[34] Pigs infected by a PRCV showed virus-specific IgG Ab-secreting cells and lymphoproliferative responses in the bronchial lymph nodes with low Ab responses in the gut, whereas the TGEV induced more IgA Ab-secreting cells in gut tissues and T cell responses in mesenteric lymph nodes, which illustrates the importance of the route of antigen or vaccine administration for inducing local immune effector mechanisms.[35,36]

These results show that specific antiviral effector mechanisms, including IgG and IgA Ab production, lymphoproliferative responses and CD8+ T cell (presumably CTL) recruitment, are induced at mucosal sites of virus replication following infection and/or vaccination, with either influenza virus or coronavirus, in the pig respiratory tract. Local immunity is more appropriate for controlling virus spreading and airborne transmission from animals to animals and from animal reservoirs to human targets.

CONCLUSION

In conclusion, pigs are valuable animal models for evaluating the respiratory mucosal immune parameters, and the preventive or therapeutic strategies, that are important for controlling the spreading of zoonotic viral respiratory infections.

REFERENCES

1. VAN DER GIESSEN, J.W.B., L.D. ISKEN & E.W. TIEMERSMA. 2004. Zoonoses in Europe: a risk to public health. RIVM Rapport.
2. PALESE, P. 2004. Influenza: old and new threats. Nat. Med. **10:** S82–S87.
3. CHEN, W. *et al.* 2005. SARS-associated coronavirus transmitted from human to pig. Emerg. Infect. Dis. **11:** 446–448.
4. TU, C. *et al.* 2004. Antibodies to SARS coronavirus in civets. Emerg. Infect. Dis. **10:** 2244–2248.
5. PEIRIS, J.S., Y. GUAN & K.Y. YUEN. 2004. Severe acute respiratory syndrome. Nat. Med. **10:** S88-S97.
6. LAUDE, H., K. VAN REETH & M. PENSAERT. 1993. Porcine respiratory coronavirus: molecular features and virus-host interactions. Vet. Res. **24:** 125–150.
7. PESTKA, S., C.D. KRAUSE & M.R. WALTER. 2004. Interferons, interferon-like cytokines, and their receptors. Immunol. Rev. **202:** 8–32.
8. LE BON, A. & D.F. TOUGH. 2002. Links between innate and adaptive immunity via type I interferon. Curr. Opin. Immunol. **14:** 432–436.
9. TUDOR, D. *et al.* 2001. Type I IFN modulates the immune response induced by DNA vaccination to pseudorabies virus glycoprotein C. Virology **286:** 197–205.
10. VAN REETH, K. 2000. Cytokines in the pathogenesis of influenza. Vet. Microbiol. **74:** 109–116.
11. VAN REETH, K., S. VAN GUCHT & M. PENSAERT. 2002. Correlations between lung proinflammatory cytokine levels, virus replication, and disease after swine influenza virus challenge of vaccination-immune pigs. Viral. Immunol. **15:** 583–594.
12. VAN REETH, K. *et al.* 2001. Characterization of the IFN-a producing cell in the lung of swine influenza virus-infected pigs. Symposium Towards Understanding Microbial Interactions. Louvain-la-Neuve.
13. VAN REETH, K. & H. NAUWYNCK. 2000. Proinflammatory cytokines and viral respiratory disease in pigs. Vet. Res. **31:** 187–213.
14. RIFFAULT, S. *et al.* 2001. Interferon-alpha-producing cells are localized in gut-associated lymphoid tissues in transmissible gastroenteritis virus (TGEV) infected piglets. Vet. Res. **32:** 71–79.
15. LA BONNARDIÈRE, C. & H. LAUDE. 1981. High interferon titer in newborn pig intestine during experimentally induced viral enteritis. Infect. Immun. **32:** 28–31.

16. LAUDE, H. *et al*. 1992. Single amino acid changes in the viral glycoprotein M affect induction of alpha interferon by the coronavirus transmissible gastroenteritis virus. J. Virol. **66:** 743–749.

17. RIFFAULT, S. *et al*. 1997. Reconstituted coronavirus TGEV virosomes lose the virus ability to induce porcine interferon-alpha production. Vet. Res. **28:** 105–114.

18. BAUDOUX, P. *et al*. 1998. Coronavirus pseudoparticles formed with recombinant M and E proteins induce alpha interferon synthesis by leukocytes. J. Virol. **72:** 8636–8643.

19. FITZGERALD-BOCARSLY, P. 1993. Human natural interferon-α producing cells. Pharmacol. Ther. **60:** 39–62.

20. ASSELIN-PATUREL, C. *et al*. 2001. Mouse type I IFN-producing cells are immature APCs with plasmacytoid morphology. Nat. Immunol. **2:** 1144–1150.

21. SIEGAL, F.P. *et al*. 1999. The nature of the principal type I interferon-producing cells in human blood. Science **284:** 1835–1837.

22. SUMMERFIELD, A. *et al*. 2003. Porcine peripheral blood dendritic cells and natural interferon-producing cells. Immunology **110:** 440–449.

23. LIU, Y.J. 2005. IPC: professional type I interferon-producing cells and plasmacytoid dendritic cell precursors. Annu. Rev. Immunol. **23:** 275–306.

24. RIFFAULT, S. *et al*. 1997. In vivo induction of interferon-alpha in pig by non-infectious coronavirus: tissue localization and in situ phenotypic characterization of interferon-alpha-producing cells. J. Gen. Virol. **78:** 2483–2487.

25. HAVERSON, K. & S. RIFFAULT. 2006. Antigen presenting cells in mucosal sites of veterinary species. Vete. Res. **37:** 339–358.

26. GUZYLACK-PIRIOU, L. *et al*. 2004. Type-A CpG oligonucleotides activate exclusively porcine natural interferon-producing cells to secrete interferon-alpha, tumour necrosis factor-alpha and interleukin-12. Immunology. **112:** 28–37.

27. ROTHENFUSSER, S. *et al*. 2002. Plasmacytoid dendritic cells: the key to CpG. Hum. Immunol. **63:** 1111–1119.

28. CHINSANGARAM, J. *et al*. 2003. Novel viral disease control strategy: adenovirus expressing alpha interferon rapidly protects swine from foot-and-mouth disease. J. Virol. **77:** 1621–1625.

29. CHARLEY, B. *et al*. 1983. Myxovirus and coronavirus induced "in vitro" stimulation of spontaneous cell-mediated cytotoxicity by porcine blood leukocytes. Ann. Virol. **134:** 119–126.

30. CHARLEY, B. & G. CORTHIER. 1977. Local immunity in the pig respiratory tract. II. – Relationship of serum and local antibodies. Ann. Microbiol. (Paris) **128B:** 109–119.

31. CORTHIER, G., B. CHARLEY & J. FRANZ. 1980. Local immunity in the pig respiratory tract. III. Immunoenzymatic determination of local immunoglobulin classes sharing anti-influenza activity. Ann. Virol. (Inst. Pasteur) **131:** 355–363.

32. LIM, Y.K. *et al*. 2001. Mucosal vaccination against influenza: protection of pigs immunized with inactivated virus and ether-split vaccine. Jpn J. Vet. Res. **48:** 197–203.

33. CHARLEY, B. 1977. Local immunity in the pig respiratory tract. I. – Cellular and humoral immune responses following swine influenza infection. Ann. Microbiol. (Paris) **128B:** 95–107.

34. HEINEN, P.P., E.A. DE BOER-LUIJTZE & A.T. BIANCHI. 2001. Respiratory and systemic humoral and cellular immune responses of pigs to a heterosubtypic influenza A virus infection. J. Gen. Virol. **82:** 2697–2707.

35. SAIF, L.J., J.L. VAN COTT & T.A. BRIM. 1994. Immunity to transmissible gastroenteritis virus and porcine respiratory coronavirus infections in swine. Vet. Immunol. Immunopathol. **43:** 89–97.
36. BRIM, T.A. *et al*. 1995. Cellular immune responses of pigs after primary inoculation with porcine respiratory coronavirus or transmissible gastroenteritis virus and challenge with transmissible gastroenteritis virus. Vet. Immunol. Immunopathol. **48:** 35–54.

Ecopathological Approach in Tropical Countries

A Challenge in Intensified Production Systems

BERNARD FAYE AND RENAUD LANCELOT

CIRAD-EMVT, Campus International de Baillarguet TA 30/A, 34398, Montpellier, France

ABSTRACT: From the 1960s, in developed countries, epidemiological approach widened in veterinary sciences in order to understand and analyze the emergence of "production diseases" in "modern farms" where animal management was compared to industrial process. This approach was linked to "productivism" in livestock farming system. In France, this approach included formerly the understanding of farmers' practices and considered the health disorders as an output of farming system. This theory was known as "ecopathological approach." Since 2000, the main purpose for veterinary sciences seems to be now emerging diseases. In tropical countries, a high intensification of livestock production is expected, especially in periurban areas. This intensification linked to a general better control of main infectious diseases (i.e., Rinderpest, CBPP, anthrax) in such farming system leads to many changes in the farming practices and is associated to the emergence of production diseases as mastitis or infertility in dairy farms, respiratory diseases in pig farms and so on. In those conditions, it is suggested to initiate ecopathological approach in these intensified systems in order to identify the main risk factors due to farmers' practices, environmental conditions, and herd characteristics. The general methodology and some examples in tropical countries (Chad, Brazil, and Senegal) are proposed in the present article.

KEYWORDS: farming system; intensification; health disorders; production; epidemiology

INTRODUCTION

The epidemiological revolution of the 1960s arose in response to the inability of reductionist methods to provide practical solutions to the complex problems of health and production in livestock systems. The epidemiological revolution

Address for correspondence: Bernard Faye, CIRAD-EMVT, Campus International de Baillarguet TA 30/A, 34398 Montpellier, France. Voice: 33-4-67-59-37-03; fax: 33-4-67-59-37-95.
e-mail: faye@cirad.fr

Ann. N.Y. Acad. Sci. 1081: 137–146 (2006). © 2006 New York Academy of Sciences.
doi: 10.1196/annals.1373.015

was described in an overview paper published in the first issue of *Preventive Veterinary Medicine.*[1] Because (*a*) the persistence of health in herds even after many named infectious diseases had been substantially controlled, (*b*) the increasing demands of governments to estimate the costs and benefits of animal health, (*c*) the absence of appropriate research methods understand and control etiologically complex diseases affecting production, and (*d*) the inability of veterinarians and producers to develop programs to control health and production constraints associated with intensive farming practices, there was an interest for an holistic approach of the causality of the diseases.

This revolution arose especially in northern countries where those "production diseases" appeared as the main health constraints in farms. In France, especially, the holistic approach of such diseases in farms was called "ecopathology" since the 1970s. We can consider that in tropical countries, the main infectious diseases (i.e., Rinderpest, CBPP, anthrax) are the main health constraints of the herds. However, the intensification linked to a general better control of these diseases especially in periurban farming system leads to many changes in the farming practices and contributes to the emergence of production diseases.[2,3] In this context, we can consider that production diseases in intensified tropical livestock systems are emerging diseases for which the ecopathological approach is an interesting challenge.

ECOPATHOLOGICAL ASSESSMENT OF HEALTH IN FARMING SYSTEMS

Formally, the farming systems research considers the interactions between three elements: the *farmer* who makes the decisions in accord with both technical and/or behavior criteria, the *herd* with its characteristics and performances in quantity and quality, and the *resources* available in their particular farming systems which greatly influence the herd productivity. The farmers' decisions are made operational through farming practices. The performances of the farming systems have been assessed by indicators which can be used in whole-farm decision making. In this conceptual model,[4] the animal health is a component of the performances and of the indicators. The basis of the epidemiological approach to explain animal health performance within the farming system was developed in France under the name *ecopathology.*[5]

Just as farmers make decisions based on technical criteria within the farming systems paradigm, ecopathologists seek to define herd health *referentials* as criteria for supporting preventive medicine and herd management decisions to improve *health performance*. These decisions will also depend, as in the farming system paradigm, on the farmer's behavior attitudes with respect to disease occurrence and risk and they will be implemented through various practices (e.g., management, culling, feeding practices, and vaccination) which, separately or in combination, will influence the risk of disease. In that sense, disease or health performance is interpreted as just another output of the farming system, like production performance, which can vary depending on environmental conditions (animal housing, climatic factors) and available resources (feeding resources). For routine decision making, it can be beneficial to define easily measurable and important health indicators to reflect both health performances (e.g., somatic cell count as a subclinical mastitis indicator) and risk status (e.g., cleanliness score as a hygiene indicator). However, as in any complex system, the development of useful indicators can be both very rewarding as well as difficult. In some circumstances, health indicators have been particularly useful in identifying, at an early stage, imbalances, and malfunctions in livestock production systems.

Ecopathologists integrate epidemiological principles into a systematic method for studying health status within farming systems using an ecopathological survey. Such a survey consists of several distinct but complementary stages.[6]

DIFFERENT STAGES OF AN ECOPATHOLOGICAL STUDY

Five main stages can be described:

1. The sampling of farms by type of farming system. Since we consider the disease as an output of the system controlled by inputs and farmers decisions, the farming system is the operational basis for future actions.
2. The use of rigorous observational study methods by multidisciplinary teams. This allows for the collection of a diversity of parameters, enlarging the frame of epidemiological information with concepts and methods from nonmedical disciplines (animal husbandry, economics, and sociology). In terms of herd health delivery, this also allows veterinary inputs to be better integrated into herd management (feeding, reproduction, and production). Thus, the ecopathological approach is both multidisciplinary and multiprofessional.
3. The management and organization of an information system in a specific database characterized in this context by a high degree of complexity and linkages and with a great diversity of studied factors. This requires that careful attention be paid to developing preliminary conceptual models based on prior biological knowledge and subsequently revised by analysis of the assembled database. This approach has been advocated for the analysis of complex biological systems with *a priori* knowledge gaps.[7] From this, empirical models are developed using prior concepts refined in an iterative approach. So, the data organization needs to be sufficiently flexible to support unexpected applications.[8]
4. A staged approach of data analysis. This will emphasize exploratory (especially graphical methods) followed by methods to developed structured disease models reflecting both previous theory and exploratory results

and, finally modeling to estimate the relative importance of different risk factors and health indices within the structure developed. However, these analyses may be complicated by a number of problems including multicollinearity, confounding, and interaction.[9] A preliminary screening of associations between independent and dependant variables can be done by various multivariate techniques, such as collection analysis, linear or logistic regression, correspondence analysis, and others.

5. The dissemination of results to all stakeholders and key players in the system. A comprehensive program to transfer the results of the surveys includes information transfer through brochures, technical documents, newspaper and magazine articles and workshop papers, skills transfer through training, development of intervention guides and prevention manuals, raising awareness through discussion groups, meetings and other publicity, and lastly, follow-up actions for assessing opinion, refining materials and evaluating and measuring the impact of the proposed modifications.[10]

The main objective of ecopathology is very practical, to identify the risk factors and their interactions which most influence health performance in specific priority farming systems. This approach has been used in tropical countries,[2] but the main studies especially on dairy cows have been conducted in France.[11,12] The general methodology of ecopathological approach was published in Vietnamese review.[13] We can consider that the diversity of disciplines involved in ecopathology both strengthens the contribution of epidemiologists[14] and enlarges the frame of epidemiological survey.[15] This is done both by including nonmedical disciplines (e.g., animal production, economics, and sociology) and by mobilizing the practical knowledge of extensionists and farmers in management, reproduction, and feeding. These experiences in expanding the scope of studies and mobilizing stakeholders can provide a useful starting point for evaluating livestock health and production in even broader contexts.

EMERGING DISEASES IN TROPICAL-INTENSIFIED LIVESTOCK SYSTEMS

In tropical countries, two trends could be observed in livestock systems in the area of intensification.

The trend of the intensification in extensive systems: the intensification can be considered as the increase of the animal productivity per time unit or surface unit or labor unit. This intensification is necessary to answer to the high increase of animal protein demand in urban areas and to the increase of human demography.[16] This productivity increasing involves both high extensive systems and already intensive systems with land constraints (as in Vietnam).

The example of camel farming in Mauritania is quite emblematic. The camel usually devoted to arid areas from Sahel and Sahara is reared in periurban areas as a high-yield dairy cow. As this milk production became the main objective, some farmers can buy pregnant females just before parturition, keep them for milk production, and then sell them after drying off.

The trend of the development of periurban production systems.[17] As for the previous example, there is a strong trend for implementation of agricultural activities close to consumption basin. The urban market supply for animal products contributes to the development of short cycle species farms around the towns, but also dairy farms. The common points for all these livestock sectors are the use of high quantity of inputs compared to rural areas, their integration to market, and the demand for a better efficiency in term of technicity and organization.

In all the case, this intensification is linked to a general better control of main infectious diseases (i.e., Rinderpest, CBPP, anthrax, and so on) and more generally to a better use of veterinary inputs (vaccination, antiparasitic treatment) in such farming system. This leads to many changes in the farming practices and is associated to the emergence of production diseases as mastitis or metabolic diseases in dairy farms, respiratory diseases in pig farms and so on. Those emerging diseases are not new but they are common in intensified systems, represent economically a high constraint and mobilize a lot of time for prevention and treatment. They have a high influence on the quality of the animal products (milk, meat, and eggs) and depend on many factors as described previously. This trend is emphasized in tropical farming system using exotic breeds for improving productivities, for example Holstein as cow breeds in tropical countries with temperate climate due to altitude (see "modern farms" in Eastern Africa or mountainous areas in Vietnam).

Elsewhere, in the past, veterinary services were more focused on the control of main infectious diseases. With the privatization of veterinary services, it was expected a better adequacy with the farmers' needs in the animal health field. However, in the most of the cases, the veterinarians are not well prepared to be efficient face to these emerging diseases in intensified systems.[3] The main questions for the veterinary research in that way are: (*a*) what are the emerging risks in the intensified livestock system where tropical and production diseases are present, (*b*) what is the new diseases' hierarchy according to their prevalence and their economical importance,[18] and (*c*) what are the main risk factors of these emerging diseases?

In some cases, ecopathological studies were achieved in tropical conditions. It was possible when the studied disease was really multifactorial, for example pneumopathy or kid mortality in small ruminants,[19] infertility in dairy cows,[20] unspecific abortion in goat,[21] diarrhea in young camel,[22] and mortality in calf.[23] It was possible also when a producer's network was set up and when multidisciplinary working group can be organized.

ONE EXAMPLE IN TROPICAL COUNTRIES: GOAT PNEUMOPATHIES IN CHAD

In Chad, as in many other Sahelian countries, goat pneumopathies are a serious problem during the dry cold season. Some authors have pointed out that most cases are not caused by specific pathogens.[24] As goats play an increasing role in farmers' income and in human nutrition (milk and meat) around the main towns in Chad, it was decided to achieve an ecopathological survey on goat pneumopathies, the main multifactorial health constraints in the area. The different steps of this study were as follow.[25]

Sampling Design

In Chad, the goat farming system includes a hierarchical structure: goats belong to a farmer flock within village flock with a common shepherd gathering several herds. Each farmer owns a small flock which spends the night near his house. During the day, these flocks are all combined for grazing and watering. Sampling units might be goats, farmers' flock, or village flocks. As the only realistic unit is the farmer, it was decided to achieve a typology survey. After preparation of questionnaire describing the farmer and its herd, the survey was carried out during the dry cold season. Using correspondence analysis and classification, three groups of farmers were identified. One of these groups showed the following characteristics: they were predominantly young farmers, who owned at least 20 goats and no cattle. They sold milk from their goats and the goats produced at least five kids each year. Thirteen villages were sampled along three-line transects framed by asphalt roads. Sixty volunteer farmers, matching the above criteria, were sampled. All their goats were ear-tagged and included in a prospective survey. Data on 3000 goats were in the database.

Statistical Considerations

Sample selection was done at the level of herd, but responses were measured on goats. As the unit of interest was both the goat which expresses the disease or not and the farmer's flock at the level of which prevention plans will be achieved, intra-herd correlation was taken into account. It is important to measure the relative magnitudes of the effects of goat, farmer's flock and village flock. Moreover, it may be that individual variation varies among flocks which itself may be a random variable. Multilevel models can be used to deal with this: linear or nonlinear mixed effect models.[26]

Observational Procedure

Three dependent variables were defined: (1) mortality, (2) occurrence of disease, and (3) severity of disease. Disease severity was scored computing the sum of partial scores for clinical signs describing the disease (nasal discharge, cough, dyspnea, and change in general condition). Separate and global analyses were made with these dependent variables. Hypothesis for possible risk factors were developed by a multidisciplinary working group. This group included field veterinarians and zootechnicians, field technicians, a statistician, and an epidemiologist. The selected hypothesis were organized in a conceptual model of analysis. This model summarized all the presumed interactions between a dependent variable and its risk factors. It was very helpful for designing the database and modeling the data.

In the present article, only results on kid mortality linked to pneumopathies will be presented.[19] The modeling steps involved 1006 kids within 51 herds among which 48 mortality cases were recorded in 23 herds. After a first screening (analysis of the relationships between covariates and dependent variables, death, by univariate analysis), 10 covariates were retained according to their P value and included in a path diagram (FIG. 1).

This diagram shows the relationships between variables. Univariable logistic regressions were performed with each of the covariates. All the odds-ratio significantly differed from 1 were retained in the final path diagram. Finally, only five covariates were significantly linked to the kid mortality and pneumopathy (FIG. 2).

Thus, the identified risk factors for kid mortality in this study were Peste des petits ruminants (PPR), low weight, and low floor space in the night housing. The herds involved in the survey originated from a farming system in which

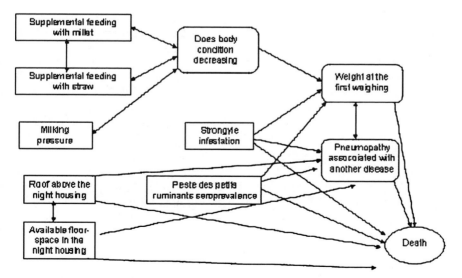

FIGURE 1. Initial path diagram for preweaning kid mortality during the dry cold season.

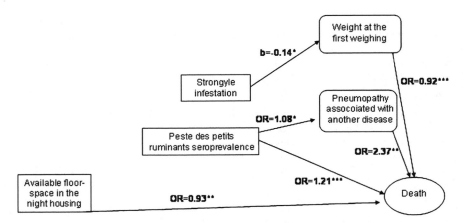

FIGURE 2. Final path diagram for the preweaning kid mortality during the dry cold season in Chad. Odds ratios (OR) or linear regression parameter (b) are those estimated by the two-level mixed effects logistic model. * $P < 0.05$; **$P > 0.01$; ***$P < 0.001$.

goats were a major importance for farmers and their families. Nevertheless, intensification was very low. This analysis highlights the fact that infectious agents as PPR explain a part of the mortality in kids during dry cold season in relation with poor housing conditions. The results obtained here and from other such surveys provide relevant tools that should help the development services to break this vicious circle.

CONCLUSION

The intensification of animal production especially in suburban areas in tropical countries represents an important deal for the research. In this context, veterinary sciences are interrogated by the new trends of health constraints in intensified farming systems. The veterinary research institutes have to manage multidisciplinary approaches to bring some responses in this complex systems were the animal health is one element of interactions between farmers' practices, resources, and animal characteristics. In Vietnam, several teams have joined their effort and competencies within a research platform called "PRISE" to contribute to a common understanding of the main consequences of animal intensification on environment, economy, quality of the products, and animal health. Such initiatives have to be encouraged for the future.

REFERENCES

1. SCHWABE, C.W. 1982. The current epidemiological revolution in veterinary medicine. Prev. Vet. Med. **1:** 5–15.

2. FAYE, B., P.C. LEFÈVRE, R. LANCELOT & R. QUIRIN. 1994. Ecopathologie animale: méthodologie; Applications en Milieu Tropical. INRA CIRAD. Versailles. 119 p.

3. LAHLOU-KASSI, A., B. REY & B. FAYE. 1994. Maladies d'élevage dans les systèmes laitiers périurbains d'Afrique sub-saharienne. L'approche du CIPEA. Actes 1er Coll. Int. Ecopathol. & Gest. Santé Anim., Clermont-Fd, 1993. Vet. Res. **25:** 331–337.

4. LANDAIS, E. 1994. Systèmes d'élevage. D'une intuition holiste à une méthode de rechjerche, le cheminement d'un concept. *In*: Dynamique Des Systèmes Agraires. A la Croisée Des Chemins: Pasteurs, éleveurs, Cultivateurs: 15–49. ORSTOM publ. Paris.

5. TUFFERY, G. 1977. Recherches sur la bucéphalose à *Bucephalus polymorphus Buer,* 1827. *In* Introduction à L'écopathologie Des Systèmes Piscicoles. Thèse Doct. Ecologie: 137 p. Université, P. and M. Curie. Paris VI, France.

6. FAYE, B., D. WALTNER-TOEWS & J. MCDERMOTT. 1999. From ecopathology to agroecosystem health. Prev. Vet. Med. **39:** 111–128.

7. MALLOWS, C. & J.W. TUKEY. 1982. An overview of techniques of data analysis emphasizing its exploratory aspects. *In* Some Recent Advances in Statistics. J. Tiago de Oliviera B. Epstein, Eds.: 111–172. Academic Press. London.

8. LESCOURRET, F., L. PÉROCHON, J.B. COULON, *et al*. 1992. Modelling an information system using the Merise method for agricultural research: the example of a database for a study on performance of dairy cows. Agric. Syst. **38:** 149–173.

9. DOHOO, I., C. DUCROT, C. FOURICHON, *et al*. 1996. An overview of techniques for dealing with large number of independent variables in epidemiologic studies. Prev. Vet. Med. **29:** 221–239.

10. ROSNER, G. 1993. The ecopatho-transfert programme of the Centre d'Ecopathologie Animale: an example of development and knowledge transfert. *In* Proc. of Int. Symp. On écopathology and Animal Health Management: 43 p. INRA, Clermont-Ferrand. France.

11. BARNOUIN, J. 1992. Approche écopathologique de la composante nutritionnelle des troubles de santé chez la vache laitière. Thèse Univ. Montpellier II. 175 p.

12. FAYE, B. & J. BARNOUIN. 1996. L'écopathologie ou comment aborder la pathologie multifactorielle. INRA Prod. Anim. Hors série, 50éme anniversaire. 127–134.

13. FAYE, B. & J. BARNOUIN. 1997. Sinh Thai Bênh ly hoc hay: tiep cân benh ly hoc da nhan to thê nao. Khoa Hoc Ky Thuat Thù y (Sciences et techniques vétérinaires), **4:** 22–43.

14. SABATIER, P., J. FORESTIER & P. MARZIN. 1994. L'élevage, le conseil et l'écopathologie. Résultats d'une approche didactique et situations de diagnostic d'élevage en production porcine. Vet. Res. **25:** 290–299.

15. CALAVAS, D., C. DUCROT & P. SABATIER. 1996. Interactions entre observateur et observé en écopathologie. Réflexions méthodologiques et épistémiologiques. Nature, Sciences et Société. **4:** 341–350.

16. DELGADO, C., M. ROSEGRANT, H. STEINFELD, *et al*. 1999. Livestock to 2020. The Next Food Revolution. Publ. IFPRI. Washington, USA. 17 p.

17. GUÉRIN, H. & B. FAYE. 1999. Spécificité de la problématique périurbaine pour les systèmes d'élevage. *In* Actes de l'atelier CIRAD-CORAF: "Agriculture périurbaine en Afrique subsaharienne. P. Moustier, A. Mbaye, H. De Bon, H. Guérin, J. Pagès (Editeurs scientifiques) Eds.: 20-24 avril 1998, Montpellier, France, 43–49.

18. MSELATTI, L. & G. TACHER. 1991. Animal health and economics. Report on the assessment of animal agriculture in sub-saharan Africa. Winrock study work group paper. IEMVT, Maisons-Alfort, France. 73 p.
19. LANCELOT, R., F. LESCOURRET & B. FAYE. 1995. Multilevel modelling of pre-weaning kid mortality during the cold, dry season 1991–1992 in the outskirts of N'Djamena, Chad. Prev. Vet. Med. **24:** 171–186.
20. DOHOO, I.R., E. TILLARD, H. STRYHN & B. FAYE. 2001. The use of multilevel models to evaluate sources of variation in reproductive performance in dairy cattle. Prev. Vet. Med. **50:** 127–144.
21. Quirin R., T.M. LEAL & B. FAYE. 1994. Analyse et prévention des troubles du cycle reproductif chez les caprins en région semi-aride dans le Nordeste brésilien. Actes 1er Coll. Int. Ecopathol. & Gest. Santé Anim., Clermont-Fd, 1993. Vet. Res. **25:** 343–348.
22. BENGOUMI, M., J.F. MICHEL, K. HIDANE, *et al.* 1998. Ecopathological study of the camel young mortality in the south of Morocco. Proc. 3rd ann. meeting for anim. prod. under arid conditions. Al-Ain, May 2–3, 1998., U.A.E.
23. LAU, H. 2000. Approche écopathologique de la mortalité des veaux dans les systèmes d'élevage de l'agriculture familiale amazonienne: les cas des régions d'Uruara et de Castanhal-Brésil. Thèse INP Toulouse. Toulouse. 177 p.
24. LEFÈVRE, P.C., J. BLANCOU & R. CHARMETTE. 2003. Principales Maladies Infec-tieuses et Parasitaires du Bétail. Ed. Med. Internat. Paris, 2 tomes. 1762 p.
25. LANCELOT, R., M. IMADINE, Y. MOPATÉ & B. FAYE. 1994. Ecopathological survey of goat pneumopathies during the dry, cold season in Chad: methodological aspects. Kenya Vet. **18:** 130–132.
26. GOLDSTEIN, H. 1987. Multilevel models in educational and social research. Griffin (Publ.). London. 98 p.

Integrated Risk Reduction along the Food Chain

ELIZABETH L. MUMFORD AND ULRICH KIHM

SAFOSO, CH-3012 Bern, Switzerland

ABSTRACT: Animal health is the crucial first part of the food chain and must be considered when developing the controls or preventative measures for an endemic or emerging zoonotic food-borne diseases. Increasing the number of complementary control measures at various points along the food processing chain results in overall risk reduction and improved safety of products for the domestic markets and trade. In addition, a risk assessment must be made and surveillance implemented. Measures require sufficient infrastructure within veterinary services, and must be controlled and re-evaluated periodically. The system must be communicated to stakeholders in order to improve compliance as well as confidence from domestic consumers, trading partners, and the international community. Bovine spongiform encephalopathy (BSE) and avian influenza (AI) can be used as examples for implementation of these control concepts.

KEYWORDS: food-borne zoonosis; risk reduction; food chain; bovine spongiform encephalopathy; avian influenza

INTRODUCTION

Integrated risk reduction along the food chain is a useful concept to apply when developing the controls or preventative measures for an endemic or emerging zoonotic food-borne disease. This approach can also be applied when examining most other zoonoses, as well as other animal diseases.

In the control of food-borne diseases, the overreaching goals are to:

1. improve animal health (or reduce prevalence in the case of subclinical disease in animals),
2. improve public health, and
3. facilitate trade.

Many integrated factors that historically have not been considered contribute to meeting these goals. It is clear that for some diseases, safe livestock feeds

Address for correspondence: Ulrich Kihm, SAFOSO, Bremgartenstrasse 109a, CH-3012 Bern, Switzerland. Voice: +41-31-631-29-31; fax: +41-31-631-29-32.
e-mail: ulrich.kihm@safoso.unibe.ch

Ann. N.Y. Acad. Sci. 1081: 147–152 (2006). © 2006 New York Academy of Sciences.
doi: 10.1196/annals.1373.016

together with appropriate animal welfare contribute to improving the overall health of animals. Healthy animals, in turn, together with safe harvesting processes and hygienic food production have two effects. First, public health is improved with the improvement in the safety of domestically produced food products. Second, the proven capability to assure that safe and hygienic harvest and post harvest processes are in place may allow countries to meet international requirements for trade in certain commodities. These requirements are most often the standards of the World Organization for Animal Health (OIE), the institution designated by the Sanitary and Phyto sanitary (SPS) agreement of the World Trade Organization (WTO) to be the international standard setting agency for issues of animal health and zoonoses. In addition, exporting countries may have to meet national requirements set by bilateral trading partners, and/or industry requirements for sale of a particular commodity to a specific market.

INTEGRATION OF THE FEED AND FOOD CHAIN

The feed and food chain can be logically divided into five steps or levels, namely animal feed, farm, harvest and processing, retail, and consumer (FIG. 1). Historically, disease control measures have been implemented only at the harvest or immediate post harvest period, ostensibly to assure that a safe product was entering the retail market. However, in our experience, the maximal effectiveness of any single control measure is only approximately 80%. Applying a single control step, therefore, means that substantial risk would still remain. Improved risk reduction can be achieved through application of a complementary system of measures at multiple steps along the food production chain.

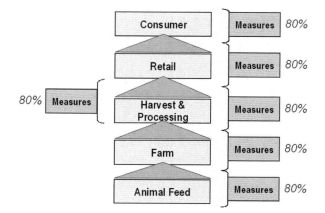

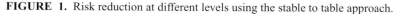

FIGURE 1. Risk reduction at different levels using the stable to table approach.

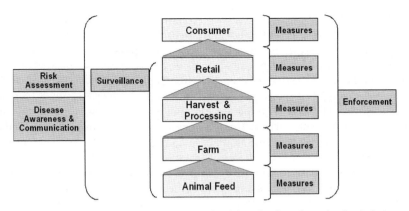

FIGURE 2. Additional tools and actions for risk reduction along the food chain.

In addition to measures directly applied at steps along the chain, other tools are required to maximally reduce risk (FIG. 2). Risk assessment, public awareness and communication, surveillance, and enforcement of measures in place are also important. All of these components must be integrated to form a coherent, national disease control policy.

Risk assessments use data from the entire national feed and food chains, including imports, to evaluate the risk of a specific hazard or scenario. They are by definition country specific, as the data used are generated by the country itself. Properly done assessments of risk are science based and should not be influenced by political factors. Therefore, properly done risk assessments allow improved efficiency of national control programs, as the most valid and appropriate measures can be identified and applied. As well, risk assessments improve the efficiency of control programs, as cost: benefit concepts can be used to evaluate which specific measures are most economical to apply. Finally, the WTO SPS agreement requires that countries provide scientific justification for any trade measures imposed that are stricter than the international standard.[1] This justification is generally provided in the form of a risk assessment.

Public awareness and communication are also tools that span the entire feed and food chains, and consist of training and education as well as use of the media. Increasing the disease awareness of stakeholders at all levels including government, veterinarians, laboratories, industry (e.g., livestock, feed, meat), and consumers leads to an increase in understanding and motivation. This in turn leads to an increase in both the ability and willingness of the stakeholders to comply with the measures that are implemented. In addition, communication must be extended to trading partners and the international community to improve transparency and boost confidence.

Surveillance is a tool that can be applied at specific steps along the chain, or at multiple steps. Generally, it is used to estimate the prevalence of a disease, but can also be used to estimate the distribution or occurrence of another concern (such as the presence of unwanted substances in livestock feed). Surveillance is important to establishing a base line, so that changes can be monitored. This monitoring is useful for early detection of disease outbreaks, but is also used to evaluate the effectiveness of measures in place.

The enforcement of measures is forgotten or its importance discounted by many countries. Often it is assumed that simply having the appropriate legislation in place is sufficient, although having legislation does not imply that the measures are actually being implemented in the field. Some agencies may rely on "paper enforcement" whereby the appropriate signature on a document is considered adequate proof of compliance. However, it is necessary to back up the implementation of measures with some additional form of enforcement whenever possible. Some examples include accreditation of operations with periodic inspections, ring trials, and periodic sampling and laboratory testing.

EXAMPLE: CONTROL OF BOVINE SPONGIFORM ENCEPHALOPATHY

The approach described above was initially conceived and developed through the experience of evaluating and controlling bovine spongiform encephalopathy (BSE) in Switzerland in the 1990s. It was found that consideration of all relevant steps was crucial to controlling this disease.[2] Since that time, this concept has been formalized and extended to apply to other diseases. Now, BSE is used as a model for the application of the approach.

As a first step in the application of the approach, as much as possible must be understood regarding the epidemiology and ecology of the disease of interest. For example, critical data about BSE include:

- Cattle are exposed through ingestion of contaminated feeds (especially meat and bone meal).
- Human variant Creutzfeldt-Jakob disease is associated with exposure to the BSE agent through contaminated food.
- It is not possible to confirm that an animal is exposed or infected ante-mortem, and the prion agent is not detectable in commodities.

Then, the integrated scheme described above can be used to identify all possible tools and actions that could be applied at each step (FIG. 3). Not all tools and actions identified will be practical to apply; therefore the next step is to prioritise the measures based on all available information according to the national risk, infrastructure, and goals.

Data collected through the risk assessment are useful to identify specific areas that hold the greatest risk for the country. Information available through sources such as the OIE can also be used, and in many cases the experiences of

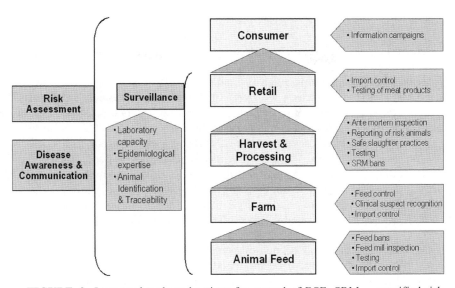

FIGURE 3. Integrated tools and actions for control of BSE. SRM = specified risk materials.

other countries is also available. It is important, however, that multiple control steps in the chain be identified through the prioritization process, in order to be able to implement a system of complementary measures.

A natural consequence of this approach is that individuals, entities, and organizations from each of the various steps and levels must cooperate and contribute to the overall control process. Communication among these groups becomes important to the success of the process, and can be facilitated through appropriate disease awareness. In general, measures also require sufficient infrastructure within veterinary services, including animal identification systems and laboratory capacity.

Using the example of BSE, effective measures for controlling animal and human exposure in most countries include import restrictions on some categories of cattle and some commodities, the implementation of feed bans and control of cross contamination (animal feed level), the identification of clinical suspects (farm level and harvest and processing level), and removal of risk materials (harvest and processing level).[3] Additionally, in order to determine the BSE status of a country and facilitate trade in BSE-relevant commodities, a national BSE risk assessment is required by the OIE.[4] Disease awareness programs, enforcement of the measures, and targeted surveillance of risk populations (including fallen stock/downer animals) optimize and allow evaluation of the risk reduction process.

EXTENSION OF THE APPROACH

Depending on the disease of interest, the levels included in the integrated scheme may be expanded, combined, or modified as appropriate. When considering highly pathogenic avian influenza (HPAI), it becomes clear that the approach applies for diseases with very different epidemiological characteristics. In contrast to BSE, HPAI is highly contagious, and is transmitted among birds by direct and indirect contact and by the airborne route. HPAI also generally causes rapid and severe on set of clinical signs in poultry, and can be diagnosed ante-mortem. As well, transmission to humans is generally through direct contact with infected birds or through contamination, and properly handled and cooked poultry is not considered to be a risk.[5] Using the integrated scheme, all relevant tools and actions can be identified and prioritized according to the national needs with the same considerations as described for BSE.

Certainly, for non-food-borne illnesses, the steps from harvest and processing through consumer must be modified completely. In the HPAI example, the animal feed level is not considered. However, the concept that a series of integrated measures, implemented at many different steps, reduces the overall risk of exposure remains valid. As well, the concepts of assessment, awareness, surveillance, and enforcement of measures remain crucial to consider when optimizing risk reduction.

REFERENCES

1. WORLD TRADE ORGANIZATION. 1994. Agreement on sanitary and phytosanitary measures. Final Act of the Uruguay Round. Article 5. Available at http://www.wto.org/english/docs_e/legal_e/15-sps.pdf
2. HEIM, D. & U. KIHM. 2003. Risk management of transmissible spongiform encephalopathies in Europe. Rev. Sci. Techn. Off. Int. Epiz. **22:** 179–199.
3. HEIM, D. & E. MUMFORD. 2005. The future of BSE from the global perspective. J. Meat. Sci. **70:** 555–562.
4. WORLD ORGANISATION FOR ANIMAL HEALTH. 2005. Bovine Spongiform Encephalopathy. Terrestrial Animal Health Code, Article 2.3.13.2 Available at http://www.oie.int/eng/normes/MCode/en_chapitre_2.3.13.htm
5. INTERNATIONAL FOOD SAFETY AUTHORITIES NETWORK. 2004. Highly pathogenic avian influenza H5N1 outbreaks in poultry and in humans: food safety implications. INFOSAN Information Note no. 2/04 – Avian Influenza. Available at http://www.who.int/foodsafety/fs_management/No_02_Avianinfluenza_Dec04_en.pdf

History and Evolution of HPAI Viruses in Southeast Asia

VINCENT MARTIN,[a] LESLIE SIMS,[b] JUAN LUBROTH,[a] SARAH KAHN,[a] JOSEPH DOMENECH,[a] AND CAROLYN BEGNINO[c]

[a]Animal Health Service of FAO 00100, Rome, Italy

[b]Asia Pacific Veterinary Information Services, Cairns, Qld 4870, Australia

[c]Animal Health Production and Health Division of FAO, Regional Office for Asia and the Pacific, Bangkok 10200, Thailand

ABSTRACT: Highly pathogenic avian influenza (HPAI) has been recognized as a serious viral disease of poultry since 1878. The number of outbreaks of this disease globally has increased in the past 10 years culminating in 2004 with the unprecedented outbreak of H5N1 HPAI involving nine countries in East and South East Asia. Apart from the geographical extent of this outbreak and apparent rapid spread, this epidemic has a number of unique features, among which is the carriage of highly pathogenic AI viruses by asymptomatic domestic waterfowl. When this disease first emerged it was recognized almost simultaneously in a number of countries for the first time. This created considerable concern among both veterinary and public health authorities especially as the virus was also shown to cause fatal disease in humans. This article brings together a range of information on H5N1 HPAI viruses in Asia that were collected by FAO during the past year through field projects and explores possible reasons for the emergence of the disease in late 2003 and early 2004. Key epidemiological features of the disease in different Asian countries are described in an attempt to look for, and where possible, explain similarities and differences. This includes assessment of factors that could have contributed to the spread of the disease. Molecular aspects of the viruses are examined to assess relationships between isolates from different locations and times so as to gain insights into the origins of viruses in various countries. It is apparent that the coincidence and grouping of the reports declaring the outbreaks of HPAI did not truly reflect the time course of disease emergence, which was widespread well before the outbreak. The factors that could have led to a change from infection to emergence of widespread disease in 2003–2004 are discussed. There are still some questions that remain unanswered regarding the origins of the 2004 outbreak. This article does not provide answers to all of these, but brings together what is currently known about these outbreaks and the viruses that have caused them.

Address for correspondence: Vincent Martin, Food and Agriculture Organization of the United Nations (FAO), Viale delle Terme di Caracalla, 00100 Rome, Italy. Voice: 39 06 570 55428; fax: 39 06 570 53023.

e-mail: vincent.martin@fao.org

Ann. N.Y. Acad. Sci. 1081: 153–162 (2006). © 2006 New York Academy of Sciences.
doi: 10.1196/annals.1373.017

INTRODUCTION

The highly pathogenic avian influenza (HPAI) epidemic in 2004–2005 is unsurpassed historically by its magnitude and the scale of its geographical distribution, requiring countries to order massive stamping out exercises, strengthen control and surveillance activities as well as initiate analytical epidemiological studies to better understand the ecology of the disease and related agroecological risk factors.

It is noteworthy that, even though countries in the region and the international community had considerable information on the existence of H5N1 HPAI viruses in the region by 2003, disease preparedness, management, and surveillance systems remained inadequate to prevent the occurrence of this major epidemic.[1]

It is now clearly understood that the disease is endemic in some ecosystems of Asia and that epidemics will reoccur unless risk management strategies implemented at source can stop virus cycling between reservoir species (domestic and probably wild water birds) and spillover hosts (chicken, quail, and other poultry).

A retrospective analysis of the evolution of H5N1 viruses in South East Asia is presented in this article and shows that one of the most significant changes responsible for the increased number of cases of HPAI in Asia is the ability of H5N1 HPAI viruses to be carried, at least for short periods of time, by domestic waterfowl. This is regarded as a key factor leading to the widespread Asian outbreaks, especially given that the affected region is home to the majority of the world's domestic waterfowl.[1]

HISTORY OF H5N1 HPAI VIRUSES IN SOUTHEAST AND EAST ASIA 1996–2004

A study of the recent history of H5N1 HPAI viruses in Asia is essential for a proper understanding of the events surrounding the 2003–2005 epidemics and the viruses associated with these outbreaks.

The Emergence of Highly Pathogenic H5N1 Virus in Asia

The known evolution of H5N1 HPAI viruses in Asia began in 1996 with the discovery of an HPAI virus that killed some geese in Guangdong province in China (Goose/GD/96).[2] The hemagglutinin (HA) gene of all subsequent isolates of H5N1 virus in Asia is related to this or similar viruses, although considerable genetic variation within this viral lineage has occurred as the viruses evolved.[3,4] Similarly, the NA genes for all but the 1997 Hong Kong H5N1 viruses are also related to that of the Goose/GD/96-like lineage.

All H5N1 viruses isolated so far have been highly pathogenic although at least some of the earlier viruses from domestic waterfowl, while still highly pathogenic, appear to be less so than those associated with outbreaks of disease from 2002 to 2004.[5,6]

Presumably Goose/GD/96 originated from an LPAI virus in aquatic birds given that these birds are regarded as the source of all AI viruses,[7] but the precise origin of this virus remains obscure. No low pathogenicity precursor for this virus has been found, probably reflecting the limited surveillance conducted in the early to mid 1990s for influenza viruses in wild birds and domestic waterfowl in Asia.

H5N1 in Hong Kong in 1997

The 1997 outbreak of H5N1 HPAI in Hong Kong was the first occasion that cases of serious disease associated with an AI virus occurred in both terrestrial poultry and man.[8] It was caused by a viral reassortment.

A goose/GD/96-like virus is considered to be the donor of the HA gene[1] of the 1997 viruses. The other seven genes were probably derived from other avian influenza viruses circulating at the time, with the most likely candidates being viruses isolated from quail (H9N2) and teal (H6N1).[9,10] Internal genes of a quail origin H9N2 virus were all at least 98% homologous with internal genes of an H5N1 virus from humans.[9] The neuraminidase (NA) of an H6N1 virus from duck was found to contain the same 19 amino acid deletion found in H5N1 viruses in Hong Kong, although it is not entirely clear whether this virus donated its NA gene to the H5N1 viruses in Hong Kong or whether the teal virus derived the gene from the 1997 H5N1 viruses.[10]

It is also not clear how or where this reassortment occurred as no Goose/GD/96-like viruses were isolated in Hong Kong prior to or during the outbreak. The earliest isolates of H5N1 virus, detected in dead poultry on a farm in Hong Kong in March 1997, already had the same complement of internal genes and the NA gene with the gene deletion typical of the 1997 Hong Kong viruses. The markets of Hong Kong, where mixed species of poultry were housed together, are one possible site.

No cases of infection with the 1997 genotype of H5N1 HPAI virus have been reported since December 1997[11] when drastic action was taken to stem the infection (a total cull of all poultry in markets and all chickens in farms).

Not all H5N1 HPAI viruses isolated during 1997 were identical. Some differences were detected between isolates, involving all genes.[12] This outbreak provided the first demonstration of the mutability of H5N1 HPAI viruses, a feature of these viruses that has been reconfirmed in subsequent years.

Emergence of Multiple Genotypes of H5N1 Virus in Domestic Waterfowl 1999–2004

By 1999 it was apparent that goose viruses similar to Goose/GD/96 continued to circulate in China[13] as a number of viruses were isolated from geese imported for slaughter in Hong Kong that originated in mainland China. Another H5N1 virus with a novel nonstructural protein gene, presumably derived from another influenza virus from an aquatic avian species, was also identified in Guangxi province[5] in samples collected in 1999 from a duck.

Over the next 3 years, multiple genotypes of H5N1 virus were detected in ducks and geese from southern China, including several with genetic constellations similar to viruses found in terrestrial poultry in 2001.[3]

Two H5N1 HPAI viruses were also detected in geese in markets in one small surveillance study in live poultry markets in Vietnam.[14] Genetic characterization of these viruses is continuing but the HA of these viruses differs considerably from that found in viruses in Vietnam in 2004. Based on the HA gene it appears to be similar to other viruses found in domestic waterfowl elsewhere in Asia in 2001–2002.

The genotype of one of the viruses isolated from a duck in Guangxi in 2001 (A/Duck/Guangxi/50/2001)[14] was very similar genetically (>99% homology for all genes) to that of viruses that subsequently emerged as the dominant genotype in the region—the so-called "Z" genotype.[1]

Samples collected from live bird markets in southern China from 2002 to 2004 confirmed that "Z" genotype viruses persisted in domestic waterfowl throughout this period.

Emergence of Multiple Genotypes of H5N1 HPAI in Terrestrial Poultry 2001–2004

In 2001, multiple H5N1 HPAI viruses were detected in terrestrial poultry through surveillance of live bird markets in Hong Kong and southern China. In total, seven different genotypes were detected, including one Goose/GD/96-like virus and six other genotypes that contained genes from other type A influenza viruses, presumed to be from aquatic birds. Of these genotypes at least three were very similar to viruses isolated previously from ducks and/or geese from southern China.[3,15,16]

Markets in Hong Kong were depopulated to eliminate these viruses locally after elevated mortality was detected in infected markets.[16] Similar depopulation was not done elsewhere.

In 2002 another five genotypes emerged in terrestrial poultry in live bird markets and farms in southern China, including Hong Kong SAR. Only two of the seven genotypes found in 2001 were detected in 2002.[14,15]

The genotype isolated most frequently was the so-called "Z" genotype. This continued to be the dominant (but not the only) genotype through 2003 and 2004, although the HA and, to a certain extent, the NA and genes coding for the internal proteins continued to change largely via mutation of existing genes and not reassortment.[1,4]

These findings demonstrated that the "Z" genotype had been evolving for several years in terrestrial and aquatic poultry before the widespread outbreaks of disease in 2004.

Detection of HPAI Viruses in Pigs 2001 and 2003

H5N1 HPAI virus was isolated from pigs in Fujian province in 2001 and 2003. Serological evidence of infection with H5 virus was also detected in pigs in Guangdong province in 2003.[17]

The virus isolated from a pig from Fujian province in 2003 was related to, but not identical with a virus isolated from a duck in Zhejiang province in the year 2000. Based on sequences in GenBank the NS protein of this pig virus differed from that of other H5N1 viruses in that it contained a five amino acid deletion additional to the one found in most recent strains.

It is not clear how these pigs were exposed to the virus but contact with infected terrestrial poultry or domestic waterfowl either directly or indirectly (e.g., via contaminated water) are the most likely possibilities. This discovery provides further evidence of the continued evolution and circulation of these viruses in southern China in the absence of reported cases of disease.

Cases of Disease in Man in 2003

At least two human cases of disease associated with H5N1 HPAI virus occurred in southern China/Hong Kong SAR in 2003. These two cases were diagnosed in Hong Kong in patients who had a history of recent travel to Fujian Province. As infected domestic poultry have been shown to be the most likely source of infection for humans it is reasonable to suspect that they were the source of infection in these cases as well. Again these cases indicate that H5N1 HPAI viruses were circulating in this area at the time.

These cases were associated with the Z+ genotype virus—a virus similar to the Z genotype except for the absence of a deletion in the NA gene.[18]

The Known Occurrence of HP H5N1 Viruses from 1996 to 2004

Based on the above information FIGURE 1 contains a series of maps showing the known locations of HPAI viruses in each year from 1996 (note: there are no reports of isolation of H5N1 viruses in 1998). This is broken down by province (China), island (Indonesia), and country (other Asian countries). It is important to remember that some countries and parts of countries did not have effective surveillance strategies for H5N1 virus until after the 2004 outbreaks and these maps only display what is known on the basis of the limited surveillance that was performed.

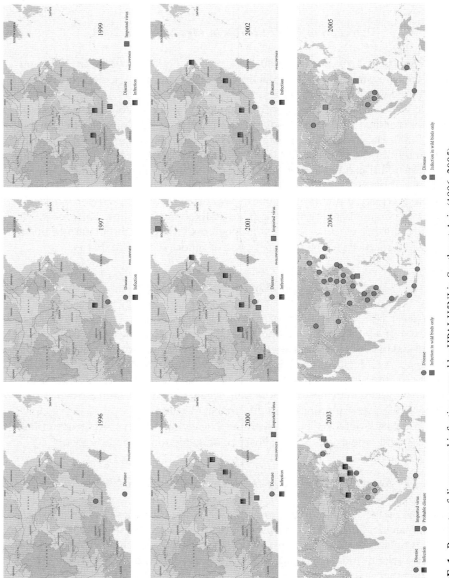

FIGURE 1. Reports of disease and infection caused by HPAI-H5N1 in Southeast Asia (1996–2005)

What Does Genetic Analysis Tell Us about the Relationships between HPAI H5N1 Viruses in Asia

Significant genetic variation has occurred in the Asian H5N1 viruses from 1996 to 2004. The changes that have occurred include:

- Changes in the HA genes and antigenic properties of the HA due to multiple point mutations.
- Changes in the internal genes and NA gene due to reassortment and point mutations.
- Variations in pathogenicity in waterfowl and experimental mammalian hosts.[1]

The striking feature of phylogenetic trees generated for these viruses is the extent of diversity that has developed in these viruses over a comparatively short space of time. This suggests that these viruses have been multiplying widely, possibly in aberrant avian hosts allowing such changes to accumulate through successive cycles of infection. It is well recognized that the replication of most RNA viruses is error prone and that this leads to a high mutation frequency.[19] This is probably one of the key factors driving change.

Several authors have identified broad patterns in the genetic composition of these viruses, based largely on the origins/lineage of the eight genes. This has resulted in the recognition of specific genotypes (e.g., the "Z" genotype). However, within these genotypes there has also been considerable temporal and spatial variation. For example, the 'Z' genotype viruses isolated from the same area in 2002 and 2004 differ. Similarly, the 'Z' genotype viruses isolated from China in 2004 differ from those in Thailand and Vietnam in the same year.[4,5,15]

In some cases, viruses associated with epidemics in the same geographic area were genetically very similar suggesting that they shared a common origin. This occurred with the epidemics in Thailand and Vietnam in which a unique "Z" genotype virus was found in these countries. The outbreaks in South Korea and Japan also appear to be linked and were due to a virus of the so-called 'V' genotype. The precise origin of these viruses is not known because identical precursor viruses have yet to be identified.

The situation in China is somewhat different from that seen elsewhere. Viruses isolated from markets and domestic waterfowl in southern China, including Hong Kong SAR, displayed quite wide genetic variation. This is also the case with the viruses from the 2004 outbreak. Even viruses isolated from the same province in the same year showed significant genetic differences. This indicates the presence of multiple sources of infection although again all are linked to the goose GD/96 lineage and are highly pathogenic.[1]

This demonstrates that a large pool of AI viruses exists in Asia and a large number of H5N1 HPAI virus genotypes have emerged from this pool over a relatively short time period.

Although many of the reassortant H5N1 viruses were first found in domestic waterfowl we do not know with certainty whether all reassortment occurred in these birds or whether it also occurred in wild aquatic birds or even in terrestrial poultry. Potentially, it could have occurred in all three types of birds.

MAIN EPIDEMIOLOGICAL FINDINGS

The study on HPAI H5N1 virus' origin and behavior was completed by field epidemiological studies conducted by the Food and Agriculture Organization and several collaborative centers to explore the risk factors responsible for the emergence of the disease. Domestic waterfowl, specific farming practices, and agroecological environments have been identified to play a key role in the occurrence, maintenance, and spread of HPAI.

It is now understood that the disease is endemic in specific ecosystems of Asia and that epidemics will reoccur, as observed this year, unless risk management strategies implemented at source can stop virus cycling between reservoir species (wild and domestic water birds) and spill-over hosts (chicken, domestic ducks, and quails).

In Vietnam and Thailand, the source of infection has been recognized to be closely related to specific husbandry practices and more particularly to free-ranging duck raising systems. This finding has been recently confirmed in Vietnam by serological and virological investigations that revealed a high level of seropositivity along with important viral excretion in this subpopulation.

Local and national trade practices also play a major role in the secondary dissemination of the disease from reservoir species. Indeed, the New Year festival in winter creates ideal conditions for epidemic generation through a significant increase in poultry production and trade volumes while a relatively cooler climate possibly favors the survival of the virus.

CONCLUSION

This study illustrates the structural changes and adaptation of H5N1 HPAI viruses that occurred since the first detection of the HPAI H5N1 virus in Geese in 1996. Prior to 1999, HPAI viruses were detected rarely in domestic ducks. Genetic changes to viruses at this time appear to have led to an expansion of host range to both domestic and wild waterbirds. By 2004, waterbirds were excreting considerable quantities of virus for an extended period of time.

H5N1 HPAI viruses in Asia will continue to circulate and mutate, and the emergence of newly reassorted H5N1 viruses cannot be ruled out. The implementation of effective control measures coupled with enhanced programs for surveillance and diagnosis of infection will help to reduce animal and human health risks associated with H5N1 HPAI viruses. However, despite the considerable gains made in the past year toward enhanced surveillance, reporting and disease management, some countries in the region still lack the animal health and veterinary public health infrastructure to support effective implementation of the required measures. These countries need a sustained commitment of resources and help to achieve these important objectives.[1]

REFERENCES

1. Sims, L.D. *et al.* 2005. The origins and evolution of H5N1 highly pathogenic avian influenza in Asia. Vet. Rec. **157**: 159–164.
2. Xu, X. *et al.* 1999. Genetic characterization of the pathogenic influenza A/Goose/Guangdong/1/96 (H5N1) virus: similarity of its hemagglutinin gene to those of H5N1 viruses from the 1997 outbreaks in Hong Kong. Virology **261**: 15–19.
3. Guan, Y. *et al.* 2002. H5N1 influenza viruses isolated from geese in southeastern China: evidence for genetic reassortment and interspecies transmission to ducks. Virology **292**: 16–23.
4. Li, K.S. *et al.* 2004. Genesis of a highly pathogenic and potentially pandemic H5N1 influenza virus in eastern Asia. Nature **430**: 209–213.
5. Chen, H. *et al.* 2004. The evolution of H5N1 influenza viruses in ducks in southern China. Proc. Natl. Acad. Sci. USA **101**: 10452–10457.
6. Hulse, D.J. *et al.* 2004. Molecular determinants within the surface proteins involved in the pathogenicity of H5N1 influenza viruses in chickens. J. Virol. **78**: 9954–9964.
7. Alexander, D.J. 2000. A review of avian influenza indifferent bird species. Vet. Microbiol. **74**: 3–13
8. Claas, E.C. *et al.* 1998. Human influenza A H5N1 virus related to a highly pathogenic avian influenza virus. Lancet **351**: 472–477.
9. Guan, Y. *et al.* 1999. Molecular characterization of H9N2 influenza viruses: were they the donors of the "internal" genes of H5N1 viruses in Hong Kong? Proc. Natl. Acad. Sci. USA **96**: 9363–9367.
10. Chin, P.S. *et al.* 2002. Molecular evolution of H6 influenza viruses from poultry in southeastern China: prevalence of H6N1 influenza viruses possessing seven A/Hong Kong/156/97 (H5N1)-like genes in poultry. J. Virol. **76**: 507–516.
11. Sims, L.D. *et al.* 2003. Avian influenza in Hong Kong 1997-2002. Avian Dis. **47** (Suppl 3): 832–838
12. Zhou, N.N. *et al.* 1999. Rapid evolution of H5N1 influenza viruses in chickens in Hong Kong. J. Virol. **73**: 3366–3374.
13. Cauthen, A.N. *et al.* 2000. Continued circulation in China of highly pathogenic avian influenza viruses encoding the hemagglutinin gene associated with the 1997 H5N1 outbreak in poultry and humans. J. Virol. **74**: 6592–9.
14. Nguyen, D.C. *et al.* 2005. Isolation and characterization of avian influenza viruses, including highly pathogenic H5N1, from poultry in live bird markets in Hanoi, Vietnam, in 2001. J. Virol. **79**: 4201–4212.
15. Guan, Y. *et al.* 2004. H5N1 influenza: a protean pandemic threat. Proc. Natl. Acad. Sci. USA **101**: 8156–8161.
16. Sims, L.D. *et al.* 2003. An update on avian influenza in Hong Kong 2002. Avian Dis. **47**(3 Suppl): 1083–1086.

17. LI, H.Y. *et al*. 2004. Isolation and characterization of H5N1 and H9N2 viruses from pigs in China. Chin. J. Prev. Vet. Med. **26:** 1–6
18. PEIRIS, J.S. *et al*. 2004. Re-emergence of fatal human influenza A subtype H5N1 disease. Lancet **363:** 617–619
19. HOLLAND, J.J. *et al*. 1999. Quantitation of relative fitness and great adaptability of clonal populations of RNA viruses. J. Virol. **65:** 2960–2967.

Surveillance for Avian Influenza in the United States

BOB H. BOKMA,[a] CHERYL HALL,[a] LYNNE M. SIEGFRIED,[a]
AND J. TODD WEAVER[b]

[a] United States Department of Agriculture, Animal and Plant Health Inspection Service, , Riverdale, Maryland 20737, USA

[b] Centers for Epidemiology and Animal Health, National Center for Animal Health Surveillance, National Surveillance Unit, Fort Collins, Colorado 80526, USA

ABSTRACT: In the United States, some 1.7 million agar gel immuno diffusion (AGID) tests for avian influenza (AI) are conducted yearly by various poultry groups, governmental sectors, and private industry. In addition to the AGID test, additional testing includes virus isolations, enzyme-linked immunosorbent assays, real-time reverse transcriptase polymerase chain reactions, and hemagglutination inhibition (HI) tests. HI and neuraminidase inhibition tests are conducted on positive AGID samples to determine the subtype. Directigen, a type of antigen capture test, is used in the field in some cases. If monitoring and surveillance activities give rise to a suspicious test result, the accredited veterinarian and official State laboratory are required to report these to the governmental authorities. A thorough investigation in collaboration with the National Veterinary Services Laboratories (a World Organization for Animal Health—AI reference laboratory), State and Federal veterinarians, and others is conducted. Testing conducted as part of the National Poultry Improvement Plan (NPIP) effectively monitors the status of breeder and multiplier flocks. A new commercial poultry program is being added and will expand NPIP AI testing to all commercial flocks. Private poultry companies conduct additional tests; and in the poultry-producing States, there are active state-wide programs to monitor poultry health. All components of the live-bird market system (source flocks, haulers, dealers, and markets) are tested under the Low Pathogenicity AI Live-Bird Market Program.

KEYWORDS: avian influenza; AGID test; surveillance; live-bird market; biosecurity; HI; NPIP

Address for correspondence: Cheryl Hall, United States Department of Agriculture, Animal and Plant Health Inspection Service, National Center for Import and Export, 4700 River Road, Unit 38, Riverdale, MD 20737. Voice: 301-734-4356; fax: 301-734-3222.
e-mail: Cheryl.I.Hall@aphis.usda.gov

Ann. N.Y. Acad. Sci. 1081: 163–168 (2006). © 2006 New York Academy of Sciences.
doi: 10.1196/annals.1373.018

INTRODUCTION

Effective surveillance for avian influenza (AI) is critical to establish a country's status with respect to notifiable AI. Subtypes H5 and H7 and any AI with an intravenous pathogenicity index greater than 1.2 (or alternatively at least 75% mortality) are now notifiable to the World Organization for Animal Health (OIE). Moreover, importing countries may have imposed restrictions in excess of international guidance and thus require evidence that poultry and poultry products are from flocks negative to additional testing requirements.

SURVEILLANCE

AI monitoring and surveillance are conducted by various poultry groups and sectors of the government and private industry. Accredited veterinarians, trained and authorized to perform certain duties by the United States Department of Agriculture's (USDA) Animal and Plant Health Inspection Service (APHIS) and the chief regulatory animal health official in the State where the individuals practice, and laboratory systems funded by and operating under the direct control of each State government, are required to report any birds showing signs that could be those of AI to the State Veterinarian and the USDA Area Veterinarian in Charge in the State.[1] The National Veterinary Services Laboratories (NVSL) is notified when the State laboratory has a positive test result, and a thorough investigation of each case is conducted. This investigation involves collaboration with NVSL (an OIE-AI reference laboratory), State and Federal veterinarians, and others depending on the location, size, and type of flock.

During 2004, NVSL produced antigen for about 1.7 million serological tests by agar gel immunodiffusion (AGID). This antigen is distributed to laboratories approved by the National Poultry Improvement Plan (NPIP), described below, poultry industry laboratories, and other State and university laboratory systems. In addition to the 1.7 million AGID tests, approximately 300,000 virus isolations, enzyme-linked immunosorbent assays, real-time reverse transcriptase polymerase chain reactions (RT-PCR), and hemagglutination inhibition (HI) tests were performed. The HI and neuraminidase inhibition tests are routinely conducted on positive AGID samples to further determine the subtype. Directigen, a type of antigen capture test, is used in the field in cases where rapid diagnosis is imperative. Summary data from State diagnostic laboratories are generally captured by the National Animal Reporting System and available for further characterization.[2,3] Results of the testing conducted by the NVSL,

---

[1] National Veterinary Accreditation Program. USDA APHIS VS (Available on http://www.aphis. usda.gov/vs/nvap/)

[2] USDA APHIS VS. National Animal Health Reporting System. (Available on http://www.aphis. usda.gov/vs/ceah/ncahs/nahms/index.htm)

[3] USDA APHIS VS. National Animal Health Reporting System (NAHRS) Online Reporting

from the referrals by State laboratories and laboratory work up of positive serology are reported annually in the proceedings of the Transmissible Diseases of Poultry and Other Avian Diseases of the United States Animal Health Association, an industry-governmental consultative group.[4]

USDA APHIS Veterinary Services also reports on surveys conducted as part of the National Animal Health Monitoring System Unit. A poultry survey was conducted in 2004 and a layer survey in 1999.[5]

NATIONAL POULTRY IMPROVEMENT PLAN

NPIP monitors the health status of commercial flocks through monitoring of genetic stock and multiplier flocks. NPIP is implemented by State authorities in cooperation with the USDA and the poultry industry. NPIP establishes the regulatory standards for sample collection, diagnostic tests performed, and the laboratory protocols for conducting tests. (Standards are contained in Title 9, *Code of Federal Regulations*.)[6]

Forty-eight States participate in the NPIP; and grandparent, parent, and multiplier flocks are registered in the program. NPIP coordinates ongoing sample collection and testing to ensure that flocks meet the certification standards for freedom from disease. For AI, NPIP requires sampling of 30 birds every 90 days for primary breeder flocks and 30 birds every 180 days for parent flocks.

A new commercial poultry program is being added and will expand NPIP AI testing to all commercial flocks.[7]

TESTING IN THE STATES

State laboratories perform AI testing on any bird presenting with respiratory or nervous system signs and also randomly on poultry submissions. Any positive finding in a State laboratory triggers reporting of the case, a determination of the circumstances, and the submission of follow-up samples to NVSL for confirmation and further identification.

Tool. October 2004. (Available on http://www.aphis.usda.gov/vs/ceah/ncahs/nsu/outlook/issue2/NAHRS_Online_Reporting_Tool.pdf)

[4] Committee on Transmissible Diseases of Poultry and Other Avian Species, United States Animal Health Association (Available on http://www.usaha.org/committees/pad/pad.shtml)

[5] National Animal Health Monitoring System (NAHMS) Unit. USDA APHIS VS. (Available on http://www.aphis.usda.gov/vs/ceah/ncahs/nahms/index.htm)

[6] USDA APHIS VS. National Poultry Improvement Plan. (Available on http://www.aphis.usda.gov/vs/npip/)

[7] USDA APHIS VS. Proposed NPIP H5/H7 Low Path Avian Influenza Control Program for Commercial Table-Egg Layers, Broilers, and Turkeys. National Poultry Improvement Program. June 2005. (Available on http://www.aphis.usda.gov/vs/ceah/ncahs/nsu/outlook/issue6/NPIP_AI_program.pdf)

Several States with large poultry populations have state-wide surveillance programs and mandatory monitoring programs. For example, the high pathogenicity AI case in 2004 in Gonzales County, Texas, was discovered through the State's surveillance program.[8] The original positive sample that was detected in routine surveillance and additional samples collected were sent to NVSL for confirmation, while the flock was held under quarantine. An intense effort in this region did not detect any further infection. In our assessment, the positive samples detected prove the program to be effective and valuable to both industry and government.

In addition to government programs, the poultry industry performs constant monitoring, usually using slaughter blood in serological testing. Many high-tech commercial farms continually analyze serology from flocks to monitor the general flock health status. Any positive sample discovered during this testing is reported to the State government for further investigation. This is how the index case of low pathogenic H7N2 was found in turkeys in Virginia during 2001.[9]

Most States have regulations requiring AI testing of any live poultry or hatching eggs to be moved into the State from other States, and all ratites must be tested before inter-state movement. State regulations require import permits and negative test results before the movement of these birds.

LIVE-BIRD MARKET PROGRAMS

The Low Pathogenicity Program for the Control and Prevention of H5 and H7 AI in the Live-Bird Markets has participation by California, Delaware, Florida, Maryland, New Jersey, New York, Pennsylvania, Texas, and the New England States of Connecticut, Maine, Massachusetts, and Vermont. These States have produced regulations to meet program standards that include registration of all live-bird market producers and businesses, including dealers, haulers, auctions markets, wholesalers, and live-bird markets.[10, 11] All birds entering the live-bird marketing system (producers, dealers, haulers, auctions, markets, wholesalers, and live-bird markets) must be tested negative using the AGID or PCR test at government laboratories for AI.

[8] Avian Influenza web page. Texas Animal Health Commission. (Available on http://www.tahc.state.tx.us/animal_health/diseases/ai/ai.shtml)

[9] Low Pathogenic Avian Influenza web page. Virginia Regulatory Services, Animal Health and Welfare. (Available on http://www.vdacs.virginia.gov/animals/avian.html)

[10] USDA APHIS Veterinary Services (VS). Prevention and Control of H5 and H7 Low Pathogenicity Avian Influenza in the Live Bird Marketing System. Uniform Standards for a State-Federal-Industry Cooperative Program. Effective October 20, 2004. (Available from USDA APHIS VS, National Center for Animal Health Programs, 4700 River Road, Unit 46, Riverdale, MD 20737, USA, or email Fidelis.N.Hegngi@aphis.usda.gov)

[11] USDA APHIS VS. Surveillance for Low Pathogenicity H5 and H7 Subtypes of Avian Influenza Virus through the Prevention and Control Program in the Live Bird Marketing System. Siegfried L. April 2005. (Available on http://www.aphis.usda.gov/vs/ceah/ncahs/nsu/outlook/issue5/surv_for_LPAI.pdf)

Further, States must fulfill requirements of regular inspections of all facilities with testing of birds and the premises environments, biosecurity training and protocols, recordkeeping of origins and health certificates of birds entering the markets, regular closures with cleaning and disinfection, and trace back and trace forward when positive test results are found. State and Federal employees routinely monitor the markets for compliance and cleanliness and take environmental samples to test for AI by RT-PCR.

EFFECTIVENESS OF SURVEILLANCE

Recently, the need for a comprehensive, coordinated, integrated, animal disease surveillance system was identified.[12] The National Surveillance Unit, part of the Centers for Epidemiology and Animal Health is largely responsible for coordinating the development of a National Animal Health Surveillance System (NAHSS).[13] Under the NAHSS umbrella, previously disparate animal disease surveillance programs are being linked in order to provide infrastructure for early detection of emerging and foreign animal diseases (Ref. 1). Data from disease surveillance programs relevant to the poultry industry are being networked through laboratory and web-based reporting systems and will be available to Veterinary Services (VS) epidemiologists for analysis and reporting.

In January 2005, the Committee for the Development of a National Surveillance Plan for Poultry Diseases held its inaugural meeting at the International Poultry Exposition in Atlanta, Georgia. The Committee includes representation form APHIS-VS, NVSL, NPIP, and industry. The Committee maintains oversight of the development of surveillance initiatives relevant to the poultry industry. Such activities include planning for the first phase of development of an Internet (WWW) based, automated NPIP System for use by NPIP staff, Official State Agency, Authorized Labs, and participants of the NPIP program. Quarterly AI reporting requirements for state cooperators participating in the Program for the Control and Prevention of Low Pathogenicity H5 and H7 AI in Live-Bird Markets were recently established, and plans to move required reporting from a paper based form to an Internet-based reporting system are being developed. Separate from the NPIP and Live-Bird Market reporting systems, the VS Application Information Management Team is working with VS Center for Import Export to develop criteria for a web-based application that would allow laboratories conducting AI testing to easily submit summary level

---

[12] The National Association of State Departments of Agriculture Research Foundation. Animal Health Safeguarding Review. October 2001. (Available on http://www.aphis.usda.gov/vs/safeguarding/)

[13] USDA APHIS VS. National Surveillance Unit. (Available on http://www.aphis.usda.gov/vs/ceah/ncahs/nsu/index.htm)

AI test data. As this new system becomes operational, the reporting system will be expanded to bring in all State and private laboratories.

Intuitively, the significant number of samples tested by the different sectors gives a level of assurance that surveillance for AI has been efficient. Formal assessment of AI surveillance in the United States has relied heavily on the data available from the NPIP on great-grandparent (meat-type, layer, and turkey), grandparent (meat-type, layer, and turkey), and parent (principally layers only) flocks. Generally, information from commercial poultry companies has been difficult to include, as these data have been considered proprietary. Nevertheless, such analyses to determine risk have been favorable and corroborate the field experience that when a flock is discovered to be affected with a form of AI, these are frequently singleton findings with little to no evidence of clinical disease. The proposal to test commercial poultry under the NPIP H5/H7 Low Pathogenicity AI Control Program for Commercial Table-Egg Layers, Broilers, and Turkeys will make commercial poultry AI test data available and permit more complete assessment of the effectiveness of surveillance. Such a result will address the needs identified.[14]

REFERENCE

1. LYNN, T., N., MARANO, T., TREADWELL, & B. BOKMA. Linking Human and Animal Health Surveillance for Emerging Diseases in the United States: Achievements and Challenges. Submitted for Annals of the New York Academy of Sciences as part of the proceedings of the biennial meeting of the Society for Tropical Veterinary Medicine, Hanoi, Vietnam, June 2005.

[14] The National Association of State Departments of Agriculture Research Foundation. Animal Health Safeguarding Review. October 2001 (Available on http://www.aphis.usda.gov/vs/safeguarding/)

Influenza A Virus Surveillance of Migratory Waterfowl in Barbados, West Indies

KIRK O. DOUGLAS, DAVID L. SUAREZ AND MARC C. LAVOIE

Department of Biological and Chemical Sciences, University of the West Indies, Barbados, West Indies

INTRODUCTION

Migratory waterfowl and shorebirds are regarded as the primordial reservoir of all influenza A viral subtypes and have been repeatedly implicated in avian influenza outbreaks in domestic poultry and swine. Avian influenza zoonotic transmission events have generated increased public health-related and scientific interest in the prevalence and variability of influenza viruses in feral birds and their potential role in human health.

All of the 16 hemagglutinin (HA) and 9 neuraminidase (NA) influenza subtypes have been isolated from approximately 90 species of wild birds with the widest distribution in waterfowl of the Order Anseriformes. Barbados is the most easterly of the Caribbean islands, located at 13° 6′ N, 59° 37′ W, having a tropical climate with temperatures ranging from 22°C to 31°C.

MATERIALS AND METHODS

Cloacal swabs were obtained from varied migratory avian species ($n = 168$) wintering in Barbados during May to October 2003 and 2004. Virus isolation attempts using 9- to 11-day-old embryonated egg culture (ECE) were conducted. Allantoic fluids were tested using hemagglutination test and hemagglutinating viruses were subjected to matrix gene-specific reverse transcriptase polymerase chain reaction (RT-PCR) previously described by Fouchier *et al.*[1]

Address for correspondence: Marc Lavoie. Department of Biological and Chemical Sciences, University of the West Indies, Barbados, West Indies.
e-mail: douglas.o.k@medscape.com

Ann. N.Y. Acad. Sci. 1081: 169–170 (2006). © 2006 New York Academy of Sciences.
doi: 10.1196/annals.1373.019

RESULTS

Two influenza A viruses and one Newcastle Disease virus were isolated. An influenza virus isolation rate of 2.6% (1/38) was observed in ducks (Anatidae).

DISCUSSION

These data (*a*) confirm the presence of influenza A viruses in migratory waterfowl wintering in the Caribbean, (*b*) confirm a higher virus isolation from ducks than shorebirds, and (*c*) the possible risk of transmission of these viruses to local and regional poultry, swine, and wildlife.

REFERENCE

1. FOUCHIER, R.A., T.M. BESTEBROER, S. HERFST, *et al.* 2000. Detection of influenza A viruses from different species by PCR amplification of conserved sequences in the matrix gene. J. Clin. Microbiol. **38:** 4096–4101.

Isolation of Avian Influenza Virus A Subtype H5N1 from Internal Contents (Albumen and Allantoic Fluid) of Japanese Quail (*Coturnix coturnix japonica*) Eggs and Oviduct during a Natural Outbreak

NARUEPOL PROMKUNTOD, CHONGMAS ANTARASENA,
PORNTIP PROMMUANG, AND PRAISON PROMMUANG

Southern Veterinary Research and Development Center, Thungsong, Nakhon Si Thammarat, Thailand 80110

ABSTRACT: Avian influenza virus (AIV) was recovered from the internal contents of eggs, including mixture of albumen and allantoic fluid, and from the oviduct of naturally infected Japanese quail (*Coturnix coturnix japonica*) flocks in the southern part of Thailand. The virus titers of $10^{4.6}$-$10^{6.2}$ ELD$_{50}$/mL were directly measured from the internal content of infected eggs. The virus was isolated by chorioallantoic sac inoculation of embryonating chicken eggs. Infected allantoic fluid was identified as hemagglutinating virus and then was indicated the presence of H5 hemagglutinin. The virus was confirmed to be H5N1 subtype influenza A virus by reverse transcriptase-polymerase chain reaction. Additionally, real-time reverse transcriptase-polymerase chain reaction assay could specifically detect influenza virus subtype H5. Furthermore, indirect fluorescent antibody (IFA) test by using specific anti-influenza A monoclonal antibody indicated that virus antigens were detected in the parenchyma of multiple tissues. Systemic localization of viral antigen detected was certainly considered to be viremic stage. In addition, influenza virus antigen was also detected by IFA in allantoic fluid sediments isolated from internal content of egg or oviduct. The conclusion of isolated AIV type A subtype H5N1 from these two infected materials was correlated to the viremic stage of infection because the virus antigens could be observed in almost all tissues. Conclusively, the need for adequate safeguards to prevent contamination and spread of the virus to the environment during movement of eggs—including hatching eggs, cracked eggs, and other relevant infected materials— or egg consumption from area of outbreak is emphasized and must not be ignored for the reasons of animal, public, and environmental health.

Address for correspondence: Naruepol Promkuntod, Southern Veterinary Research and Development Center, Thungsong, Nakhon Si Thammarat, Thailand 80110.
e-mail: naruepol_p@yahoo.com

Ann. N.Y. Acad. Sci. 1081: 171–173 (2006). © 2006 New York Academy of Sciences.
doi: 10.1196/annals.1373.020

KEYWORDS: influenza virus; Japanese quail; subtype H5N1; albumen; allantoic fluid; oviduct

INTRODUCTION

Avian influenza virus (AIV), a pathogen of social and economical importance, can infect many species of birds and mammals, but the natural host and reservoir are believed to be free-living aquatic birds. For instance, quail can also provide an environment in which the adaptation of influenza viruses from duck generate novel variants that can cross the species barrier. Moreover, wider distributions by infected migrating birds are causes for pandemic concern.[1] In late 2003 and early 2004, huge outbreaks of highly pathogenic avian influenza (HPAI; H5N1) virus infection were reported to cause lethal illness among poultry in East and South-East Asian countries including Thailand (officially reported January 23, 2004). This article describes isolation, identification, and characterization of infectious pathogen caused by AIV type A subtype H5N1 from internal content of naturally infected Japanese quail egg and oviduct.

METHODS AND RESULTS

AIV was recovered from the internal contents of eggs, including both mixture of albumen and allantoic fluid, and from the oviduct of naturally infected Japanese quail flocks in the southern part of Thailand. The virus titers of $10^{4.6}$–$10^{6.2}$ ELD_{50}/mL were directly measured from infected internal content. Indirect fluorescent antibody (IFA) test using acetone-fixed visceral tissues of naturally infected Japanese quail incubated with anti-influenza A (nucleoprotein) monoclonal antibody demonstrates large amount of positive cells typically exhibited bright apple-green reaction products in nucleus and cytoplasm of those clinical tissues. By chorioallantoic sac inoculation, the isolated virus made the embryo die within 1–4 days *PI* and gave positive result of influenza A virus infection by rapid immunochromatographic assay. The virus was subsequently identified as AIV subtype H5 by using HA&HI test specific for H5 antibody. The virus was confirmed to be H5N1 subtype by reverse transcriptase-polymerase chain reaction (RT-PCR) using type and subtype-specific primers of matrix, HA, and NA genes. Additionally, the virus was detected as H5 subtype by real-time RT-PCR (RRT-PCR) using H5 subtype-specific probe sets.

DISCUSSION

Virus isolation in chicken embryo inoculation is the gold standard for diagnosis of AIV. Rapid immunoassay should serve as a preliminary screening test. In this study, the ability of IFA test could distinguish the virus as HPAI based on systemic detection of influenza A antigen in the internal organs.[1] Evaluation of RT-PCR and RRT-PCR was very sensitive and specific for demonstration of AIV in clinical specimens along with speed and reduced chance of cross-contamination among samples. The possibility of egg-borne transmission must be seriously considered. Eggs could be contaminated with AIV before or after ovoposition and therefore could have internal and external contamination. Accordingly, for animal, public, and environmental health, adequate safeguards to prevent contamination and virus spreading to the environment during an outbreak by movement of eggs and infected materials or egg consumption from area of outbreak must be emphasized.[2]

REFERENCES

1. SWANE, D.E. & D.A. HALVORSON. 2003. Influenza. *In* Disease of Poultry, 11th ed. Y.M. Saif, *et al.*, Eds.: 135–160. Iowa State Press. Ames, Iowa.
2. CAPPUCCI, D.T., D.C. JOHNSON, M. BRUGH, *et al.* 1985. Isolation of avian influenza virus (subtype H5N2) from chickens eggs during a natural outbreak. Avian Dis. **29:** 1195–1200.

Principles for Vaccine Protection in Chickens and Domestic Waterfowl against Avian Influenza

Emphasis on Asian H5N1 High Pathogenicity Avian Influenza

DAVID E. SWAYNE

U.S. Department of Agriculture, Agricultural Research Service, Southeast Poultry Research Laboratory, Athens, Georgia, USA

ABSTRACT: The H5N1 highly pathogenic (HP) avian influenza (AI) epizootic began with reports of mortality from China in 1996 and, by June 2005, caused outbreaks of disease in nine additional Asian countries, affecting or resulting in culling of over 200 million birds. Vaccines can be used in programs to prevent, manage, or eradicate AI. However, vaccines should only be used as part of a comprehensive control strategy that also includes biosecurity, quarantine, surveillance and diagnostics, education, and elimination of infected poultry. Potent AI vaccines, when properly used, can prevent disease and death, increase resistance to infection, reduce field virus replication and shedding, and reduce virus transmission, but do not provide "sterilizing immunity" in the field; i.e., vaccination does not completely prevent AI virus replication. Inactivated AI vaccines and a recombinant fowlpox-H5-AI vaccine are licensed and used in various countries. Vaccines have been shown to protect chickens, geese, and ducks from H5 HPAI. The inactivated vaccines prevented disease and mortality in chickens and geese, and reduced the ability of the field virus to replicate in gastrointestinal and respiratory tracts. Although the Asian H5N1 HPAI virus did not cause disease or mortality in ducks, the use of inactivated vaccine did reduce field virus replication in the respiratory and intestinal tracts. The inactivated vaccine protected geese from morbidity and mortality, and reduced challenge virus replication. The recombinant fowlpox-H5-AI vaccine has provided similar protection, but the vaccine is used only in chickens and with the advantage of application at 1 day of age in the hatchery.

KEYWORDS: avian influenza; control; vaccine

Address of correspondence: David E. Swayne, U.S. Department of Agriculture, Agricultural Research Service, Southeast Poultry Research Laboratory, 934 College Station Road, Athens, GA 30605. Voice: 706-546-3433; fax: 706-546-3161.
e-mail: dswayne@seprl.usda.gov

Ann. N.Y. Acad. Sci. 1081: 174–181 (2006). © 2006 New York Academy of Sciences.
doi: 10.1196/annals.1373.021

INTRODUCTION

The H5N1 highly pathogenic (HP) avian influenza (AI) epizootic began with reports of mortality from China in 1996 and, by June 2005, caused outbreaks of disease in nine additional Asian countries, affecting or resulting in culling of over 200 million birds. Traditional stamping-out programs used in previous HPAI epizootics have not been effective at eradication of the virus from the region and vaccine usage can be a valuable part of a control program. Vaccination should be viewed and used only as a single tool in a comprehensive control strategy that includes: (a) biosecurity, (b) education, (c) surveillance and diagnostics, and (d) elimination of AI virus-infected poultry. One or more of these components are used to develop AI control strategies to achieve one of three goals or outcomes[1]: (a) *prevention*—preventing introduction of AI; (b) *management*—reducing losses by minimizing negative economic impact through management practices; or (c) *eradication*—total elimination of AI.

VACCINES

Protection against AI is the result of immune response against the hemagglutinin protein (HA), of which there are 16 different HA subtypes, and to a lesser extent against the neuraminidase protein (NA), of which there are 9 different NA subtypes.[2,3] Immune responses to the internal proteins, such as nucleoprotein or matrix protein, are insufficient to provide field protection. Therefore, there is no one universal AI vaccine. Practically, protection is provided against the individual HA subtype(s) included in the vaccine.

A wide variety of vaccines have been developed and examined in the laboratory for potential use in the field. However, only vaccines from two technologies are licensed around the world and used in poultry: inactivated whole AI virus vaccines and a recombinant fowlpox virus vectored vaccine with an H5 AI gene insert (from AI virus A/turkey/Ireland/83 [H5N8]). These two vaccine technologies have been shown to produce safe, pure, and potent vaccines. Both vaccine technologies require handling and injection of individual birds. The inactivated vaccine can provide protection in multiple species of poultry. The recombinant fowlpox-H5-AI vaccine can only be used in chickens, but has the advantage of application at 1 day of age in the hatchery, the most biosecure portion of commercial poultry production.

Historically, AI virus strains selected for manufacturing of inactivated vaccines have been based on low pathogenicity (LP) AI viruses obtained from field outbreaks that have homologous HA protein; i.e., H5 vaccine virus obtained from an H5 LPAI outbreak. Rarely, HPAI strains have been used to manufacture inactivated vaccines, because to be done properly, these require specialized, high biocontainment manufacturing facilities which are uncommon in the world. Contrary to rumor, HPAI strains do replicate to sufficient titer in embryonating eggs to be used in inactivated AI vaccines, but their use has been discouraged due to biosecurity and biosafety manufacturing concerns. Furthermore, LPAI strains, with fewer biosecurity and biosafety concerns for manufacturing, protect against HPAI viruses of the same HA subtype.

The quantity of AI vaccine used around the world in poultry is not well documented, but reliable information suggests that the largest use has been 2 billion doses of inactivated H5N2 AI vaccine in China (December 2003 to early 2005). During the same period, Indonesia also has used H5 inactivated AI vaccine. In Mexico, since January 1995, and more recently in Guatemala and El Salvador, the AI vaccination programs have used over 1.5 billion doses of inactivated and over 1.6 million doses of recombinant fowlpox vaccines. The H5N2 HPAI has been eradicated (last isolate was in June 1995), but H5N2 LPAI still circulates in central Mexico, Guatemala, and El Salvador. Pakistan began using H7 inactivated AI vaccine in 1995, with use in three regions following epizootics of H7N3 HPAI (1995, 2001, and 2004). Vaccines for the control of LPAI have been used sporadically. H9N2 inactivated vaccines have been and are used to control LPAI in many countries within Asia, the Middle East, and Eastern Europe, but the number of doses is unknown. Recently, H7 inactivated vaccines have been used in a high-risk area of northern Italy and in one chicken layer company in the United States to control LPAI.

Recently, two new vaccines for use in China have been reported (PROMED 20050207.0415 and 20050210.0456): (*a*) recombinant fowlpox-H5N1 AI vaccine and (*b*) a reverse-genetically produced influenza A inactivated vaccine. The new recombinant fowlpox vaccine is a live, injectible vaccine for chickens and uses the same technology as the previously licensed recombinant fowlpox virus-AI-H5 vaccine (cDNA copy of the AI HA gene from A/turkey/Ireland/83 [H5N8]), but includes inserted cDNA copies of AI HA (H5) and NA (N1) genes (both from A/goose/Guangdong/3/96 [H5N1]).[4] This type of vaccine can only be used in 1-day-old chickens and not in older birds where immunity to fowlpox virus will inhibit replication of the vaccine virus and prevent development of effective immunity.[5] The other new vaccine is a traditional inactivated oil emulsion AI vaccine, but unlike current inactivated AI vaccines, the new vaccine virus is not an H5 LP or HPAI field virus. The vaccine virus was produced by reverse genetics using the six internal genes from a human influenza vaccine strain (PR8) and the HA and NA genes from A/goose/Guangdong/3/96 (H5N1) AI virus. The use of PR8 internal genes imparts the characteristic of growth to high virus content in embryonating chicken eggs used in the manufacturing process, and thus produces a high concentration of the protective HA protein in the vaccine. Another change in the vaccine virus is the portion of the gene that codes for the HA proteolytic cleavage site which has been changed from an HP sequence to an LP sequence; thus the vaccine virus is an LPAI virus and can be manufactured at lower levels of biosafety. Both vaccines require handling and injection of individual birds. Data published or presented at scientific meetings indicate that these new vaccines are as efficacious as the existing licensed vaccines, but no data have been presented to demonstrate that they provide superior protection.

VACCINE PROTECTION

Experimental and field studies have shown that properly used vaccines will accomplish several goals: (*a*) protect against clinical signs and death, (*b*) reduce shedding of field virus if vaccinated poultry become infected, (*c*) prevent contact transmission of the field virus, (*d*) provide at least 20 weeks' protection following a single vaccination for chickens (this may require two or more injections in turkeys or longer-lived chickens), (*e*) protect against challenges by low to high doses of field virus, (*f*) protect against a changing virus, and (*g*) increase a bird's resistance to AI virus infection.[6,7] These positive qualities are essential in contributing to AI control strategies. Most AI vaccine studies and field use have concentrated on chickens and turkeys because of the high death rates following infection by HPAI viruses and the high concentrations of virus excretion in the environment by these species. However, with the changing epidemiology of the H5N1 HPAI virus in Asia, the infection of domestic ducks and geese has become a very important contributor to the maintenance and spread of the H5N1 HPAI virus. Experimentally, vaccines have been shown to protect chickens, geese, and ducks from H5 HPAI. The inactivated vaccines prevented disease and mortality in chickens, and reduced the ability of the field virus to replicate in gastrointestinal (GI) and respiratory tracts. The recombinant fowlpox-H5-AI vaccine has provided similar protection. Although the Asian H5N1 HPAI virus did not cause disease or mortality in ducks, the inactivated vaccine did reduce field virus replication in the respiratory and intestinal tracts. By contrast, the inactivated vaccine protected geese from morbidity and mortality, and reduced challenge virus replication. Thus, proper vaccine use will decrease environmental contamination (especially in ponds, lakes, and rivers) and reduce contact transmission. Proper vaccination of domestic chickens, ducks, geese, and other poultry species will have a positive impact on control of H5N1 HPAI in Asia.

The vaccine strains used in inactivated AI vaccines have been shown to provide protection against diverse field viruses (88–100% similarity to the challenge virus HA) isolated over a 38-year period.[8] Recently, both North American and Eurasian lineages of AI vaccine viruses from 1968 to 1986 have been shown to be protective against the most recent 2003–2004 Asian H5N1 HPAI viruses.[1] This broad and longer-term protection efficacy of poultry AI vaccines is in contrast to the frequent changes of human influenza vaccine strains which have been necessary. The discrepancy can be explained as follows: (*a*) poultry vaccines use proprietary oil-emulsion-adjuvant technology which elicits more intense and longer-lived immune response in poultry than alum-adjuvant influenza vaccines in humans, (*b*) the AI virus immune response in poultry appears to be broader than in humans, (*c*) the immunity in domestic poultry population is more consistent because of greater host genetic homogeneity than is present in the human population, and (*d*) the vaccine use in poultry is targeted to a relatively young, healthy population as compared to humans where the vaccine is optimized for groups with the highest risk of severe illness and death.

However, the protection efficacy of individual poultry AI vaccines should be evaluated every 2–3 years to assure that they are still protective against circulating virus strains. For example, a recent study demonstrated that the 1994 Mexican H5N2 vaccine strain is no longer protective against circulating H5N2 LPAI viruses in Central America and that a change in vaccine strains is needed.[9] With the H5N1 AI virus in Asia circulating as only an HP strain, future vaccines may require use of reverse genetics[10,11] to generate new LPAI vaccine strains or other molecular techniques to produce vectored vaccine products, such as new recombinant fowlpox virus vaccines. Some of these products use patented technologies and will require legal clarification before use in the field.

VACCINE USE IN CONTROL STRATEGY

"Sterilizing immunity" is not feasible in the field. Some experiments have reported "sterilizing immunity," but closer examination indicated that such studies used very few experimental birds without statistical evaluation, used a very low virus challenge, or used low sensitivity virus isolation/detection methods. In the field, vaccines will reduce replication of challenge virus in respiratory and GI tracts, and thus reduce environmental load of virus and virus transmission. However, the protection in conventional poultry in the field will always be less than that seen in specific-pathogen-free poultry under laboratory conditions because of other factors, such as improper vaccination technique, reduced vaccine dose, immunosuppressive viral infections, and improper storage and handling of vaccines. The other four components of a control strategy (biosecurity, education, surveillance and diagnostics, and elimination of AI virus-infected poultry) are essential because vaccines and their use are not perfect.

Economics and animal health control drive the use of vaccines in poultry. Vaccines are used in geographic areas of highest risk and in the agricultural sector affected or at greatest risk to be affected. In the United States, inactivated AI vaccines cost on an average $0.05/dose and another $0.05–0.07 for labor and equipment to administer. In examining new vaccine technologies, such adoption will only occur if protection is as good as or better than the existing technologies and the product is cost effective.[1] If the cost is prohibitively high, the farmer or the company will not use the vaccine.

When deciding to use AI vaccine in poultry, a simple animal health algorithm, in decreasing order of application, should be used: (*a*) high-risk situations, for example, as a suppressor vaccine in the outbreak or high-risk zone, or as ring vaccination outside the outbreak zone when compartmentalization is effective for geographic quarantine, (*b*) rare captive birds, such as in zoological collections, (*c*) valuable genetic poultry stock, such as pure lines or grandparent stocks whose individual value is high, (*d*) long-lived poultry, such as egg layers or parent breeders, and, last (*e*) meat production poultry. In addition, issues which must be resolved before deciding to use AI vaccines include the following: (*a*) the vaccine strain must be of the same HA subtype and be shown in poultry studies to be protective against the circulating field virus, (*b*) standardized manufacturing of vaccines must be followed to produce consistent and efficacious vaccines, (*c*) policies must be established for proper storage, distribution, and administration of the vaccine, (*d*) adequate serological or virological surveillance must be done to determine if the field virus is circulating in vaccinated flocks, and (*e*) an exit strategy must be developed to prevent permanent use of the vaccine. In addition, for inactivated whole AI vaccines, the following should be addressed: (*a*) the need for adequate AI viral antigen content to elicit a protective immune response either by establishing a minimum HA protein content in the vaccine (e.g., a minimum of 1–5 μg/dose if using generic adjuvant system, less antigen is needed if a proprietary system gives higher titers), or by demonstrating a high level of protection as measured by *in vivo* challenge studies or presence of a minimal hemagglutination inhibition (HI) antibody titer in vaccinated birds (e.g., a minimum of 1:32–1:40 HI test), (*b*) the need for a good oil-emulsion-adjuvant system, and (*c*) the establishment of a high level of biosecurity practice for vaccination crews that enter farms to prevent accidental spreading of field virus. If using recombinant fowlpox vaccine, the vaccine should only be administered to 1-day-old chickens in hatchery, which will give good protection, improved biosecurity, and a high degree of quality control. Before new vaccine technologies are used in the field, assessment of safety in target species, environmental impact to nontarget species, purity, and efficacy must be demonstrated.

SURVEILLANCE FOR INFECTION IN VACCINATED POPULATION

Surveillance must be conducted on vaccinated flocks to determine if the field virus is circulating and the control strategy is working. This should be done by both serological and virological surveillance of vaccinated and nonvaccinated flocks. For serological surveillance, several methods can be used to identify infections by field virus in vaccinated populations: (*a*) placement of unvaccinated sentinel birds and looking for antibodies against AI viruses, such as in ducks, (*b*) if using inactivated vaccine, looking for specific antibodies against NA of the circulating field virus in vaccinated birds (if using an inactivated vaccine strain with different NA subtypes than circulating field virus[12]), or looking for antibodies against the nonstructural protein,[13] or (*c*) if using recombinant fowlpox vaccine, looking for antibodies to nucleoprotein/matrix protein. For virological surveillance, examination for specific AI viral nucleic acids or proteins, or isolation of the virus may be used to determine if the field virus is circulating. This is best done on sentinel birds that are showing clinical signs or that die. Alternatively, examination of dead poultry from vaccinated populations will give an indication if the field virus is circulating.

ACKNOWLEDGMENT

Some concepts in this article were originally presented in PROMED 20050307.0680.

REFERENCES

1. SWAYNE, D.E. 2004. Application of new vaccine technologies for the control of transboundary diseases. Dev. Biol. (Basel) **119:** 219–228.
2. SWAYNE, D.E. & D.A. HALVORSON. 2003. Influenza. *In* Diseases of Poultry. Y.M. Saif, H.J. Barnes, A.M. Fadly, J.R. Glisson, L.R. McDougald & D.E. Swayne, Eds.: 135–160. Iowa State University Press. Ames, IA.
3. SUAREZ, D.L. & C.S. SCHULTZ. 2000. Immunology of avian influenza virus: a review. Dev. Comp. Immunol. **24:** 269–283.
4. QIAO, C.L., K.Z. YU, Y.P. JIANG, *et al.* 2003. Protection of chickens against highly lethal H5N1 and H7N1 avian influenza viruses with a recombinant fowlpox virus co-expressing H5 haemagglutinin and N1 neuraminidase genes. Avian Pathol. **32:** 25–32.
5. SWAYNE, D.E., J.R. BECK & N. KINNEY. 2000. Failure of a recombinant fowl poxvirus vaccine containing an avian influenza hemagglutinin gene to provide consistent protection against influenza in chickens preimmunized with a fowl pox vaccine. Avian Dis. **44:** 132–137.
6. SWAYNE, D.E. 2003. Vaccines for list A poultry diseases: emphasis on avian influenza. Dev. Biol. (Basel) **114:** 201–212.
7. CAPUA, I., C. TERREGINO, G. CATTOLI & A. TOFFAN. 2004. Increased resistance of vaccinated turkeys to experimental infection with an H7N3 low-pathogenicity avian influenza virus. Avian Pathol. **33:** 158–163.
8. SWAYNE, D.E., M.L. PERDUE, J.R. BECK, *et al.* 2000. Vaccines protect chickens against H5 highly pathogenic avian influenza in the face of genetic changes in field viruses over multiple years. Vet. Microbiol. **74:** 165–172.
9. LEE, C.W., D.A. SENNE & D.L. SUAREZ. 2004. Effect of vaccine use in the evolution of Mexican lineage H5N2 avian influenza virus. J. Virol. **78:** 8372–8381.
10. LEE, C.W., D.A. SENNE & D.L. SUAREZ. 2004. Generation of reassortant influenza vaccines by reverse genetics that allows utilization of a DIVA (differentiating infected from vaccinated animals). Vaccine **22:** 3175–3181.

11. LIU, M., J.M. WOOD, T. ELLIS, *et al*. 2003. Preparation of a standardized, efficacious agricultural H5N3 vaccine by reverse genetics. Virology **314:** 580–590.
12. CAPUA, I., C. TERREGINO, G. CATTOLI, *et al*. 2003. Development of a DIVA (differentiating infected from vaccinated animals) strategy using a vaccine containing a heterologous neuraminidase for the control of avian influenza. Avian Pathol. **32:** 47–55.
13. TUMPEY, T.M., R. ALVAREZ, D.E. SWAYNE & D.L. SUAREZ. 2005. A diagnostic aid for differentiating infected from vaccinated poultry based on antibodies to the nonstructural (NS1) protein of influenza A virus. J. Clin. Microbiol. **43:** 676–683.

Vaccines Developed for H5 Highly Pathogenic Avian Influenza in China

CHUANLING QIAO,[a,b] GUOBIN TIAN,[a,b] YONGPING JIANG,[a,b] YANBING LI,[a,b] JIANZHONG SHI,[a,b] KANGZHEN YU,[a*] AND HUALAN CHEN[a,b**]

[a]Animal Influenza Laboratory of the Ministry of Agriculture, Harbin 150001, People's Republic of China

[b]National Kay Laboratory of Veterinary Biotechnology, Harbin Veterinary Research Institute, Chinese Academy of Agricultural Sciences, Harbin 150001, People's Republic of China

ABSTRACT: Since the first detection of highly pathogenic H5N1 avian influenza virus from sick goose in Guangdong province in China in 1996, scientists in China started to develop vaccines for avian influenza pandemic preparedness. An H5N2 inactivated vaccine was produced from a low pathogenic virus, A/turkey/England/N-28/73, and was used for the buffer zone vaccination in the H5N1 outbreaks in 2004 in China. We also generated a low pathogenic H5N1 reassortant virus A/Harbin/Re-1/2003 (Re-1) that derives its HA and NA genes from GSGD/96 virus and six internal genes from the high-growth A/Puerto Rico/8/34 (PR8) virus by using plasmid-based reverse genetics. The inactivated vaccine derived from Re-1 strain could induce more than 10 months protective immune response in chickens after one dose inoculation, and most importantly, this vaccine is immunogenic for geese and ducks. An H5N1 fowlpox vectored live vaccine was also generated by inserting the HA and NA genes of GSGD/96 virus in the genome of a fowlpox vaccine strain. Laboratory tests indicated that after one dose of immunization of this vaccine, chickens could develop an over than 40 weeks protective immune response against H5N1 virus challenge.

KEYWORDS: vaccines; H5 subtype; highly pathogenic avian influenza

INTRODUCTION

An H5N1 avian influenza virus A/goose/Guangdong/1/96(GSGD/96) was first isolated from geese in Guangdong province in China in 1996.[1,2] In 1997,

**Address for correspondence: Hualan Chen, Harbin Veterinary Research Institute, CAAS, 427 Maduan Street, Harbin 150001, People's Republic of China. Voice: 86-451-82761925; fax: 86-451-82733132.

e-mail: hlchen1@yahoo.com

*Current address: Kangzhen Yu, National Animal Husbandry and Veterinary Service of the Ministry of Agriculture, 20 Maizidian Street, Beijing 100026, People's Republic of China.

Ann. N.Y. Acad. Sci. 1081: 182–192 (2006). © 2006 New York Academy of Sciences.
doi: 10.1196/annals.1373.022

H5N1 avian influenza virus caused disease outbreaks in poultry in Hong Kong[3,4] and a reassortant virus bearing the hemagglutinin (HA) gene of the GSGD/96-like virus and the NA gene, and six internal genes from H6N1-subtype A/teal/Hong Kong/W312/97-like virus[5] was transmitted to humans and caused six deaths in 18 infected people.[6,7] Continuing outbreaks of highly pathogenic avian influenza (HPAI) in a number of countries emphasize that the H5N1 viruses are not only pathogens disastrous for domestic poultry but also bears a substantial threat to public health.

An inactivated vaccine derived from A/turkey/England/N-28/73 (H5N2) was used for the buffer zone vaccination in the H5N1 outbreaks in 2004 in China. And now a genetically modified reassortant H5N1 low pathogenic avian influenza A/Harbin/Re-1/2003 (Re-1) virus that derives its HA and NA genes from GSGD/96 virus and six internal genes from the high-growth A/Puerto Rico/8/34 (PR8) virus by plasmid-based reverse genetics, was generated as described previously.[8] Furthermore, a recombinant fowlpox virus co-expressing HA and NA genes of GSGD/96 virus has been proved to be very immunogenic in specific-pathogen-free (SPF) chickens in the previous study.[9]

In the present article, the efficacies of a formalin-inactivated vaccine derived from A/Harbin/Re-1/2003 (Re-1) and an H5N1 fowlpox vectored live vaccine were evaluated. We also demonstrated that this inactivated vaccine is immunogenic in ducks and geese and is able to completely protect these waterfowl from highly pathogenic H5N1 virus challenge.

MATERIALS AND METHODS

Viruses

A PR8-based reassortant virus, A/Harbin/Re-1/2003 (Re-1), which contains the HA and NA genes of GSGD/96, was generated as described previously.[10]

A recombinant fowlpox rFPV-HA-NA virus co-expressing HA and NA genes of GSGD/96 virus was constructed as previously reported.[9]

GSGD/96 was the first H5N1 HPAI virus isolated in China and has been characterized as previously reported.[1,2] CKTJ/04 and DKSH/04 were isolated during the 2004 outbreaks. The viruses were propagated in the allantoic cavity of 10-day-old SPF chicken embryonated eggs and kept in a $-70°C$ freezer before use for challenge study.

Efficacy of a Formalin-Inactivated Re-1 Virus Vaccine in Chickens, Geese, and Ducks

All the laboratory and field tests were conducted as previously reported.[10]

Immune Efficacy of a Fowlpox Virus Vectored Vaccine in Chickens

A total of 80 4-week-old white Leghorn SPF chickens were randomly alloc-ated into eight groups. Eight chickens of each group were vaccinated with one dose of vaccine containing 2×10^3 PFU of rFPV-HA-NA. Another two chickens were kept as control for challenge. Serum was firstly collected at 3 days after vaccination, and then sera were collected on a weekly base to check the dynamic changes in the hemagglutinin inhibition (HI) antibody titer after immunization. Challenge experiment was carried out, respectively, 3 days, and 1, 2, 10, 20, 30, 35, and 40 weeks after immunization.

Challenge Experiments

The experimental animals were challenged with 10^7 EID$_{50}$ (or 100 CLD$_{50}$) of the homologous virus GSGD/96 intranasally. Oropharyngeal and cloacal swabs were collected on day 3, 5, and 7 post challenge (p.c.) for virus titration, and animals were observed for disease signs and death for 2 weeks after challenge experiments. And these experiments were conducted in a P3 facility.

Serologic Tests and Virus Titration

Hemagglutination inhibition assays were performed by following the WHO standard. Each swab was washed in 1 mL cold PBS and virus titration was conducted in 10-day-old SPF embryonated chickens' eggs and calculated by the method of Reed and Muench.[11]

RESULTS

Immunogenicity and Protective Efficacy of Re-1 Formalin-Inactivated Vaccine in Chickens

The 0.3 mL of formalin-inactivated vaccines (containing 2.8 μg of the HA protein) prepared from the Re-1 virus were intramuscularly (i.m.) injected into 3-week-old SPF chickens, and sera was collected on a weekly base to check the dynamic changes in the HI antibody titer. As shown in FIGURE 1, the HI antibody was detected at 1-week post vaccination (p.v.) and reached the peak of 10 log 2 at 6 weeks p.v., then very slowly declined to 4 log 2 at 43 weeks p.v.

To determine whether the long-lasting HI antibody of the immunized chickens still correlated with protection, groups of chickens were challenged with the homologous highly pathogenic virus GSGD/96 at the different

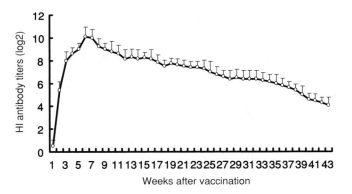

FIGURE 1. HI antibody duration induced by inactivated vaccine derived from Re-1 strain in SPF chickens. Three-week-old white Leghorn SPF chickens were injected i.m. with 0.3 mL of formalin-inactivated vaccine, and sera were collected randomly from eight chickens on a weekly base for HI antibody detection. The bars indicate the standard deviation.

time points of 2, 3, and 43 weeks p.v., respectively. The results (shown in TABLE 1) indicate that the vaccinated chickens were completely protected from GSGD/96 challenge at 2, 3, and 43 weeks p.v. When we challenged the chickens at 3 weeks p.v. with A/chicken/Tianjing/65/2004 (H5N1) (CKTJ/04) and A/duck/Shanghai/16/2004 (H5N1) (DKSH/04), respectively. The results show that the chickens were completely protected from death and disease (TABLE 1).

The Vaccine Efficacy in Geese

Laboratory Studies

Three-week-old geese were immunized with 0.5 mL of the vaccine, and challenge was conducted 2 and 3 weeks after immunization. The results shown in TABLE 2 indicated that the geese were completely protected from the challenge at 3 weeks after vaccination.

Field Studies

The HI antibody duration in the geese vaccinated in the field are shown in FIGURE 2 A. During the 36 weeks investigation period, the geese were given three shots in total. Geese developed HI antibody very slowly after the first shot. However, the antibody increased sharply and reached the peak of 10 log 2 at 3 weeks after the second immunization and then gradually declined to 4

TABLE 1. Protective efficacy of the H5N1 formalin-inactivated vaccines in SPF chickens

Administration			Virus isolation from the swabs on different days p.c.: shedding/total ($\log_{10}EID_{50}$)						
			Day 3		Day 5		Day 7		Survival/total
Vaccines	Challenge virus	Challenge time (weeks p.v.)	Oropharyngeal	Cloacal	Oropharyngeal	Cloacal	Oropharyngeal	Cloacal	
Experiment I									
Re-1	GSGD/96	2	1/8 (0.9)	0/8	0/8	0/8	0/8	0/8	8/8
Control	GSGD/96	2	8/8 (3.1 ± 0.6)	8/8 (2.4 ± 1.2)	5/5 (2.4 ± 0.6)	5/5 (2.9 ± 0.5)	[b]	[b]	0/8
Re-1	GSGD/96	3	0/8	0/8	0/8	0/8	0/8	0/8	8/8
Control	GSGD/96	3	8/8 (3.3 ± 0.9)	8/8 (2.2 ± 1.3)	6/6 (2.4 ± 0.7)	6/6 (2.7 ± 0.6)	[b]	[b]	0/8
Re-1	GSGD/96	43	0/8	0/8	0/8	0/8	0/8	0/8	8/8
Control	GSGD/96	43	8/8 (3.1 ± 0.6)	8/8 (2.6 ± 0.6)	1/1 (1.9)	1/1 (1.4)	[b]	[b]	0/8
Experiment II									
Re-1	CKTJ/04	3	2/8 (1.0 ± 0.9)	0/8	0/8	0/8	0/8	0/8	8/8
Control	CKTJ/04	3	8/8 (4.1 ± 0.5)	8/8 (3.8 ± 0.8)	[b]	[b]	[b]	[b]	0/8
Re-1	DKNH/04	3	0/8	0/8	0/8	0/8	0/8	0/8	8/8
Control	DKNH/04	3	8/8 (3.9 ± 0.7)	8/8 (4.3 ± 0.3)	[b]	[b]	[b]	[b]	0/8

[a]Groups of 3-week-old SPF chickens were vaccinated with 0.3 mL of the vaccine preparations and challenged with GSGD/96 at different time points of 2, 3, 26, and 43 weeks p.v. respectively, in experiment I. In experiment II, groups of vaccinated chickens were challenged with two H5N1 avian influenza viruses isolated in China in 2004 at 3 weeks p.v.
[b]Chickens died.

TABLE 2. Vaccine efficacy of the H5N1 inactivated vaccine in geese and ducks

Administration[a]			Virus isolation from the swabs collected on different days after challenge: positive/total (titers, $\log_{10}EID_{50}$)						
Group and vaccination schedule		Challenge time (weeks p.v.)	Day 3		Day 5		Day 7		Survival /total
			Oropharyngeal	Cloacal	Oropharyngeal	Cloacal	Oropharyngeal	Cloacal	
Geese[a]	Vaccinated	2	1/5 (0.9)	0/5 (<)	4/5 (2.0 ± 1.4)	3/5 (0.8 ± 0.4)	1/3 (2.0)	2/3 (2.1 ± 1.4)	3/5
	Control	2	3/5 (1.6 ± 1.3)	0/5 (<)	5/5 (2.4 ± 0.1)	3/5 (1.8 ± 1.0)	[b]	[b]	0/5
	Vaccinated	3	0/5 (<)[g]	0/5 (<)	0/5 (<)	0/5 (<)	0/5 (<)	0/5 (<)	5/5
	Control	3	0/5 (<)	1/5 (1.5)	5/5 (1.7 ± 0.4)	3/5 (1.1 ± 0.5)	2/2 (2.4 ± 0.2)	2/2 (1.7 ± 0.3)	0/5
Field geese	Vaccinated	34[c]	0/10	0/10	0/10	0/10	0/10	0/10	10/10
	Control	[d]	9/10 (1.4 ± 1.1)	4/10 (0.9 ± 0.7)	9/9 (3.2 ± 0.7)	3/9 (0.9 ± 0.7)	1/1 (3.3)	[b]	0/10
Ducks[a]	Vaccinated	3	0/30 (<)	0/30 (<)	0/30 (<)	0/30 (<)	0/30 (<)	0/30 (<)	30/30
	Control	3	13/15 (2.1 ± 0.8)	8/15 (1.8 ± 0.6)	7/15 (2.1 ± 1.0)	5/15 (0.8 ± 0.3)	0/2 (<)	0/2 (<)	2/15
Field ducks	Vaccinated	51[e]	2/10 (0.6 ± 0.1)	0/10 (<)	0/10 (<)	0/10 (<)	0/10 (<)	0/10 (<)	10/10
	Control	[f]	10/10 (3.0 ± 0.6)	3/10 (1.2 ± 1.1)	5/9 (1.8 ± 1.2)	1/9 (0.7 ± 0.5)	0/9 (<)	0/9 (<)	9/10

[a] Three-week-old avian influenza serological negative geese or ducks were vaccinated with 0.5 mL of the Re-1 vaccine preparations and were challenged with $10^{7.5}$ EID$_{50}$ of the highly pathogenic virus DKSH/04 in 0.1 mL volume intranasally at 2 or 3 weeks p.v.
[b] All geese in that group died.
[c] Geese were challenged at 34 weeks after the first shot (20 weeks after the third shot).
[d] Eight-month-old avian influenza negative geese were used as a control.
[e] Ducks were challenged 52 weeks after the first shot (38 weeks after the second shot).
[f] Ten-month-old avian influenza negative ducks were used as a control.
[g] "<" means virus was not detected from undiluted samples.

log 2 by 13 weeks (17 weeks after the first immunization). The pattern of the antibody titers after the third shot is similar to that induced by the second shot, but the antibody duration was 4 weeks longer than the previous one.

When the HI antibody declined to 4 log 2 (17 weeks after the third shot), 10 geese were transferred to negative pressure isolates in the laboratory and challenged with $10^{7.5}$ EID_{50} of highly pathogenic H5N1 avian influenza virus DKSH/2004. As shown in TABLE 2, all of the vaccinated geese were completely protected from the virus challenge.

Vaccine Efficacy in Ducks

Laboratory Studies

Three-week-old avian influenza serological negative ducks were immunized with 0.5 mL of the Re-1 vaccine preparations and were challenged 3 weeks after immunization with HPAI virus. As shown in TABLE 2, all the vaccinated ducks were completely protected during the 1-month observation period.

Field Studies

To investigate the antibody kinetics induced by vaccination in ducks, sera were collected randomly from 20 of the vaccinated ducks in the field on a weekly base for HI antibody detection. As shown in FIGURE 2 B, the average HI antibody titer of 3 log 2 was detected 1 week p.v., reached the peak of 8 log 2 at 4 weeks p.v., and then gradually declined to 4 log 2 by 14 weeks p.v. The antibody titers increased rapidly to 10 log 2 1 week after the second shot, and remained at 6 log 2 38 weeks later (52 weeks after first dose, the end of the observation period) (FIG. 2 B).

At 38 weeks after the second shot, 10 ducks from the field were transferred to the laboratory and challenged with $10^{7.5}$ EID_{50} of the H5N1 highly pathogenic virus DKSH/04 intranasally The results shown in TABLE 2 indicated that the vaccinated ducks were protected from clinical disease and death, though low titers of virus (from undiluted samples) were detected from the oropharyngeal swabs of two ducks on day 3 after challenge. Only one duck in the control group died during the 2 weeks observation period, indicating that adult ducks are much more resistant to the H5N1 avian influenza viruses compared with the young ducks.

Immune Efficacy of a Fowlpox Virus Vectored Vaccine in Chickens

Four-week-old chickens were vaccinated with one dose of vaccine containing 2×10^3 PFU of rFPV-HA-NA. Sera were collected on a weekly base to check

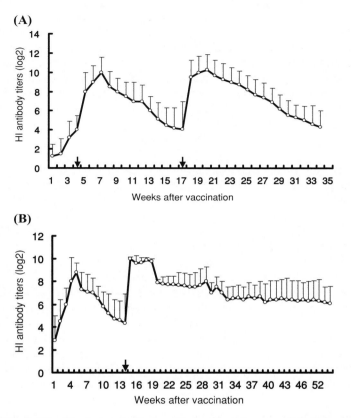

FIGURE 2. HI antibody duration induced by inactivated vaccine derived from the Re-1 strain in geese (**A**) and ducks (**B**). Field geese were vaccinated two more times with 1.5 mL of the vaccine preparation with 13.8 μg HA protein at 4 and 17 weeks, respectively, after the first shot with 0.5 mL of the vaccine preparation containing 4.6 μg HA protein. Ducks received the second shot of 1.0 mL of the vaccine preparation with 9.2 μg HA protein at 14 weeks after the first shot with 0.5 mL of the vaccine preparation containing 4.6 μg HA protein. Sera were collected randomly from 20 of each type of birds on a weekly base for the HI antibody detection. The bars indicate the standard deviation and the arrows indicate the time points for the second or third shots.

the dynamic changes in the HI antibody titer. The HI antibody was detected 1 week after vaccination and rise up to about 7.0 log 2 2 weeks p.v. The HI antibody titer keeps above 4 log 2 till 30 weeks p.v., then it slowly declined to about 3 log 2 40 weeks after immunization.

To determine whether the long-lasting HI antibody of the immunized chickens still correlated with protection, groups of chickens were challenged with GSGD/96 at the different time points of 3 days, and 1, 2, 10, 20, 30, 35, and 40 weeks after immunization. The results indicate that all the vaccinated chickens were protected from virus-shedding, clinical disease signs, and death after challenged with GSGD/96 1, 2, 10, 20, 30, 35, and 40 weeks after immunization, while the control chickens died within 2 weeks (data not shown). These results demonstrated that one-dose of the recombinant virus vaccine could induce complete protection against challenge with H5N1 HPAI virus 1 week after immunization and the immunity could last for at least 40 weeks.

DISCUSSION

The efficacy of the inactivated whole virus vaccines for avian influenza in chickens and turkeys have been confirmed and this kind of vaccines have been used to control the outbreaks caused by highly pathogenic H5 and H7 viruses.[12,13] Using plasmid-based reverse genetics, we have generated the low-pathogenicity/high growth H5N1 virus Re-1 strain, which is antigenically well-matched with the H5N1 highly pathogenic viruses found in China. The animal studies indicate that the H5N1 vaccine derived from the Re-1 strain is immunogenic and efficient in chickens, ducks, and geese.

Though the inactivated whole virus AI vaccines have shown efficacy against the outbreak of HPAI, it would induce immune responses to the group-specific influenza A nucleoprotein (NP) antigen that negates detection of natural infection.[14] Several studies were conducted on the basis of development of a novel vaccine strategy. HA and NA are the major surface glycoproteins of influenza A virus primarily involved in the induction of specific humoral immunity. Functionally, distinct roles have been attributed to the humoral response elicited by these two viral proteins. A variety of vaccines derived from HA and NA genes of AIV, including recombinant virus vaccine,[15] subunit hemagglutinin protein,[16] and DNA vaccines[17] have been shown experimentally to be effective for immunization against influenza. In this study, the immunogenicity and efficacy of a recombinant fowlpox virus expressing HA and NA genes of avian influenza virus was evaluated in SPF and commercial chickens. One-dose of the recombinant virus vaccine could induce complete protection against challenge with H5N1 highly pathogenic avian influenza virus. The immune efficacy, protecting chickens from the clinical signs and death after challenge, was obtained 1 week after immunization and the immunity could last for 40 weeks.

In summary, we generated a high-growth H5N1 reassortant as an inactivated vaccine seed virus by plasmid-based reverse genetics and demonstrated that one dose of inactivated oil-emulsion vaccine could induce 10 months of protective immune response in chickens. Moreover, we first provided evidence that the oil emulsion inactivated vaccine is indeed immunogenic and then proved the efficacy in domestic ducks and geese, which demonstrates that it is actually feasible to apply vaccines to protecting domestic waterfowl from H5N1 influenza virus infection. And an H5N1 fowlpox vectored live vaccine was also generated by inserting the HA and NA genes of GSGD/96 virus in the genome of a fowlpox vaccine strain. Laboratory tests indicated that after one dose of immunization of this vaccine, chickens could develop an over than 40 weeks protective immune response against H5N1 virus challenge. This vaccine is much cheaper than the inactivated vaccines, and the application of this vaccine will not interfere with the NP-based antibody avian influenza serological surveillance. The proper application of these vaccines is expected to play key role in the eradication of HPAI viruses in China.

REFERENCES

1. CHEN, H., G. DENG, Z. LI, *et al.* 2004. The evolution of H5N1 influenza viruses in ducks in southern China. Proc. Natl. Acad. Sci. USA **101:** 10452–10457.
2. XU, X.Y., K. SUBBARAO, N.J. COX & Y.J. GUO. 1999. Genetic characterization of the pathogenic influenza A/Goose/Guangdong/1/96 (H5N1) virus: similarity of its hemagglutinin gene to those of H5N1 viruses from the 1997 outbreaks in Hong Kong. Virology **261:** 15–19.
3. SIMS, L.D., Y. GUAN, T.M. ELLIS, *et al.* 2003. An update on avian influenza in Hong Kong 2002. Avian. Dis. **47**(Suppl): 1083–1086.
4. SHORTRIDGE, K.F., N.N. ZHOU, Y. GUAN, *et al.* 1998. Characterization of avian H5N1 influenza viruses from poultry in Hong Kong. Virology **252:** 331–342.
5. CHIN, P.S., E. HOFFMANN, R. WEBBY, *et al.* 2002. Molecular evolution of H6 influenza viruses from poultry in southeastern China: prevalence of H6N1 influenza viruses possessing seven A/Hong Kong/156/97 (H5N1)-like genes in poultry. J. Virol. **76:** 507–516.
6. CLAAS, E.C., A.D. OSTERHAUS, R. VAN BEEK, *et al.* 1998. Human influenza A H5N1 virus related to a highly pathogenic avian influenza virus. Lancet **351:** 472–477.
7. SUBBARAO, K., A. KLIMOV, J. KATZ, *et al.* 1998. Characterization of an avian influenza A (H5N1) virus isolated from a child with a fatal respiratory illness. Science **279:** 393–396.
8. SUBBARAO, K., H. CHEN, D. SWAYNE, *et al.* 2003. Evaluation of a genetically modified reassortant H5N1 influenza A virus vaccine candidate generated by plasmid-based reverse genetics. Virology **305:** 192–200.
9. QIAO, C.L., K.Z. YU, Y.P. JIANG, *et al.* 2003. Protection of chickens against highly lethal H5N1 and H7N1 avian influenza viruses with a recombinant fowlpox virus co-expressing H5 haemagglutinin and N1 neuraminidase genes. Avian. Pathol. **32:** 25–32.
10. TIAN, G.B., S.H. ZHANG, Y.B. LI, *et al.* 2005. Protective efficacy in chickens, geese and ducks of an H5N1-inactivated vaccine developed by reverse genetics. Virology **341:** 153–162.
11. REED, L.J. & H. MUENCH. 1938. A simple method of estimating fifty percent endpoints. Am. J. Hyg. **27:** 493–497.
12. CAPUA, I., C. TERREGINO, G. CATTOLI, *et al.* 2003. Development of a differentiating infected from vaccinated animals (DIVA) strategy using a vaccine containing a heterologous neuraminidase for the control of avian influenza. Avian. Pathol. **32:** 47–55.

13. ELLIS, T.M., C.Y. LEUNG, M.K. CHOW, *et al*. 2004. Vaccination of chickens against H5N1 avian influenza in the face of an outbreak interrupts virus transmission. Avian. Pathol. **33:** 405–412.
14. BEARD, C.W., W.M. SCHNITZLEIN & D.N. TRIPATHY. 1991. Protection of chickens against highly pathogenic avian influenza virus(H5N2) by recombinant fowlpox viruses. Avian. Dis. **35:** 356–359.
15. CHAMBER, T., Y. KAWAOKA & R.G. WEBSTER. 1988. Protection of chickens from lethal influenza infection by vaccinia expressed hemagglutinin. Virology **167:** 414–421.
16. KODIHALLI, S., V. SIVANANDAN, K.V. NAGARAJA, *et al*. 1994. A type-specific avian influenza virus subunit vaccine for turkeys: induction of protective immunity to challenge infection. Vaccine **12:** 1467–1472.
17. CHEN, Z., S. KADOWAKI, Y. HAGIWARA, *et al*. 2000. Cross-protection against a lethal influenza virus infection by DNA vaccine to neuraminidase. Vaccine **18:** 3214–3222.

Development and Use of Fowlpox Vectored Vaccines for Avian Influenza

MICHEL BUBLOT,[a] NIKKI PRITCHARD,[b] DAVID E. SWAYNE,[c]
PAUL SELLECK,[d] KEMAL KARACA,[e] DAVID L. SUAREZ,[c]
JEAN-CHRISTOPHE AUDONNET,[a] AND THOMAS R. MICKLE[f]

[a]Merial SAS, Discovery Research, 69007 Lyon, France

[b]Merial Select, Inc. Gainesville, Georgia 30503, USA

[c]Southeast Poultry Research Laboratory, Agricultural Research Service, U.S.
Department of Agriculture, Athens, Georgia 30605, USA

[d]Commonwealth Scientific and Industrial Research Organization, Geelong
3220, Australia

[e]Merial Limited Inc., Athens, Georgia 30601, USA

[f]Merial Avian Global Enterprise, Gainesville, Georgia 30503, USA

ABSTRACT: The avian influenza (AI) vaccine designated TROVAC™-AIV H5 (TROVAC-H5) contains a live recombinant fowlpox rec. (FP) recombinant (recFP), expressing the hemagglutinin (HA) gene of an AI H5 subtype isolate. This recombinant vaccine was granted a license in the United States for emergency use in 1998 and full registration in Mexico, Guatemala, and El Salvador where over 2 billion doses have been administered. One injection of TROVAC-H5 protects chickens against AI-induced mortality and morbidity for at least 20 weeks, and significantly decreases shedding after challenge with a wide panel of H5-subtype AI strains, regardless of neuraminidase subtype. Recently, excellent protection was demonstrated against 2003 and 2004 Asian highly pathogenic H5N1 isolates. Whereas TROVAC-H5 AI H5 efficacy was not inhibited by anti-AI or anti-fowlpox maternal antibodies (passive immunity), protection to AI was significantly decreased in chickens previously vaccinated or infected with FP (active immunity). Advantages of the TROVAC-H5 vaccine over inactivated AI vaccines are: (*a*) single administration at 1 day of age and early onset (1 week) of protection, (*b*) easy monitoring of AI infection in vaccinated flocks with agar gel precipitation (AGP) and enzyme-linked immunosorbent assay (ELISA) used as tests to differentiate infected from vaccinated animals (DIVA tests), and (*c*) no residue problem due to adjuvant. These features make TROVAC-H5 an ideal AI vaccine for routine administration of day-of-age chicks in hatcheries.

Address for correspondence: Michel Bublot, Merial SAS, Discovery Research, 254, rue Marcel Mérieux, 69007 Lyon, France. Voice: 33-4-7272-5973; fax: 33-4-7272-3316.
  e-mail: michel.bublot@merial.com

Ann. N.Y. Acad. Sci. 1081: 193–201 (2006). © 2006 New York Academy of Sciences.
doi: 10.1196/annals.1373.023

RecFP expressing HA from three lineages of H7 subtype (Eurasian, American, and Australian) were also tested for efficacy against a highly pathogenic avian influenza (HPAI) Eurasian HPAI H7N1. Only the recFP expressing the Eurasian H7 gene provided sufficient protection indicating that the breadth of protection induced by recFP is apparently restricted for H7 isolates. The fowlpox vector technology can also be used for the production of an emergency vaccine: once the HA sequence of an emerging AI virus is known, recFP can be rapidly generated. TROVAC-H5 has recently been shown to be immunogenic in cats and could therefore also be considered for use in mammals.

KEYWORDS: avian influenza; recombinant vaccine; fowlpox vector; DIVA vaccine

INTRODUCTION

Biosecurity is the first line of defense against avian influenza (AI), but controlled vaccination has been recognized as a useful tool to help eradication. There are currently two types of licensed AI vaccines: inactivated vaccines and recombinant fowlpox vaccines (recFP). Inactivated vaccines are the most widely used vaccines in AI vaccination programs. They are particularly well suited to protect adult chickens, turkeys, and other birds in emergency situations, e.g., when ring vaccination is used in an outbreak area. However, in young chicks, their efficacy is optimal only at 2–3 weeks of age, and they cannot induce optimal protection in one-day-old birds. Other problems with inactivated vaccines are that (a) they require individual administration by parenteral route, (b) there is currently no serology test commercially available that can differentiate infected from noninfected birds in a vaccinated population (i.e., DIVA test), and (c) reactions to the killed vaccines may cause a drop in performance when given at one day of age. Thus, monitoring infection in vaccinated flocks requires the use of unvaccinated sentinel birds, or ad hoc heterologous neuraminidase tests can be developed and used if vaccine and field strains have different neuraminidase subtypes.[1] Alternative AI vaccines are needed to overcome these problems.

Fowlpox-based AI vaccines have been generated and evaluated by several laboratories.[2–15] The AI vaccine designated TROVAC[TM]-AIV H5 (TROVAC-H5) contains a live recFP, expressing the hemagglutinin (HA) gene of an AI H5 subtype isolate, and it has been widely used in Central America with over 1.6 billion doses used in the field. The current information on the TROVAC-H5 vaccine will be reviewed. Furthermore, recent data obtained with recFP for the H7 subtype, as well as potential applications of the recFP technology as emergency AI vaccine for chickens or mammals, will be presented.

TROVAC™-AIV H5 VACCINE

TROVAC™-AIV H5 Vaccine Description and Administration

TROVAC-H5 is a recFP expressing the HA of the A/turkey/Ireland/1378/83 H5N8 isolate. The fowlpox vector was derived from the vaccine strain contained in the DIFTOSEC fowlpox vaccine.[2] TROVAC-H5 received license in the United States in 1998 and has since been used in Mexico, Guatemala, and El Salvador, and was recently authorized in Vietnam.

TROVAC-H5 is adapted to administration one-day-old in the hatchery where the environment is clean, biosecurity is optimal, and the vaccination equipment is available with qualified operators. The aqueous solution of TROVAC-H5 is easier to inject than the oily emulsion of inactivated vaccines. It is administered by subcutaneous (SC) injection into the nape of the neck using Marek's disease automatic or semiautomatic injection machines. The vaccine is approved for combination with Marek's and Bursal disease vaccine. The control of AI vaccination in a specific area may be better achieved by vaccination in hatcheries rather than at the farms. TROVAC-H5 vaccine may also be used to vaccinate any age bird as long as a live fowlpox vaccine or natural infection with fowlpox has not preceded the use of TROVAC-H5 (see below).

TROVAC™-AIV H5 Vaccine Safety

The fowlpox virus is host species specific and replicates poorly, if at all, in non-gallinaceous avian species. Injection of cats and mice with the TROVAC-H5 vaccine did not result in any adverse reactions. Attempts to isolate the fowlpox virus from the skin at the injection site or from internal organs of mice have been unsuccessful.

Safety experiments have been conducted in chickens (100 × dose) as well as in several nontarget avian species including ducks, pigeons, quails, and turkeys. No adverse reactions were reported. In chicken studies, TROVAC-H5 did not spread from bird to bird when vaccinates were commingled with unvaccinated susceptible birds.

In contrast to inactivated vaccines, the manufacturing of TROVAC-H5 does not involve the production of a pathogenic agent and therefore, the risks of accidental release into the environment and incomplete inactivation during production of the vaccine are nonexistent.

Field trials have been performed in three states in the United States (Georgia, Maryland, and Texas) as well as in Mexico (two trials with 48,000 and 32,000 chicks). No adverse reactions were reported.[16] Limited field trials were also performed recently in Vietnam in three farms (total of 30,000 chicks). Again, TROVAC-H5 vaccine was shown to be safe under Vietnamese field conditions.

The vaccine has been used routinely to vaccinate broiler chickens and one-day-old pullets for 7 years in Mexico, and more recently in Guatemala and El Salvador. More than 2 billion doses have been used so far, and no adverse reactions or vaccine failures have been reported, indicating safety in different field conditions.

TROVAC^(TM)-AIV H5 Vaccine Efficacy against Mexican and Other HPAI Strains Isolated before 1998

Studies aimed at evaluating the efficacy of the TROVAC-H5 vaccine were performed using a highly pathogenic avian influenza (HPAI) Mexican H5N2 isolate. The minimum protective dose of TROVAC-H5 using the SC route of administration to one-day-old specific pathogen free (SPF) chickens was shown to be as low as 1.5 $\log_{10}$ $TCID_{50}$.[10] The TROVAC-H5 vaccine protected against mortality (90–100%), and morbidity (90–100%), and cloacal (reduction of 50–75% of positive chickens), and respiratory (significant reduction of 1.0–2.1 $\log_{10}$) shedding of challenge virus.[7,10] Vaccination reduced in-contact transmission of HP AI challenge virus to both TROVAC-H5- and vector-control-vaccinated chickens.[7,10] Furthermore, the duration of immunity was at least 20 weeks after a single injection at one day of age.[10] Combined administration of TROVAC-H5 with Marek's disease vaccine at one day of age did not interfere with protection against Marek's, AI or fowlpox disease.[10]

TROVAC-H5 has been shown to be efficacious in field conditions and more particularly, in commercial chickens hatched from breeders vaccinated with fowlpox and/or inactivated AI vaccines.[16] Results have shown that significant protection (>70%) can be achieved in SPF or commercial chickens 1-week postvaccination, indicating rapid onset of protection even in commercial chickens with maternal antibodies. Full protection after challenge was obtained at 7 weeks of age (usual slaughtering age of broilers) (TABLE 1).[16] These data indicate that the presence of maternal immunity against fowlpox and maternal antibodies to AIV (passive immunity) does not significantly interfere with the induction of immunity in progeny vaccinated at one day of age with TROVAC-H5. However, protection levels decreased in birds preimmunized with a fowlpox vaccine (active immunity); hence, TROVAC-H5 is not recommended for birds previously immunized against or infected with fowlpox.[13]

TROVAC-H5 has been evaluated for efficacy against other HPAI isolates: it provided a broad-based protection (100%) against clinical signs and death following challenge by nine different HP H5 AI viruses collected over a period of 38 years that had 87.3–100% HA protein sequence similarity with vaccine HA. This result suggested that frequent updating of the HA gene in the vaccine may not be necessary.[11,12] However, some association between the HA protein sequence homology of vaccine and challenge virus and the ability to reduce shedding from the oropharynx but not from the cloaca has been observed.

TABLE 1. Morbidity, mortality, and protection observed in nonvaccinated (mock) and TROVACH-vaccinated chickens (TROVAC) after HPAI H5N2 Mexican challenge 7, 21, and 49 days after vaccination.

Type of chickens	d7		d21		d49	
	Mock	TROVAC	Mock	TROVAC	Mock	TROVAC
Control SPF	7/6/7[a]	2/0/8	6/5/7	0/0/8	7/5/7	0/0/8
	(0%[b])	(75%)	(14%)	(100%)	(0%)	(100%)
Without Mab	15/14/15	4/0/15	15/13/15	0/0/15	15/1/15	0/0/15
	(0%)	(73%)	(0%)	(100%)	(0%)	(100%)
With Mab	8/2/15	2/1/15	6/1/15	2/2/15	10/2/15	0/0/15
	(47%)	(87%)	(60%)	(87%)	(33%)	(100%)

[a]Number of sick/number of dead/total.
[b]Percentage of protection against morbidity.
[c]Three types of chickens were used: control SPF, and commercial chickens with and without AI maternal antibodies (Mab). The commercial chickens were hatched from breeders regularly vaccinated against fowlpox (adapted from Ref. 16)

Furthermore, the reduction in oropharyngeal viral titers was most consistent for challenge viruses within the same lineage (i.e., Eurasian lineage) as the vaccine.[11,12]

TROVAC[TM]-AIV H5 Vaccine Efficacy against Recent Asian H5N1 HPAI Isolates

The TROVAC-H5 vaccine has recently been evaluated for efficacy against two recent HPAI H5N1 Asian isolates: A/chicken/South Korea/03 (SK/03) and A/chicken/Vietnam/04 at South East Poultry Research Laboratory (SEPRL, USDA, ARS, Athens, Georgia, USA) and at CSIRO (Geelong, Australia), respectively.

The results of the first trial performed at SEPRL indicated levels of 100% and 92% of clinical protection against a SK/03 challenge were induced with a $1\times$ and $10\times$ dose of TROVAC-H5 administered to 1-day-old SPF chicks, respectively.[17] The amount of virus shed via the cloacal route was reduced below the detectable level for both doses of TROVAC-H5, and shedding via the oral route was reduced below the detectable level (group receiving the 10 $\times$ dose) or by 1.4 $\log_{10}$ (group receiving the $1\times$ dose), but this 1.4 $\log_{10}$ was not significantly different from the controls.[17]

The second trial performed at SEPRL compared the SK/03 chicken infectious dose 50 (CID_{50}) in unvaccinated SPF chicks or chicks vaccinated with TROVAC-H5. The SK/03 challenge virus at a concentration of $10^{3.5}$ EID_{50}/dose caused 80% mortality in the unvaccinated group. All unvaccinated chickens challenged with higher concentrations ($10^{5.0}$, $10^{6.5}$, and $10^{8.0}$) of the SK/03 virus died (mean death time of 2.4, 2.0, and 2.0 days post challenge, respectively). TROVAC-H5 vaccination protected all chickens from mortality and morbidity challenged with $\leq 6.5 \log_{10} EID_{50}$ of the SK/03, and 80%

chickens challenged with $10^{8.0}$ EID_{50}. Cloacal and oral shedding were reduced by ≥ 4 and 2–4 $\log_{10}$ in the vaccinated groups, respectively.

The efficacy of TROVAC-H5 against a A/chicken/Vietnam/04 H5N1 HPAI challenge was also evaluated in SPF chickens at CSIRO. All unvaccinated chickens died within 48 h after exposure, whereas all TROVAC-H5-vaccinated chickens were protected against both mortality and morbidity.

These three studies demonstrate that the pox vectored AI vaccine is highly efficacious against the current HPAI H5N1 isolates circulating in East Asia and are therefore a potentially valuable part of a vaccine and surveillance program to eradicate the HPAI H5 virus circulating in Asia.

The amino acid sequence of the A/turkey/Ireland/1378/83 HA expressed by TROVAC-H5 was compared to that of recent Asian H5N1 isolates. Conservation of an important antigenic site overlapping the receptor binding site (including aa 129–133)[18] was unexpectedly observed: the TROVAC-H5 HA sequence HEASLGVSS (aa125-133) was found in recent HPAI H5N1 Thailand 04, Vietnam 04, Hong Kong 03 and 02 isolates, whereas most sequences from other H5 isolates (including the Hong Kong 97 H5N1 human isolate) were HDASSGVSS. H5N1 Indonesia 04, South Korea 03, and Hong Kong 01 had the intermediate sequence HEASSGVSS. Further studies need to be done to show whether this homology plays a role in the proven efficacy of TROVAC-H5 against recent H5N1 Asian strains.

Monitoring of Vaccination and Infection in TROVAC^TM-AIV H5 Vaccinated Flocks

When using vaccination as part of an AI control strategy, it is important to be able (*a*) to check whether the birds were correctly vaccinated, and (*b*) to detect infection in a vaccinated flock.

Chickens vaccinated with TROVAC-H5 will develop high levels of antibodies (7–8 $\log_2$) detectable by the hemagglutinin inhibition (HI) test using A/turkey/Ireland/1378/83 H5N8 homologous antigen (titers up to 7-8 $\log_z$ when using ether-treated antigen). In contrast, HI titers against heterologous antigens will be very low or undetectable. In the first trial with the SK/03 challenge, only one out of 24 TROVAC-H5 vaccinated chickens had detectable HI antibodies against the SK/03 antigen before challenge, whereas 23/24 were protected. This result confirms the fact that TROVAC-H5 vaccine protects chickens even in the absence of HI antibody against the challenge virus.

TROVAC-H5 vaccine expresses the HA only. Vaccinated chickens will not produce antibodies against the matrix or nucleoprotein, detectable by common serological tests, such as agar gel precipitation (AGP; also called agar gel immunodiffusion test [AGID]) and enzyme-linked immunosorbent assay (ELISA). These tests can be used as differentiate infected from vaccinated animals (DIVA tests)[1] in order to detect infection in a vaccinated flock, and therefore, the use of sentinel birds in a TROVAC-H5-vaccinated flock may not be necessary.

FOWLPOX-H7 RECOMBINANT VACCINE

RecFP viruses (TROVAC vector) expressing the HA of H7 AI isolates belonging to each of the three lineages of H7 subtype (Eurasian, American, and Australian) were generated. A study comparing the efficacy of these three vaccine candidates against a Eurasian HPAI H7N1 challenge has shown that only the recFP expressing the Eurasian HA type provided sufficient protection (90%) against the Eurasian HPAI challenge. Australian and American HA induced partial (20%) protection in this model. This finding contrasts with the wide protection provided by the AI H5 recFP. Homologous HI titers induced by the fowlpox-H7 Eurasian recombinant were also very low (3–4 $\log_2$) compared to those induced by TROVAC-H5 (7–8 $\log_2$).

FOWLPOX RECOMBINANTS AS EMERGENCY VACCINES AND FOR MAMMALS

The fowlpox vector technology can also be used for the production of an emergency vaccine: once the HA sequence of an emerging AI virus is known, a synthetic gene can be rapidly produced and cloned into a fowlpox vector (e.g., TROVAC vector). The synthesis of the HA gene allows generation of an AI vaccine without having to import or manipulate the pathogen. A synthetic nucleotide sequence coding the HA can be designed for optimal expression and cloning, and the cleavage site can easily be modified to match that of low pathogenicity AI strains. This concept has been tested for the H5N1 Asian outbreak before knowing the excellent level of protection provided by the existing TROVAC[TM]-ANHS vaccine. The process of the receipt of the sequence to the production of a premaster seed of the fowlpox virus recombinant took place over approximately 4 months, demonstrating the feasibility to use recFPs as emergency vaccines.

RecFPs have been used also as nonreplicative vectors in mammals.[19] Reports of cats as well as of other felids (tiger and panther) becoming ill and dying from AI H5N1 were published;[20] therefore TROVAC-H5 was evaluated in cats. After one administration of 6 $\log_{10}$ TCID$_{50}$, TROVAC-H5 induced an HI titer approximately 5 $\log2$ against homologous antigen. This titer was boosted by a second administration, and significant heterologous HI titers against a recent H5N1 antigen could be detected after the second administration.[21] These data clearly show that the TROVAC-H5 vaccine is immunogenic in cats, and could therefore be considered for this and potentially other mammalian species.

CONCLUSIONS

The AI-fowlpox TROVAC^{TM}-AIV H5 vaccine has shown to be safe and efficacious against a panel of different H5 isolates including recent HPAI H5N1 isolates from East Asia. The administration of TROVAC-H5 to one-day-old chicks can be performed at the hatchery. Hatchery vaccination is an advantageous over vaccination at the farms because (*a*) commercially used vaccination devices/practices designed for one-day-old chicks can be used, (*b*) vaccination can be more easily performed, controlled, and centralized (hatcheries are less numerous than farms), and (*c*) it allows early onset of immunity. In addition, control of infection in TROVAC-H5-vaccinated flocks can easily be achieved using classical AGP or ELISA as DIVA tests.

Preliminary data obtained with recFP-H7 (TROVAC vector) indicated that the protection provided by HA gene of the H7 subtype may not be as broad as the one provided by H5 gene. In certain instances, the rapid development of homologous fowlpox-based AI vaccines may be needed and can be achieved rapidly by using a synthetic gene without having to manipulate the pathogen. Furthermore, recFPs may have application as nonreplicative vectored vaccine for influenza in mammals species.

REFERENCES

1. CAPUA, I. *et al*. 2003. Development of a DIVA (differentiating infected from vaccinated animals) strategy using a vaccine containing a heterologous neuraminidase for the control of avian influenza. Avian Pathol. **32:** 47–55.
2. TAYLOR, J. *et al*. 1988. Protective immunity against avian influenza induced by a fowlpox virus recombinant. Vaccine **6:** 504–508.
3. TRIPATHY, D.N. & W.M. SCHNITZLEIN. 1991. Expression of avian influenza virus hemagglutinin by recombinant fowlpox virus. Avian Dis. **35:** 186–191.
4. BEARD, C.W., W.M. SCHNITZLEIN & D.N. TRIPATHY. 1991. Protection of chickens against highly pathogenic avian influenza virus (H5N2) by recombinant fowlpox viruses. Avian Dis. **35:** 356–359.
5. BEARD, C.W., W.M. SCHNITZLEIN & D.N. TRIPATHY. 1992. Effect of route of administration on the efficacy of a recombinant fowlpox virus against H5N2 avian influenza. Avian Dis. **36:** 1052–1055.
6. WEBSTER, R.G. *et al*. 1991. Efficacy of nucleoprotein and haemagglutinin antigens expressed in fowlpox virus as vaccine for influenza in chickens. Vaccine **9:** 303–308.
7. WEBSTER, R.G. *et al*. 1996. Immunity to Mexican H5N2 avian influenza viruses induced by a fowlpox-H5 recombinant. Avian Dis. **40:** 461–465.
8. BOYLE, D.B. & H.G. HEINE. 1994. Influence of dose and route of inoculation on responses of chickens to recombinant fowlpox virus vaccines. Vet. Microbiol. **41:** 173–181.
9. BOYLE, D.B., P. SELLECK & H.G. HEINE. 2000. Vaccinating chickens against avian influenza with fowlpox recombinants expressing the H7 haemagglutinin. Aust Vet J. **78:** 44–48.

10. SWAYNE, D.E., J.R. BECK & T.R. MICKLE. 1997. Efficacy of recombinant fowl poxvirus vaccine in protecting chickens against a highly pathogenic Mexican-origin H5N2 avian influenza virus. Avian Dis. **41:** 910–922.
11. SWAYNE, D.E. *et al.* 2000. Protection against diverse highly pathogenic H5 avian influenza viruses in chickens immunized with a recombinant fowlpox vaccine containing an H5 avian influenza hemagglutinin gene insert. Vaccine **18:** 1088–1095.
12. SWAYNE, D.E. *et al.* 2000. Vaccines protect chickens against H5 highly pathogenic avian influenza in the face of genetic changes in field viruses over multiple years. Vet. Microbiol. **74:** 165–172.
13. SWAYNE, D.E., J.R. BECK & N. KINNEY. 2000. Failure of a recombinant fowl poxvirus vaccine containing an avian influenza hemagglutinin gene to provide consistent protection against influenza in chickens preimmunized with a fowl pox vaccine. Avian Dis. **44:** 132–137.
14. QIAO, C.L. *et al.* 2003. Protection of chickens against highly lethal H5N1 and H7N1 avian influenza viruses with a recombinant fowlpox virus co-expressing H5 haemagglutinin and N1 neuraminidase genes. Avian Pathol. **32:** 25–32.
15. CHENG, J. *et al.* 2002. Recombinant fowlpox virus expressing HA from subtype H9N2 of avian influenza virus and its protective immunity against homologous challenge in chickens. Wei Sheng Wu Xue Bao **42:** 442–447.
16. GARCIA-GARCIA, J. *et al.* 1998. Experimental studies and field trials with recombinant fowlpox vaccine in broilers in Mexico. *In* Proceedings of the Fourth International Symposium on avian influenza. Athens, Georgia, USA. D.E. Swayne & R.D. Slemons, Eds. U.S. Animal Health Association, 245–252.
17. SWAYNE, D.E. 2004. Application of new vaccine technologies for the control of transboundary diseases. *In* Control of Infectious Animal diseases by Vaccination, Vol. 119. A. Schudel & M. Lombard, Eds.: 219–228. Karger. Basel.
18. GARCIA, M. *et al.* 1997. Evolution of the H5 subtype avian influenza A viruses in North America. Virus Res. **51:** 115–124.
19. TAYLOR, J. & E. PAOLETTI. 1988. Fowlpox virus as a vector in non-avian species. Vaccine **6:** 466–468.
20. KUIKEN, T. *et al.* 2004. Avian H5N1 influenza in cats. Science **306:** 241.
21. KARACA, K. *et al.* 2005. Immunogenicity of fowlpox virus expressing the avian influenza H5 gene (TROVAC-AIV H5) in Cats. Clin. Diagn. Lab. Immunol. **12:** 1340–1342.

SEPPIC Vaccine Adjuvants for Poultry

L. DUPUIS, S. ASCARATEIL, J. AUCOUTURIER, AND V. GANNE

SEPPIC, 75321 Paris, Cedex 07, France

ABSTRACT: Two inactivated antigens (Newcastle and *Pasteurella Multocida*) were formulated with different adjuvants and tested in two separate experiments in poultry. Oil formulations constituting water in oil (W/O) or water in oil in water (W/O/W) emulsions were assessed for antibody response, protection, local reactions, and vaccine physicochemical parameters. Robust, efficacious, and safe formulations were obtained with W/O formulations whereas W/O/W was especially safe with maintained efficacy. Results show that it is possible to improve traditional Tween Span formulations for safety and efficacy parameters by using Montanide™ ISA 70 for W/O formulations and Montanide™ ISA 206 for W/O/W when safety is the priority.

KEYWORDS: adjuvants; poultry vaccine; Montanide

INTRODUCTION

Inactivated antigens require an oily formulation for the production of efficacious vaccines. Two different animal experiments were carried out to test several oily adjuvants for poultry vaccines. Vaccine efficacy, safety, and formulation robustness were compared.

MATERIAL AND METHODS

Vaccination Experiment 1

ISA Brown layers aged 16 weeks and maintained under conventional conditions at the Ecole Nationale Vétérinaire de Nantes (France) were inoculated with different vaccines. Antigen included in vaccinal preparations resulted from inactivation of a *Pasteurella multocida* strain (serotype 3) (PMS3). Protection and safety were assessed.

Address for correspondence: Laurent Dupuis, SEPPIC, 75 quai d'Orsay, 75321 Paris, Cedex 07, France. Voice: +33-0-1-40-62-53-45; fax: +33-0-1-40-62-52-53.
  email: laurent.dupuis@airliquide.com

Ann. N.Y. Acad. Sci. 1081: 202–205 (2006). © 2006 New York Academy of Sciences.
doi: 10.1196/annals.1373.024

Vaccination Experiment 2

Five hundred SPF Leghorn chicks distributed in different cages were inoculated with different vaccine formulations or different vaccine doses. The antigen is an inactivated Newcastle Disease (ND) virus. Four-week-old chicks were vaccinated intramuscularly with either complete 0.5 mL doses or 1/25th, 1/50th, or 1/100th fractional doses using micro-syringes. Three weeks after vaccination, all of the vaccinated chicks and 10 SPF nonvaccinated control subjects were inoculated with 106 LD 50 of a virulent ND virus strain via a 0.5 mL intramuscular injection on the left side of the breastbone. Protection and safety were assessed.

Adjuvants

A classical Tween Span mineral oil water in oil (W/O) emulsion was compared with different SEPPIC adjuvants (TABLE 1). W/O emulsions were prepared under high shear (rotor stator equipment). One step process water in oil in water (W/O/W) emulsion was prepared under low shear.

RESULTS

Experiment 1 (PMS3)

Antibody titers after 28 and 56 days were similar for the three W/O formulations in intensity (7000) and significantly higher than the control (FIG. 1). Local reactions were detected at all injection sites for Tween Span formulations whereas none were found in either the Montanide™ (Paris, France) ISA 70 and ISA 775 adjuvant groups or with the control antigen alone (FIG. 2).

Experiment 2 (ND)

Approximately 100% protection was obtained for 0.5 mL doses whatever the adjuvant system (FIG. 3). When the vaccine dose was reduced to 1/25th of

TABLE 1. MONTANIDE™ SEPPIC adjuvants tested in poultry vaccines

MONTANIDE™	Oil	ADJ/ANTIG (w/w)	Emulsion	Viscosity (mPa.s)
ISA 70	MINERAL	70/30	W/O	30
ISA 775	MINERAL + NONMINERAL	70/30	W/O	25
ISA 206	MINERAL	50/50	W/O/W	10

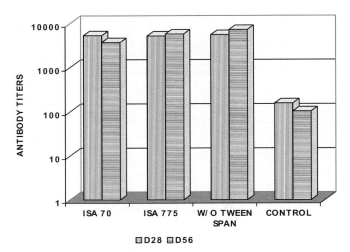

FIGURE 1. PMS3 vaccine antibody titers.

the dose, protection with ISA 70 remained 100% but dropped down to 0% for ISA 206 and to 40% for Tween Span formulation. ISA 70 conserved 100% protection for 1/50 and 1/100 volume doses, whereas ISA 206 and Tween Span no longer induced a protection. No local reactions were observed with any of the vaccines.

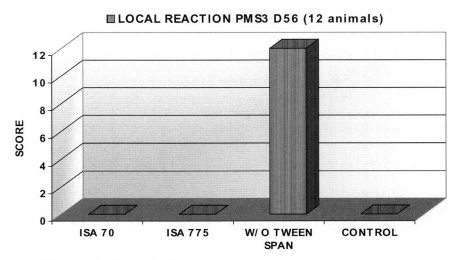

FIGURE 2. PMS3 vaccine local reactions.

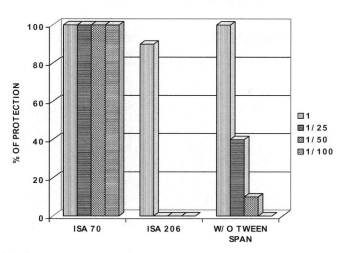

PROTECTION NEWCASTLE : DOSE EFFECT

FIGURE 3. ND vaccine dose effect.

DISCUSSION AND CONCLUSION

Different oily adjuvants were compared with a bacterial and viral antigen in poultry. Efficacy and safety were assessed and compared to classic water in mineral oil Tween Span formulation. The bacterial antigen, more immunogenic but also reactogenic, proved that a selected W/O formulation could maintain the same level of antibody response with disappearance of local reactions. For a conventional viral antigen (ND), the same formulation proved its superiority by keeping the same protection level even when the dose volume is reduced by 100 times. In this experiment, a W/O/W formulation was tested and gave a similar protection to the reference with the advantage of safety linked to aqueous fluid formulations. Furthermore, aqueous formulations can be used to dilute lyophilized live vaccines and are easy to inject. High tech adjuvants (for W/O or W/O/W) can help to reformulate existing vaccines with a cost effectiveness (reduction of the antigen load or vaccinal dose), a safety efficiency (when antigens are reactogenic or for sensitive animals), and an outstanding efficacy when a strong protection is needed. The possibility of adjusting adjuvant formulation according to antigens for efficacy, safety, and stability of the vaccine even for high antigen ratio and stability disturbing antigens is a specificity of the Montanide™ range.

West Nile Virus in Guadeloupe

Introduction, Spread, and Decrease in Circulation Level: 2002–2005

THIERRY LEFRANÇOIS,[a] BRADLEY J. BLITVICH,[b] JENNIFER PRADEL,[a]
SOPHIE MOLIA,[a] NATHALIE VACHIÉRY,[a] DOMINIQUE MARTINEZ,[a]

[a]Centre de Coopération Internationale en Recherche Agronomique pour le
Développement, Département Elevage et Médecine Vétérinaire Tropicale
(CIRAD, EMVT Department), 97170 Petit Bourg Guadeloupe

[b]Arthropod-borne and Infectious Diseases Laboratory, Department of
Microbiology, Immunology and Pathology, Colorado State University,
Fort Collins, Colorado 80523, USA

ABSTRACT: In July 2002, a surveillance system was implemented on
Guadeloupe to detect for the potential introduction and monitor the
spread of West Nile virus (WNV). From 2002 to 2004, equines and chickens were serologically assayed for antibodies to WNV by IgG and IgM
enzyme-linked immunosorbent assay (ELISA), epitope-blocking ELISA,
and plaque reduction neutralization tests. After introduction, probably
through migratory birds at the end of 2001, many seroconversions occurred between July and October 2002 resulting in a high seroprevalence
(19.3%) in equines in 2003. WNV circulation levels decreased dramatically in 2003 and 2004 as assessed by the absence of seroconversion in
equine and the very low prevalence in chickens. This decrease coincided
with a 7-month drought that presumably caused a decrease in vector
populations. In 2005, a sentinel survey was implemented in equines and
chickens placed in areas at high risk and the very low rate of seroconversion (1 equine out of 106, no chicken) demonstrated that WNV circulation
is now occurring at a very low level.

KEYWORDS: West Nile virus; *flavivirus*; Guadeloupe; Caribbean; equine;
avian; ELISA; epidemiology; public health

INTRODUCTION

West Nile virus (WNV) was introduced in the United States in September
1999 in New York state[1] and subsequently spread to the South and the West.

Address for correspondence: Thierry Lefrançois, CIRAD, EMVT Department Guadeloupe, Domaine
de Duclos, Prise d'eau, 97170 Petit Bourg, Guadeloupe, FWI. Voice: +590-590-25-5995; fax: +590-
590-94-0396.
e-mail: thierry.lefrancois@cirad.fr

Ann. N.Y. Acad. Sci. 1081: 206–215 (2006). © 2006 New York Academy of Sciences.
doi: 10.1196/annals.1373.025

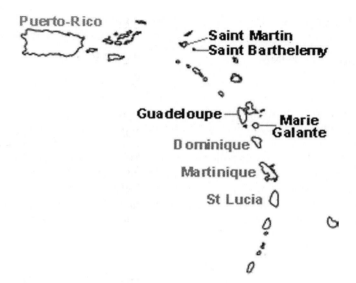

FIGURE 1. Map of the Caribbean showing the studied islands (Guadeloupe main island, Marie Galante, Saint Martin, and Saint Barthelemy).

In 2002 antibodies to WNV were detected in horses and birds in Mexico[2–4] and Guadeloupe,[5,6] and in birds in Jamaica, Puerto Rico,[7] and the Dominican Republic.[8] Migratory birds are suspected to play a major role in the long-distance trafficking of WNV into new areas.[9,10] The Caribbean Islands are a principal landfall for many species of birds migrating from the northeastern, midwestern, and southern United States.[11] In the Caribbean, and more generally in the Neotropics, transmission of WNV probably occurs year-round because the high temperature and humidity is favorable to mosquito proliferation. The purpose of this article is to report and discuss the temporal evolution of WNV circulation in Guadeloupe in order to increase our understanding of WNV epidemiology in the Neotropics.

MATERIAL AND METHODS

Equine and Avian Serologic Surveys

The surveys were conducted in the Guadeloupe archipelago, which includes Guadeloupe (the main island), Marie Galante, Saint Martin, and Saint Barthelemy (FIG. 1).

In July 2002, sera were collected from 360 horses and in December 2002, sera were collected from 136 horses at study sites where WNV activity was detected in July 2002. Exhaustive equine surveys were conducted afterwards in

July 2003 and August 2004, with sera collected from 487 equines (437 horses, 34 donkeys, and 16 ponies) and 431 equines (386 horses, 27 donkeys, and 18 ponies), respectively.

In 2005, a longitudinal survey was implemented in seven study sites considered to be at high risk for WNV activity because of their geographic location and high abundance of mosquitoes and wild birds. All together, 106 seronegative equines were sampled and monitored every 6 months for seroconversion.

In December 2002, 20 chickens from two farms neighboring a horse-riding center were bled. Comprehensive surveys of chickens were performed in July 2003 and July 2004 with sera collected from 656 and 801 chickens, respectively. The farms were selected to cover most parts of the Guadeloupe Island. The ages of the chickens ranged from 1 month to 2 years.

In 2005, a sentinel survey was implemented in four places considered to be at high risk (presence of many mosquitoes and wild birds). All together, 40 seronegative chickens were sampled every month for seroconversion.

Serologic Assays

In 2002, enzyme linked immunosorbent assays (ELISA) were performed to detect specific IgG anti-WNV in equines and chickens. Immunocapture IgM ELISA was performed on WNV IgG ELISA positive equines.[12]

Epitope-blocking ELISA were performed to test all sera collected in 2003–2005 using the WNV-specific monoclonal antibody (MAb) 3.1112G (Chemicon Temecula, CA) as previously described.[6,13]

Plaque reduction neutralization tests (PRNTs) were performed on all serum samples that had blocking ELISA antibodies to WNV. PRNTs were performed using Vero cells and WNV (strain NY99-35261-11) and Saint Louis encephalitis virus (SLEV; strain TBH-28) as previously described.[3]

A serum sample was considered to have antibodies to WNV if it significantly inhibited the binding of MAb 3.1112G by blocking ELISA and had a $PRNT_{90}$ titer to WNV that was at least fourfold greater than the corresponding SLEV $PRNT_{90}$ titer.

RESULTS

Cross-Sectional Serologic Surveys in Equines

In July 2002, 10 of 360 (2.8%) horses had antibodies to WNV by IgG ELISA, and two were also positive by IgM ELISA. Seven horses had PRNT confirmed WNV infections. The seropositive horses were located in Guadeloupe main island and Marie Galante (TABLE 1). In December 2002, 68 of 136 horses from seven equine centers (the equine center tested were those where seropositive equines were detected in July 2002), had IgG antibodies to WNV but none had IgM antibodies (TABLE 1).

TABLE 1. WNV seroprevalence in equines and chickens in Guadeloupe 2002–2004

	Equine				Chicken		
	July 2002	December 2002	July 2003	August 2004	December 2002	July 2003	July 2004
	10*	68*	94	70	11*	11	5
WNV positive	(2.8%)	(50.0%)	(19.3%)	(16.2%)	(52.4%)	(1.7%)	(0.6%)
Total tested	360	136	487	431	21	656	801

* Determined by IgG ELISA.

In July 2003, serum samples were obtained from 487 equines (437 horses, 34 donkeys, and 16 ponies). Ninety-four (19.3%) equines had antibodies to WNV by both blocking ELISA and PRNT (TABLE 1).

In August 2004, serum samples were obtained from 431 equines (386 horses, 27 donkeys, and 18 ponies). Seventy (16.2%) equines had antibodies to WNV by both blocking ELISA and PRNT (TABLE 1).

No significant differences in WNV seroprevalence were found in mares, stallions, and geldings (19%, 27%, and 17%, respectively in 2003, χ^2 test $P = 0.3$; and 17%, 24% and 15%, respectively in 2004, χ^2 test $P = 0.5$).

In the July 2003 survey, age had no significant effect on WNV seroprevalence (data not provided). However, none of the 14 equines born in 2003 was seropositive. In August 2004, none of the six equines born in 2004 and only one of 23 equines born in 2003 was seropositive. Equines born in 2001 or later were significantly less likely to be infected with WNV than equines born prior to 2001 (TABLE 2).

In 2003, seroprevalences were related to the farm location and were highly heterogeneous by county (TABLE 3). In six of the 13 counties of the Guadeloupe main island examined, the seroprevalence for WNV in equines was less than 8%. In the other seven counties of the Guadeloupe main island, the seroprevalence ranged from 15.4% to 55.6%. In Marie Galante, seroprevalence ranged from 16.7% to 71.4%. One horse (2.9%) in Saint Martin was seropositive for WNV. No seropositive equines were found in Saint Barthelemy. Most WNV seropositive equines were located in evergreen forests (characterized by a low altitude [0–100 m] and farming of sugar cane), near mangroves, back-mangroves (consisting of marshy forests mainly with *Pterocarpus* sp.), and soft to brackish water swamps.

TABLE 2. WNV seroprevalence in equines by age, Guadeloupe August 2004

Year of birth	WNV positive	Total tested
2001–2004	2 (3.0%)*	66
<2001	63 (19.9%)	316

* $P < 0.01$.

TABLE 3. WNV seroprevalence in equines by county, Guadeloupe July 2003

County	WNV positive	Total equine
Guadeloupe main Island		
Deshaies	0 (0%)	9
Gosier	0 (0%)	16
Saint Claude	0 (0%)	44
Saint François	0 (0%)	19
Anse Bertrand	3 (4.4%)	68
Moule	1 (7.7%)	13
Sainte Rose	10 (15.4%)	65
Abymes	10 (29.4%)	34
Petit Bourg	14 (36.8%)	38
Baie Mahault	29 (37.7%)	77
Sainte Anne	5 (45.5%)	11
Morne à l'Eau	3 (50%)	6
Goyave	5 (55.6%)	9
Sub-total Guadeloupe main Island	80 (19.6%)	409
Marie Galante		
Capesterre	2 (16.7%)	12
Grand-Bourg	6 (54.4%)	11
Saint Louis	5 (71.4%)	7
Sub-total Marie Galante	13 (43.3%)	30
Saint Martin	1 (2.9%)	34
Saint Barthélémy	0 (0%)	14
TOTAL	94 (19.3%)	487

Cross-Sectional Serologic Surveys in Chicken

In December 2002, sera were collected from chickens in two backyards (10 per site) neighboring a horse-riding club where seropositive animals were detected. Eleven of these chickens were positive by IgG ELISA (TABLE 1).

In July 2003, 656 chicken serum samples were collected from 25 farms comprising 17 to 20,000 chickens (between 16 and 30 chickens were bled per farm). Eleven chickens had antibodies to WNV by both epitope-blocking ELISA and PRNT (TABLE 1).

TABLE 4 shows the 2003 and 2004 seroprevalences in farms containing at least one seropositive chicken. A total of three WNV seropositive chickens were found in two farms (average apparent seroprevalence in these farms 4.7%, TABLE 4) giving an apparent seroprevalence of 0.5% (3/602) in Guadeloupe main island. A total of eight seropositive chickens were located in the two farms of Marie Galante giving an average apparent seroprevalence of 14.8% (8/54) in this small island (TABLE 4).

In July 2004, 801 chicken samples were collected from 27 farms comprising 15 to 20,000 chickens (between 6 and 45 chickens were bled per farm). Five chickens had antibodies to WNV by both epitope-blocking ELISA and PRNT. All of the seropositive chickens were in Guadeloupe main island. In

TABLE 4. Chicken farms with WNV positive chickens in Guadeloupe, 2003–2004

Year	Farm code	County	WNV positive	Number tested
July 2003	A	Goyave	2 (5.6%)	36
	B	Sainte Anne	1 (3.6%)	28
	C	Grand bourg (Marie Galante)	5 (20.8%)	24
	D	Capesterre (Marie Galante)	3 (10%)	30
July 2004	E	Petit Bourg	1 (3.3%)	30
	F	Petit Bourg	2 (10.0%)	20
	G	Baie Mahault	1 (4.0%)	25
	H	Port Louis	1 (16.7%)	6

the four farms containing seropositive chickens, the average apparent WNV seroprevalence was 6.2% (TABLE 4).

In 2003, seven WNV seropositive chickens were at least 1 year old and four (all from one farm in Marie Galante) were 4 months old. In 2004, one seropositive chicken was 7 months old; the other four were at least 1 year old (TABLE 5).

Longitudinal Study and Seroconversion

Analysis of the paired serum samples collected from equines in July 2002 and December 2002 revealed that 54 of 114 (47.4%) horses seroconverted.

The 62 seronegative horses tested in December 2002, and retested in July 2003 remained seronegative.

The 257 seronegative horses in 2003 and tested again in July 2003 remained WNV seronegative in July 2004. Thus, no WNV seroconversions were observed in equines between 2003 and 2004.

In 2005, one equine sampled in May 2005 was seropositive for WNV. None of the sentinel chickens seroconverted during the first semester of 2005.

Persistence of WNV Antibodies

Seven of the 10 WNV seropositive equines in July 2002 were tested in August 2004. All were still seropositive 25 months later. The 36 WNV seropositive equines in December 2002 which were tested in August 2004 (20 months later),

TABLE 5. Chicken WNV seroprevalence according to age categories, Guadeloupe

Age	July 2003		July 2004	
	WNV positive	Number tested	WNV positive	Number tested
0-6 months	4 (1.2%)	339	(0%)	465
6-12 months	2 (1.0%)	204	1 (0.7%)	148
> 12 months	5 (4.4%)	113	4 (2.1%)	188
Total	11 (1.7%)	656	5 (0.6%)	801

remained seropositive. Sixty-one WNV seropositive equines in July 2003 were still WNV seropositive in 2004.

DISCUSSION

The first serologic evidence of WNV activity in Guadeloupe was the detection of IgG in 10 horses sampled in July 2002. A likely mode of introduction of WNV into Guadeloupe is by infected migratory birds.[14,15] Indeed, many species of migratory birds migrate from the eastern coast of the United States into the Caribbean.[15,16] We speculate that WNV was introduced into Guadeloupe in the fall of the year 2001, during the bird migration period.

In July 2002, the WNV seroprevalence in equines was 2.8%. The majority of seroconversions occurred between July 2002 and December 2002 and a high seroprevalence was found in equines in 2003 (19.3%). The exact comparison of seroprevalences obtained in July 2002 and July 2003 cannot be performed since different serologic tests were used. The seroprevalence observed in 2003 is presumably a good representation of the overall WNV seroprevalence in equines in Guadeloupe because a comprehensive serosurvey was conducted. The seroprevalence is similar to that found in Mexico (29%).[17]

Seropositive equines and chickens were found mainly near evergreen forests with sugar cane culture, characterized by a minimum annual rainfall of 1250 mm and low elevation (0–100 m). Mangroves, back-mangroves, and swamps are located nearby. Mangrove areas contain many species of wild birds and mosquitoes potentially involved in WNV circulation in Guadeloupe. The area of Baie Mahault is also a breeding place for cattle egret, a very common wild bird in Guadeloupe. The most common mosquito species in Guadeloupe are *Culex quinquefasciatus*, *Culex nigripalpus*, *Ochlerotatus taeniorhynchus*, and *Aedes aegypti*. *C. nigripalpus* and *Oc. taeniorhynchus* are particularly common in mangrove areas (Joël Gustave, personal communication). *Culex* species are considered to be the major amplification vectors of WNV in the United States, whereas *Culex, Aedes,* and *Ochlerotatus* species are the major bridging vectors of this virus.[18,19] Moreover *C. nigripalpus* feeds mainly on birds but is very opportunistic and can also feed on mammals.[20] It is therefore a good candidate for WNV amplification and transmission in Guadeloupe.

Equine and avian serosurveys suggest that the transmission of WNV dramatically decreased in 2003 and 2004 in comparison to 2002. No seroconversion occurred between January and August 2003. In 2004, young equines ($\leq$3 years of age) were significantly less likely to be infected than older equines. In 2002, 10 out of 21 chickens were found seropositive. Afterwards, the seroprevalence in chickens was very low in 2003 (1.7%) and 2004 (0.6%). The low seroprevalence found in 2003 and 2004 could be because most chickens tested were born in 2003 and 2004 when the virus circulation was low as shown by equine studies. Similarly, in July 2004 only one seropositive chicken was less than a year old.

Weather exerts profound effect on mosquito populations and therefore arboviral recrudescence or disappearance. In the tropics where the temperature is favorable for mosquito proliferation year-round, changes in rainfalls could significantly effect vector populations.[21] *C. nigripalpus* and *Oc. taeniorhynchus* need heavy rains or changes in the water level to develop. These mosquito species are usually abundant during the rainy season (July–November), but their populations decrease during the dry season. Between November 2002 and May 2003 less than half of the normal rains occurred. These 7 months should have affected the population of these mosquito species. Precipitation appeared to be more important than temperature in predicting arboviral activity in Rhode Island.[22] If we consider that *C. nigripalpus* is a major species involved in WNV transmission in Guadeloupe, a decrease of its population could have induced a drop in virus circulation level. However, from June 2003, weather has been exceptionally humid (twice the normal rains), and one could have expected an increase in mosquito populations with an increase of virus circulation. The reasons why the virus circulation was not then reamplified at the end of 2003 or in 2004 are unknown. A decrease in the number of non immune resident birds could account for the reduction in virus circulation. However, reintroduction could have occurred through migratory birds between August and November 2003 and 2004. The exact American origin of migratory birds remains to be determined to know if they are originating from locations where a lower level of virus circulation was observed in 2003 and 2004, than in 2001 and 2002.

If the serosurveys pointed out a drop in virus circulation, several results show that the circulation even at a low level is still present: one equine born in May 2003 was found seropositive in August 2004, four 4-month old chickens of Marie Galante tested positive in July 2004 and finally the longitudinal survey on seronegative equines in 2005 allowed us to detect one seroconversion in Petit Bourg.

The persistence of antibodies to WNV in serum is not well defined. IgG are detectable for several months or years, and IgM persist for approximately 2 months, although they have been found in humans up to 17 months after illness onset.[23] In addition, neutralizing antibodies to WNV have been found in horses 15 months after onset.[24] Our longitudinal serologic studies demonstrate that antibodies to WNV can persist in equines for at least 2 years.

Entomological studies have to be implemented to confirm our hypothesis on WNV amplification and bridging vectors in Guadeloupe. The sentinel survey on equine and chickens has to be continued to point out any reintroduction of the virus or amplification of the virus circulation.

ACKNOWLEDGMENTS

We thank Guillaume Pallavicini, Rosalie Aprelon, Carène Pagesy, and Valérie Pinarello for technical assistance and the veterinarians of Guadeloupe for the equine serum sampling. We thank Direction des services veterinaries (DSV) hospital, Cellule Inter-Regionale d'Epidémiologie (CIRE Antilles-Guyane), and Direction de la Santé et du Développement Social (DSDS) for their active collaboration on WNV surveillance. We are grateful to Barry Beaty (Colorado State University, Fort Collins, CO, USA) for helpful advice. Equine IgG and IgM ELISA were performed by AFSSA, France. PRNTs were performed thanks to grant U50 CCU820510 from the Centers for Disease Control and Prevention.

REFERENCES

1. CENTERS FOR DISEASE CONTROL AND PREVENTION. 1999. Outbreak of West Nile-like viral encephalitis – New York. MMWR Morb Mortal Wkly Rep **48:** 845–849.
2. BLITVICH, B.J., I. FERNANDEZ-SALAS, J.F. CONTRERAS-CORDERO, *et al.* 2003. Serologic evidence of West Nile virus infection in horses, Coahuila State, Mexico. Emerg. Infect. Dis. **9:** 853–856.
3. FERNANDEZ-SALAS, I., J.F. CONTRERAS-CORDERO, B.J. BLITVICH, *et al.* 2003. Serologic evidence of West Nile Virus infection in birds, Tamaulipas State, Mexico. Vector Borne Zoonotic Dis. **3:** 209–213.
4. ESTRADA-FRANCO, J.G., R. NAVARRO-LOPEZ, D.W. BEASLEY, *et al.* 2003. West Nile virus in Mexico: evidence of widespread circulation since July 2002. Emerg. Infect. Dis. **9:** 1604–1607.
5. QUIRIN, R., M. SALAS, S. ZIENTARA, *et al.* 2004. West Nile virus, Guadeloupe. Emerg. Infect. Dis. **10:** 706–708.
6. LEFRANÇOIS, T., B.J. BLITVICH, J. PRADEL, *et al.* 2005. West Nile virus surveillance, Guadeloupe, 2003 – 2004. Emerg. Infect. Dis. **11:** 1100–1103.
7. DUPUIS, A.P. II, MARRA, P.P., L.D. KRAMER. 2003. Serologic evidence of West Nile virus transmission, Jamaica, West Indies. Emerg. Infect. Dis. **9:** 860–863.
8. KOMAR, O., M.B. ROBBINS, K. KLENK, *et al.* 2003. West Nile virus transmission in resident birds, Dominican Republic. Emerg. Infect. Dis. **9:** 1299–1302.
9. MALKINSON, M., C. BANET, Y. WEISMAN, *et al.* 2002. Introduction of West Nile virus in the Middle East by migrating storks. Emerg. Infect. Dis. **8:** 392–397.
10. RAPPOLE, J.H., S.R. DERRICKSON, Z. HUBALEK. 2000. Migratory birds and spread of West Nile virus in the Western Hemisphere. Emerg. Infect. Dis. **6:** 319–328.
11. RAFFAELE, H., J. WILEY, O. GARRIDO, *et al.* 1998. A Guide to The Birds of the West Indies. Princeton University Press, Princeton, NJ.
12. MURGUE, B., S. MURRI, S. ZIENTARA, *et al.* 2001. West Nile in France in 2000 : the return 38 years later. Emerg. Infect. Dis. **7:** 692–696.
13. BLITVICH, B.J., N.L. MARLENEE, R.A. HALL, *et al.* 2003. Epitope-blocking enzyme-linked immunosorbent assays for the detection of serum antibodies to West Nile virus in multiple avian species. J. Clin. Microbiol. **41:** 1041–1047.
14. PETERSON, A.T., D.A. VIEGLAIS, J.K. ANDREASEN. 2003. Migratory birds modeled as critical transport agents for West Nile Virus in North America. Vector Borne Zoonotic Dis. **3:** 27–37.
15. RAPPOLE, J.H., S.R. DERRICKSON, Z. HUBALEK. 2000. Migratory birds and spread of West Nile virus in the Western Hemisphere. Emerg. Infect. Dis. **6:** 319–328.
16. USGS, NORTHERN PRAIRIE WILDLIFE RESEARCH CENTER, Migration of Birds, Routes of Migration. Available from http://www.npwrc.usgs.gov/resource/birds/migratio/routes.htm.

17. CENTRO NATIONAL DE VIGILENCIA EPIDEMIOLOGICA. Diagnostico de laboratorio para VOM hasta el 9 de diciembre de 2004. Available from http://www.cenave.gob.mx/von/archivos/ResumenCASOSVON.xls

18. GOULD, L.H., E. FIKRIG. 2004. West Nile virus: a growing concern? [review] J. Clin. Invest. **113:** 1102–1107.

19. GODDARD, L.B., A.E. ROTH, W.K. REISEN & T.W. SCOTT. 2002. Vector competence of California mosquitoes for West Nile virus. Emerg. Infect. Dis. **8:** 1385–1391.

20. EDMAN, J. & D. TAYLOR 1968. Culex nigripalpus: seasonal shift in the bird mammal feeding ratio in a mosquito vector of human encephalitis. Science **161:** 67–68.

21. REITER, P. 1988. Weather, vector biology, and arboviral recrudescence. *In* The Arboviruses: Epidemiology and Ecology, Vol. 1. T.P. Monath Ed.: 245–255. CRC Press. Florida.

22. TAKEDA, T., C.A. WHITEHOUSE, M. BREWER, *et al.* 2003. Arbovirus surveillance in Rhode Island: assessing potential ecologic and climatic correlates. J. Am. Mosq. Control Assoc. **19:** 179–189.

23. ROEHRIG, J.T., D. NASH, B. MALDIN, *et al.* 2003. Persistence of virus-reactive serum immunoglobulin M antibody in confirmed West Nile virus encephalitis cases. Emerg. Infect. Dis. **9:** 376–379.

24. OSTLUND, E.N., R.L. CROM, D.D. PEDERSEN, *et al.* 2001. Equine West Nile encephalitis, United States. Emerg. Infect. Dis. **7:** 665–669.

Serological Assessment of West Nile Fever Virus Activity in the Pastoral System of Ferlo, Senegal

VÉRONIQUE CHEVALIER,[a] RENAUD LANCELOT,[b] AMADOU DIAITÉ,[c] BERNARD MONDET,[d] BABA SALL,[e] AND XAVIER DE LAMBALLERIE[f]

[a] Centre International de Recherche Agronomique pour le Développement (CIRAD), 34398 Montpellier Cedex 5, France

[b] Ambassade de France–SCAC-RE BP 834, Antananarivo 101, Madagascar

[c] Institut Sénégalais de Recherche Agricole (ISRA), BP 2057 Dakar-Hann, Sénégal

[d] Institut de Recherche pour le Développement (IRD), BP 1386 Dakar-Hann, Sénégal

[e] Direction de l'Élevage, BP 67 Dakar, Sénégal

[f] Unité des Virus Émergents, Faculté de Médecine de Marseille, 13005 Marseille, France

ABSTRACT: The Ferlo area (north-central Senegal) is characterized by a system of temporary ponds favorable to arboviruses among which West Nile fever (WNF) was already identified. During the rainy season in 2003, a serological study was undertaken on horses to assess the activity of the WNF virus (WNFV) in Barkedji (Ferlo). The observed serological prevalence rate was 78.3% for neutralizing antibodies, with a 95% confidence interval (CI) of [64.0, 92.7]. This prevalence rate significantly increased with age ($P = 10^{-5}$). This study confirmed that WNF was endemic in the Ferlo. The transmission risks depended on the introduction of the WNFV in the ecosystem—probably with migrating birds, on its amplification in hosts and on the vector-population dynamic. Further studies are needed to investigate how the cycle is initiated in Barkedji at the beginning of the rainy season and the impact of climatic variations on the risk of transmission of WNF. A surveillance system should be implemented: (a) to assess the clinical impact of the WNF on human and equine populations, (b) to provide an early detection of virulent strains, and (c) to assess the risk of WNF transmission to disease-free ecosystems via migrating birds.

KEYWORDS: epidemiology; horse; Senegal; West Nile fever virus

Address for correspondence: V. Chevalier, Centre International de Recherche Agronomique pour le Développement (CIRAD), 34398 Montpellier Cedex 5, France. Voice: 00 (33) 4 67 59 38 29; fax: 00 (33) 4 67 59 37 54.
e-mail: chevalier@cirad.fr

Ann. N.Y. Acad. Sci. 1081: 216–225 (2006). © 2006 New York Academy of Sciences.
doi: 10.1196/annals.1373.026

INTRODUCTION

West Nile fever (WNF) is an arthropod-borne disease and an anthropozoono-sis caused by a *Flavivirus* (*Flaviviridae*). Its epidemiological cycle involves birds (reservoirs) and mosquitoes (vectors)—mainly from the *Culex* genus.[1] Humans or horses may be infected by mosquitoes. Infection is often unappar-ent or mild (flue-like syndrome in humans) in birds, humans, and horses. Some virus strains are lethal for different bird species. Though relatively rare, se-vere clinical forms (meningo-encephalitis) are observed in these populations.[2] Heavy losses were reported in naïve horse populations in different parts of the world.[3,4]

West Nile fever virus (WNFV) was isolated from *Aedes* and *Culex* mosquitoes in the Senegal valley[5] and in the Ferlo[6] (northern and central Senegal) between 1988 and 1995. A serological survey in humans also showed that the infection was endemic in this semi-arid area.[2]

A research program was implemented in the Ferlo to assess human and animal health risks related to the use of this ecosystem.

This article reports the WNF study. Its specific goals were (*a*) to assess the activity pattern of WNFV in the Ferlo and (*b*) to propose possible improvements of WNF surveillance.

MATERIALS AND METHODS

The study was carried out in the village of Barkedji (14°52' W, 15°16' N), in the central Ferlo (FIG. 1). This region is a large lateritic plateau chiseled by a fossil valley (a former affluent of the Senegal River), which gave its name to the area. Annual rainfalls range from 300 to 500 mm, occurring between July and September.

During the rainy season, temporary ponds fill up and constitute a favor-able biotope for many mosquito species, mainly from *Culex* or *Aedes* genus. Based on repeated isolations, high field infection rates and abundance, *Culex* mosquitoes were considered as the main vectors of WNFV (among other viruses).[6] Many species of endemic and migratory birds are attracted by these ponds and allow the amplification of the epidemiological cycle.

During the rainy season, farmers are settled close to the ponds. Most of them own horses which are used for transportation and animal traction. They live close to farmers' housing and share the same exposure factors to WNF.

A cross-sectional survey in horses was undertaken to assess the WNF trans-mission risk in this ecosystem.

Horse Data

WNF was never reported in horses by the Senegalese veterinary services. It was assumed that local horse breeds were somewhat resistant to this disease.

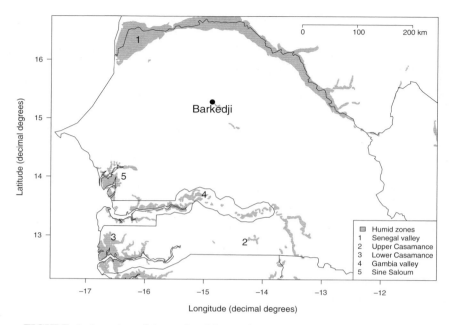

FIGURE 1. Location of the study of the serological prevalence of West Nile fever in Barkedji (Senegal) during the rainy season 2003.

Life expectancy is long in horses and circulating antibodies are found in their blood years after a WNF infection.[3] Therefore, a point prevalence survey on a sample of horses showing a broad range of ages should provide valuable information on the time pattern of WNF incidence.

Meetings were organized with horse owners in Barkedji and neighbor villages to explain the goals of the study. During July 2003, jugular blood was sampled in any horse visiting the veterinary post of Barkedji for vaccination. Their origin (village) and age were recorded, according to owners' declarations. Foals were not sampled to avoid colostral antibodies.

Serological Analysis

Blood samples were centrifuged and the resulting sera were frozen. At the end of the field survey, sera were sent to the Laboratory of Emerging Viruses (University of Marseille, France).

Horse sera were tested for anti-WNFV neutralizing antibodies with the plaque reduction neutralization test (PRNT) following a modified Buckley's procedure.[7] Sera were inactivated at 56°C during 30 min. Twofold dilutions were made from 1/10 to 1/320. Serum and virus dilutions (containing 50 plaque-forming units for the latter) were mixed and incubated at 37°C for

1 h. The mixture was added to human SW13 cell monolayers and incubated at 37°C for 1 h. Agarose was added and plates were incubated for 5 days at 37°C. Cells were fixed with formaldehyde and stained with naphthalene black. The number of plaques was then counted.

Sera were also tested for immunoglobulins M (IgM) using an immunocapture enzyme-linked immunosorbent assay (ELISA).

Data Analysis

The dependant variables were prevalence rates, thus proportions. Because of the sampling frame (horses clustered in villages), responses from the same cluster (village) were possibly correlated: so-called "overdispersion" caused by unobserved features common to individuals of the same cluster, and different from cluster to cluster.[8]

Empirical rates and their variance were first computed using the ratio method for cluster sampling.[9] The intra-class correlation was computed using the maximum-likelihood (ML) method.[10] A beta-binomial regression model was then used to account for this correlation in the estimation of the prevalence rate and its standard error, with the age categorized in age-classes as the explanatory variable.[11]

Three different correlation structures were compared: (*a*) no correlation (regular logistic-regression model), (*b*) correlation common to all groups, and (*c*) age-specific correlation. They were compared with the Akaike information criterion (AIC): AIC $= -2 *$ log (maximized likelihood) $+ 2 *k$, where k was the number of parameters in the models. The best model was the one with the lowest AIC.[12]

Prevalence data were used to estimate the annual incidence rate (IR) in horses, assuming (*a*) a constant annual incidence, (*b*) a lifelong persistence of neutralizing antibodies, and (*c*) that mortality related to WNF was null. Under these hypotheses, the prevalence rate at age n (starting from 0 for age <1 year) was a function of IR: PR $_n = 1 - (1 - \text{IR})^n$. Given the sample age structure, the overall prevalence rate was a linear combination of the age-specific prevalence rates, i.e., a polynomial function of IR with annual class sizes as the coefficients; the root of this polynomial, constrained to lie between 0 and 1, was an estimate of IR.

The R software was used for data analysis and graphics[13] with an add-on package gathering the statistical methods used in this article.[14]

RESULTS

One hundred and twenty horses were sampled, their age ranging from 1 to 21 years (mean = 7.5 years). Their age structure is shown in FIGURE 2. Sixty percent of the horses came from the village of Barkedji. The observed

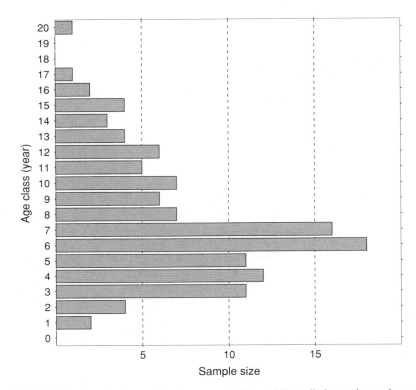

FIGURE 2. Age structure of the horse sample ($n = 120$) studied to estimate the sero-logical prevalence of West Nile fever in Barkedji during the rainy season 2003.

serological prevalence rate was 78.3% for neutralizing antibodies, with a 95% confidence interval (CI) of [64.0, 92.7]. Three sera (2.5%) were tested positive with the IgM ELISA.

Three age classes were considered (in years): [1, 4), [4, 7), and [7, +). Data were grouped by village and age class. The ML intra-cluster correlation was close to 0 within each age class. This result was confirmed by the regression step: the model with the lowest AIC was the logistic regression model (no correlation structure).

Estimated prevalence rates and their CI are displayed in TABLE 1. The prevalence rate increased with age and this increase was highly significant (likelihood ratio test: $\chi^2 = 23$, df $= 2$, $P(> \chi^2) = 10^{-5}$).

The estimated constant annual IR was 19.2%. The fitted serological prevalence and its residuals are shown in FIGURE 3. Negative residuals were observed for the first 3 annual classes (2-, 3- and 4-year old) but class size was small for two of them (FIG. 2). They were followed by three positive residuals (5-, 6- and 7-year old).

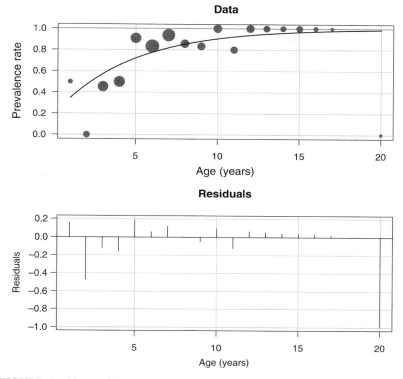

FIGURE 3. Observed (*grey points*) and predicted (*curves*) West Nile fever serological prevalence in a sample of 120 horses from Barkedji (Senegal) during the rainy season 2003. The size of points was proportional to the number of horses. The curves were obtained assuming a constant annual incidence rate derived from the prevalence rate: the solid curve corresponded to the average rate; the dashed curves corresponded to its 95% upper and lower limits computed with a bootstrap procedure.

DISCUSSION

The overall serological prevalence rate of WNF neutralizing antibodies was high in horses (78.3%). This result corroborates previous observations made in

TABLE 1. Serological prevalence of West Nile fever according to age in 120 horses from Barkedji (Senegal) during the 2003 rainy season, as estimated from a logistic-regression model

Age class (years)	*n*	Prevalence rate (%) and 95% CI (in brackets)
[1, 4)	17	35.3 [16.8, 59.6]
[4, 7)	41	75.6 [60.3, 86.3]
[7, +)	62	91.9 [82.0, 96.6]

the same area: a high serological prevalence was observed in human population; 45% in children < 5 years ($n = 20$), 80% in the age group [5, 15) years ($n = 20$), and 98% in adults >15 years ($n = 50$).[2] In Egypt, where WNF was endemic, high serological prevalence rates were also detected in horses, ranging from 36% to 80%.[15]

The logistic-regression results showed that horse serological prevalence rate significantly increased with age ($P = 10^{-5}$). Moreover, the annual IR derived from the overall prevalence rate, was high (19.2%). The general pattern of prevalence according to age was compatible with an assumption of WNF transmission occurring each year (FIG. 3, upper graph). However, there were some indications of between-year variations (FIG. 3, lower graph). The detection of three early infections in July also showed that WNF transmission already occurred at the beginning of the rainy season.

During the rainy season, many farmers were settled close to the temporary ponds with little protection against mosquito bites: they were exposed to a high risk of WNFV transmission. WNF surveillance in horses and humans should be implemented in the Ferlo and other risky areas of Senegal. It might consist in reporting and investigating any case of encephalitis in dispensaries, hospitals, and veterinary posts located in areas selected according to their high WNF exposure risk: Senegal valley and delta, upper and lower Casamance, Sine Saloum, and Ferlo valley. For this purpose, training programs should be designed for human and veterinary staff, and specific procedures should be elaborated for specimen collection and laboratory analysis.

Two main goals should be assigned to this surveillance system: (*a*) assess the actual clinical incidence of WNF in human and horses to evaluate the need for prevention and control measures; and (*b*) monitor the virulence of WNFV strains to prevent and manage local outbreaks and provide early-warning information for the transmission risk from Senegalese to European ecosystems through bird migrations. As a matter of fact, some WNFV strains isolated in Senegal had a neuro-invasive capacity in baby mice, which was considered as a human virulence criterion during the recent north-American epidemic.[16]

The three IgM-positive horse sera observed in July 2003 showed that WNFV transmission occurred in Barkedji when the abundance of *Culex* mosquitoes was still low.[17] How was this transmission initiated?

Vertical transmission of WNFV was observed in *Culex* spp.[18–20] This feature might be important during the amplification of WNFV transmission. Because *Culex* eggs and larvae do not survive during the dry season, it did not explain the occurrence of early serological incidence in Barkedji horses.

In New York (USA), WNFV was able to survive over the winter in *Culex* mosquitoes.[18,21] In Barkedji, a few *Culex* mosquitoes were present at the beginning of the rainy season.[17] Despite the small size of this population, its role in the maintenance of WNF infection cannot be excluded.

The virus was isolated from *Aedes vexans* in the Ferlo[6] and this mosquito species was dominant at the beginning of the rainy season.[17] Vertical transmission of different arboviruses (e.g., Rift Valley fever) was reported in female mosquitoes of different *Aedes* species.[22] Infected eggs survived in the dried mud and infected neonates hatched at the beginning of the next rainy season, initiating a new virus cycle.[23] As far as we know, this phenomenon was not reported for WNFV.

WNF infections were experimentally obtained with *Argas persicus* and *A. hermani*, two ornithophilic soft-body ticks previously described in Barkedji. Life expectancy of these ticks is long and they may harbor the virus for years.[15] However, no WNFV transmission was obtained with these ticks.

Two species of hard-body ticks, *Ixodides scapularis* and *Dermacentor Andersoni* were able to acquire the WNF virus from viremic hosts and the virus was transmitted from nymph to adult phases. However, vector competency of these ticks was not demonstrated[24] and their presence was not reported in Barkedji.

At last, WNFV might be borne from infected to virus-free areas, either with viremic migratory birds or with infected ticks hosted by these birds.[25] The Ferlo is a crossroad between wet areas: Senegal valley, upper and lower Casamance, Gambia valley and Sine Saloum (FIG. 1). *Culex* populations use to persist during the dry season (Mondet, personal communication) in these ecosystems which are frequented by large populations of birds migrating from other parts of Africa and Europe for wintering.[26] Therefore, these wet areas are good candidates for a year-long WNFV activity. The virus might be disseminated by birds from these places to the Ferlo and more remote regions such as Europe.

CONCLUSION

This study confirmed that WNF was endemic in the Ferlo. Several mechanisms may be involved to explain the virus persistence in this ecosystem, the most likely being bird-borne dissemination. However, this assumption is difficult to demonstrate, because thousands of bird captures and samplings would be needed to analyze the transmission risk of WNF between distant ecosystems.

The high estimated serological incidence observed in the Ferlo—and probably in other parts of Senegal, highlighted the need for an improved surveillance system for early detection of potentially dangerous WNFV strains. Beyond the report and investigation of horse and human encephalitis cases, this surveillance system should rely on the monitoring of sentinel chick flocks in areas of ornithological importance, to reveal seasonal and annual changes in incidence rates. It should also be associated with an international information system on bird migration sharing data from European and African ecosystems. Such actions will be carried out in the frame of an international research project funded by the European Union (Emerging Diseases European Network—EDEN).

The assessment of clinical risk associated with WNFV infection should be used to define a set of control measures, from application of insect repellents to vaccination in humans and horses. The popularization and implementation of such measures should involve the local populations exposed to a high risk of WNF infection as well as the increasing number of tourists visiting areas of ornithological interest in Senegal.

ACKNOWLEDGMENTS

We wish to thank M. Lesnoff (CIRAD), R. Pin (IRD), D.A. Sow (ISRA), T. Manga (veterinary officer), the horse owners and local authorities of Barkedji. The study was supported by the grant "ACI Écologie Quantitative" funded by the French Ministry of Research, the grant "CORUS" funded by the French Ministry of Foreign Affairs, and CIRAD.

REFERENCES

1. KOMAR, N. 2000. West Nile viral encephalitis. Rev. Sci. Tech. Off. Int. Epiz. **19:** 166–176.
2. MURGUE, B., H. ZELLER & V. DEUBEL. 2002. The ecology and epidemiology of West Nile Virus in Africa, Europe and Asia. Curr. Top. Microbiol. Immunol. **267:** 195–221.
3. DURAND, B., V. CHEVALIER, R. POUILLOT, et al. 2002. West Nile virus outbreak in horses, southern France, 2000: results of a serosurvey. Emerg. Infect. Dis. **8:** 777–782.
4. SCHULER, L., M. KHAITSA, N. DYER, et al. 2004. Evaluation of an outbreak of West Nile virus infection in horses: 569 cases (2002). J. Am. Vet. Med. Assoc. **225:** 1084–1089.
5. GORDON, S., R. TAMMARIELLO, K. LINTHICUM, et al. 1992. Arbovirus isolations from mosquitoes collected during 1988 in the Senegal River basin. Am. J. Trop. Med. Hyg. **47:** 742–748.
6. TRAORE-LAMIZANA, M., H.G. ZELLER, M. MONDO, et al. 1994. Isolations of West Nile and Bagaza viruses from mosquitoes (*Diptera: Culicidae*) in central Senegal (Ferlo). J. Med. Entomol. **31:** 934–938.
7. BUCKLEY, A.D.A., S.R. MOSS & S.A. HINSLEY. 2003. Serological evidence of West Nile virus, Usutu virus and Sindbis virus infection of birds in the UK. J. Gen. Virol. **84:** 2807–2817.
8. MCDERMOTT, J.J., Y.Y. SCHUKKEN & M.M. SHOUKRI. 1994. Study design and analytic methods for data collected from clusters of animals. Prev. Vet. Med. **18:** 175–191.
9. COCHRAN, W.G. 1999. Sampling Techniques, 3rd ed. Wiley. New York.
10. ZOU, G. & A. DONNER. 2004. Confidence interval estimation of the intraclass correlation coefficient for binary outcome data. Biometrics **60:** 807–811.
11. GRIFFITHS, D.A. 1973. Maximum likelihood estimation for the beta-binomial distribution and an application to the household distribution of the total number of cases of disease. Biometrics **29:** 637–648.

12. BURNHAM, K.P. & D.R. ANDERSON. 2002. Model Selection and Multimodel Inference: a Practical Information-Theoretic Approach. Springer-Verlag. New York.
13. R DEVELOPMENT CORE TEAM. 2005. R: A language and environment for statistical computing. R Foundation for Statistical Computing, Vienna, Austria. ISBN 3-900051-07-0, URL http://www.R-project.org.
14. LESNOFF, M. & R. LANCELOT. 2005. aod: Analysis of Overdispersed Data. R package version 1.1–2. http://cran.r-project.org
15. SCHMIDT, J.R. & H.K. EL MANSOURY. 1963. Natural and experimental infection of Egyptian equines with West Nile virus. Ann. Trop. Med. Parasitol. **57:** 415–427.
16. BEASLEY, D.W.C., L. LI, M.T. SUDERMAN, *et al.* 2002. Mouse neuroinvasive phenotype of West Nile virus strains varies depending upon virus genotype. Virology **296:** 17–23.
17. MONDET, B., A. DIAÏTÉ, A.G. FALL, *et al.* 2005. Relations entre la pluviomètrie et le risque de transmission virale par les moustiques : cas du virus de la Rift Valley Fever (RVF) dans le Ferlo (Sénégal). Environnement, Risques et Santé **4:** 125–129.
18. BAQAR, S., C.G. HAYES, J.R. MURPHY, *et al.* 1993. Vertical transmission of West Nile virus by *Culex* and *Aedes* species mosquitoes. Am. J. Trop. Med. Hyg. **48:** 757–762.
19. MILLER, B.R., R.S. NASCI, M.S. GODSEY, *et al.* 2000. First field evidence for natural vertical transmission of West Nile virus in *Culex univittatus* complex mosquitoes from Rift Valley province, Kenya. Am. J. Trop. Med. Hyg. **62:** 240–246.
20. DOHM, D.J., M.R. SARDELIS & M.J. TURELL. 2002. Experimental vertical transmission of West Nile virus by *Culex pipiens* (*Diptera: Culicidae*). J. Med. Entomol. **39:** 640–644.
21. DOHM, D., M. O'GUINN & M.J. TURELL. 2002. Effect of environmental temperature on the ability of *Culex pipiens* (*Diptera: Culicidae*) to transmit West Nile virus. J. Med. Entomol. **39:** 221–225.
22. LINTHICUM, K.J., F.G. DAVIES, A. KAIRO, *et al.* 1985. Rift Valley fever virus (family Bunyaviridae, genus Phlebovirus). Isolations from *Diptera* collected during an inter-epizootic period in Kenya. J. Hyg. (Lond.) **95:** 197–209.
23. HARWOOD, R.F. & W.R. HORSFALL. 1959. Development, structure, and function of coverings of eggs of floodwater mosquitoes. III. Functions of coverings. Ann. Entomol. Soc. Am. **52:** 113–116.
24. ANDERSON, J., A. MAIN, T. ANDREADIS, *et al.* 2003. Transstadial transfer of West Nile virus by three species of ixodid ticks (*Acari: Ixodidae*). J. Med. Entomol. **40:** 528–533.
25. MALKINSON, M. & C. BANET. 2002. The role of birds in the ecology of West Nile virus in Europe and Africa. Curr. Top. Microbiol. Immunol. **267:** 309–322.
26. ZELLER, H.G. & B. MURGUE. 2001. Rôle des oiseaux migrateurs dans l'épidémiologie du virus West Nile. Médecine et maladies infectieuses **31:** 168s–174s.

Recommendations from the Avian Influenza Vaccine Workshop

DAVID E. SWAYNE

U.S. Department of Agriculture, Agricultural Research Service, Southeast Poultry Research Laboratory, Athens, Georgia 30605, USA

The following recommendations were compiled from a workshop on the development of vaccines against avian influenza held in conjuction with the STVM-05 Symposium on Trends in Avian Zoonoses, June 30, 2005.

1. Use of high quality, properly administered vaccines in association with the existing components of biosecurity, movement controls, surveillance, and education will greatly enhance the success of the comprehensive avian influenza control strategy of Vietnam.
2. Vaccination should focus on raising the immunity of domestic poultry, especially ducks and geese, within poultry production sectors 3 and 4 such that infection rates in poultry will decrease and result in lower environmental contamination. This immunity should be reached in a minimum of 95% of the poultry in a geographic region.
3. Vaccination of commercial poultry in production sectors 1 and 2 in high-risk geographic areas will provide addition avian influenza control and protect the economic value of the commercial industries.
4. The Vietnamese government is commended for designing an initial implementation vaccination program in four provinces for August 2005, followed by full vaccination programs in 40 additional provinces in September and October 2005. Lessons learned from this early study on administration methods and logistics will assist in developing the full vaccination implementation plan.
5. Surveillance by sentinels and dead birds should be implemented in vaccinated flocks to monitor the effect of vaccination in control. The success of the vaccination program should be based on surveillance data with ongoing changes to optimize the program's success by reducing infection rates.

Address of correspondence: David E. Swayne, U.S. Department of Agriculture, Agricultural Research Service, Southeast Poultry Research Laboratory, 934 College Station Road, Athens, GA 30605. Voice: 706-546-3433; fax: 706-546-3161.
e-mail: dswayne@seprl.usda.gov

Ann. N.Y. Acad. Sci. 1081: 226–227 (2006). © 2006 New York Academy of Sciences.
doi: 10.1196/annals.1373.008

6. Financial and human resources should be committed to the vaccination program to allow ongoing and broad use of vaccine for 2 to 3 years.
7. The efficacy of the vaccines used in the field should be evaluated annually or biennially to determine if the vaccines are still protective from antigen drift of field viruses. If protection is inadequate, vaccine strains should be updated.
8. Additional research is needed to develop and license new vaccine technologies that can be applied by *in ovo*, *per os,* and spray administration.

Genotyping of Newcastle Disease Viruses Isolated from 2002 to 2004 in China

ZHILIANG WANG, HUALEI LIU, JIANGTAO XU, JINGYUE BAO, DONGXIA ZHENG, CHENGYING SUN, RONG WEI, CUIPING SONG, AND JIMING CHEN

National Reference Laboratory for Newcastle Diseases, Animal Quarantine Institute, Ministry of Agriculture, Qingdao 266032, People's Republic of China

ABSTRACT: The main function region of the fusion (F) protein gene of 124 strains of Newcastle disease virus isolated from 2002 to 2004 in China was amplified and sequenced for further phylogenetic and residue substitutive analysis. Most of the isolates were classified into genotype VIIc, VIId, VIf, and VIb, while others into genotype IX, III, or II. The genotype IX, a unique genotype which includes strain F48, the first Chinese virulent NDV strain isolated in 1948, were still found inducing sporadic infections in certain areas. Subgenotype VIIc, VIId, and VIIe viruses, which were distributed in clusters in the phylogenetic tree distinct from members of subgenotypes VIIa and VIIb, were responsible for most outbreaks in China and circulated predominantly in China in recent years. Strain NDV03-026, an isolate of the genotype II which was normally lentogenic, was found carrying ^{112}RRQKRF^{117} motif at the cleavage site of F protein as the virulent strain.

KEYWORDS: Newcastle disease virus; phylogenetic tree; genotype

INTRODUCTION

Newcastle disease (ND), one of the most important diseases of poultry caused by *Newcastle disease virus* (NDV), is divided into five pathotypes based on the virulence and clinical signs, namely viscerotropic velogenic, neurotropic velogenic, mesogenic, lentogenic, and asymptomatic.[1] It was also classified as an A list disease by the World Animal Health Organization (Office International des Epizooties, OIE).[2] NDV has been placed in the genus *Avulavirus*, sub-family *Paramyxovirinae*, family *Paramyxoviridae*, order *Mononegavirales* in the current taxonomy,[3,4] which has a negative-sense, single-stranded RNA

Address for correspondence: Zhiliang Wang, National Diagnostic Center for Exotic Animal Diseases, Animal Quarantine Institute, Ministry of Agriculture, 369 Nanjing Road, Qingdao, P.C. 266032, People's Republic of China. Voice: 86532-7839188; fax: 86532-7839922.
e-mail: zlwang111@yahoo.com.cn

Ann. N.Y. Acad. Sci. 1081: 228–239 (2006). © 2006 New York Academy of Sciences.
doi: 10.1196/annals.1373.027

genome of 15 kb that contains six genes in the order of 3′-NP-P-M-F-HN-L-5′, encoding six proteins (nucleoprotein, phosphorprotein, matrix protein, fusion protein, hemagglutinin-neuraminidase protein, and large protein, respectively).[5–9] The F glycoprotein that mediated fusion of viral and cellular membranes is synthesized as an inactive precursor, F_0, containing 553 amino acids. The precursor is proteolytically cleaved at the peptide bond between residues 116 and 117, to generate active polypeptides F1 and F2, which are linked by disulphide bonds. The virulent type of NDV has multiple basic amino acid sequence at the C terminus of the F2 protein. These multiple basic amino acid sequences can be recognized by ubiquitous host proteinases. Pathotype prediction and diagnosis of the virulence of NDV can be performed using the F protein cleavage site sequence analysis.[11–14] Various methods have been used to identify and analysis of NDV including differences in pathogenicity,[10] antigenicity,[11,15] and genomes.[11–13,16–18] Several epidemiological studies of NDV have been carried out using molecular-based methods.

There have been three main panzootics of ND in the world.[10,19] Major panzootic strains of NDV could be divided into three lineages or seven genotypes by comparing the nucleotide sequences and phylogenetic analysis.[19–22] Genotypes II and IV were involved in the first epizotic of ND, genotypes V and VI might have caused the second and third panzootics.[19,22] It was also suggested that genotypes VI and VII, isolates of the Middle East in the late 1960s and isolates of Indonesia in the late 1980s, caused epizootic infection of Europe in the 1990s. Recently, there were several reports concerning molecular characterization of NDV in East Asia.[23–28]

ND has been endemic for decades in China since it was first described in rural chicken flocks in 1946. In China, the epidemiological situation is complex. There are many genotypes in addition to genotype VII, which is in vogue in all over the world, as well as older genotypes, such as genotype II, genotype III. In particular, there is genotype IX which is only found in China.[23,25,29,30] In order to efficiently control this high variability and reduce economic loses, it is necessary to research the prevalence of NDV. In the current study, we carried out genotypical characterization of NDV strains derived from different regions of China during the period of 2002–2004, to determine the phylogenetic relationships of these viruses and epidemiological relationships of ND outbreaks. We were particularly interested in obtaining information on NDV isolates that caused epizootics in recent years.

MATERIALS AND METHODS

Virus Isolation and Identification

All viral samples were isolated from clinical cases in China. NDV strains were isolated in specific-pathogen-free (SPF) chicken embryonated eggs by standard procedures. Virus identification was performed using hemagglutination (HA) and hemagglutination inhibition (HI) assays according to the method with OIE standard.[31]

Viral RNA Preparation

Viral RNA was extracted from allantoic fluids of SPF chicken embroys using the TRIzol reagent (Gibco, Invitrogen Carlsbad, CA). The viral RNA was resuspended in diethylpyrocarbonate (DEPC)—treated water and stored at $-70°C$ before use.

Reverse Transcriptase Polymerase Chain Reaction (RT-PCR)

Primers for the RT-PCR amplification for the main function region of the fusion protein gene were designed on the basis of published NDV sequence data.[23] Two primers P1: 5′-ATGGGCYCCAGAYCTTCTAC-3′ (sense, from nt 47-66 of the F gene) and P2: 5′-CTGCCACTGCTAGTTGTGATAATCC-3′ (antisense, from nt 557-581 of the F gene) were synthesized in TakaRa Biotechnology (Dalian, China). The two primers could generate a 535 bp fragment of the F gene. The RT-PCR protocol was used by the Ready-to-Go RT-PCR Beads kit (Amersham Biosciences Piscataway, NJ). The reaction mixture was incubated at 42°C for 40 min. The PCR reaction mixture was then cycled 36 times at 94°C for 30 s, 50°C for 30 s, 72°C for 45 s and finally at 72°C for 5 min.

Nucleotide Sequencing

The purified PCR products were cloned into pMD18-T vector (TakaRa). Recombinant plasmids were identified by digestion with restriction endonuclease. The F gene clones were sequenced by TakaRa Biotechnology.

Analysis of Sequence Date

Nucleotide sequence editing, analysis, and prediction of amino acid sequences were conducted using the Editseq and MegAlign program in the Lasergene package (DNASTAR Inc. Madison, WI). Phylogenetic trees were constructed with the Jotun Hein Method of the Program by comparison of the nucleotide sequences of F gene from nt 47 to 420.

RESULTS

Virus Isolation and Identification

One hundred and twenty-four strains were isolated from the tissue specimens, and identified by HA and HI tests. All the isolates were saved as infected allantoic fluid samples in the National Reference Laboratory for Newcastle Disease, Animal Quarantine Institute, Ministry of Agriculture.

Phylogenetic Relationships among NDV Isolates

Phylogenetic analysis of all the NDV strains characterized in this study and representative strains from the literature was performed using the variable region of the F gene (nt 47–420) (FIGS. 1 and 2). The phylogenetic tree showed that 124 isolates from this study and 45 representative strains from the literature were distributed in nine distinct clusters corresponding to the different genotypes of NDV. Among these genotypes, eight groups (genotype I–VIII) have been reported previously. A novel group recognized as genotype IX composed by nine viruses (NDV02-032, NDV03-061, NDV04-23, NDV02-445, NDV03-011, NDV032-023, NDV03-009, NDV03-045, and F48E8), which were isolated exclusively in mainland China was reported more recently in China (FIG. 2). Nine strains characterized in this study were assigned to genotype VI, within which six strains (NDV03-007, NDV03-001, NDV02-054, NDV02-069, NDV03-003, and NDV03-006) belonged to the established subgroup VIf and other three strains fell into two subgroups, which we designated VIb and VIg (FIG. 2). Most of genotype II isolates (21 strains) were shown to be derived from commercial vaccines, but one strain, NDV03-026 shown distinct from the vaccine strain LaSota/26, which normally lentogenic, were found to have the characterization of virulent strains, whose cleavage site of F protein was ^{112}RRQKRF^{117}. This was the first report of this strain which will be sequenced to study the characterization and origin of the virus. Eighty-four strains were assigned to genotype VII, within which 74 of these strains belonged to the established subgroups VIId, nine strains were subgroups VIIc, while one strain (NDV04-21) diverged from VIIc and VIId viruses by 4.4–6.9% were assigned to a novel subgroup VIIe (FIG. 1).

Alignment of the Predicted Amino Acid Sequences

Protein sequences corresponding to amino acid residues 1-129 of the F protein of different genotypes and subtypes were aligned (FIG. 3). The cleavage sites of all isolated were analyzed. In the 84 strains of genotype VII, most of them (77 strains) had the residues ^{112}RRQKRF^{117}, three (NDV03-044, NDV03-018, and NDV02-047) possessing ^{112}KRQKRF^{117}, two (NDV02-040 and

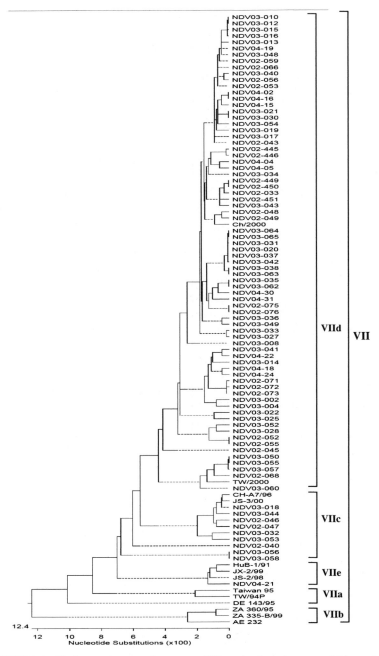

FIGURE 1. Phylogenetic tree of genotype VII strains based on a variable region (nt 47–420) of the F gene.

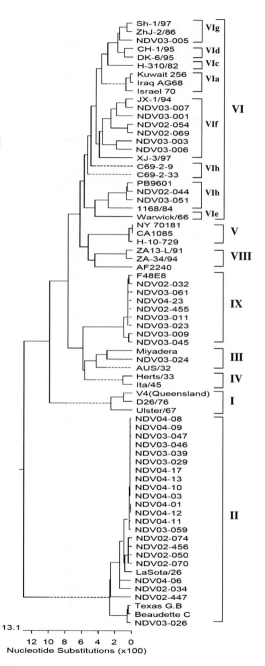

FIGURE 2. Phylogenetic tree of other genotype isolates apart from VII based on a variable region (nt 47–420) of the F gene.

```
Majority         M G S R S S T R I P V P L M L I T R I M L I L S C I C L T S S L D G R P L A A A G I V
                                    10                  20                  30                  40

V4(Queensland)-I . . . . . . . . . . . . . . . . T V . V . . . A . . . V . P . . A . . . . . . . . . . . 43
NDV03-026-II     . . . . . . . K N . T . M . . T V . V A . V . . . . P A N . I . . . . . . . . 43
NDV02-034-II     . . . . . . . . . . A . . . . T I Q . A . V . . . . P A N . . . . . . . . . . 43
NDV03-024-III    . . . . . . . . . . . . . . . T I . . T . A . . Y V R . . . . . . . . . . . . 43
Herts/33-IV      . . . . . . . . . . . . . P . . I . V . T . . . . R . . . . . . . . . . . . . 43
CA1085-V         . . . K P . . . . S . . . . . . . . . T . . . . . . . . . . . . . . . . . . . 43
Kuwait 256-VIa   . . K P . . . . . . . . . . . . . . . . . . . . . . . . . . . . . . . . . . . 43
NDV02-044-VIb    . . . . . . A . P . . V . . . . . . . . . . . . P . G . . . . . . . . . . . . 43
H-310/82-VIc     . . . K P . . . V S . . . . . . . . T . . . . . . . . . . . . . . . . . . . . 43
CH-1/95-VId      . . . K P P . . . S . . P . . . . . . . . . . . . . . . . . . . . . . . . . . 43
Warwick/66-VIe   . . . K P . . . . . . . . . . . . . . . . . . . . . . . . . . . . . . . . . . 43
NDV03-001-VIf    . . . . L P . . . . P . . . . . . . . . . . . . . . . . . . . . . . . . . . . 43
NDV03-005-VIg    . . . . L P . . . S L . P . . . . . T . . S . . . . . . . . . . . . . . . . . 43
Taiwan 95-VIIa   . . . E P . . . V . . . . . . . . . . . N . . . . . . . . . . . . . . . . . . 43
AE 232-VIIb      . . . K P . . . . A . . . . . . V . . . S . . . R S . . . . . . . . . . . . . 43
NDV03-044-VIIc   . . . . . . . . . A . P . . . . . . . . . . . . . A . . . . . . . . . . . . . 43
NDV04-22-VIId    . . . . . . . . . A . . . . . . . . . . R . . . . . . . . . . . . . . . . . . 43
NDV02-449-VIId   . . . . . . . . . A . . . . . . . . G . . R P . . . . . . R . . . . . . . . . 43
HuB-1/91-VIIe    . . . K P . . . . . S . . . . . . . . . . . . . . . . . . . . . . . . . . . . 43
AF2240-VIII      . . . K . . . . T . . . . T . . . . . T . . . . . . . . . . . . . . . . . . . 43
NDV02-032-IX     . . . . . . . . N V . A . P . . T V . . A . A . . . V R . . N . . . . . . . . 43
NDV04-23-IX      . . . . . . . . N V . A . . . . T V . . A . A . . . V R . . N . . . . . . . . 43
```

```
Majority         V T G D K A V N I Y T S S Q T G S I I V K L L P N M P K D K E A C A K A P L E A Y N R
                                    50                  60                  70                  80

V4(Queensland)-I . . . . . . . . . . . . . . . . . . . I . . . . . . . . . . . . . . . . . . . . . 86
NDV03-026-II     . . . . . . . . . . . . . . . . . . . . . . . . . L . . . . . . . . . . D . . . . 86
NDV02-034-II     . . . . . . . . . . . . . . . . . . . . . . . . . L . . . . . . . . . . D . . . . 86
NDV03-024-III    . . . . . . . . . . . . . . . . . . . . . . . . . . . . . . . . . . . . . . . . . 86
Herts/33-IV      . . . . . . . . . . . . . . . . . . . . . . . . . . . . . . . . . . . . . . . . . 86
CA1085-V         . . . . . . . . . . . . . . . . . . . . . . . . . . . . . . . . . . . . . . . . . 86
Kuwait 256-VIa   . . . . . . . . . . . . . . . . . . . . . . . . . . . . . . . . . . . . . . . . . 86
NDV02-044-VIb    . . . . . . I . . . . . . . . . . . . . . . . . . . . . . . . . . . . . . . . . . 86
H-310/82-VIc     . . . . . . . . . . . . . . . . . . . I . . . . . . . . . . . . . . . . . . . . . 86
CH-1/95-VId      . . . . . . . . . . . . . . . . . . . I . . . . . . . . . . . . . . . . . . . . . 86
Warwick/66-VIe   . . . . . . . . . . . . . . . . . . . . . . . . . . . . . . . . . R . . . . . . . 86
NDV03-001-VIf    . . . . . . . . . . . . . . . . . . . . . . . . . . . . . . . . . . . . . . . . . 86
NDV03-005-VIg    . . . . . . . . . . . . . . . . . . . I . . . . . . . . . . . . . . . . . . . . . 86
Taiwan 95-VIIa   . . . . . . . . . . . . . . . . . . . . . . . . . . . . . . . . . . T . . . . . . 86
AE 232-VIIb      . . . E . . . . . . . . . . . . . . . . . . . . . . . . . . . . . . . . . . . . . 86
NDV03-044-VIIc   . . . . . . . . . . . . . . . . . . . . . . . . . . . . . . . . . . . . . . . . . 86
NDV04-22-VIId    . . . . . . . V . . . . . . . . . . . . . . R . . . . . . . . . . . . . . . . . . 86
NDV02-449-VIId   . . . . . . . V . . . . . . . . . . . . . . R . . . . . . . . . . . . . . . . . . 86
HuB-1/91-VIIe    . . . . . . . . . . . . . . . . . . . . . . . . . . . . . . . . . . . . . . . . . 86
AF2240-VIII      . . . . . . . . . . . . . . . . . . . . . . . . . . . . . . . . . P . V . . . . . 86
NDV02-032-IX     . . . . . . . . . . . . . . . . . . . . . . . . . . . . . . . . . . . . . . . . . 86
NDV04-23-IX      . . . . . . . . . . . . . . . . . . . . . . . . . . . . . . . . . . . . . . . . . 86
```

```
Majority         T L T T L L T P L G D S I R R I Q G S V S T S G G R R Q K R F I G A I I G S V A L G V
                                    90                 100                 110                 120

V4(Queensland)-I . . . . . . . . . . . . . . . E . T . . . . . G K . G . L . . . . . . G . . . . 129
NDV03-026-II     . . . . . . . . . . . . . . . E . T . . . . . . . . . . . . . . . . . . G . . . . 129
NDV02-034-II     . . . . . . . . . . . . . . . E . T . . . . . G . . G . L . . . . . . G . . . . 129
NDV03-024-III    . . . . . . . . . . . . . . . E . T . . . . . . R . . . . . . . . . . . . . . . 129
Herts/33-IV      . . . . . . . . . . . . . K . E . T . . . . . R . . . . . . . . . . . . . . . . 129
CA1085-V         . . . . . . . . . . . . A T . . . . . . . . . . . . . . . . V . . . . . . . . . 129
Kuwait 256-VIa   . . . . . . . . . . . . . . . . . . . . . . . . . . . . . . . . . . . . . . . . 129
NDV02-044-VIb    . . . . . . . . . . . . . . . . . . . . . W E K . . . . . . . . . . . . . . . . 129
H-310/82-VIc     . . . . . S . . . . . . . . . . . . . . . . . . . . . . . . . . . . . . . . . . 129
CH-1/95-VId      . . . . . S . . . . . . . . . . . . . . . . . . . . . . . . . . . . . . . . . . 129
Warwick/66-VIe   . P . . . . . . . . . . . . . . . T . . . . . . . . . . . . . V . . . . . . . . 129
NDV03-001-VIf    . . . . . . . . . . . . . K . . . . . . . . R . . . . . . . . . . . . . . . . . 129
NDV03-005-VIg    . . . . . S . . . . . . . . . . . . . . . . . . . . . . . . . V . . . . . . . . 129
Taiwan 95-VIIa   . . . . . . . . . . . . . K . . . . . . . . . . . . . . . . . V . . . . . . . . 129
AE 232-VIIb      . . . . . . . . . . . . . . . E . . . . . . K . R . . . . . V . . . . . . . . . 129
NDV03-044-VIIc   . . . . . . . . . . . . . K . . . . . . . . K . . . . . . . V . . . . . . . . . 129
NDV04-22-VIId    . . . . . . . . . . . . . K . . . . . . . . . . . . . . . . . V . . . . . . . . 129
NDV02-449-VIId   . . . . . A . . . . . . . K . . . . . . . . . . . . . . . . . V . . . . . . . . 129
HuB-1/91-VIIe    . . . . . . . . . . . . . K . . . . . . . . R . . . . . . . V . . . . . . . . . 129
AF2240-VIII      . . . . . . . . . . . . . . . T . . . . . . . . . . . . . . . V . . . . . . . . 129
NDV02-032-IX     . . . . . . . . . . . . . . . E . A T . . . . . . R . . . . . . . . . . . . . . 129
NDV04-23-IX      . . . . . . . . . . . . . . . E . A T . . . . . . R . . . . . . . . . . . . . . 129
```

Decoration 'Decoration #1': Hide (as '.') residues that match the Consensus exactly.

FIGURE 3. Alignment of the predicted amino acid sequences of F proteins of different genotypes and subgenotype.

NDV04-21) having ^{112}RRRKRF^{117}, and one (NDV04-24) having the characterization of ^{112}RRQRRF^{117}, which indicated that all the isolates were velogenic. In the 22 strains of genotype II, most of them have the same residues, which were identical to the vaccine of LaSota/26, showing they were lentogenic strains, but only one strain (NDV03-026) had the motif of ^{112}RRQKRF^{117}, which was identical with the mesogenic strain of Beaudette C and velogenic strain of Texas G.B., indicated that it may be a virulent strains. Because there were no similar strains used in China, its origin and characteristic would be interested to study, we would sequence the complete genome of strain NDV03-026 for further characterization. All the isolates of genotype IX isolated in China only have identical cleavage site ^{112} RRQRRF^{117}, indicated that all of them were velogenic.

DISCUSSION

Sequence analysis of the F protein cleavage site were used for determining the pathogenicity of NDV instead of conventional methods such as mean death time (MDT) and intracerebral pathogenic index tests (ICPI).[11–14] In the present study, the phylogenetic analysis of partial F gene nucleotide sequence produced similar tree topology compared with those from entire gene sequences as shown in previous studies.[12,17,19–21,23,25] In this research, we isolated and collected 124 strains from 2002 to 2004 in China, and successfully amplified and sequenced the main function region of F gene with cleavage site by use of the one-step RT-PCR technique. From the results, we concluded that the prevalence of NDV genotypes in China is complex including genotype II, III, VI, and VII (but mostly isolates belong to the genotype VII). These results indicated that the prevalence was in accordance with the fourth epizootic in the world.[19,23,32] The sequence distances were biggest among the different genotype isolates. The vaccine strains used in China belonged to genotype I, II, and IX. Obviously, it was not in accordance with the prevalent genotype. We cannot ensure that the difference was relative to the ND outbreaks in China. At present, there are ongoing studies to evaluate new vaccines to control the disease, but some researchers continue to use traditional vaccines. A recent study at the National Laboratory for Newcastle Disease of Animal Quarantine Institute, Ministry of Agriculture indicated the LaSota/26 vaccine can effectively safeguard artificial infection with some genotype isolates.

In this article, we identified a novel genotype IX (include 8 strains, together with the traditional vaccine strain F48E8 in China). All genotype IX strains had residue substitutions of I $\rightarrow$ V at 9 position and V $\rightarrow$ A at the 106 position that distinguished them from all other genotypes. Residue substitutions of R $\rightarrow$ K at the 101 position and I $\rightarrow$ V at the 121 position, unique to subgenotype VIIa, was shared by subgroups VIIc, VIId, and VIIe. The ^{101}K and ^{121}V were the characteristic of genotype VII virus (TABLE 1).

TABLE 1. Unique residue substitutions of deduced amino acid sequences of F gene for NDV strains of different genotypes or subgenotypes

Genotype and subgenotype	4	5	9	10	13	16	17	23	28	63	93	101	104	106	107	109	112	113	114	115	116	117	118	121
	R	S	I	P	L	T	V	L	P	V	T	R	E	V	T	S	R	R	Q	K	R	F	I	I
I	–	–	–	–	–	–	–	–	–	I	–	–	–	–	–	–	G	K	–	G	–	L	–	–
II	–	–	–	–	–	–	I	–	–	–	–	–	–	–	–	–	G	–	–	G	–	L	–	–
III	–	–	–	–	–/P	–	I	–	–	–/I	–	–	–	–	–	–	–	–	–	–/R	–	–	–	–
IV	K	P	–	S	–	I	I	–	L	–	–	–	G	A	–	–	–	–	–	R	–	–	–	–
V	K	P	–	–	–	I	T	–	L	–/I	–	–	G	–	–	–	–	–	–	–	–	–	V	–
VI a	K	P	–	–	–	I	T	–	L	–	–	–	G	–	S	–	–	–	–	–	–	–	–	–
b	K	P	–	S	–	I	T	–	L	I	–	–	G	–	S	–	G	–	–	–	–	–	–	–
c	K	P	V/–	S	P	I	T	–	L	I	S	–	G	–	S	–	–	–	–	–	–	–	–	–
d	K	P	–/T	–	P	I	T	–	L	I	S	–	G	–	S	–	–	–	–	–	–	–	–	–
f	–	–	–	–	–	–	T	–	–/Q	–	S	–/K	G	–	S	–	–	–	–/R	–	–	–	–/V	–
g	–	–	–	–	P	–	T	–	–	I	–	–	G	–	S	–	–	–	–	–	–	–	–	–
h	–	–	–	–	–	–	–	–	–	–	S	K	G	–	S	–	–	–	–	–	–	–	–	–
VII a	K	P	T	–	–	I	T	S	L	–	–	K	G	–	S	P	–	–	–	–	–	–	–	–/v
b	K	P	–	–	–	I	T	–	L	–	–	K	G	–	S	–	–	–	–	–	–	–	–	–/v
c	–	P	–	–	–	–	T	–	L	–	–	K	G	–	S	–	–	–	–	–	–	–	–	–/v
d	–/R	P	–	–	–	–	T	–	L	–	–	K	G	–	S	–	–	–	–	–	–	–	–	–/v
e	–	P	–	–	–	V	–	–	L	–	–	K	G	–	S	–	–	–	–	–	–	–	–	–/v
VIII	K	–	–	–	–	–	–	–	L	–	–	–	G	A	–	–	–	–	R/–	–	–	–	–	L/–
IX	–	–	V	–	P	–	–	–	–	–	–	–	–	–	–	–	–	–	–	R	–	–	–	–

In this article, we also described the occurrence of the genotype II. Genotype II had been isolated in 1945 in China and was the traditional vaccine strain (La-Sota/26 strains) used popularly in China. We isolated a strain, namely NDV03-026, which was different from other isolates at the cleavage site of F protein of genotype II isolates. The motif of the sequence was ^{112}RRQKRF^{117}, which was consistent with the characterization of velogenic strain, indicating it may be a virulent strain. The genome of the strain NDV03-026 will be sequenced to analyze its characterization and origin.

The efficient proteolytic activation of the F protein and virulence of NDV is related to the presence of two pairs of basic amino acids at the C terminus of the F2 polypeptide. To date variations of amino acid sequences of cleavage site of F protein have been reported. Among the 84 genotype VII strains, 77 possessed the motif of ^{112}RRQKRF^{117}, 3 were ^{112}KRQKRF^{117}, 2 were ^{112}RRRKRF^{117}, and only one possessed ^{112}RRQRRF^{117} motif, showing that all the isolates were velogenic. In the 22 strains of genotype II, 21 isolates have the same residues ^{112}GRQGRL^{117}, suggesting that they were lentogenic strains. The only exceptional strain, NDV03-026, had the motif of ^{112}RRQKRF^{117}, indicated that it might be a virulent strain, and this was confirmed in a subsequent study. Approach to the origin of this isolate would be interesting since no similar strains have ever been reported in China.

CONCLUSION

According to the phylogenetic analysis, we have shown that multiple genotypes of NDV have co-circulated in China, and the genotype VIId has been maintained by enzootic infectious in recent years in China.

REFERENCES

1. AHLERT, T. *et al.* 1997. Tumor-cell number and viability as quality and efficacy parameters of autologous virus-modified cancer vaccines in patients with breast or ovarian cancer. J. Clin. Oncol. **15:** 1354–1366.
2. ALEXANDER, D.J. 2001. Gordon memorial lecture. Newcastle disease. Br. Poult. Sci. 5–22.
3. MA, M. 2002. A summary of taxonomic changes recently approved by ICTV. Arch. Virol. **147:** 1655–1663.
4. MA, M. 2002. Virus taxonomy-Houston. Arch. Virol. **147:** 1071–1076.
5. HUANG, Z. *et al.* 2003. Recombinant Newcastle disease virus as a vaccine vector. Poult. Sci. **82:** 899–906.
6. PEETERS, B.P. *et al.* 2000. Genome replication of Newcastle disease virus: involvement of the rule-of-six. Arch. Virol. **145:** 1829–1845.
7. KRISHNAMURTHY, S. & S.K. SAMAL. 1998. Nucleotide sequences of the trailer, nucleocapsid protein gene and intergenic regions of Newcastle disease virus strain Beaudette C and completion of the entire genome sequence. J. Gen. Virol. **79:** 2419–2424.

8. DE LEEUW, O. & B. PEETERS. 1999. Complete nucleotide sequence of Newcastle disease virus: evidence for the existence of a new genus within the subfamily Paramyxovirinae. J. Gen. Virol. **80:** 131–136.

9. ROMER-OBERDORFER, A. *et al.* 1999. Generation of recombinant lentogenic Newcastle disease virus from cDNA. J. Gen. Virol. **80:** 2987–2995.

10. COLLINS, M.S., J.B. BASHIRUDDIN & D.J. ALEXANDER. 1993. Deduced amino acid sequences at the fusion protein cleavage site of Newcastle disease viruses showing variation in antigenicity and pathogenicity. Arch. Virol. **128:** 363–370.

11. ALEXANDER, D.J. *et al.* 1997. Newcastle disease outbreak in pheasants in Great Britain in May 1996. Vet. Rec. **140:** 20–22.

12. SEAL, B.S., D.J. KING & J.D. BENNETT. 1995. Characterization of Newcastle disease virus isolates by reverse transcription PCR coupled to direct nucleotide sequencing and development of sequence database for pathotype prediction and molecular epidemiological analysis. J. Clin. Microbiol. **33:** 2624–2630.

13. MARIN, M.C. *et al.* 1996. Virus characterization and sequence of the fusion protein gene cleavage site of recent Newcastle disease virus field isolates from the southeastern United States and Puerto Rico. Avian Dis. **40:** 382–390.

14. GOULD, A.R. *et al.* 2001. Virulent Newcastle disease in Australia: molecular epidemiological analysis of viruses isolated prior to and during the outbreaks of 1998-2000. Virus Res. **77:** 51–60.

15. RUSSELL, P.H. & D.J. ALEXANDER.1983. Antigenic variation of Newcastle disease virus strains detected by monoclonal antibodies. Arch. Virol. **75:** 243–253.

16. JARECKI-BLACK, J.C. & D.J. KING. 1993. An oligonucleotide probe that distinguishes isolates of low virulence from the more pathogenic strains of Newcastle disease virus. Avian Dis. **37:** 724–730.

17. SEAL, B.S., D.J. KING & J.D. BENNETT. 1996. Characterization of Newcastle disease virus vaccines by biological properties and sequence analysis of the hemagglutinin-neuraminidase protein gene. Vaccine **14:** 761–766.

18. SEAL, B.S., D.J. KING & R.J. MEINERSMANN. 2000. Molecular evolution of the Newcastle disease virus matrix protein gene and phylogenetic relationships among the paramyxoviridae. Virus Res. **66:** 1–11.

19. LOMNICZI, B. *et al.* 1998. Newcastle disease outbreaks in recent years in western Europe were caused by an old (VI) and a novel genotype (VII). Arch. Virol. **143:** 49–64.

20. SAKAGUCHI, T. *et al.* 1989. Newcastle disease virus evolution. I. Multiple lineages defined by sequence variability of the hemagglutinin-neuraminidase gene. Virology **169:** 260–72.

21. TOYODA, T. *et al.* 1989. Newcastle disease virus evolution. II. Lack of gene recombination in generating virulent and avirulent strains. Virology **169:** 273–282.

22. BALLAGI-PORDANY, A. *et al.* 1996. Identification and grouping of Newcastle disease virus strains by restriction site analysis of a region from the F gene. Arch. Virol. **141:** 243–261.

23. YANG, C.Y. *et al.* 1999. Newcastle disease virus isolated from recent outbreaks in Taiwan phylogenetically related to viruses (genotype VII) from recent outbreaks in Western Europe. Avian Dis. **43:** 125–130.

24. KE, G.M. *et al.* 2001. Molecular characterization of Newcastle disease viruses isolated from recent outbreaks in Taiwan. J. Virol. Methods **97:** 1–11.

25. YU, L. *et al.* 2001. Characterization of newly emerging Newcastle disease virus isolates from the People's Republic of China and Taiwan. J. Clin. Microbiol. **39:** 3512–3519.

26. LIANG, R. *et al.* 2002. Newcastle disease outbreaks in western China were caused by the genotypes VIIa and VIII. Vet. Microbiol. **87:** 193–203.

27. MASE, M. *et al.* 2002. Phylogenetic analysis of Newcastle disease virus genotypes isolated in Japan. J. Clin. Microbiol. **40:** 3826–3830.

28. LIU, X.F. *et al.* 2003. Pathotypical and genotypical characterization of strains of Newcastle disease virus isolated from outbreaks in chicken and goose flocks in some regions of China during 1985-2001. Arch. Virol. **148:** 1387–1403.

29. WANG, J. *et al.* 2001. Study of Newcastle disease virus in the treatment of human laryngeal squamous carcinoma. Zhonghua Er Bi Yan Hou Ke Za Zhi **36:** 138–141.

30. WANG, Z.L. *et al.* 2000. Isolation and genotyping of Newcastle disease. Chinese J. Prev. Vet. Med. **22:** 69–71.

31. EPIZOOTIES, O.I.D. 1996. LIST A AND B DISEASES OF MAMMALS, BIRDS AND BEES MUNAL OF STANDARDS FOR DIAGNOSTIC TESTS AND VACCINES.

32. HERCZEG, J. *et al.* 1999. Two novel genetic groups (VIIb and VIII) responsible for recent Newcastle disease outbreaks in Southern Africa, one (VIIb) of which reached Southern Europe. Arch. Virol. **144:** 2087–2099.

Descriptive and Spatial Epidemiology of Rift Valley Fever Outbreak in Yemen 2000–2001

S. ABDO-SALEM,[a,b] G. GERBIER,[a] P. BONNET,[a] M. AL-QADASI,[c]
A. TRAN,[a] E. THIRY,[d] G. AL-ERYNI,[b] AND F. ROGER[a]

[a]CIRAD-EMVT, Montpellier, France

[b]College of Veterinary Sciences, University of Dhamar, Dhamar, Yemen

[c]Ministry of Agriculture, Sana'a, Yemen

[d]Faculty of Veterinary Medicine, University of Liege, Liège B-4000, Belgium

ABSTRACT: Rift valley fever (RVF) is an arboviral disease produced by a bunyavirus belonging to the genus Phlebovirus. Several species of *Aedes* and *Culex* are the vectors of this virus that affects sheep, goats, buffalos, cattle, camels and human beings. The human disease is well known, especially during periods of intense epizootic activity. The initial description of the disease dates back to 1930, when animals and human outbreaks appeared on a farm in Lake Naivasha, in the Great Rift Valley of Kenya. Until 2000, this disease was only described in Africa, and then outbreaks were also declared in the Kingdom of Saudi Arabia (2000–2001 and 2004) and in Yemen (2000–2001). Animal and human cases were recorded. This work presents a retrospective summary of the data collected on animal RVF cases during this epidemic in Yemen. Results from several RVF surveys were gathered from the Yemeni vet services and FAO experts. Geographical data (topographic maps and data freely available on internet) were used for the location of outbreaks. After cleaning and standardization of location names, all the data were introduced into a GIS database. The spatial distribution of outbreaks was then studied at two scales: at the national level and at a local scale in the particular area of Wadi Mawr in the Tihama plain, Western coast of Yemen.

KEYWORDS: Rift valley fever; Yemen; vector-borne disease; zoonosis

INTRODUCTION

Rift valley fever (RVF) is an arboviral disease produced by Bunyavirus belonging to the genus Phlebovirus. Several species of *Aedes* and *Culex*

Address for correspondence: Dr. Shaif Abdo-Salem, TA30/E, Campus international de Baillarguet, 34398 Montpellier Cedex 5, France. Voice: +33 4 67 59 38 33; fax: +33 4 67 59 37 54.
e-mail: abdo-salem.shaif@cirad.fr

Ann. N.Y. Acad. Sci. 1081: 240–242 (2006). © 2006 New York Academy of Sciences.
doi: 10.1196/annals.1373.028

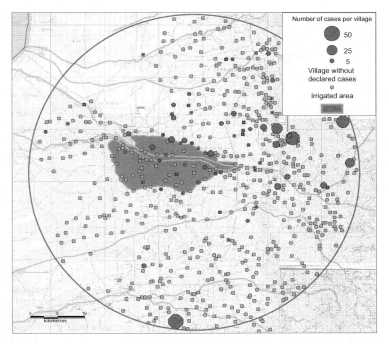

FIGURE 1. Villages infected around Bajilah from September 23, 2000 to February 3, 2001.

mosquitoes are the vectors of this virus, which not only affects sheep, goat, buffalo, cattle, and camels but also human beings. The human disease is well known, especially during the period of intense epizootic activity. Until 2000 this disease was only described in Africa; then outbreaks were declared for the first time outside Africa,[1,2] in the Kingdom of Saudi Arabia (2000–2001 and 2004) and in Yemen (2000–2001); animal and human cases were recorded. This work presents a retrospective summary of the data collected on animal RVF during the epidemics in Yemen.

METHODS

Results from several surveys were gathered and standardized from Yemen epidemiology unit Sana'a and FAO experts. The data used were from September 23, 2000 to February 3, 2001. An RVF case was defined as a village with at least one death or abortion in cattle, sheep, goat, or camel during this period. A 30 km radius area around the village of Bajilah was chosen in the Wadi Mawr (coast of Tihama). This intersects the districts of Az-Zuhrah, Al-Qanawis, Al-Luhayah, Az-Zaydiyah in the Governorates of Al-Hodeidah, Al-Tur, Kuaydinah, and Abs in Hajjah. In this area, 612 villages were pointed on 1:50,000 scale paper maps and compared with the epidemiological data set.

RESULTS AND DISCUSSION

Out of these villages, 67 were found infected with the RVF (FIG. 1). Most of these villages were located around the irrigation canal Wadi Mawr. The analyses of the precipitation data in the three meteorological stations (Az-Zuhrah, Kadamat Malaryah, and Jabal Al-Malah) from 1975 to 2002, showed no significant difference. No countrywide entomological studies were conducted nor were sentinel herds set up during the epidemics.[3] A first interpretation of a vegetation index derived from satellite imagery (NDVI: normalized difference vegetation index) showed a spatial heterogeneity in the cases location but no significant difference between the years 1999 and 2000. In the future the passive surveillance should be continued and quality of data should be improved. Landscape studies and entomology surveys in the area should be performed.

REFERENCES

1. ANONYMOUS. 2000. Outbreak of Rift Valley fever-Yemen, August-October 2000. MMWR Morb. Mortal Wkly Rep. **49:** 1065–1066.
2. WORLD ORGANIZATION ANIMAL HEALTH. 2004. Rift Valley fever in Saudia Arabia—serological findings. OIE Disease information. **17:** 40.
3. LINTHICUM, K.J., C.L. BAILEY, et al. 1987. Detection of Rift Valley fever viral activity in Kenya by satellite remote sensing imagery. Science **235:** 1656–1659.

Efficacy of DNA Immunization with F and G Protein Genes of Nipah Virus

XIJUN WANG,[a] JINYING GE,[a,b] SEN HU,[a] QINGHUA WANG,[a]
ZHIYUN WEN,[a] HUALAN CHEN,[a] AND ZHIGAO BU[a]

[a]*National Key Laboratory of Veterinary Biotechnology, Harbin Veterinary Research Institute, Chinese Academy of Agricultural Science, Harbin 150001, People's Republic of China*

[b]*College of Veterinary Medicine, Nanjing Agricultural University, Nanjing 210095, People's Republic of China*

ABSTRACT: We investigated the antibody response of DNA immunization with two mammalian codon optimized envelope glycoprotein genes, F and G, of Nipah virus in a mouse model. The results indicated that G gene immunization elicited more significant specific serum IgG response and neutralization antibody response than F gene did, suggesting that the G gene DNA immunization is a potential vaccine strategy against Nipah virus.

KEYWORDS: Nipah virus; DNA immunization; F protein; G protein

INTRODUCTION

In late 1998 and early 1999, an outbreak of acute encephalitis with 40% mortality of pig handlers in Malaysia and Singapore led to the discovery of a novel paramyxovirus named Nipah virus (NiV). Pigs are susceptible to NiV, and may get infection by contacting with the Pteropus fruit bat, the nature host for NiV.[1] Both fusion glycoprotein (F) and attachment glycoprotein (G) of NiV are required to mediate fusion with host target cell membranes and key structure proteins for inducing protective immune responses.[2] In this study, we investigated the antibody response induced by DNA immunization in mouse model with F and G glycoproteins of NiV.

METHODS

Two mammalian codon optimized F and G genes were generated by assembly PCR and inserted into mammalian expression vector pCAGGS.[3–5]

Address for correspondence: Zhigao Bu, Ph.D., National Key Laboratory of Veterinary Biotechnology, Harbin Veterinary Research Institute, Chinese Academy of Agricultural Science, 427 Maduan Street, Harbin 150001, P.R. China. Voice: 86-451-85935062; fax: 86-451-82733132.
e-mail: zgb@hvri.ac.cn

Ann. N.Y. Acad. Sci. 1081: 243–245 (2006). © 2006 New York Academy of Sciences.
doi: 10.1196/annals.1373.029

The resulting plasmids were named as pCAGGS-F and pCAGGS-G. Co-transfection with pCAGGS-F and pCAGGS-G in BHK-21 caused cell fusion, and the F and G expressions were confirmed by Western blot. Six-week-old female BALB/c mice were intramuscularly primed with 100 μg of plasmids pCAGGS-F, pCAGGS-G, or pCAGGS-F + pCAGGS-G and boosted with the same dose after 4 weeks. The sera were collected at 3 weeks post priming and boost, respectively. The serum IgG against NiV F and G proteins was detected by indirect enzyme-linked immunosorbent assay using recombinant Baculovirus expressed NiV F and G glycoproteins. For serum neutralization antibody detection, an NiV F and G protein pseudotyped recombinant Vesicular Stomatitis Virus (VSV), VSVΔG*F/G, in which the VSV envelope protein G gene was replaced by the green fluorescent protein (GFP) gene (VSVΔG*G), was generated to replace live NiV.[6,7] Serial twofold diluted heat-inactivated serum from mouse immunized with different plasmids or NiV immunized rabbit serum, nonimmunized rabbits serum, and naïve mice serum were mixed with 1.5×10^5 IU (infectious unit) of VSVΔG*F/G. After incubation at 37°C for 1 hour, the mixtures containing 5×10^4 IU of VSVΔG*F/G were added to PBS rinsed Vero E6 mono-layers in triplicate wells of 24-well plate. Neutralizing titers were expressed as the reciprocal of the highest serum dilution that fully inhibited GFP expression in cells infected with VSVΔG*F/G. The GFP positive cells were counted at 16 hours postinfection under a fluorescence microscope.

RESULTS AND DISCUSSION

DNA immunization with pCAGGS-G elicited more significant, specific IgG response than pCAGGS-F did in mice. pCAGGS-G induced 16 times higher titer of neutralization antibody response than pCAGGS-F in mice. Co-immunization with pCAGGS-F and pCAGGS-G does not enhance the specific IgG antibody and neutralization antibody response induced by pCAGGS-G alone. DNA immunizations with NiV envelope glycoprotein (especially G protein) efficiently elicit specific antibody responses and these antibodies are able to block NiV to entry susceptible cells. DNA immunization is a potential vaccine strategy for the prevention of NiV.

ACKNOWLEDGMENTS

We thank Dr. Whitt M. for providing VSVΔG*G system and Drs. Bryan Eaton and Linfa Wang for providing the rabbit antiserum to NiV. This study was supported by the Chinese 10th five-year plan 2005BA711A10 and Chinese national basic research 973 program 2005CB523200.

REFERENCES

1. CHUA, K.B., W.J. BELLINI, P.A. ROTA, *et al*. 2000. Nipah virus: a recently emergent deadly paramyxovirus. Science **288:** 1432–1435.
2. GUILLAUME, V., H. CONTAMIN, P. LOTH, *et al*. 2004. Nipah virus: vaccination and passive protection studies in a hamster model. J. Virol. **78:** 834–840.
3. CHAN, Y.P., K.B. CHUA, C.L. KOH, *et al*. 2001. Complete nucleotide sequences of Nipah virus isolates from Malaysia. J. Gen. Virol. **82**(Pt 9): 2151–2155.
4. BU, Z., L. YE, R.W. COMPANS, *et al*. 2003. Enhanced cellular immune response against SIV Gag induced by immunization with DNA vaccines expressing assembly and release-defective SIV Gag proteins. Virology **309:** 272–281.
5. NIWA, H., K. YAMAMURA, J. MIYAZAKI, *et al*. 1991. Efficient selection for high-expression transfectants with a novel eukaryotic vector. Gene **108:** 193–199.
6. TAKADA, A., C. ROBISON, H. GOTO, *et al*. 1997. A system for functional analysis of Ebola virus glycoprotein. Proc. Natl. Acad. Sci. USA **94:** 14764–14769.
7. OGINO, M., H. EBIHARA, B.H. LEE, *et al*. Use of vesicular stomatitis virus pseudotypes bearing hantaan or seoul virus envelope proteins in a rapid and safe neutralization test. Clin. Diagn. Lab. Immunol. **10:** 154–160.

Generating Vesicular Stomatitis Virus Pseudotype Bearing the Severe Acute Respiratory Syndrome Coronavirus Spike Envelope Glycoprotein for Rapid and Safe Neutralization Test or Cell-Entry Assay

JINYING GE,[a,b] ZHIYUN WEN,[a] XIJUN WANG,[a] SEN HU,[a]
YONGGANG LIU,[a] XIANGANG KONG,[a] HUALAN CHEN,[a]
AND ZHIGAO BU[a]

[a] *National Key Laboratory of Veterinary Biotechnology, Harbin Veterinary Research Institute, Chinese Academy of Agricultural Science, Harbin 150001, People's Republic of China*

[b] *College of Veterinary Medicine, Nanjing Agricultural University, Nanjing 210095, People's Republic of China*

ABSTRACT: We generated a recombinant vesicular stomatitis virus (VSV) pseudotype (VSV Δ G*SG) by replacing the envelope G gene with the GFP gene and complementing with spike glycoprotein (S) of SARS-CoV *in trans*. The neutralization and infection blocking tests showed that the VSV Δ G*SG and SARS-CoV reacted similarly to SARS-CoV specific antiserum, suggesting the VSVΔ G*SG can be a safe replacement of the live SARS-CoV for neutralization test and cell-entry assay.

KEYWORDS: SARS coronavirus; spike protein; VSV; pseudotype

INTRODUCTION

The handling of severe acute respiratory syndrome coronavirus (SARS CoV) is strictly restricted in bio-safety level 3 plus laboratory facility, which limits the relative research and vaccine development.[1] The spike glycoprotein (S) mediates SARS CoV to attach the receptor, enter the host cells by membrane fusion, and induce neutralization antibodies.[2–4] In this study, the vesicular

Address for correspondence: Zhigao Bu, Ph.D., National Key Laboratory of Veterinary Biotechnology, Harbin Veterinary Research Institute, Chinese Academy of Agricultural Sciences, 427 Maduan Street, Harbin 150001, P.R. China. Voice: 86-451-85935062; fax: 86-451-82733132.
e-mail: zgb@hvri.ac.cn

Ann. N.Y. Acad. Sci. 1081: 246–248 (2006). © 2006 New York Academy of Sciences.
doi: 10.1196/annals.1373.030

stomatitis virus (VSV) pseudotype bearing the S of SARS CoV was generated to replace the live virus to establish a novel, rapid, and safe neutralization test or cell-entry assay.

METHODS

The leader sequence of CD5 and residues 12 to 1,255 of the codon optimized S gene of SARS CoV which contains 17 residues of the cytoplasmic tail, and attaches 9 amino acids within the cytoplasmic tail mostly close to the transmembrane domain of VSV G protein, was cloned into pCAGGS.[2,4,5] The resulting plasmid pCAGGS-SG was used to transfect cells and the surface expression of S was confirmed by indirect fluorescence assay and Western blot. To generate pseudotype recombinant VSV with S of SARS CoV (VSVΔG*SG), 293T cells were transfected with pCAGGS-SG, and then infected with a recombinant VSV (VSVΔG*G), in which the open reading frame of G was replaced with the green fluorescent protein (GFP) gene and complemented with G *in trans*.[5,6] Three hundred $TCID_{50}$ of SARS CoV or 300 infectious units (IU) of VSVΔG*-SG was added to twofold diluted SARS CoV specific chicken antisera. After incubation for 1 hour, the mixtures containing 100 $TCID_{50}$ of virus or 100 IU VSVΔG*SG were added to the rinsed Vero E6 cells in triplicate wells of 96-well plates. Serum from specific pathogen free (SPF) chickens was included as negative controls. The cells infected with SARS CoV were monitored daily for the cytopathic effect for 5 days. Neutralizing titers were expressed as the reciprocal of the highest serum dilution that fully inhibited the virus replication in cells infected with SARS CoV or fully inhibited GFP expression in cells infected with VSVΔG*-SG. The GFP-positive cells were counted at 16 hours post infection under a fluorescence microscope.

RESULTS AND DISCUSSION

The GFP expression in the infected Vero E6 cells confirmed the infectious ability of the VSVΔG*-SG and also indicated that the virus titers ranged from 10^5 to 10^6 IU/mL in the 293T cells supernatant. A polyclone serum against SARS CoV blocks the infectivity of the VSVΔG*SGG in Vero E6 virus, and the blocking titer is similar to the titer blocking the live SARS CoV. These results indicated that the VSVΔG*SG will be a safe and useful replacement of the live SARS CoV for SARS neutralization test, cell-entry assay, and novel vaccine or antiviral drugs development.

ACKNOWLEDGMENTS

We thank Dr. Michael F. for providing signal sequence of CD5 and codon optimized S gene of SARS CoV, Dr. Kawaoka Y. for providing pCAGGS, and

Dr. Whitt M. for providing VSVΔG*G systems. This study was supported by the Chinese 10th five-year plan 2005BA711A10 and Chinese national basic research 973 program 2005CB523200.

REFERENCES

1. ROTA, P.A., M.S. OBERSTE, S.S. MONROE, *et al.* 2003. Characterization of a novel coronavirus associated with severe acute respiratory syndrome. Science **300:** 1394–1399.
2. LI, W., M.J. MOORE, N. VASILIEVA, *et al.* 2003. Angiotensin-converting enzyme 2 is a functional receptor for the SARS coronavirus. Nature **426:** 450–454.
3. YANG, Z.Y., W.P. KONG, Y. HUANG, *et al.* 2004. A DNA vaccine induces SARS coronavirus neutralization and protective immunity in mice. Nature **428:** 561–564.
4. MOORE, M.J., T. DORFMAN, W. LI, *et al.* 2004. Retroviruses pseudotyped with the severe acute respiratory syndrome coronavirus spike protein efficiently infect cells expressing angiotensin-converting enzyme 2. J. Virol. **78:** 10628–10635.
5. TAKADA, A., C. ROBISON, H. GOTO, *et al.* 1997. A system for functional analysis of ebola virus glycoprotein. Proc. Natl. Acad. Sci. USA **94:** 14764–14769.
6. OGINO, M., H. EBIHARA, B.H. LEE, *et al.* Use of vesicular stomatitis virus pseudotypes bearing hantaan or seoul virus envelope proteins in a rapid and safe neutralization test. Clin. Diagn. Lab. Immunol. **10:** 154–160.

Prevalence of *Salmonella* Species in Various Raw Meat Samples of a Local Market in Kathmandu

MAHENDRA MAHARJAN,[a] VANDANA JOSHI,[a] DURGA D. JOSHI,[b] AND POORNIMA MANANDHAR[c]

[a]*Central Department of Zoology (Parasitology), Tribhuvan University, Kathmandu, Nepal*

[b]*National Zoonoses and Food Hygiene Research Centre, Tahachal, Kathmandu, Nepal*

[c]*Central Veterinary Laboratory, Veterinary Complex, Tripureshor, Kathmandu, Nepal*

ABSTRACT: A cross-sectional study of raw meat samples from the local meat market of Kathmandu Metropolitan City was carried out during September 2002 to May 2003 with special emphasis on isolation and identification of *Salmonella* bacteria. A total of 123 raw meat samples (55 chicken, 37 buffalo, and 31 goat) were collected and analyzed relative to season. *Salmonella* spp was found in 11.4% (14/123) meat samples. Eight samples of chicken, that is, 14.5%, five samples of buffalo (13.5%), and one sample of goat (3.3%) were found to be positive for *Salmonella*. *Salmonella* prevalence revealed *Salmonella (S.) pullorum* in 3.3% samples, *S. gallinarum* in 0.8%, *S. typhi* in 1.6%, *S. choleraesuis* in 0.8%, and *Salmonella* of subgenus I or II group in 4.9% samples. More than 80% meat samples microbiologically processed indicated coliform contamination. Seasonal prevalence of *Salmonella* was highest in the months of April/May. Surveys revealed unsatisfactory conditions of sanitation in the local meat markets of Kathmandu.

KEYWORDS: *Salmonella*; chicken; buffalo; goat; local market; Nepal

INTRODUCTION

Meat is one of the most widely used animal origin food item. Its high nutritive value having both essential macro- and micronutrients makes it an important part of a balanced diet for most people. Unfortunately, meat is also a suitable media for growth of different micro-organisms. Among food-borne diseases of

Address for correspondence: Mahendra Maharjan, Central Department of Zoology (Parasitology), Tribhuvan University, Kirtipur, GPO Box: 23414, Kathmandu, Nepal. Voice: +977-1-4312314; fax: +977-1-4331896.

e-mail: mahendra_maharjan@yahoo.ca

Ann. N.Y. Acad. Sci. 1081: 249–256 (2006). © 2006 New York Academy of Sciences.
doi: 10.1196/annals.1373.031

animal origin, salmonellosis is considered as one of the main cause of bacterial gastroenteritides in humans.[1] Worldwide, salmonellosis is a leading cause of enteric infectious disease attributable to foods. *Salmonella (S.)* is one of the major meat and meat product-associated bacterial pathogen in relation to the increased salmonellosis cases in the world during the last 20 years.[2]

Improperly cooked chicken, eggs, and other chicken products are responsible for about 50% of common vehicle epidemics, other associated food include improperly cooked meats particularly beef and pork, that is, 13%.[3] Other than infected cases, in general the muscle of live, healthy animals is sterile. Intrinsic bacteria may be present in low levels in muscle tissue, but these are not the most common source of contamination. Extrinsic factors are by far the greatest contributors to carcass and meat contamination. Poor slaughtering facilities and meat handling practices contribute greatly to the spread of this disease. Meat carcasses may become contaminated from fecal material, paunch content, and from the hide.[4] Additional sources of cross-contamination exist in slaughtering process, such as tools, equipments, human contact, and carcass to carcass contact.[5] Large meat animals undergo a significant amount of cutting and boning in order to result finished products. Each time the carcass is cut, fresh new surfaces are exposed, which are highly susceptible to contamination. Immediately after slaughtering, the principal types of bacteria found on carcasses are animal strains; by the time the final cuts reach the retail consumer level, however, human strains become prevalent.[6]

Eggs, chicken, meat, and meat products are the most common food vehicles of salmonellosis to humans. In America and Europe *S. enteritidis* has become the predominant strain and outbreaks are related to eating of chicken or eggs from hens whose ovaries are colonized by *S. enteritidis*.[7]

In Nepal, buffalo contribute about 64% of meat consumed, followed by goat 20%, pork 7%, and chicken 6%.[8] The subtropical climate, poor sanitary conditions, improper storage facilities, poor food hygiene practices, and lack of prevention against diseases in Nepal have all contributed to a number of diseases originating from meat.

Consumption of meat is highest in Kathmandu, a capital city where more than 90% people are nonvegetarian. Due to lack of sufficiently well-organized slaughter houses, poor hygiene in the meat shops, and shortage of clean water, meat in Kathmandu is subject to contamination. Enteric fever is endemic in the Kathmandu valley. The disease flares to epidemic proportion from time to time.[9] This article deals with the slaughtering facilities and practices in a typical market place in Kathmandu and reports the isolation of *Salmonella* spp. in consumable meat.

MATERIALS AND METHODS

A total of 123 different raw meat samples were collected from 40 identified meat shops (28 registered and 12 not registered) in a Kathmandu local market in three different seasons during September/October, 2002; November/December, 2002; and April/May, 2003.

Approximately 1–2 mL of chicken, buffalo, and goat meat samples were collected using the sterile knives from all the identified meat shops, transported to the laboratory in sterile vials, and examined for bacteria.

Sample Processing

Pre-enrichment/Enrichment

Samples were pre-enriched in peptone water for about 6 h at 37°C by adding 10 mL of strontium chloride enrichment broth and incubated at 43°C for 24 h.[10]

Primary Culture

After pre-enrichment, one loopful sample of the peptone water was taken and streaked on eosin methylene blue media for the detection of *E. coli* and on MacConkey agar to detect lactose fermenting and nonlactose fermenting bacteria. The inoculated plates were incubated for 24 h at 37°C.

A loopful of enriched samples (incubated at 43°C for 24 h) were taken and streaked on bismuth sulphite agar (BSA) by the quadrant streak method for isolation of *Salmonella*. The inoculated plates incubated at 37°C were observed daily for 7 days unless the culture was obtained.

Subculture

Isolates from BSA agar were streaked onto brilliant green agar (BGA) and xylose lysine deoxycholate (XLD) agar. The inoculated plates were incubated for 48 h at 37°C. The colonies of *Salmonella* were streaked from sub-culture agar to nutrient agar for pure culture and incubated at 37°C for 24 h for the further test.

Identification of Isolated Salmonella *Species*

The typical colonies of *Salmonella* on BSA, BGA, and XLD were identified by their morphological characteristics and biochemical tests.[11,12] The primary test includes motility, Gram's stain, catalase, oxidase, and oxidation/fermentation test followed by secondary/biochemical tests.

To confirm the *Salmonella* obtained in culture media during the process of identification, agglutination test was carried out by using two types of antiserums: Poly O sera and Oxoid Latex Test Reagent.

TABLE 1. Species wise prevalence of *Salmonella* in Kathmandu local market

Isolates	Positive cases out of 123 samples	Percentage
S. pullorum	4	3.3%
S. gallinarum	1	0.8%
S. typhi	2	1.6%
S. choleraesuis	1	0.8%
Salmonella of subgenus I or II group	6	4.9%

RESULTS

In Kathmandu meat markets, various kinds of meat are sold. Some shops sell meat from one species only. Samples were collected from 12 goat shops, 24 chicken shops, and 14 buffalo shops with 10 shops keeping both chicken and goat. During the survey, it was found that the chickens and goats were slaughtered either in or around shops and sometimes along the roads. Buffalo were slaughtered outside the shop and only carcasses were brought to the shop for sale.

Most shops (24) used hot water for cleaning chicken and goats, but repeated use of water was found to be common. Cold water was used generally for buffalo meat. An irregular water supply to most of the shops made washing practices more difficult and consequently, washing utensils and knives were infrequently practiced. Out of 40 shops only 16 shops (40%) had refrigeration available. Covering and hanging of carcass was unusual.

Prevalence of Salmonella *Species in Various Raw Meat Samples*

Out of 123 samples tested 14 (11.4%) samples were found to be positive for various species of *Salmonella. S. pullorum* was found in 3.3% samples, *S. gallinarum* in 0.8%, *S. typhi* in 1.6%, *S. choleraesuis* in 0.8%, and S*almonella* of subgenus I and II in 4.9% samples (TABLE 1). *Salmonella* prevalence in various raw meat samples collected from the market showed that 14.5% in chicken, 13.5% in buffalo, and 3.2% in goats (TABLE 2).

Out of 55 chicken samples, 8 were found to be positive for *Salmonella,* among them 4 were *S. pullorum,* 1 was *S. gallinarum,* and 3 isolates were of *Salmonella* of subgenus I or II type. Most of the *Salmonella* isolates from poultry samples were found to be of the contaminant type, since *S. pullorum* and *S. gallinarum* are *Salmonella* types adapted to poultry. Among 5 buffalo isolates, 2 were *S. typhi* 1 was *S. choleraesuis,* and 2 were *Salmonella* of subgenus I and II group. *S. typhi* and *S. choleraesuis* are *Salmonella* types not adapted to cattle. *S. typhi* is human adapted type and *S. choleraesuis* is swine adapted type. Thus their presence in buffalo samples may be the case of extrinsic contamination. *Salmonella* of subgenus I or II group were isolated

TABLE 2. Prevalence of *Salmonella* in various raw meat samples of Kathmandu local market

Type of meat sample	Total sample processed	Primary culture							Sub culture			Total percentage
		Growth in EMB agar		Growth in MacConkey agar				Growth in BSA agar +ve	Growth in BGA +ve	Growth in XLD +ve	Total positive	
				Lac. fer.		Non lac.fer.						
		+ve	%	+ve	%	+ve	%					
Chicken	55	44	80	55	100	16	29	9	8	7	8	14.5%
Buffalo	37	33	89	37	100	11	29	6	3	5	5	13.5%
Goat	31	22	70	31	100	7	22	2	1	1	1	3.2%
Total	123	99	80	123	100	34	27	17			14	11.4%

Lac. fer. = lactose fermenting; Non lac. fer. = nonlactose fermenting; +ve = positive.

TABLE 3. Species wise prevalence of *Salmonella* in various raw meat samples

Types of sample	Total sample processed	Total positive	Isolates	Positive cases	Percentage
Chicken	55	8	*S. pullorum*	4	7.3%
			S. gallinarum	1	1.8%
			Salmonella of subgenus I or II	3	5.5%
Buffalo	37	5	*S. typhi*	2	5.4%
			S. choleraesuis	1	2.7%
			Salmonella of subgenus I or II	2	5.4%
Goat	31	1	*Salmonella* of subgenus I or II	1	3.2%

from all species and could not be differentiated, but subgenus I includes type species like *S. entiritidis* that is a very prevalent species(TABLE 3).

Seasonal Variation of Salmonella *Species Contamination in Various Raw Meat Samples*

The presence of *Salmonella* in meat samples were found to be highest in the months of April/May (summer season) at 18% while in September/October (autumn) it was found to be only 4.3%. *Salmonella* was isolated from 13.15% of samples in the months of November/December (FIG. 1).

DISCUSSION AND CONCLUSION

Meat is an important source of protein and a valuable commodity in resource poor communities, such as Nepal. In concert with the intensification of animal husbandry in developing countries and development of different types of food of animal origin, new problems of food-borne zoonotic diseases are arising.

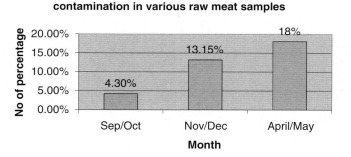

FIGURE 1. Seasonal variation of the *Salmonella* contamination in various raw meat samples.

Parasitic and zoonotic food-borne diseases are particularly prevalent in tropical and subtropical countries. There are a number of factors responsible for the spread of zoonotic disease, such as salmonellosis. Clean washing water is critical. Sanitation and clean water use during the slaughtering and processing of meat can protect the meat from contamination. This study of meat shops in Kathmandu revealed that most of the shops do not operate in a safe and clean environment. Covering and hanging carcasses were rarely practiced. Further, the chopping blocks were found to be same for different meat types. Thus, if any prior carcass happens to be infected, further chances of cross-contamination of uninfected carcass increases. It is well documented that *Listeria* spp. *staphylococcus aureus, yersinea enterocolitica, Salmonella,* and *Aeromonas* spp. may be detected in slaughter house environment, for example, on floor and walls, cold room floor, hand basins, splitting saws, chopping blocks, etc. The processing of carcass into parts further spreads contamination by exposing more carcass surface and susceptible fleshy parts to the contaminants if the same cutting tables and knives are used.[6]

The shops using cold water were at high risk of using contaminated water for the processing of meat. A survey of the ground water quality of an urban area of the Lalitpur district of Nepal showed that 85.6% samples of water from different sources were positive for fecal contamination. *Salmonella* species were detected in 10.8% of the sources.[13]

ACKNOWLEDGMENTS

We are very much thankful to the Royal Nepal Science and Technology (RONAST) for providing partial grant to Vandana Joshi. The Head of the Central Department of Zoology, the Director of the Central Veterinary Laboratory, and the National Zoonoses and Food Hygiene Research Centre are also acknowledged for providing laboratory facilities during the study period.

REFERENCES

1. STEELE, J.H. & M.M. GALTON. 1998. Epidemiology of food borne salmonellosis. Health Lab. Sci. **4:** 207–212.
2. WHO. 1982. Bacterial and viral zoonoses. Tech. Report Series. **682:** 7–9.
3. CENTER FOR DISEASE CONTROL AND PREVENTION. 1999. Outbreak of *Salmonella* serotype muenchen infection associated with unpasteurized orange juice. US. Canada **48:** 582–585.
4. LAHR, J.A. 1996. Beef carcass microbial contamination-post slaughter number of bacteria, sources of contamination and variability. Proceeding of 49th Annual Reciprocal Meats Conference. 132–137. Provo, Utah.
5. HUFFMAN, R.D. 2002. Current and future technologies for the decontamination of carcass and fresh meat. ICoMST-Rome **1:** 9–14.
6. MORTON, S. 2002. Use of irradiation for microbial decontamination of meat: situation and perspective. 48th ICoMST Room **1:** 3–7.

7. MORRIS, E.P., M. YASMIN & K.K. FRITZ. 1997. Emerging of foodborne diseases. World Health Organization. Geneva, Switzerland **1:** 16–17.
8. JOSHI, D.D., M. MAHARJAN, M.V. JOHNSEN, *et al*. 2003. Improving meat inspection and control in resources poor communities. The Nepal example. Acta Tropica **87:** 119–127.
9. MALLA, F.B. & G.M. SAKYA. 1984. Enteric fever—a review of clinical records. J. Nep. Med. Assoc. **22:** 9–15.
10. ELIZABETH, O.K. 1975. The identification of unusual pathogenic gram negative bacteria. First edition. U.S. Department of Health, Education and Welfare Public Health Service, Atlanta, Georgia.
11. COWAN, S.T. 1974. Cowan and Steele's Manual for the Identification of Medical Bacteria, 2nd ed. Cambridge University Press. London.
12. HOLT, J.G., N.R. KRIEG, P.H.A. SNEATH, *et al*., Eds. 1994. Bergey's Manual of Determinative Bacteriology London. 9th ed. The Williams and Wilkins Company. Baltimore, Maryland.
13. MAHARJAN, M. & A.P. SHARMA. 2000. Bacteriological quality of ground water in urban Patan and antibiotic sensitivity against isolated enteric bacteria. J. Nep. Med. Assoc. **39:** 269–274.

Prevalence of *Salmonella* in Retail Chicken Meat in Hanoi, Vietnam

LUU QUYNH HUONG,[a] REINHARD FRIES,[b] PAWIN PADUNGTOD,[c]
TRAN THI HANH,[a] MOSES N. KYULE,[d] MAXIMILIAN P.O. BAUMANN,[d]
AND KARL H. ZESSIN[d]

[a]*National Institute of Veterinary Research, Hanoi, Vietnam*

[b]*Institute of Meat Hygiene, Freie Universität, Berlin D14195, Germany*

[c]*Chiang Mai University, Chiang Mai, 50100 Thailand, Thailand*

[d]*Department of International Animal Health, Freie Universität Berlin, Germany*

ABSTRACT: Infection with *Salmonella (S.)* is the most frequently reported
cause of bacterial food-borne illness worldwide. Poultry are a common
source and, in recent years, much attention has been focused in determining the prevalence of *Salmonella* during the different stages in the
poultry production chain. This article was designed to investigate the
prevalence of *Salmonella* serovars in retail chicken meat sold in Hanoi.
A total of 262 samples were randomly collected from retail markets and
examined for the presence of *Salmonella*. Of these samples, 48.9% were
found to be contaminated with *Salmonella*. Predominant serotypes were
S. Agona, S. Emek, S. London. The prevalence of *S. Enteritidis* and
S. Typhimurium was considered. These findings have highlighted the
magnitude of *Salmonella* contamination in retail chicken meat in Hanoi.
On the basis of these preliminary survey results, it is recommended that a
cost-effective monitoring and surveillance system for *Salmonella* should
be established in Hanoi. This system should be augmented by good agricultural and hygienic practices and well-designed longitudinal research
activities on the whole poultry production chain.

KEYWORDS: *Salmonella*; serotyping; Vietnam; poultry; retail

INTRODUCTION

Most information on the prevalence of zoonotic agents is available from
European and Northern American countries. In developing countries, enteric
infections are a major cause of morbidity and also mortality. However, there

Address for correspondence: Prof. Dr. Reinhard Fries, Scientific Panel Veterinary Public Health,
Institute of Meat Hygiene, Faculty of Veterinary Medicine, Freie Universität, Berlin D 14195, Germany.
Voice: +49-30-8385-2790; fax: +49-30-8385-2792.
e-mail: fries.reinhard@vetmed.fu-berlin.de

Ann. N.Y. Acad. Sci. 1081: 257–261 (2006). © 2006 New York Academy of Sciences.
doi: 10.1196/annals.1373.032

is a lack of information on the identity of the agents and their prevalence in particular areas.

The aim of this article was to collect information from Hanoi as this is one of the most highly populated urban/suburban areas of South East Asia, where production and consumption overlap. Data were collected on the prevalence of *Salmonella* (*S.*) contamination of chicken meat on sale at several markets.

MATERIALS AND METHODS

For this survey, only smaller shops were chosen. Two hundred sixty-two samples were collected from 16 markets in 5 districts of the capital of Hanoi as detailed in TABLE 1. From each of these districts, 4 markets (in district 1) and 3 markets (in districts 2, 3, 4, and 5) were randomly selected for sample collection. In each market, 4 shops were conveniently selected and 4 chicken pieces were collected from each shop (5 chicken pieces were collected from each shop in district 1).

The processing of the meat, from slaughter of the bird to preparation for the customer, was generally done by one person. In this survey, no tracing back to the source of the poultry was performed. Samples were taken between December 2004 and April 2005 (TABLE 1). Each sample consisted of approximately 300 g of meat. Each sample was handled separately and kept at 4°C prior to analysis. After arrival at the laboratory, the samples were stored in a refrigerator and processed within 6 h of collection.

Twenty-five grams of the sample were examined using protocol ISO 6579.[1] Isolates were stored as a pure culture on agar and serotyped using omnivalent serum. All isolates were further identified using polyvalent (I, II), somatic (O), and flagellar (H) antisera[2,3] (manufacturer of all reagents: Sifin, Berlin, Germany). Results were statistically calculated using the χ^2-test.

TABLE 1. Number and distribution of samples

Sampling time	District	Market	Shop	Sample/shop	Total
1st sampling	D1	4	14	5	70
	D2	3	12	4	48
2nd sampling	D3	3	12	4	48
	D4	3	12	4	48
	D5	3	12	4	48
Total					$n = 262$

TABLE 2. Proportion of *Salmonella* contaminated sample

Prevalence of *Salmonella* contaminated	n	No. of positive	Percent
Overall	262	128	48.9

RESULTS

Of the 262 samples, 128 (48.9%) were positive (TABLE 2).

A total of 128 *Salmonella* positive samples were tested for serogrouping using polyvalent antisera I and II. Out of these samples 129 isolates were obtained (2 isolates from sample 44-D2M1S2). All the 129 *Salmonella* isolates belonged to 5 somatic groups. The main somatic groups were B (42.6%), C (27.9%), and E (25.6%) (TABLE 3).

Most isolates belonged to main group B, among them in particular *S. Agona*. In group C, the most important serotype was *S. Emek*, and in group E, the predominant serotype was *S. London*.

S. Enteritidis played a minor role (2 isolates), perhaps reflecting the remote and individual character of chicken supply in the north of Vietnam. The same was true with *S. Typhimurium* (10 isolates). TABLE 4 gives the results of serotyping, overall, 12 serotypes were identified from 129 isolates. Most (31.01%) isolates were *S. Agona*, followed by *S. London* (18.6%) and *S. Emek* (17.83%). The prevalence of *Salmonella* differed by area. For example, in D2, 62.5% of samples were positive, but in D4, only 37.5% of samples

TABLE 3. Isolates and their main group distribution

Group	No. of isolates in group	Percent
Group B	55	42.6
Group C	36	27.9
Group E	33	25.6
Group D	2	1.6
Group F-67	3	2.3
Total	129	100

TABLE 4. Somatic and flagellar antigens of the isolates

Serotypes	Group	Total *n*	Percent %
S. Agona	B	40	31.01
S. London	E	24	18.6
S. Emek	C	23	17.83
S. Typhimurium	B	10	7.75
S. Brunei	C	8	6.2
S. Senftenberg	E	5	3.87
S. Derby	B	5	3.87
S. Wetevreden	E	4	3.1
S. Haardt	C	4	3.1
S. F-67	F-67	3	2.33
S. Enteritidis	D	2	1.55
S. Newport	C	1	0.78
No. of serotypes			100
No. of isolates		129	

TABLE 5. Results from districts, markets, and shops (samples)

Result	n	No. of positive	Percent	P value	Serotypes identified
By districts ($n = 5$)					
- D1	70	29	41.42		
- D2	48	30	62.5	$P = 0.0698$	
- D3	48	27	56.25		
- D4	48	18	37.5		
- D5	48	24	50		
By markets in district					
D1					
M1	20	10	50		
M2	20	8	40		
M3	20	8	40	$P = 0.7584$	5
M4	10	3	30		
D2					
M1	16	10	61.2		
M2	16	13	81.2	$P = 0.0907$	5
M3	16	7	43.7		
D3					
M1	16	11	68.7		
M2	16	8	50	$P = 0.4667$	5
M3	16	8	50		
D4					
M1	16	6	37.5		
M2	16	7	43.7	$P = 0.7659$	1
M3	16	5	31.2		
D5					
M1	16	8	50		
M2	16	9	56.2	$P = 0.7788$	8
M3	16	7	43.75		
Total	262	128	48.9		

were positive. However, this finding was not statistically significant ($P = 0.169$) (TABLE 5). From the markets in district 4, only one serotype (*S. Agona*) was obtained. Only one of the shops was negative for *Salmonella* and one shop with 100% sample positive with *Salmonella*.

With respect to the markets, the lowest number of positive samples came from M4 in D1 (30%) and the highest rate was found in D2 with M2 (81.2%). Also here no significant difference was obtained between the markets.

DISCUSSION

The aim of this study was to establish the prevalence of the contamination rates of poultry meat with *Salmonella* in Hanoi, a large city where production and consumption overlap.

A total of 262 samples of poultry meat were collected from small shops operating in 16 markets in 5 districts of Hanoi and examined for *Salmonella*. The salmonellae were investigated in the presence/absence of test.

Mainly *S. Agona* (group B), *S. Emek* (group C), *S. London* (group E), and *S. Typhimurium* (group B) were obtained. In a similar study,[4] Phan *et al.* collected samples from markets (from beef, chicken, duck, and shrimp) in the Mekong Delta, Vietnam. Predominant serotypes were S. Weltevreden (group E), *S. Derby* (group B), *S. London* (group E), *S. Lexington* (group E), and *S. Tennessee* (group C). Isolates from chicken meat were more broadly distributed, among them *S. Emek* (group C), *S. Typhimurium* (group B), and *S. Dessau* (group E).

It is interesting that data from the EU[5,6] clearly show a different pattern of Salmonella serotypes from that detected in Vietnam. From the Zoonoses Report (2005), the range of predominant serotypes was *S. Enteritidis* (group D), *S. Typhimurium* (group B), *S. Saintpaul* (group B), and *S. Heidelberg* (group B). In the EU, most isolates were from group D.

REFERENCES

1. ISO 6579 2002E: International Standard. Microbiology of food and animal feeding stuffs–Horizontal method for the detection of *Salmonella* spp. Fourth edition.
2. POPOFF, M.Y. 2001. Antigenic formulas of the *Salmonella* serovars. WHO Collaborative Centre for Reference and Research on *Salmonella*. Institut Pasteur, 75724 Paris Cedex, France.
3. SIFIN. 2000, 2005. Fachinformation *Salmonella*- Diagnostik. Sifin Institut für Immunpräparate. 13188 Berlin, Germany.
4. PHAN, T.T., L.T.L. KHAI, N. OGASAWARA, *et al.* 2005. Contamination of *Salmonella* in retail meats and shrimps in the Mekong Delta, Vietnam. J. Food Prot. **68:** 1077–1080.
5. EUROPEAN COMMISSION. 2005. Trends and sources of zoonotic agents in animals. Feeding stuffs, food and man in the European Union and Norway 2003.
6. HEALTH & CONSUMER PROTECTION DIRECTORATE-GENERAL. Directorate D, Biological Risks. Sanco/339/2005, Brussels. 102.

Study of *Salmonella, Campylobacter,* and *Escherichia coli* Contamination in Raw Food Available in Factories, Schools, and Hospital Canteens in Hanoi, Vietnam

HA THI ANH DAO AND PHAM THANH YEN

The National Institute of Nutrition, Department of Food Science and Food Safety, Hanoi, Vietnam

ABSTRACT: This study on the contamination rates of raw foods available in factory, school, and hospital canteens in Hanoi, Vietnam, with the bacteria of *Salmonella, Campylobacter,* and *Escherichia coli (E. coli)* was carried out between 2003 and 2004. A total of 177 raw food samples of vegetables, meat (beef and pork), fish, and poultry were examined to provide baseline data for evaluation of microbiological risks in general, and identification of potential vehicles for pathogenic cross-contamination in canteens. The study confirmed that unprocessed fish and poultry are likely to be contaminated with *Salmonella* and in the absence of proper kitchen hygiene and may contaminate processed foods. Raw poultry samples were highly contaminated with *E. coli* (45%), *Campylobacter jejuni (C. jejuni)* (28.3%), and S*almonella* (8.3%) and classified as high-risk food. *E. coli* was also detected in raw meat, fish, and vegetables with the rate of 21.3%, 6.6%, and 18.5%, respectively. This article confirmed the importance of hygienic working practices when preparing food.

KEYWORDS: raw food; cross-contamination; high-risk food

INTRODUCTION

Worldwide diarrhea diseases are an important cause of morbidity and mortality. About 3 million children die each year from diarrhea diseases and hundreds of millions more suffer from frequent episodes of diarrhea and its debilitating consequences.[1] Food is thought to be a major route of transmission of micro-organisms causing diarrhea diseases and other food-borne illness. Current statistics of food-borne illness in Vietnam found that up to 50% of cases may be caused by microbiologically contaminated food. In addition, a serious

Address for correspondence: Ha Thi Anh Dao, M.Sc., Ph.D., Head of Food Science and Food Safety Department, The National Institute of Nutrition, Ministry of Health, 48B Tang Bat Ho Street, Hanoi, Vietnam. Voice: 84-4-8211413; fax: 84-4-9717885.
 e-mail: Dao.atvstp@nutrition.org.vn

Ann. N.Y. Acad. Sci. 1081: 262–265 (2006). © 2006 New York Academy of Sciences.
doi: 10.1196/annals.1373.033

threat exists to the health and welfare of people as food-related diseases has an impact on economic productivity, consumer confidence, and food production.[2]

Today, in Vietnam, more and more people are eating out on a daily basis often in food establishments with mass catering services. When food is contaminated with *Salmonella, Campylobacter jejuni (C. jejuni),* and *Escherichia coli (E. coli)* it looks and smells normal. Among known sources of infection food, raw meat, and vegetables are likely to be contaminated. The aim of this article was to provide data on microbiological contamination of raw food available in factory, school, and hospital canteens with respect to *Salmonella, C. jejuni,* and *E. coli* contamination. A selection of potential high-risk raw foods was screened in the study. The results provided valuable baseline data for the identification of fresh high-risk foods.

MATERIALS AND METHODS

Samples

A total of 177 raw food samples of poultry, meat (pork, beef), fish and vegetables were collected from six canteens in Hanoi. Each canteen served more than 100 customers per day. Four of the canteens were in schools (1 primary school and 3 preschools) and the other two were a factory and a hospital.

Sampling Procedure

The samples were collected immediately after the food had been prepared. A sample of approximately 250 g was collected into a sterile plastic bag, and transported, as soon as possible, on dry ice to the Microbiological Laboratory at the National Institute of Nutrition.

Microbiological Examination of Food Samples

Salmonella spp. and *E.coli* in raw food samples were determined using FAO procedure.[3] Testing for the presence of *Campylobacter* was undertaken using the WHO procedure.[4] In this study, we used the classical microbiological methods and culturing parameters.

In each determination reference strains were used as controls namely, *S. enteritidis* (ATCC 13076), *S. typhimurium* (ATCC 14028), *C. jejuni* (ATCC 33291), and *E. coli* (ATCC 25922).

Statistical Analysis

The χ^2 test was used to compare the prevalence of microbiological contamination between samples obtained from different foods and canteens. The level of significance was set at $P < 0.05$.

RESULTS AND DISCUSSION

Among the four types of raw foods, poultry samples were highly contaminated with *E.coli*, *C. jejuni*, and S*almonella*. *Salmonella* spp. was found in 8.3% of poultry, 1.2% of meat, and 6.6% of fish. Vegetables were found to be free of contamination with *Salmonella* spp. The *E. coli* counts ranged from 0 to 10^2 per gram and were most frequently found in poultry with 45% of samples being contaminated. Twenty one percent of meat, 6.6% of fish, and 18.5% of vegetables were found to be contaminated with *E. coli*. Meat can become contaminated during slaughter, and organisms can be thoroughly mixed into meat when it is ground. *C. jejuni* was not found in meat, fish, and vegetables. The contamination rates of raw foods available in the canteens are given in TABLES 1 and 2. There was no significant difference between the prevalence of pathogenic bacteria in raw food at different canteens.

CONCLUSION

This study on the contamination rates of raw food available in canteens in Hanoi with *Salmonella* spp., *Campylobacter* spp., and *E. coli* established that fish and poultry were likely to be contaminated with *Salmonella* spp., while vegetables were free. Poultry samples were highly contaminated with *E.coli* (45%), *C. jejuni* (28.3%), S*almonella* (8.3%) and thus can be classified as a high-risk food.

TABLE 1. Prevalence of pathogenic bacteria in raw food at canteens

Name of canteen	Type of food	N	Number of contaminated food samples	Percentage of contaminated food samples
1. Hospital	Poultry	15	9	60
	Meat (pork, beef)	15	6	40
	Fish	5	1	20
	Vegetables	9	2	22.2
Subtotal		44	18	40.9
2. Factory	Poultry	15	9	60
	Meat (pork, beef)	15	5	33.33
	Fish	5	1	20
	Vegetables	9	2	22.22
Subtotal		44	17	38.6
3. Schools	Poultry	30	18	60.0
	Meat (pork, beef)	45	12	26.66
	Fish	5	0	0
	Vegetables	9	1	11.1
Subtotal		89	31	34.8
Total		177	66	37.3%

TABLE 2. Contamination degree of raw materials used at canteens ($N = 177$)

Type of food	Contaminants examined	Level of microbial counts/g food	Number and percentage of contaminated food
1. Poultry	*Salmonella* spp.	(+)	5 (8.3%)
($n = 60$)	*E. coli*	$0-10^2$	27 (45%)
	C. jejuni	(+)	17 (28.3%)
2. Meat	*Salmonella* spp.	(+)	1 (1.2%)
($n = 75$)	*E. coli*	0–10	16 (21.3%)
	C. jejuni	(+)	0
3. Fish	*Salmonella* spp.	(+)	1 (6.6%)
($n = 15$)	*E. coli*	0–10	1 (6.6%)
	C. jejuni	(+)	0
4. Vegetable	*Salmonella* spp.	(+)	0
($n = 27$)	*E. coli*	0–10	5 (18.5%)
	C. jejuni	(+)	0

Positive result (+).

ACKNOWLEDGMENTS

The authors wish to express sincere thanks to the World Health Organization and the National Institute of Nutrition in Vietnam for financial support. We are thankful to the Microbiological Laboratory, Department of Food Science, and Food Safety for the productive cooperation.

REFERENCES

1. WHO. 2000. Food Borne Disease: a Focus for Health Education. Word Health Organization. Geneva, Switzerland.
2. MOH. 2004. Vietnam Country Report of Food Administration.
3. FAO. Manual of Food Quality Control. 4.Rev-1. 1992. Microbiological Analysis. Rome.
4. WHO, Global Salm-Surv. Identification of themotolerant. 2003. Campylobacter.

Prevalence of *Salmonella* spp. in Poultry in Vietnam

TRAN T. HANH,[a] NGUYEN T. THANH,[a] HOANG Q. THOA,[b] LE T. THI,[c] LAM M. THUAN,[d] AND NGUYEN T.H. LY[e]

[a]*National Institute of Veterinary Research, Hanoi, Vietnam*

[b]*Hanoi Regional Animal Health Center, Hanoi, Vietnam*

[c]*Sub of National Institute of Veterinary Research, Khanhhoa, Vietnam*

[d]*Thu Duc Agricultural and Forest University, Hochiminh, Vietnam*

[e]*National Center for Veterinary Hygiene Inspection N02, Hanoi, Vietnam*

ABSTRACT: The prevalence of *Salmonella* spp. in chickens and ducks from North, Central, and South Vietnam was followed over a 4 year period. Several different analyses were employed and the current prevalence was shown to be less than in previous studies.

KEYWORDS: *Salmonella*; prevalence; poultry

INTRODUCTION

The aim of this article is to present the prevalence of *Salmonella* spp. in poultry in Vietnam. Investigations of bacterial food poisoning outbreaks in Alexandria, Egypt in 1999 detected *Salmonella* spp. in 16 outbreaks with 43 cases. *S. enteritidis* (5 out of 16 outbreaks with 13 cases) was the most prevalent serovar. Japan registered 1217 outbreaks of all types of food poisoning in 1996, involving 46,327 cases. In Vietnam from 1997 to 2000 there were 1364 food poisoning outbreaks with 24,541 cases, 207 died.[1] In Ho Chi Minh city in 1994, 370 cases of food poisoning following consumption of contaminated soup were identified as Salmonellosis. Another food-borne poisoning of 300 cases caused by *S. enteritidis* in Thai Binh in North Vietnam was reported. There was no information about the reservoir and routes for food poisoning agents.

MATERIALS AND METHODS

The study was carried out to determine the prevalence of *Salmonella* spp. in chicken and ducks in the North, Central, and South Vietnam in a period of

Address for correspondence: Tran Thi Hanh, National Institute of Veterinary Research, Hanoi, Vietnam.
e-mail: edmour.blouin@okstate.edu

Ann. N.Y. Acad. Sci. 1081: 266–268 (2006). © 2006 New York Academy of Sciences.
doi: 10.1196/annals.1373.034

4 years from 2001 to 2004. In total 6557 samples were analyzed during this period. Samples were randomly collected in various breeding farms as fecal samples, rectal swabs, collected floor feces, inner organs (intestine, cecum, liver) from dead chicken of any age, and dead embryos from unhatched eggs.

Bacteriological analyses were developed as follows[2,3]: (*a*) pre-enrichment on buffered peptone water (BPW); (*b*) selective enrichment using Rapport Vassiliadis (RV); (*c*) plating on XLD agar and MacConkey agar; and (*d*) biochemical confirmation using Kligler, API 20, or micro-ID3; 5-serotyping by poly OH.

RESULTS

In North Vietnam, *Salmonella* spp. were isolated in chicken samples from 113/2824 (4%) of the feces, from 28/907 (3.09%) of the organ samples, and from 26/412 (6.31%) of the dead embryos. In ducks, *Salmonella* positive samples were found in 5.57% (53/950) of the feces, in 9.52% (12/126) of the organs, and in 10.12% (16/158) of the dead embryos. In Central Vietnam, 6 out of 100 (6%) duck organ samples were found positive with *Salmonella* spp. Feces and organ samples were not taken. In chickens, none of the samples were positive out of 70 fecal, 50 organ, and 80 dead embryos samples. In South Vietnam, fecal samples were not taken. In chicken, 22/326 (6.7%) of organ samples, 6/200 (3%) of dead embryos were found positive for *Salmonella* spp., whereas in duck, 6/42 (14.3%) of the organ samples and 10/312 (3.2%) of the dead embryos were positive. These results are summarized in TABLE 1.

DISCUSSION AND CONCLUSION

In previous studies, such as in 1998 on 502 samples of feces and eggs collected from 7 duck farms in Ho Chi Minh city and surrounding areas, Tran Xuan Hanh[4] reported a *Salmonella* spp. prevalence of 8.8% on duck hens, 24.7% on duckling, and 31.7% on dead embryos. In 1999, Tran Thi Hanh[5] found 30.91% *Salmonella* spp. in a week old infected chicken.

TABLE 1. Prevalence of *Salmonella* spp. in three areas of Vietnam

Areas	Breeding farms	Number of samples (*n*)	Number of positive samples	Percentage (%)
North	Chicken	4,143	167	4.00
	Duck	1,234	81	6.56
Central	Chicken	200	0	0.00
	Duck	100	6	6.00
South	Chicken	526	28	5.32
	Duck	354	16	4.51
Total		6,557	298	4.60

In conclusion, the *Salmonella* spp. prevalence found in our recent investigation is lower than the above mentioned authors.

REFERENCES

1. KIM, PHAN T. 2001. Foodborne Diseases. 5–38.Youth Publisher.
2. SELBITZ, H.-J., H.-J. SINELL & A. SZIEGOLAIT. 1995. Das Salmonella – Problem. Gustav-Fischer Verlag. Jena-Stuttgart.
3. SELBITZ, H.-J. 2001. Grundsaetzliche Sicherheitsanforderungen beim Einsatz von lebend impfstoffen bei lebensmittelliefernden Tieren. Berl. Munch. Tieraurzl. Wschr. **114:** 428–432.
4. HANH, T.X. 1998. Preliminary results of duck Salmonellosis studies in vicinity of Ho Chi Minh city. Vet. Sci. Tech. **V:** 61–67.
5. HANH, T.T. 1999. Pollution by *Salmonella* in the environment and in the products of industrial poultry rearing. Vet. Sci. Tech. **V:** 7–11.

Prevalence and Epidemiology of *Salmonella* spp. in Small Pig Abattoirs of Hanoi, Vietnam

CÉDRIC LE BAS,[a] TRAN T. HANH,[b] NGUYEN T. THANH,[b]
DANG D. THUONG,[b] AND NGO C. THUY[b]

[a]*CIRAD, International Cooperation Center on Research for Development, 34398 Montpellier Cedex 5, France*

[b]*NIVR, National Institute of Veterinary Research, Hanoi, Vietnam*

ABSTRACT: The prevalence of *Salmonella* spp. in pigs was evaluated in a survey of small abattoirs in Hanoi, Vietnam. Cecal contents, carcass swabs, and tank water samples were collected for bacterial isolation in various media. Prevalence rates exceeded 50% in pig samples and 62% in water samples. This increased prevalence indicates the need for risk assessment evaluations along the entire production chain.

KEYWORDS: *Salmonella*; prevalence; epidemiology; risk assessment

INTRODUCTION

Food safety is an emerging research topic of preliminary importance in Vietnam,[1,2] mainly because of the foreseen World Trade Organization (WTO) membership, the increase of consumer demand for quality and safety,[3,4] and the need for a global public health improvement. In this context, risk analysis research is urgently needed. Slaughtering is an essential step in the risk assessment of zoonotic food pathogens in animal production. This step gives information on upstream and downstream hygienic status for live animals or carcasses.[3,5] Small abattoirs (10 to 30 pigs/day) are still the most common structure for slaughtering pigs in North Vietnam.[6] *Salmonella* spp. remains one of the most frequent zoonotic food pathogens reported in the world and pigs are known to be asymptomatic carriers. The *Salmonella* spp. shedding pigs are most likely to contaminate carcasses and slaughtering environments, and follow the entire production chain downstream.[5] This article aimed to make a preliminary assessment of *Salmonella* spp. prevalence and epidemiology in some pig slaughtering units in Hanoi.

Address for correspondence: Cedric le Bas, CIRAD, International Research Institute in Agronomy for Tropical Countries, Montpellier, France.
e-mail: edmour.blouin@okstate.edu

Ann. N.Y. Acad. Sci. 1081: 269–272 (2006). © 2006 New York Academy of Sciences.
doi: 10.1196/annals.1373.035

MATERIALS AND METHODS

Sampling

Cecal contents were chosen to provide an estimation of the upstream load with *Salmonella* spp. (farm, transport, and lairage). The carcass swabs, taken a short time prior to the expedition to the market, give a picture of the cross-contamination during the slaughtering process. Tank water samples allow an estimation of the water contamination, which can represent an important vehicle of contamination. Prior to the sampling, an analysis of the slaughtering practices was performed in different units. Cecal content of slaughtered pigs, carcass swabs, and tank water samples were taken randomly among 15 slaughtering units. Slaughtering practices are identical in the 15 units. Units and pigs were chosen at random. Water and swab samples were taken aseptically. Ceca were tied up with two strings, cut, and transported in plastic bags. All samples were transported to the laboratory at 5°C. The 15 g of ceca were cauterized and incised with sterile chisels.

Analysis

Samples were diluted to one-tenth with buffered peptone water and incubated 16–20 h at 37°C for pre-enrichment: 15 g cecum content up to 150 g, cotton swabs up to 150 g, and 15 g water up to 150 g. One hundred microliters of pre-enrichment broth were added to 10 mL of Rappaport-Vassiliadis broth, incubated 24 h at 42°C for selective enrichment. Isolation was performed through streaking out 1 μL of the enrichment broth onto the XLT4 agar, incubated 24 h at 37°C. At least one *Salmonella* spp. characteristic colony was identified on the Kligler Iron tubes, incubated 24 h at 37°C. Each characteristic *Salmonella* spp. strain on Kligler Iron was confirmed through additional biochemical tests—manitol, motility, urease, indol, Lysin decarboxylase, ONPG, ADH, ODC, and serotyping—results of serotyping not presented.

Statistical Analysis

Prevalence estimates are given for each sample type with the corresponding absolute precision at a confidence level of 95%. The absolute precision was calculated following the One Mean procedure of Poisson analysis: $i^2 = \varepsilon$ pq/n (i, absolute precision, ε depending on the confidence level, p, estimated prevalence, q = 1-p, and n, number of samples).

RESULTS AND DISCUSSION

Prevalence results are listed in TABLE 1. More than 50% of the pigs are *Salmonella* spp. carriers—presence of *Salmonella* spp. in cecal content and potential shedders at the time of slaughtering, which represents a high contamination pressure for the slaughtering environment and therefore downstream the production chain. This prevalence rate is higher than reported in other studies, usually between 6% and 23% for cecal samples at slaughterhouse.[7,8] This seems to indicate that practices at farm, transport, and lairage in the study area are favorable for a *Salmonella* spp. dissemination between pigs. Compared to the international literature, usually reporting a carcass contamination rate from 1.4% to 11.2%,[8–10] the percentage (95%) of positive swabs samples of our study is extremely high. This can be explained by several factors: first because of the high contamination pressure from the pigs, then because of the slaughtering practices. Indeed, in the studied units, there are no strictly separated areas for the different slaughtering steps and after evisceration carcasses are lying on the ground with many manipulations by the workers, allowing cross-contaminations before their transport to the market. Moreover, the workers use tank water to rinse carcasses after evisceration, and we showed that this water is highly contaminated, with 62% of positive samples. This contamination seems to be due to the occasional use of tank water for washing hands or material and due to the absence of cleaning and disinfection every slaughtering day. Besides this, we found some positive well water samples—the water used as a source for boiling or filled in the tank—although we have not enough samples to give a statistically valid picture of this contamination rate. Thus, the water source could also potentially play a role in the epidemiology of *Salmonella* spp. at those slaughter places. Whereas evisceration has been described in Europe as the major cause of carcass contamination,[5] this study in some abattoir places of Hanoi shows the central role played by the lack of good hygienic slaughtering practices and by the contamination of water used for rinsing carcasses. Thus, it is interesting to note that a little improvement of the practices could considerably reduce the carcass contamination rate. If this hygienic context is not necessarily a cause of public health concern for sufficiently cooked traditional pork products, the risk is now growing because of the rising industrial processed products and implementation of cold chains. Besides this, the contamination rate of some traditional products still should be assessed,

TABLE 1. Positive samples for *Salmonella* spp. and confidence intervals

Sample type	Positive samples for *Salmonella* spp.	Confidence interval at 95% confidence level
Ceca	52.1% (61/117)	43.1–61.2%
Swabs	95.7% (44/46)	89.8–100%
Water (tank)	62.5% (20/32)	45.7–79.3%

like raw fermented meat or traditional sausages. This study shows the need to perform risk assessment for specific issues on the entire production chain with a farm-to-fork approach. This should be led with a multidisciplinary approach involving socioeconomical researches on production and consumption levels.

REFERENCES

1. ANONYMOUS. 2002. Capacity Building for the Prevention of Foodborne Diseases – Final Report. 32. World Health Organization, Hanoi.
2. KIM, P.T. 2002. Food Safety Activities in Vietnam. FAO/WHO Global Forum of Food Safety Regulators, Marrakech, Morocco.
3. ANONYMOUS. 2000. Opinion of the Scientific Committee on Veterinary Measures Relating to Public Health on Food-Borne Zoonoses. 34. European Commission.
4. GINHOUX, V. 2001. Etude de la sensibilité des consommateurs urbains de viande porcine. 79.
5. BERENDS, B.R., F. VAN KNAPEN, J.M.A. SNIJDERS & D.A.A. MOSSEL. 1997. Identification and quantification of risk factors regarding *Salmonella* spp. on pork carcasses. Int. J. Food Microbiol. **36:** 199–206.
6. WEGENER, H.C. 1999. The Hygiene Inspection System of the Veterinary Services in Vietnam. Consultancy Mission, 6–10 June 1999. Strengthening of Veterinary Services in Vietnam (SVSV). 73. Ministry of Agriculture and Rural Development in Vietnam, European Commission.
7. DAVIES, R.H., R. DALZIEL, J.W. WILESMITH, *et al.* 2001. National survey for *Salmonella* in pigs at slaughter in Great Britain. Proceedings of the 4th International Symposium on the Epidemiology and Control of *Salmonella* and Other Food Pathogens in Pork. 2–5 September 2001, Leipzig, Germany.
8. WRAY, C. 2001. Review of research into *Salmonella* infections in pigs. Meat and Livestock Commission, 63.
9. ALBAN, L. & K.D.C. STARK. 2005. Where should the effort be put to reduce the *salmonella* prevalence in the slaughtered swine carcass effectively? Prevent. Vet. Med. **68:** 63–79.
10. KORSAK, N., B. JACOB, B. GROVEN, *et al.* 2003. *Salmonella* contamination of pigs and pork in an integrated pig production system. J. Food Protect. **66:** 1126–1133.

Study on the Prevalence of *Campylobacter* spp. from Chicken Meat in Hanoi, Vietnam

LUU QUYNH HUONG,[a] TRAN THI HANH,[a] PHUNG DAC CAM,[b] AND NGUYEN THI BE[b]

[a]*National Institute of Veterinary Research, Hanoi, Vietnam*

[b]*National Institute of Epidemiology and Hygiene, Hanoi, Vietnam*

ABSTRACT: *Campylobacter* spp. is considered to be the most common bacterial cause of human gastroenteritis worldwide. In developing countries, *Campylobacter* spp. diarrhea is an important cause of childhood morbidity. Chicken meat is known to be a major source of Campylobacteriosis infection in the world. The purpose of this study was to investigate the prevalence of *Campylobacter* spp. in chicken meat. A total of 100 samples from breast part of chicken carcass were collected from retail market in Hanoi. The samples were taken for bacteriological analysis following the ISO 10272 standards. Thirty one samples (31%) were found positive for *Campylobacter* spp. The most frequently isolated Campylobacter was *Campylobacter jejuni* (45.2%) followed by *Campylobacter coli* (25.8%). Due to high contamination rates of retail chicken products, special attention must be paid to good manufacturing practices of food processors and vendors. Further studies should be done to assess the risk factors of *Campylobacter* spp. contamination in the Vietnamese fowl production chain.

KEYWORDS: prevalence; chicken meat; *Campylobacter jejuni*; *Campylobacter coli*

INTRODUCTION

Campylobacters are bacteria that are a major cause of diarrhea in humans and are generally regarded as the most common bacterial cause of gastroenteritis worldwide.[1] The only form of Campylobacteriosis of major public health importance is *Campylobacter* enteritis due to *C. jejuni* and *C. coli*.[2] The purpose of this article was to investigate the prevalence of *Campylobacter* spp. in chicken meat.

Address for correspondnce: Luu Quynh Huong, National Institute of Veterinary Research, 86 Truong chinh road, Dong Da dist., Hanoi, Vietnam. Voice: 00-84-4-8695544; fax: 00-84-4-8694082.
e-mail: lqhuongvet@yahoo.com

Ann. N.Y. Acad. Sci. 1081: 273–275 (2006). © 2006 New York Academy of Sciences.
doi: 10.1196/annals.1373.036

TABLE 1. Number of *campylobacter*-positive samples isolated from chickens

No. of samples examined	No. of *Campylobacter*-positive samples	Percentage (%)
100	31	31

TABLE 2. Proportion of *campylobacter*-positive samples by season

Time	No. of samples examined	No. of *Campylobacter*-positive samples	Percentage (%)
Winter time	60	17	28.33
Spring time	40	14	35

(2p = 0.627

TABLE 3. Identification of *campylobacter* spp. isolated from chicken samples

	Serotype	No. of isolates	%
1	*C. jejuni*	14	45.2
2	*C. coli*	8	25.8
3	Unknown	9	29.0
	Total	31	100

MATERIALS AND METHODS

A total of 100 samples from the breast part of chicken carcasses were collected from five retail markets (four shops were visited in each market) in two districts in Hanoi by random sampling methods. The first sampling: January, 2005: winter time in Hanoi and the second sampling: April, 2005: spring time in Hanoi. The samples were taken for bacteriological analysis following ISO 10272 standards.

RESULTS AND DISCUSSION

A total of 100 samples were examined for a contamination rate of *Campylobacter*; 31 samples were positive with *Salmonella* yielding 31% of positive samples (TABLE 1).

Our results are in agreement with those observed in other countries as 49.50% of the chicken meat in Spain (2002)[3] and 45.9% in broiler carcasses in Germany (1999).[4] However, the contamination rate in the present study was generally much lower than in other studies: 83% in UK (2002)[5]; 83.3% of chicken portions in UK (2000).[6] In winter, the percentage of *Campylobacter*-contaminated chicken (28.33%) is lower than in spring (35%). With χ^2 $P = 0.627$, the differently contaminated proportion of chicken was not significant (TABLE 2). In the present study, the most common serotype identified from chicken meat in Hanoi was *C. jejuni* (45.2%) followed by *C. coli* (25.8%) (TABLE 3).

These serotypes were also found in other surveys in Germany with 43% *C. jejuni* and 13% *C. coli* from broiler carcasses (1999).[4] In the UK 77.3% *C. jejuni* and 10.7% *C. coli* were identified from chicken portions (2000).[6] Due to high contamination rates of retail chicken products, special attention must be paid to good manufacturing practices of food processors and vendors. Further studies should be done to assess the risk factors of *Campylobacter* spp. contamination in the Vietnamese fowl production chain.

REFERENCES

1. BAN MISHU, A. 2001. *Campylobacter jejuni* infections: update on emerging issues and trends. Food safety. Clin. Infect. Dis. **32:** 1201–1206.
2. NACHAMKIN, I. & M.J. BLASER. 2000. Campylobacter, 2nd ed. American Society for Microbiology. Washington.
3. DOMINGUEZ, C., I. GOMEZ & J. ZUMALACARREGUI. 2002. Prevalence of Salmonella and Campylobacter in retail chicken meat in Spain. Int. J. Food Microbiol. **72:** 165–168.
4. ATANASSOVA, V. & C. RING. 1999. Prevalence of Campylobacter spp. in poultry and poultry meat in Germany. Int. J. Food Microbiol. **51:** 187–190.
5. JORGENSEN, F. *et al.* 2002. Prevalence and numbers of Salmonella and Campylobacter spp. on raw, whole chickens in relation to sampling methods. Int. J. Food Microbiol. **76:** 151–164.
6. KRAMER, J.M. *et al.* 2000. Campylobacter contamination of raw meat and poultry at retail sale: identification of multiple types and comparison with isolated from human infection. J. Food Prot. **63:** 1654–1659.

Characterization of Lactic Acid Bacteria and Other Gut Bacteria in Pigs by a Macroarraying Method

NARUT THANANTONG, SANDRA EDWARDS, AND OLIVIER A.E. SPARAGANO

Newcastle University, School of Agriculture, Food and Rural Development, Newcastle upon Tyne, NE1 7RU, United Kingdom

ABSTRACT: Lactic acid bacteria (LAB) consist of many genera, Gram-positive, and nonspore-forming micro-organisms; some members being used as probiotics while some others have negative effects on pig health. Bacterial species in the gastrointestinal tract can produce antibacterial substances, reduce serum cholesterol in their host, or can be responsible for growth reduction, diarrhea, and intestinal epithelial damage. It is therefore important for the pig industry to evaluate the impact of food and farm management on the presence of "good" or "bad" bacteria and the risk for consumers. This articles focuses on the molecular identification of gut microflora species following different diets given to pigs in UK and correlating the data on growth, health, and welfare. First of all, pig feces were individually collected from sows before and after farrowing and also from piglets before and after weaning over several months. Bacteria colonies were grown on MRS agar plates from feces and DNA was extracted (QIAamp DNA stool kit) and amplified using 16S rDNA (27f and 519r) primers. DNA sequencing and sequence alignment allowed us to identify species-specific zones, which were used as probes in a macroarray system also known as reverse line blot hybridization. Some probes were found to be species specific for the following species: *Lactobacillus acidophilus, L. animalis, L. gallinarum, L. kitasanotis, L salivarius, Streptococcus alactolyticus, S. hyointestinalis,* and *Sarcina ventriculi.* Actual studies are now focusing on the impact of diets of the microflora in different gut parts and at different stages of the animal's life.

KEYWORDS: pig; gut; *Lactobacillus*; diet; RLB

Address for correspondence: Dr. Olivier A.E. Sparagano, School of Agriculture, Food and Rural Development, Newcastle University, Agriculture Building, Newcastle upon Tyne NE1 7RU, UK. Voice: 44-191-2225071; fax: 44-191-2226720.
e-mail: Olivier.sparagano@ncl.ac.uk

Ann. N.Y. Acad. Sci. 1081: 276–279 (2006). © 2006 New York Academy of Sciences.
doi: 10.1196/annals.1373.037

INTRODUCTION

The pig gastrointestinal tract harbors various populations of micro-organisms. Lactic acid bacteria (LAB) are one of the most dominant groups of bacteria found in the gastrointestinal tract. LAB produce lactic acid as a byproduct from their usual growth and also bacteriocins (antibiotic-like com-pounds).[1] Knowledge of the LAB in the gut may provide a way to encourage good animal health and control pathogenic bacteria. Their antibacterial[2,3] and antifungal[4] activity has already been well established. LAB have been exten-sively used in food processing for meat,[5] cheese,[6,7] or wheat-derived[8] products. The current classification of LAB combines both phenotypic properties and genotypic examination. Molecular methods using specific genetic material of LAB are increasingly being applied as an identification tool. The 16S ribo-somal RNA (rRNA) gene has been identified as a molecule whose sequence reflects the phylogenetic position of a given bacterial species. 16S rRNA gene sequences have been used to detect certain bacterial groups or species without the necessity to grow them.[9,10] Reverse line blot (RLB) assay is used as a tool to simultaneously identify several species.

MATERIALS AND METHODS

Two experiments were conducted in this study. For experiment 1, 55 pig fecal samples from different animals were collected. LAB and coliforms were grown on specific media and one colony per plate was isolated. DNA was extracted (QIAamp DNA stool kit; Qiagen, Crawley UK) and amplified us-ing the REDExtract_N_amp polymerase chain reaction (PCR) kit from Sigma (Warrington, UK). PCR was performed by using two universal primers (27f and 519r) targeting the 16S rRNA gene. For each PCR reaction, positive and negative controls were used.

Amplified PCR fragments were sequenced by Lark Technologies, Inc. (Essex, UK) and sequences were compared with the GenBank Database. Then, species-specific probes were identified and validated in an RLB hybridization as previously used.[10–13] During the second experiment, two replicate samples from the digesta and wall of the ileum, cecum, and colon of 10 pigs were used (feces for each animal were also collected).

RESULTS

Phylogenetic analysis of the 16S rDNA sequence of isolates revealed the presence of *Lactobacillus acidophilus, L. reuteri, L. animalis, L. murinus, L. gallinarum, L. kitasatonis, L. salivarius, Streptococcus alactolyticus, S. hyointestinalis,* and *Sarcina ventriculi.*

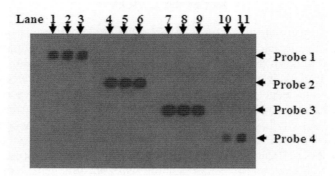

FIGURE 1. RLB validation. Lanes 1–3 = *L. reuteri* amplified DNA samples; Lanes 4–6 = *L. murinus* amplified DNA samples; Lanes 7–9 = *L. acidophilus* amplified DNA samples; Lanes 10–11 = *L. kitasatonis* amplified DNA samples. Probe 1 = probe for *L. reuteri*; Probe 2 = probe for *L. murinus;* Probe 3 = probe for *L. acidophilus;* Probe 4 = probe for *L. kitasatonis.*

Twenty-four (44%) representative colonies of the bacterial isolates were identified as *L. reuteri.*

The designed probes were shown to be species specific and not to cross-react with DNA of other species (FIG. 1).

CONCLUSION

It is evident from the 16S rDNA sequences that the majority of the isolates were *L. reuteri,* suggesting that this species predominates in the population of pigs investigated. However, this observation is not correlated by a previous study[14] showing that *L. ruminis* was the dominant species in pig guts.

These species-specific probes may be used to identify LAB in pig digesta samples and, as more probes are validated, it will become possible to identify many of the LAB in the pig gastrointestinal tract. These oligonucleotide probes can then provide a tool to evaluate the impact of different pig diets on LAB microflora in relation to health and performance.

Although in our study we could see variations in RLB dot intensities showing a change in the targeted species populations and sometimes showing a correlation between the presence of one species and the disappearance of another, it is not yet a quantitative method. However, a real-time PCR based on RNA extraction coupled together with RLB would give a higher evaluation of the population size and its viability for coliforms and LAB, for instance.

ACKNOWLEDGMENTS

This study was partially supported by a Royal Thai Government studentship and by the Yorkshire Agricultural Society.

REFERENCES

1. TODOROV, S.D. & L.M.T. DICKS. 2004. Partial characterization of bacteriocins produced by four lactic acid bacteria isolated from regional South African barley beer. Ann. Microbiol. **54:** 403–413.
2. ARQUES, J.L., E. RODRIGUEZ, P. GAYA, *et al.* 2005. Inactivation of *Staphylococcus aureus* in raw milk cheese by combinations of high-pressure treatments and bacteriocin-producing lactic acid bacteria. J. Appl. Microbiol. **98:** 254–260.
3. GOLLOP, N., V. ZAKIN & Z.G. WEINBERG. 2005. Antibacterial activity of lactic acid bacteria included in inoculants for silage and in silages treated with these inoculants. J. Appl. Microbiol. **98:** 662–666.
4. SCHNURER, J. & J. MAGNUSSON. 2005. Antifungal lactic acid bacteria as biopreservatives. Trends Food Sc. Technol. **16:** 70–78.
5. GRECO, M., R. MAZZETTE, E.P.L. DE SANTIS, *et al.* 2005. Evolution and identification of lactic acid bacteria isolated during the ripening of Sardinian sausages. Meat Sc., **69:** 733–739.
6. FLOREZ, A.B., S. DELGADO & B. MAYO. 2005. Antimicrobial susceptibility of lactic acid bacteria isolated from a cheese environment. Can. J. Microbiol. **51:** 51–58.
7. KUNG, H.F., Y.H. TSAI, C.C. HWANG, *et al.* 2005. Hygienic quality and incidence of histamine-forming lactobacillus species in natural and processed cheese in Taiwan. J. Food Drug Analysis **13:** 51–56.
8. VANCANNEYT, M., P. NEYSENS, M. DE WACHTER, *et al.* 2005. *Lactobacillus acidifarinae sp nov* and *Lactobacillus zymae sp nov.,* from wheat sourdoughs. Intern. J. Syst. Evol. Microbiol. **55:** 615–620.
9. HANNIFFY, S., U. WIDERMANN, A. REPA, *et al.* 2004. Potential and opportunities for use of recombinant lactic acid bacteria in human health. Adv. Appl. Microbiol. **56:** 1–64.
10. MOREIRA, J.L.S., R.M. MOTA, M.F. HORTA, *et al.* 2005. Identification to the species level of *Lactobacillus* isolated in probiotic prospecting studies of human, animal or food origin by 16S-23S rRNA restriction profiling. BMC Microbiol. **5(1):** 15.
11. BEKKER, C.P.J., S. DE VOS, A. TAOUFIK, *et al.* 2000. Simultaneous detection of *Anaplasma* and *Ehrlichia* species in ruminants and detection of *Ehrlichia ruminantium* in *Amblyomma variegatum* ticks by reverse line blot hybridization. Vet. Microbiol. **89:** 223–238.
12. GUBBELS, M.J., A.P. DE VOS, M. VAN DER WEID, *et al.* 1999. Simultaneous detection of bovine *Theileria* and *Babesia* species by reverse line blot hybridization. J. Clin. Microbiol. **37:** 1782–1789.
13. SCHNITTGER, L., H. YIN, B. QI, *et al.* 2004. Simultaneous detection and differentiation of *Theileria* and *Babesia* parasites infecting small ruminants by reverse line blotting. Parasitol. Res. **92:** 189–196.
14. YIN, Q.Q. & Q.H. ZHENG. 2005. Isolation and identification of the dominant *Lactobacillus* in gut and faeces of pigs using carbohydrate fermentation and 16S rDNA analysis. J. Biosc. Bioeng. **99:** 68–71.

Porcine Eperythrozoonosis in China

JIANSAN WU,[a] JIANMIN YU,[a] CUIPING SONG,[a] SHENGJUN SUN,[a,b] AND ZHILIANG WANG[a]

[a]National Exotic Animal Disease Center, Animal Quarantine Institute, Ministry of Agriculture, Qingdao 266032, P.R. China

[b]Department of Animal Medicine, Laiyang Agriculture College, Qingdao 266109, P.R. China

ABSTRACT: Eperythrozoonosis of swine (also designated as porcine mycoplasmosis) is a disease of swine under stress, expressed as a febrile condition with development of an acute ictero-anemia. It is caused by *Eperythrozoon suis* and usually causes a subclinical infection with a latent carrier state that persists for extended periods. In China, this disease has gradually developed as an important intercurrent disease and an emerging swine disease that, in recent years, has spread throughout all provinces except Tibet. Classical swine fever (hog cholera), porcine influenza, swine enzootic pneumonia, porcine reproductive and respiratory syndrome (blue ear disease), streptococci, and toxoplasmosis were detected in *Eperythrozoonosis*-infected pig herds, and caused serious economic losses. National epidemiology surveillance in 2002 revealed that this disease caused a total morbidity of 30% and a mortality of 10–20%. Total mortality (which includes culling sick pigs) was more than 60%. The morbidity within infected herds was near 100%, has spread throughout with a total mortality rate usually over 50%. Mortality of piglets in some districts was as high as 50%. The highest infection rate on pig farms was more than 90%. The farms with higher infection rates occurred in pig-raising areas during epidemic seasons. New diagnostic tests, such as ELISA and PCR, have been developed for the detection of porcine eperythrozoonosis, but traditionally the diagnosis of the disease is still based on clinical history and optical microscopic examination of the causative agent in blood smears. Efficient preventive and control measures include the detection of carriers in pig herds and treatment of sick pigs with drugs, such as long-acting oxytetracycline, doxycycline, or aceturate of diminazene. Oxytetracyclines as feed additives have been introduced for eperythrozoonosis prevention in uninfected pig herds, and pig producers have taken measures to reduce stress and improve sanitary conditions.

KEYWORDS: porcine eperythrozoonosis; epidemiology surveillance; diagnosis; therapeneutics

Address for correspondence: Prof. Jiansan Wu, National Exotic Animal Disease Center, National Animal Quarantine Institute, Ministry of Agriculture, 266032, Qingdao, P.R. China. Voice: +86-532-85631530; fax: +86-532-85621552.

e-mail: wujians@public.qd.sd.cn

Ann. N.Y. Acad. Sci. 1081: 280–285 (2006). © 2006 New York Academy of Sciences.

doi: 10.1196/annals.1373.038

INTRODUCTION

Porcine eperythrozoonosis is a zoonotic disease caused by *Eperythrozoon suis,* and is likely to have worldwide distribution. Splitter and Williamson first recognized it in 1950.[1] *E. suis* was formerly classified in the order *Rickettsiales.* Recently, on the basis of a comparison of 16s rRNA gene sequences, it has been shown to belong to the *Mycoplasmatales* and has been included in the genus *Mycoplasma,*[2] but this classification at the genus level is disputed.[3]

The disease is usually subclinical, but can on occasion produce a disease characterized by icterus, hemolytic anemia, fever, and weakness in neonatal and stressed feeder pigs; delayed estrus, early embryonic death, and abortions in late gestation. On most occasions the incidence of the clinical disease is low. Under stress, porcine eperythrozoonosis is expressed as a febrile condition with development of an acute ictero-anemia and observed in animals of all ages, from piglets to pregnant sows.[4–7]

Swine eperythrozoonosis has been endemic in swineherds in China since the last century, and has been well recognized, especially since the 1990s. It has become an important new emerging intercurrent swine disease, causing serious economic losses to the swine industry in most provinces in China.[8–11] To date, swine eperythrozoonosis outbreaks have spread through most provinces except Tibet, and reports of epidemiology surveillance, clinical investigations, and research have greatly increased. Disease syndromes have been well recognized and it caused heavy morbidity and mortality in pig herds, resulting in serious economic losses to the swine industry. The present article intends to introduce briefly some information on prevalence and comprehensive control of swine eperythrozoonosis in recent years in China.

MATERIALS AND METHODS

Swine eperythrozoonosis was investigated through clinical symptoms and epidemiological surveillance combined with microscopical blood smear examination, and serology tests, such as IHA, ELISA, and PCR. The disease was controlled by treatment with several chemicals or prophylactic measures. Historical animal health records in the surveyed area were consulted, and national or regional epidemiological surveillances were carried out. Scientific research reports on swine eperythrozoonosis were consulted as a basis for the analysis.

RESULTS

The Pathogen

The shape of the cell-wall-less organisms is round to oval, with disc and ring forms being common. The average diameter of 0.8–1.0 μM, and multiple organisms (of 10 or more) on one erythrocyte may be observed. Free organisms are sometimes seen in the blood plasma, tissue fluids, and cerebrospinal fluids. According to the observation with scanning and transmission electron microscopy, the surface of the erythrocyte membrane was affected and became rough with the erythrocyte appearing to have a hole in it.[12]

Epidemiology

This cell-wall-less uncultivated parasitic bacterium is thought to be transmitted from pig to pig by bloodsucking insects, including mosquitoes, ticks, and midges. Infection is usually subclinical, but on occasion it produces a disease characterized by icterus, hemolytic anemia, fever, and weakness in neonatal and stressed feeder pigs; delayed estrus, early embryonic death, and abortions. In most porcine eperythrozoonosis-affected herds other diseases were found, including classical swine fever (hog cholera), or other co-infections, such as porcine influenza, streptococci, swine enzootic pneumonia, pasteurellosis, porcine reproductive and respiratory syndrome (PRRS) (blue ear disease), or toxoplasmosis. A surveillance reported from 2002 revealed that *E. suis* infection was combined with classical swine fever (hog cholera), porcine influenza, or PRRS (blue ear disease) in Zhejiang, Fujian, Jiangsu, Anhui, Shan-dong, and Hebei provinces; as a main co-infection with classical swine fever and PRRS in Hunan, Hubei, Jangxi, Si-chuan, Chongqing, Shanxi, and Liaoning provinces and municipalities. The seasons of highest prevalence were May or June to November in 2001 with peaks from July to September, or March to October in 2002 with peaks from June to September. Outbreaks would occur associated with stress, caused by weaning, movement, and castration. In some endemic areas, the average infection and mortality rates of swine eperythrozoonosis in the national surveillance in 13 provinces and municipalities, involving 57 swine farms in 27 cities in 2002, was 30% and 10–20%, respectively. The total mortality rate (including culling of sick pigs) was over 60%. In some infected herds, the morbidity was 100%, with total death rates usually over 50%. The highest infection rate on any pig farm was more than 90%. The pig farms with higher infection rate occurred in pig-raising area in epidemic seasons. For example, in a village of southern China, where pig feed lots are on a large scale, morbidity of pigs was nearly 100%, with total mortality rates of 60%. Serious economic losses have been suffered in the swine industry in China. Pigs that recovered from swine eperythrozoonosis remain carriers of the disease. Pathogens persist in the circulating bloodstream but are not detected in blood films. The climatic factors contributing to the disease are high temperatures and high humidity. Stress, caused by weaning, movement, and castration is an important factor. In addition, in most affected herds other diseases were found, including classical swine fever, as well as co-infections, such as porcine influenza, streptococci, swine enzootic pneumonia, pasteurellosis, PRRS, or toxoplasmosis. Weaning, movement, and castration may induce clinical disease. The distribution of the disease in China has increased yearly. In 1991–2001, it was distributed in most provinces and municipalities, except Zhejang, Hainan, Sichuan, Guizhou, and Tibet. In 2002, it was distributed in all provinces and municipalities, except Tibet.

Diagnosis

Diagnosis of the disease is based on clinical history, post-mortem findings, and optical microscopic examination of the causative agent in blood smears. The disadvantage of blood smear detection is that it is only effective in the acute stage, but in latent carriers the pathogen may be missed. Some tests have been developed for the detection of swine eperythrozoonosis.[14–18] The immunofluorescene assay test was reported to be 40% more sensitive than microscopic examination. An ELISA with horseradish peroxidase-staphylococcal protein as the second antibody was sensitive and specific. It is operated on nitrocellulose membranes; the result was easy to judge with the naked eye. PCR has been established for surveillance. In order to probe into the effect of *E. suis* on the immunity level in piglets, the red blood cell (RBC) C3b receptor rosette rate, the RBC immune complete rosette rate, the lymphocyte transformation rate, and the formation rate of EA rosettes and EAC rosettes were used.[19,20] All the data obtained in artificially infected piglets were significantly lower than in healthy ones ($P < 0.001$). Therefore, *E. suis* can impede the immune function of piglets. These experiments revealed that the entire immune function was diminished as the quantity of C3b receptors and T lymphocytes changed. This may explain the intercurrent infections of virus pathogens in the infected herds. Research on the effects of *E. suis* on the antioxidant function confirmed that *E. suis* could cause the low antioxidant ability, increased accumulation of NO and oxygen-free radicals, and the strengthening reaction of lipoperoxidation, which is one of the causes of serial pathological lesion.

Treatment and Control

The detection and treatment of carriers is an efficient method for the control of swine eperythrozoonosis.[11,12,21] Clinical records confirm the effect of long-acting oxytetracycline, doxycycline, and aceturate of diminazene. The cure rate with doxycycline appeared to be higher than that of aceturate of diminazene, and may be due to its ability to enter the fetus in the uterus. Hematinics are beneficial feed additives for recovery from the infection. Although injections of long-active oxytetracycline are probably the most effective, they are often not practical because of the high cost and the labor input required. Some commercial productions including traditional Chinese herb medicines have been used in the disease control, but recovered animals frequently become re-infected and the cost of treatment is higher than can be really justified. As a preventative treatment, oxytetracycline as a feed additive has been introduced for the prevention of eperythrozoonosis in clean pig herds. Individual producers and swine farm owners have increased efforts toward reducing stress, and improving pig sanitary conditions.

DISCUSSION AND CONCLUSION

Swine eperythrozoonosis has become a newly emerging disease in China. Because of significant increases in prevalence in this country except in Tibet, it has caused heavy economic losses in the swine industry and the disease poses a potential threat to pig producers. *E. suis* can cause a diminished immune function, and has become a very important factor contributing to co-infection with other pathogens in pig herds in China. *E. suis* is still an uncultivated pathogen, and protective antibodies do not develop effectively following infection. The use of live vaccines using these fragile pathogens is not an adequate control strategy and cannot be based on the development of live vaccines. New idea strategies for the current protection of pigs in endemic areas should be developed. The exact economic importance should be more accurately surveyed. Reliable diagnostic methods that are easy to operate, should be developed for field use. There is a need to establish and standardize them for the identification of pathogens and use in epidemiological investigations. Molecular analysis of *E. suis* should be persued toward the development of subunit and genetic vaccines or, if possible, multivalent vaccines.

ACKNOWLEDGMENTS

The authors gratefully thank Dr. Gerrit Uilenberg, Editor of the Newsletter on Ticks and Tick-borne diseases of Livestock in the tropics, a publication of the ICTTD-3 program, Coordination Action project No. 510561, funded by the International Cooperation Program of the EU, for his advice and manuscript review. We are very grateful to Dr. Jean-Charles Maillard for his valuable comments and suggestions. We would also like to thank Professor Hu Ouxiang, Editor of the Chinese Journal of Animal Quarantine, for his friendly manuscript checking.

REFERENCES

1. SPLITTER, E.J. & R.L. WILLIAMSON. 1950. Eperythrozoonosis in swine: a preliminary report. J. Am. Vet. Med. Assoc. **116:** 360–364.
2. NEIMARK, H., K.-E. JOHANSSON, Y. RIKIHISA & J.G. TULLY. 2001. Proposal to transfer some members of the genera *Haemobartonella* and *Eperythrozoon* to the

genus *Mycoplasma* with descriptions of '*Candidates* Mycoplasma haemofelis', '*Candidatus* Mycoplasma haemomuris', '*Candidatus* Mycoplasma haemosuis' and '*Candidatus* Mycoplasma wenyonii'. Int. J. Syst. Evol. Microbiol. **51:** 891–899.

3. UILENBERG, G., F. THIAUCOURT & F. JONGEJAN. 2004. On molecular taxonomy: what is in a name ? Exp. Appl. Acarol. **32:** 301–312.

4. SPLITTER, E.J. 1950a. *Eperythrozoon suis,* the etiologic agent of ictero-anemia or an anaplasmosis-like disease in swine. Am. J. Vet. Res. **11:** 324–330.

5. SPLITTER, E.J. 1950b. *Eperythrozoon suis* n. sp., and *Eperythrozoon parvum* n. sp., 2 new blood parasites in swine. Science **111:** 513–514.

6. BERRIER, H.H. & R.E. GOUGE. 1954. Eperythrozoonosis transmitted in utero from carrier sows to their pigs. J. Am. Vet. Med. Assoc. **124:** 98–100.

7. HENRY, S.C. 1979. Clinical observations on eperythrozoonosis. J. Am. Vet. Med. Assoc. **174:** 601–603.

8. PU, X. & Y. XU. 1982. Primary report on discovery of *Eperythrozoon suis* in pigs infected with swine red skin disease [Ch]. Chin. J. Vet. Sci. Technol. **2:** 32–35.

9. WU, Y. 2001. Eperythrozoonosis[Ch]. J. Qinghai Anim. Husbandry Vet. **31:** 47–48.

10. WU, W. *et al.* 2000. The zoonosis of eperythrozoonosis [Ch]. Guangxi Anim. Husbandry Vet. **8:** 22.

11. XU, Y. *et al.* 2001. Epidemiological investigation and control of swine eperythrozoonosis [Ch]. Chin. J. Vet. Med. **37:** 14–15.

12. ZHANG, R., F. PAN, *et al.* 2001. Infection and control for human and livestock eperythrozoonosis [Ch]. Chin. J. Zoonoses **17:** 1261–1284.

13. BEI, J. *et al.* 2002. Election microscopic feature and observation of treatment efficiency on eperythrozoonosis [Ch]. Chin. J. Zoonosis **18:** 104–107.

14. ZHANG, S., G. ZHAN, H. WANG, *et al.* 2004. Aplication of IHA for diagnosis of swine eperythrozoonosis [Ch]. Chin. J. Vet. Med. **40:** 17–18.

15. CHANG, Y.C. & W. WANG. 2000. Diagnosis and treatment of eperythrozoonosis in piglets [Ch]. Chin. J. Vet. Med. **36:** 9–22.

16. HAN, H.Y., R. MENG, H. JIA, *et al.* 2004. Development of PPA-ELISA method for detection of *Eperythrozoon suis* [Ch]. Chin. J. Vet. Sci. Technol. **35:** 49–51.

17. ZHANG, H., M. XIE, J. ZHANG, *et al.* 2004. Establishment primary application of PCR assay for eperythrozoon swine, eperythrozoon [Ch]. Proceeding of Chinese society of Animal parasitology, Guilin, P. 135–140.

18. WANG, Y., S. ZHANG & S.-G. LIU. 2005. Establishment of the PCR method for detection of swine eperythrozoonosis, [Ch]. Sci. Agric. Sin. **38:** 2153–2156.

19. CHAI, F., L. JIA & S. ZHANG. 2005. Effect of *Eperythrozoon suis* in immunity level in piglets [Ch]. J. Agric. Sci. Yanbian Univ. [Ch] **27:** 14–16.

20. LI, Q., X. ZHAI, X. ZHONG, *et al.* 2005. Research on effects of eperythrozoon on the anti-oxidant function. [Ch]. Prog. Vet. Med. **26:** 92–94.

21. WANG, J., Z. WANG, X. ZHAN, *et al.* 2003. Research progress of swine eperythrozoonosis [Ch]. Chin. J. Anim. Quarantine **20:** 44–46.

Bovine Transcriptome Analysis by SAGE Technology during an Experimental *Trypanosoma congolense* Infection

DAVID BERTHIER,[a] ISABELLE CHANTAL,[a] SOPHIE THÉVENON,[b] JACQUES MARTI,[c] DAVID PIQUEMAL,[d] AND JEAN-CHARLES MAILLARD[a]

[a] *Cirad-Emvt Baillarguet, 34098 Montpellier Cedex 5, France*

[b] *Cirdes, BP 454 01 Bobo Dioulasso, Burkina Faso*

[c] *GET, 34095 Montpellier Cedex 5, France*

[d] *Skuld-tech Cie, 34095 Montpellier Cedex 5, France*

ABSTRACT: In central and sub-Saharan Africa, trypanosomosis is a tsetse fly-transmitted disease, which is considered as the most important impediment to livestock production in the region. However, several indigenous West African taurine breeds (*Bos taurus*) present remarkable tolerance to the infection. This genetic capability, named trypanotolerance, results from numerous biological mechanisms most probably under multigenic dependences, among which are control of the trypanosome infection by limitation of parasitemia and control of severe anemia due to the pathogenic effects. Today, some postgenomic biotechnologies, such as transcriptome analyses, allow characterization of the full expressed genes involved in the majority of animal diseases under genetic control. One of them is serial analysis of gene expression (SAGE) technology, which consists of the construction of mRNA transcript libraries for qualitative and quantitative analysis of the entire genes expressed or inactivated at a particular step of cellular activation. We developed four different mRNA transcript libraries from white blood cells on a N'Dama trypanotolerant animal during an experimental *Trypanosoma congolense* (*T. congolense)* infection: one before experimental infection (ND0), one at the parasitemia peak (NDm), one at the minimal packed cell volume (NDa), and the last one at the end of the experiment after normalization (NDf). Bioinformatic comparisons in bovine genomic databases allowed us to obtain more than 75,000 sequences, among which are several known genes, some others are already described as expressed sequence tags (ESTs), and the last are completely new, but probably functional in trypanotolerance. The knowledge of all identified named or unnamed genes involved in trypanotolerance characteristics will allow us to

Address for correspondence: David Berthier, CIRAD Département EMVT UMR17, Campus International de Baillarguet TA 30/G 34398 Montpellier Cedex 5, France. Voice: +33-467-593-724; fax: +33-467-593-798.

e-mail: david.berthier@cirad.fr

Ann. N.Y. Acad. Sci. 1081: 286–299 (2006). © 2006 New York Academy of Sciences.

doi: 10.1196/annals.1373.039

use them in a field marker-assisted selections strategy and in microarrays prediction sets for bovine trypanotolerance.

KEYWORDS: sage; trypanotolerance; n'Dama; *Trypanosoma congolense*; transcriptomics

INTRODUCTION

African trypanosomosis is a parasitic infection caused by protozoan pathogens belonging to the *Trypanosomatidae* family. This disease is transmitted by a tsetse fly hematophagous vector. In central and sub-Saharan Africa, it represents an important factor that limits cattle breeding by reducing or preventing livestock production (milk, meat, fertility, culling) on a 9 million km^2 (approximately one-third of Africa) area spread over 37 countries. The United Nations estimates that at least 50 million bovine are affected and the resulting economic losses are about 1 to 1.2 billion U.S. dollars. However, certain local breeds have developed a tolerance to trypanosome infections during the centuries spent in areas strongly infested by glossines.[1–7] This ability, named trypanotolerance, results from several biological mechanisms under multigenic control. Indeed, some breeds present the remarkable capacity to control their parasitemia level,[8–11] to be opposed to the development of severe anemia[12–15] during the infection, and to remain productive in a zone strongly infested by tsetse flies.[16] These two characteristics (limited parasitemia and anemia) are known to be highly heritable and genetically linked to cattle productivity. More than one single gene, it seems probable that two pools of genes are involved but all the techniques used up to now have failed to identify them. Neither the zootechnical studies,[17–21] nor the quantitative genetic approaches,[22] the electrophoretic analysis of certain targeted proteins,[23,24] and typing MHC,[25] did not allowed to progress in trypanotolerance understanding. Quantitative trait loci (QTL) studies could give some information but until now have not succeeded in identifying the involved genes.[26,27] Moreover, these studies are complicated and expensive and the identified chromosomal location still remains too vast to allow their use in a selection-assisted marker strategy (SAM). Today, in addition to the microarrays, a biotechnology much more significant than the EST approaches allows access to an exhaustive functional analysis.[28] The serial analysis of gene expression (SAGE) is based on a "transcriptomic" strategy able to characterize the differential expression of whole expressed genes.[29–31]

Four libraries were developed with a trypanotolerant N'Dama cattle: the first one before the experimental infection (ND0), a second corresponding to the maximum parasitemia (NDm), a third at minimum packed cell volume or maximum anemia (NDa), and a final library after the recovery of the initial value for packed cell volume (PCV) and no parasite in serum (NDf). The comparison of all the libraries at different stages before and during infection will allow us to refine the results already found in our previous study.[29]

MATERIALS AND METHODS

Animals and Experimental Infection

We used one N'Dama animal, which is a "longhorn," indigenous West African taurine (*Bos taurus*) well known to be tolerant to trypanosomosis infection. This animal was selected in Burkina Faso (CIRDES) in an environment strongly infested with tsetse flies and was classified as trypanotolerant on the basis of criteria defining trypanotolerance (parasitemia, PCV, body weight). A serologic control allowed us to check for the presence of *Trypanosoma congolense (T. congolense)*-specific antibodies, a trypanotolerance character appearing after successive infections.[32–34]

The animal was then isolated in a specific environment in order to avoid tsetse bites and was treated against blood (Veriben: diminazene aceturate, 7 mg/kg) and gastrointestinal parasites (Vermitan: albendazole, 7.5 mg/kg) to guarantee the absence of parasites before the beginning of the experiment. After a few days, a first blood sample was collected using PAXgene blood RNA tubes (Qiagen SA, Courteboeuf, France; Cat. No. 762125) containing an RNA conservation solution. This first sample enabled us to develop the SAGE reference library before experimental infection (ND0) from total white blood cells (WBC). The N'Dama taurine was then infected by syringe inoculation[33–36] with a clone of *T. congolense* (Ser/71/STIB/212) of medium pathogenicity to follow the evolution of the infection without killing the animal. Moreover, this clone is not present in Burkina Faso; therefore, the animal could not develop immunity against this clone and brought us closer to a primary infection condition.

The venous inoculation route was selected to avoid cutaneous reactions and to focus on peripheral blood cell genes expression. Parasitemia and anemia were monitored every 2 days by blood examination to determine the parasitemia level and PCV values. Other samples were collected during experimentation, respectively, at the maximum of parasitemia (NDm), minimum PCV or maximum anemia (NDa), and a last one when the parasite was not detectable and PCV value was stabilized (NDf). These four libraries were constructed using I-SAGE™ kit from Invitrogen (Cat.; Cergy Pontoise, France; Cat. no. T5000-01) and were used in a differential comparison of expressed genes before and after *T. congolense* infection. The confrontation of the sequenced tags observed with the potential tags in the international databanks (Unigen, Tigr, SageMap) allowed us to identify the tags obtained and to confirm our previous results.[29]

SAGE Method

The SAGE method generates 14-bp tags derived from the 3' end of each transcript present in a cell or tissue type at a particular time. These tags can be rapidly analyzed and matched to genomic sequence data and permit identification of specific genes and their relative frequencies.[29-31,37-39] The mRNA are isolated from the whole RNA population using oligo-dT beads that retain the mRNA by their poly A^+ tail. After double-stranded cDNA synthesis and *Nla III* cutting, the sample is separated into two identical fractions and two specific adaptors are linked to both the cDNA fractions. The following step consists of cleaving with the *BsmF I* type IIS restriction enzyme and linking the two DNA fractions together. An ultimate step consists of the 110-bp amplification using specific primers and a last digestion with *Nla III* in order to release the 14-bp tags. The tags are linked together to form a long DNA molecule that is cloned and sequenced. The expression level of the transcript is quantified by the number of times (occurrence) a particular tag is observed in one library. Each library is then compared with each other in order to observe the variation level in the expression of each transcript.

RESULTS AND DISCUSSION

The four library results (ND0, NDm, NDa, and NDf) are summarized in TABLES 1 and 2. From 75,005 sequenced tags, 20,177 are distinct transcripts. Among them, 12,193 tags are identified in the international databases (Unigen, Tigr, SageMap) as EST or cDNA corresponding to 61%, of which 472 are known genes. Around 7984 tags (39%) failed to be identified and correspond to unknown tags. Due to the wide information generated by SAGE, except for immunity-related tags (TABLE 1), only the tags with a P value < 0.001 between ND0 and NDm libraries are presented in the following table (TABLE 2).

Several transcripts could be identified as molecules closely involved in the defense mechanism of the immune system (immunoglobulins, B and T cell, MHC molecules...), some others corresponded to EST ribosomal proteins, and others are unknown genes (no match).

Considering the class I molecules, we have observed a reduction of 50% in the expression level of the β-2 microglobulin gene (TABLE 1). This molecule forms an integral part of the class I molecule, located on the majority of the various cellular types. One of the main functions of the class I molecules is to present the antigenic peptides to the T $CD8^+$ cytotoxic cells in charge of the cellular mediation immunity targeted mainly against bacteria, viruses, and parasites. The reduction in these transcripts reflects the capacity, which seems to be faded here, of the antigenic-presenting cells to induce a cellular response by T cell lymphocytes. For the heavy chains of these molecules the decrease is less significant (TABLE 1). The expression level of tags coding for most of the class I heavy chain seems to be stable or decreases slightly more than the light chains after the experimental infection in the NDm library. These results confirm those already obtained with smaller quantity of tags on the first two libraries[29] and previous immunologic results.[32]

TABLE 1. Expression of the most important immunity-related tags

Sequence Tag	ND0	NDm	NDa	NDf	Id	Name
Immunity and related proteins						
CATGGCTAAGCCTA	414	209	242	210	TC289234	β-2-microglobulin
CATGTTTAGAGTAA	2	1	1	3	Bt.5269	β-2-microglobulin
CATGATAAACATTA	0	0	1	1	TC276434	
Total	416	210	244	214		
CATGATTATATTTC	1	15	3	3	Bt.11581	Platelet factor 4
CATGCCTCAATAGA	0	1	3	1	Bt.11581	
CATGGAAATATGCA	0	2	1	0	Bt.11581	
CATGCTATCAAAAC	0	3	0	2	Bt.11581	
Total	1	21	7	6		
Immunoglobulin						
CATGGACCCCTGAG	66	195	139	134	Bt.29797	Immunoglobulin light chain variable region
CATGGAGCCCGCAG	57	76	85	50	TC262246	Immunoglobulin heavy chain constant region
CATGAGTGCAGACT	6	52	27	6	TC262219	IgM heavy chain constant region, secretory
CATGGTCACCAGCT	3	6	2	6	Bt.12490	*B. taurus* mRNA for IgG1 heavy chain
CATGCAGGTGAGGC	2	1	1	0	Bt.12490	*B. taurus* mRNA for IgG1 heavy chain
CATGCAGAAGTCCA	5	5	3	6	Bt.16033	Ig C g = IgG2a heavy chain constant region
MHC class I						
CATGGCGCCCCTTC	57	44	48	39	Bt.2592	MHC class 1 (clone 6)
CATGAGGAGTTGGG	58	53	73	109	Bt.23328	MHC class I
CATGCGCTGAGTAA	22	26	26	27	Bt.27760	Class I, A (HLA-A)
CATGAGGGAAGAGA	1	0	0	1	Bt.27760	
Total	23	26	26	28		
CATGCTGCTCTTGG	0	0	2	1	Bt.28448	
CATGGAGTTTGGGG	5	1	1	0	Bt.28448	MHC class I heavy chain
Total	5	1	3	1		
CATGGGCATCATTG	39	39	29	91	Bt.4762/Bt.	MHC class I
CATGAGGGGCTTCA	0	1	0	1	Bt.29815/B	MHC class I
CATGGTGAGGAAGG	1	2	2	0	Bt.4762/Bt.	MHC class I
CATGGCACGTGTAT	0	2	0	0	Bt.28450	MHC class I
CATGTCCTGGGT CT	0	2	1	1	Bt.4762/Bt.	MHC class I
CATGATGAGGAAGG	0	0	1	1	Bt.8121/Bt.	MHC class I
CATGGGCATCATTC	0	0	1	0	Bt.33169	nonclassical MHC class I antigen
Total	40	46	34	94		
CATGTGGCCTGAGG	12	11	4	2	TC262122	nonclassical MHC class I antigen
CATGCTCCTAAAGT	7	3	4	10	TC262167	MHC class I antigen
CATGTGACCCAT CA	3	1	1	1	Bt.29284	MHC class I heavy chain
CATGGAGCTTGTGG	4	1	3	3	Bt.32652	MHC class I heavy chain
CATGGAGTTTGGGG	5	1	1	0	Bt.28448	MHC class I heavy chain
CATGACTCTACATC	6	2	7	8	TC262168	MHC class 1 precursor
CATGAAGGGGGATT	0	1	0	3	Bt.7773	MHC class I heavy chain
MHC class II						
Invariant chain Li						
CATGAGCCACCCTT	68	92	94	110	Bt.23174	CD74 chain Li
CATGGAAGTGGTGG	6	4	6	4	Bt.23174	CD74 chain Li
CATGAGAGGCTGAC	2	3	2	3	Bt.23174	CD74 chain Li
CATGCCCCCAGTTA	0	1	2	1	Bt.23174	CD74 chain Li
CATGATCTTGGAGT	0	0	1	1	Bt.23174/Bt.	CD74 chain Li
Total Li	76	100	105	119		

Continued

TABLE 1. Continued

Sequence Tag	ND0	NDm	NDa	NDf	Id	Name
DRA molecule						
CATGTAATGCCTTT	34	32	64	46	Bt.8552	DRA
CATGCTTCAGCACT	0	0	0	1	Bt.8552	DRA
CATGGCTTCGAAAT	0	2	0	0	Bt.8552	DRA
CATGTGACACTGAT	1	0	0	0	Bt.8552	DRA
Total	35	34	64	47		
DRB molecule						
CATGGAAAGGTTTC	3	2	4	6	Bt.5356	DRB
CATGGTGATGCTTG	0	1	0	1	Bt.5356	DRB
CATGCTGTGAAGAA	0	0	1	1	Bt.5356	DRB
Total	3	3	5	8		
Total *DR*	38	37	69	55		
DQ molecule						
CATGGTTGAGGAAT	0	0	1	0	Bt.22867	
CATGAATTTGATGG	0	0	0	1	Bt.4046	DQA
CATGCCAAAGAACA	0	1	0	0	TC262946	DQA
Total	0	1	1	1		
CATGATTATGAGTT	18	17	21	14	Bt.350	DQB
CATGCGCTGACTCC	6	2	2	3	Bt.350/Bt.7	DQB
CATGAGCCCCTTCT	0	0	0	1	Bt.350/Bt.7	DQB
CATGAATATAAATT	3	6	8	8	Bt.4594	DQB
CATGGTAGGCAACT	1	0	1	0	Bt.4751	DQB
CATGAGATCACTGG	0	0	0	1	Bt.4751	DQB
CATGATTATGAGTG	0	1	0	0	Bt.20925	DQB
Total	28	26	32	27		
Total *DQ*	28	27	33	28		
DM molecule						
CATGGCAGGGTTGT	0	0	1	1	Bt.344	DM alpha
CATGTCAAGGCAAT	9	9	9	6	TC292801	DM alpha
Total	9	9	10	7		
CATGACTGAGCGAC	5	6	11	15	Bt.1007/Bt.	DMB
CATGAGGTCGCAAA	0	1	1	0	Bt.28935	
CATGGGGTCACGAA	0	0	0	1	Bt.1007	DMB
Total	5	6	11	16		
Total *DM*	14	15	21	23		
B cell						
CATGGCCACTTAGT	28	38	56	29	Bt.4436	CD79a/*B. taurus* mRNA
CATGACAGAGCAGG	2	1	0	1	Bt.4436	
Total	30	39	56	30		
CATGGCCCTGTGAA	2	1	4	8	Bt.20540	CD79b
CATGATCCAGACCT	0	1	0	0	Bt.20540	
Total	2	2	4	8		
CATGTATATTGATT	10	4	9	8	Bt.4725	B cell translocation gene 1, antiproliferative
CATGACCTGGGGAA	2	0	0	3	Bt.4725	
CATGCTTACTAGTT	0	0	1	0	Bt.4725	
Total	12	4	10	11		

Continued

TABLE 1. Continued

Sequence Tag	ND0	NDm	NDa	NDf	Id	Name
T cell						
CATGTGAGGGTGCC	16	14	11	16	TC260844	TCR beta C3
CATGTGGGGAAAAA	13	4	9	10	Bt.4289	TCR alpha
CATGGATGAGAAGG	1	0	0	0	Bt.4289	TCR alpha
CATGTTGGGGAAAA	1	0	1	0	Bt.4289/ Bt.21296	TCR alpha
Total	15	4	10	10		
CATGAATGTGCTAA	7	6	14	17	Bt.5368	CD3 E
CATGTTAATAAAAG	2	2	2	3	TC276543	T cell activation protein
CATGGGGAAGGCCT	0	1	0	0	Bt.4763	CD3 Z
CATGGATGGAAACC	3	4	4	3	Bt.4763	CD3 Z
Total	3	5	4	3		
CATGGGCCATAGTA	0	1	0	0	Bt.13934	CD3 G
CATGTGAAAGAAGT	1	0	0	0	Bt.13934	CD3 G
Total	1	1	0	0		
CATGTTGACACAGA	14	15	6	3	Bt.11088	CD97 T cell activated (ligand CD55)
CATGTACCTGGAAA	3	17	9	6	Bt.4140	activation des macrophages
CATGCCAGTGAATG	0	0	0	1	Bt.4140	Cytochrome b-245, alpha polypeptide
CATGGAACAGGCGA	0	2	2	1	Bt.4140	
Total	3	19	11	8		
Lysozyme						
CATGAGTTGGTCCT	2	10	3	4	Bt.16049	Lysosomal-associated multispanning mb p5
CATGAATGCTATAA	3	15	16	11	Bt.209	Lysozyme, macrophage
CATGAAGGATATAA	1	1	1	0	Bt.209	
CATGAAACTAAGCT	1	1	1	1	Bt.209	
CATGACAGCAAGAT	1	0	1	0	Bt.209	
Total	6	17	19	12		
Complement						
CATGGCTGAGGGCG	24	18	40	24	TC262727	Complement factor D precursor
CATGTCTTGGAACT	2	3	4	2	TC289601	Complement C1q subcomponent,
CATGTTAAGTGTTG	51	28	22	4	TC279667	Decay-accelerating factor CD55
CATGTCTACACGTG	0	3	3	3	Bt.23488	

(ND0) = noninfected library; (NDm) = maximum parasitemia library; (NDa) = minimum PCV or maximun anemia; (NDf) = final library with initial values for PCV and no parasitemia.

TABLE 2. Expression of the most up- and downregulated tags with *P* value <0.0001 between ND0 and NDm.

Sequence Tag	ND0	NDm	NDa	NDf	Id	Name
EST						
CATGACAACACATA	129	267	239	142	CO879468	EST
CATGTGCTGTGCAT	28	8	4	3	Bt.31251	EST
CATGTGAGAACATT	26	56	55	37	Bt.32804/Bt.38667	
CATGACAGTAGAAA	0	1	3	1	Bt.32804/Bt.38667	
CATGGCCTTCCAAT	21	44	27	11	Bt.25265	EST
CATGTATCTCCAAA	4	22	5	2	BM258171	EST
Others genes						
CATGTAGGTTGTCT	192	320	233	126	BE664428	TPT1
CATGGCATTCAAAT	78	28	40	76	TC278419	chemokine precursor
CATGGACGACACGA	73	28	93	87	TC274657	
CATGTTGGCAAAAC	35	11	19	13	TC262646	Rattus norvegicus profilaggrin-like, partial (8%)
CATGACGAAGCCTC	6	26	6	6	Bt.4389	Spleen trypsin inhibitor
CATGGCCCCCAATA	0	14	11	10	Bt.5472	Lectin, galactoside-binding, soluble,
CATGGGGACGTCAA	1	0	0	0	Bt.5472	
CATGCGCGTTGAAA	1	0	0	0	Bt.5472	
CATGATTGGAGAGA	1	3	1	0	Bt.5472	
Total	3	17	12	10		
Ribosomal protein						
CATGGCCTGATGGG	198	128	190	127	Bt.5211	ribosomal protein
CATGAATTCATAGG	2	1	2	2	Bt.5211	
Total	200	129	192	129		
CATGGACGACACGA	73	28	93	87	TC274595	40S ribosomal protein S28
CATGCTCACCAATA	66	121	182	114	Bt.37200	ribosomal protein
CATGGTGGCAGAAA	1	0	2	1	Bt.37200	
CATGATTAAGGAGG	0	5	1	1	Bt.37200	
CATGAGTGTAGGGC	0	1	1	1	Bt.37200	
CATGTTCTCAAATT	1	0	0	1	Bt.37200	
Total	68	127	186	118		
CATGCACAAACAGT	64	6	44	17	TC262425	40S ribosomal protein S27
CATGACATCATTGA	58	16	67	56	TC276438	60S ribosomal protein L12
CATGATTCTTTGGT	49	22	25	14	TC260882	60S ribosomal protein L23
CATGTGAAAGATGC	39	18	31	24	TC262484	ribosomal protein S4
CATGAAAACAGTAG	20	5	26	20	TC275093	ribosomal protein L37a
CATGGCCTTTAAAG	14	2	5	10	TC262089	ribosomal protein S2
CATGGCGCTCTGAT	1	13	8	2	TC263267	
No match						
CATGATGTTATTTC	26	8	19	8		Not Found
CATGTTAACTGGCA	12	1	4	1		Not Found

(ND0): noninfected library; (NDm): maximum parasitemia library; (NDa): minimum PCV or maximun anemia; (NDf): final library with initial values for PCV and no parasitemia.

We can also observe a significant increase, around 32%, in the transcription of gene coding for the invariant chain "Li" between ND0 and NDm libraries, then respectively, +5% between NDm and NDa libraries, +13% between NDa and NDf libraries, so that there is a total increase of more than 50% between the beginning and the end of the experiment. For memory, this molecule links the class II molecule into the furrow formed by the association of the alpha and beta chains. This invariant chain is necessary for the association process of the alpha and beta chains for a good presentation of antigenic peptide to the cells of the immune system. The tags associated to *DR* molecules are relatively well represented in the bank, in particular the alpha chain of this molecule (*DRA*) which, although stable between ND0 and NDm, presents an increase of more than 80% between NDm and NDa libraries. The beta chain does not show the same tag proportions; this may be because of the wide possibility of potential alleles for this chain. Some other transcripts identified as *DQB* molecules seem to be stable between ND0 and NDm but increases up to 23% between NDm and NDa (minimum PCV). The class II molecules are mainly present on the antigen-presenting cell membranes and B lymphocytes. As described in several previous studies on trypanotolerance, a proliferation of the B cell population in charge of the humoral immunity by polyspecific antibody[40,41] could explain the N'Dama taurine's ability to resist the infection.

We note that the expression of some genes associated with molecules closely related to specific cellular types seems disturbed. For some surface antigens, such as CD79a, which is specifically expressed on the B lymphocyte membranes, an increase of 30% between ND0 and NDm is observed, with more than 43% between NDm and NDa, and then recovery of the initial value at the end of experiment (NDf). The total increase of the CD79 value borders at 86% between ND0 and NDa, clearly indicating a proliferation of the B cell population. It has been highlighted on mice infected by *T. brucei* and also on bovines infected by *T. congolense* that immunologic deteriorations consisting of an expansion of the B cells, an important elevation of IgM in serum, and a strong immunosuppression in the first stage of infection occur. Transcriptome analysis shows concordant results that tend to confirm the previous results.[2,3,9,30,32,42] The parasite, which is an extracellular parasite, is always exposed to the immune system of its host. To face this constraining environment it has to evolve and develop several mechanisms of protection and escape. One of the strategies used consists of the immunosuppression[43] of the host defenses by locking the T cell-dependent immune responses and also by changing its surface glycoprotein, VSG.[44]

It would seem that prevalent immunity, at least at the beginning of infection, is related to a T cell-independent response. The SAGE results seem to confirm this T cell decrease. Indeed, if we consider the expression level of the tags corresponding to the alpha TCR, we can observe a decrease of around 78% between ND0 and NDm, with a quick recovering value in the following libraries, indicating that the N'Dama cattle are able to face infection by increasing the B cell population and reducing the loss of their T cells.

On the other hand, the increase in transcripts encoding for various chains of IgM seems to confirm the previous assumption of an increase in B cell population. The expression of IgM is significantly increased and seems to be strongly regulated. The gene expression encoding for IgM light chain is not threefold higher in the NDm library than in the ND0 library and the expression of the IgM-secreted form between ND0 and NDm is eightfold higher.

The IgM are polyreactive and polyspecific in the serum of individuals infected by *T. congolense*. Most of them are not only directed against the VSG of *T. congolense* but also against specific products of the parasite. During an infection, these IgM increase considerably and constitute a primary mechanism of defense, before the establishment of the IgG-specific immunity.[45,46] It is known that these antibodies, anti-VSG, are neutralizing and protective.[47] The VSG-exposed epitopes induce mainly T cell-independent responses producing a large amount of IgM that would be sufficient to control parasitemia.[2,48] It is now well established that during a primary infection, the response involved primarily IgM immunoglobulin followed by a more specific response with IgG immunoglobulin, mainly IgG1 and IgG2 (TABLE 1).

The macrophage population seems to play an important role in the trypanotolerant character. The increase of some transcripts in the library postinfection is a good indicator of macrophage activation. Indeed, the expression level of cytochrome b-245, which reflects the macrophage cell activation, increases more than sixfold between ND0 and NDm. The expression of the gene encoding for the platelet factor 4 is 21-fold higher in NDm than in the ND0 library. This gene is well known to induct monocyte differentiation in macrophages. At the same time, the lysozyme gene presents a significant increase bordering 180% between the ND0 and NDm libraries indicating that the phagocytic system cells are really activated.

Some specific transcripts, such as the CD55 and also other complement, components seem to indicate a strong activation of the complement from the maximum of the parasitemia library (NDm). Indeed, due to the decrease of CD55 (−45% between ND0 and NDm libraries), which normally takes part in the regulation of the C3 convertase activity, the complement seems to be upregulated and this point is now well documented in some publications.[32] The CD55 antigen is present in a wide population of cells including erythrocytes and acts to prevent the abnormal destruction of the self-cell by the complement system. Although the decrease of this gene seems to be related to the decrease in the total lymphocyte population, it could also be attributed to the immunosuppressive action of the parasite. It has been demonstrated that trypanosomes are able to transfer some parasitic particles on the red blood cell membrane. This transfer allows the parasite to divert the host immune response (lysis by complement action) and is responsible to the severe anemia[49] observed in trypanosome infection.

Finally, much ribosomal proteins and several ESTs seem to be strongly up- or downregulated. A particular protein, EST, a translationally controlled tumor protein, is strongly upregulated in the course of parasitic infection with the highest level at maximum parasitemia and a value close to that before infection in the third library. This molecule, first described and isolated in human tumor cells, is involved not only in the reversion of tumoral cells, but also in several cellular functions. The role of this protein is not well understood but it would seem that its sphere of activity is as broad as cell multiplication, cellular transformation morphology, and blocking of apoptosis. This protein seems to be a good candidate that could be involved in trypanotolerance. Further analyses with trypano-susceptible animals should follow to confirm this assumption.

Many more ESTs were found with a negatively or positively regulated expression in the course of infection. The EST with the most significant P values are presented in TABLE 2. Many of them are interesting, but further developments of the bovine map will be needed to clearly identify them and the most relevant according to their expression level could be spotted on microarrays with further applications.

Finally, some tags came from *T. congolense*, but due to the poor quality of the trypanosome database, these results must be confirmed (data not shown).

Nevertheless, these results open a very interesting path to analyze host–parasite interactions by comparing the host and parasite library. In this way, in order to perform this analysis, and also to separate the specific parasite tags to the bovine tags, a *T. congolense* library will be developed.

These first interesting results obtained on a single animal must now be expanded to identify and isolate the most important tags in these first four libraries. To identify the genes involved in trypanotolerance, we need to perform other analyses using other individuals from several other cattle breeds. Others libraries for another trypanotolerant individual (Baoule/*Bos taurus*) and at least one susceptible animal (zebu/*Bos indicus*) are under construction and will allow us to compare gene expression profiles in an interbreed analysis.

REFERENCES

1. CHANDLER, R.L. 1952. Comparative tolerance of West African N'Dama cattle to trypanosomiasis. Ann. Trop. Med. Parasitol. **46:** 127–134.
2. DE RAADT, P. 1974. Immunity and antigenic variation: clinical observations suggestive of immune phenomena in trypanosomiasis. *In*: Trypanosomiasis and Leishmaniasis with Special Reference to Chaga's Disease, CIBA Foundation Symposium 20 (new series). 199–211. Elsevier, Amsterdam.
3. DESOWITZ, R.S. 1959. Studies on immunity and host-parasite relationships. I. The immunological response of resistant and susceptible breeds of cattle to trypanosomal challenge. Ann. Trop. Med. Parasitol. **53:** 293–313.

4. DESROTOUR, J., P. FINELLE, P. MARTIN & E. SINODINOS. 1967. Les bovins trypan-otolérants : leur élevage en République Centrafricaine. Rev. Elev. Méd. Vét. Pays Trop. **20:** 589–594.

5. PIERRE, C. 1906. L'élevage dans l'Afrique occidentale française. Gouvernement Général De L'afrique Occidentale Française. Inspection de l'Agriculture. Chalamel, Paris.

6. ROBERTS, C.J. & A.R. GRAY. 1973. Studies on trypanosome-resistant cattle. II. The effect of trypanosomiasis on N'Dama, Muturu and Zebu cattle. Trop. Anim. Health Prod. **5:** 220–233.

7. STEWART, J.L. 1951. The West African shorthorn cattle. Their value to Africa as trypanosomiasis-resistant animals. Vet. Rec. **63:** 454–457.

8. DOLAN, R.B. 1987. Genetics and trypanotolerance. Parasitol. Today **3:** 137–143.

9. GIBSON, J.P. 2001. Towards an understanding of genetic control of trypanotolerance. Newslett. Integ. Control Pathog. Trypanosomes Vect. **4:** 12–14.

10. MURRAY, M., W.I. MORRISON & D.D. WHITELAW. 1982. Host susceptibility to African trypanosomiasis: trypanotolerance. Adv. Parasitol. **21:** 1–68.

11. ROELANTS, G.E. 1986. Natural resistance to African Trypanosomiasis. Parasite Immunol. **8:** 1–10.

12. AGYEMANG, K., R.H. DWINGER, D.A. LITTLE, *et al.* 1992. Interaction between physiological status in N'Dama cows and trypanosome infections and its effects on health and productivity of cattle in the Gambia. Acta Trop. **50:** 91–99.

13. TRAIL, J.C.M., G.D.M. D'IETEREN, A. FERON, *et al.* 1991. Effect of trypanosome infection, control of parasitaemia and control of anaemia development on productivity of N'Dama cattle. Acta Trop. **48:** 37–45.

14. TRAIL, J.C.M., G.D.M. D'IETEREN, J.C. MAILLE & G. YANGARI. 1991. Genetic aspects of control of anaemia development in trypanotolerant N'Dama cattle. Acta Trop. **48:** 285–291.

15. TRAIL, J.C.M., G.D.M. D'IETEREN, P. VIVIANI, *et al.* 1992. Relationships between trypanosome infection measured by antigen detection enzyme immunoassays, anaemia and growth in trypanotolerant N'Dama cattle. Vet. Parasitol. **42:** 213–223.

16. DWINGER, R.H., K. AGYEMANG, W.F. SNOW, *et al.* 1994. Productivity of cattle kept under traditional management conditions in the Gambia. Vet. Q. **16:** 81–86.

17. D'IETEREN, G.D.M., E. AUTHIÉ, *et al.* 1998. Trypanotolerance, an option for sustainable livestock production in areas at risk from trypanosomosis. Rev. Sci. Techn. Off. Int. Epiz. **17:** 154–175.

18. D'IETEREN, G.D.M., E. AUTHIÉ, N. WISSOCQ & M. MURRAY. 1999. Exploitation of resistance to trypanosomes, *In* R.F.E. Axford, S.C. Bishop, F.W. Nicholas, *et al.*, Eds.: 195–216. Breeding for Disease Resistance in Farm Animals, 2nd ed. CABI Publishing. Wallingford.

19. HOSTE, C. 1992. Contribution du bétail trypanotolérant au développement des zones affectées par la trypanosomiase animale africaine. Rev. Mond. Zootech. 70–71; 21–29.

20. HOSTE, C., E. CHALON, G.D.M. D'IETEREN & J.C.M. TRAIL. 1988. Le bétail trypanotolérant en Afrique occidentale et centrale.Vol. 3: Bilan d'une décennie. Étude FAO Production et santé animale, No. 2/3, Organisation des nations unies pour l'alimentation et l'agriculture, Rome.

21. MURRAY, M., M.J. STEAR, J.C.M. TRAIL, *et al.* 1991. Trypanosomiasis in cattle: prospects for control. *In* J.B. Owen & R.F.E. Axford, Eds.: 203–223. Breeding for Disease Resistance in Farm Animals, 1st ed. CABI Publishing. Wallingford.

22. TRAIL, J.C.M., N. WISSOCQ, G.D.M. D'IETEREN, *et al*. 1994. Quantitative phenotyping of N'Dama cattle for aspects of trypanotolerance under field tsetse challenge. Vet. Parasitol. **55:** 185–195.
23. QUEVAL, R. & L. BAMBARA. 1984. Le polymorphisme de l'albumine dans la race Baoulé et une population de zébus de type soudanien. Rev. Elev. Méd. Vét. Pays Trop. **37:** 288–296.
24. QUEVAL, R. & J.-P. PETIT. 1982. Polymorphisme biochimique de l'hémoglobine de populations bovines trypanosensibles, trypanotolérantes et de leurs croisements dans l'Ouest africain. Rev. Elev. Méd. Vét. Pays Trop. **35:** 137–146.
25. MAILLARD, J.-C., S.J. KEMP, H. LEVEZIEL, *et al*. 1989. Le système majeur d'histocompatibilité de bovins ouest-africains. Typage d'antigènes lymphocytaires (*BoLA*) de taurins Baoulé (*Bos taurus*) et de zébus soudaniens (*Bos indicus*) du Burkina Faso (Afrique occidentale). Rev. Elev. Méd. Vét. Pays Trop. **42:** 275–281.
26. HANOTTE, O., Y. RONIN, M. AGABA, *et al*. 2003. Mapping of quantitative trait loci controlling trypanotolerance in a cross of tolerant West African N'Dama and susceptible East African Boran cattle. Proc. Natl. Acad. Sci. USA **13:** 7443–7448.
27. HILL, E.W., G.M. O'GORMAN, M. AGABA, *et al*. 2005. Understanding bovine trypanosomiasis and trypanotolerance: the promise of functional genomics. Vet. Immuno. Immunopathol. **105:** 247–258.
28. PIQUEMAL, D., T. COMMES, L. MANCHON, *et al*. 2002. Transcriptome analysis of monocytic leukemia cell differentiation. Genomics **80:** 316–371.
29. BERTHIER, D., R. QUÉRÉ, S. THEVENON, *et al*. 2003. Genet. Sel. Evol. **35**(Suppl 1): S35–S47.
30. MAILLARD, J.C., D. BERTHIER, S. THEVENON, *et al*. 2005. Efficiency and limits of the serial analysis of gene expression (SAGE) method: discussions based on first results in bovine trypanotolerance. Vet. Immuno. Immunopathol. **108:** 59–69.
31. MAILLARD, J.C., D. BERTHIER, S. THEVENON, *et al*. 2004. Use of the serial analysis of genes expression (SAGE) method in veterinary research: a concrete application in the study of the bovine trypanotolerance genetic control. Ann. N. Y. Acad. Sci. **1026:** 171–182.
32. AUTHIÉ, E. 1993. Contribution à l'étude des mécanismes immunologiques impliqués dans la trypanotolérance des taurins d'Afrique. Thèse doctorat ès sciences,Université Bordeaux II.
33. PALING, R.W., S.K. MOLOO, J.R. SCOTT, *et al*. 1991. Susceptibility of N'Dama and Boran cattle to tsetse-transmitted primary and rechallenge infections with a homologous serodeme of *Trypanosoma congolense*. Parasite Immunol. **13:** 413–425.
34. PALING, R.W., S.K. MOLOO, J.R. SCOTT, *et al*. 1991. Susceptibility of N'Dama and Boran cattle to sequential challenges with tsetse transmitted clones of *Trypanosoma congolense*. Parasite Immunol. **13:** 427–445.
35. DWINGER, R.H., D.J. CLIFFORD, K. AGYEMANG, *et al*. 1992. Comparative studies on N'Dama and Zebu cattle following repeated infections with *Trypanosoma congolense*. Res. Vet. Sci. **52:** 292–298.
36. NANTULYA, V.M., A.J. MUSOKE, F.R. RURANGIRWA & S.K. MOLOO. 1984. Resistance of cattle to tsetse-transmitted challenge with *Trypanosoma brucei* or *Trypanosoma congolense* after spontaneous recovery from syringe passed infections. Infect. Immun. **43:** 735–738.

37. BERTELSEN, A.H. & V.E. VELCULESCU. 1998. High-throughput gene expression analysis using SAGE. Drug Discov. Today **3:** 152–159.

38. VELCULESCU, V.E., L. ZHANG, B. VOGELSTEIN & K.W. KINZLER. 1995. Serial analysis of gene expression. Science **270:** 484–487.

39. VELCULESCU, V.E., B. VOGELSTEIN & K.W. KINZLER. 2000. Analyzing uncharted transcriptomes with SAGE. Trends Genet. **16:** 423–425.

40. ELLIS, J.A., J.R. SCOTT, N.D. MACHUGH, et al. 1987. Peripheral blood leucocytes subpopulation dynamics during *Trypanosoma congolense* infection in Boran and N'Dama cattle: an analysis using monoclonal antibodies and flow cytometry. Parasite Immunol. **9:** 363–378.

41. WILLIAMS, D.J.L., J. NAESSENS, J.R. SCOTT & F.A. MCODIMBA. 1991. Analysis of peripheral leucocytes populations in N'Dama and Boran cattle following a rechallenge infection with *Trypanosoma congolense*. Parasite Immunol. **13:** 171–185.

42. OKA, M. & I. YOSHIRITO. 1987. Polyclonal B-cell activating factors produced by spleen cells of mice stimulated with a cell homogenate of *Trypanosoma gambiense*. Infect. Immun. **55:** 3162–3167.

43. FLYNN, J.N. & M. SILEGHEM 1993. Immunosuppression in trypanotolerant N'Dama cattle following *Trypanosoma congolense* infection. Parasite Immunol. **15:** 547–552.

44. SILEGHEM, M. & J.N. FLYNN. 1992. Suppression of T-cell responsiveness during Tsetse-transmitted trypanosomiasis in cattle. Scand. J. Immunol. **36:** 37–40.

45. BUZA, J. & J. NAESSENS 1999. Trypanosome non-specific IgM antibodies detected in serum of *Trypanosoma congolense*-infected cattle are polyreactive. Vet. Immunol. Immunop. **69:** 1–9.

46. WILLIAMS, D.J.L., K. TAYLOR, J. NEWSON, et al. 1996. The role of anti-variable surface glycoprotein antibody responses in bovine trypanotolerance. Parasite Immunol. **18:** 209–218.

47. LUCKINS, A.G. 1974. The immune response of zebu cattle to infection with *Trypanosoma congolense* and *T. vivax*. Ann. Trop. Med. Parasitol. **70:** 133–145.

48. NAESSENS, J., A.J. TEALE & M. SILEGHEM. 2002. Identification of mechanisms of natural resistance to African trypanosomiasis in cattle. Vet. Immun. Immunop. **87:** 187–194.

49. RIFKIN, M.R. & F.R. LANDSBERGER. 1990. Trypanosome variant surface glycoprotein transfer to target membranes: a model for the pathogenesis of trypanosomiasis. Proc. Natl. Acad. Sci. USA **87:** 801–805.

Trypanosomosis in Goats

Current Status

CARLOS GUTIERREZ,[a] JUAN A. CORBERA,[a] MANUEL MORALES,[a]
AND PHILIPPE BÜSCHER[b]

[a]Veterinary Faculty, University of Las Palmas, Las Palmas, 35416 Canary Islands, Spain

[b]Institute of Tropical Medicine, Nationalstraat 130, Antwerp, Belgium

ABSTRACT: Trypanosomosis is a major constraint on ruminant live-stock production in Africa, Asia, and South America. The principal host species affected varies geographically, but buffalo, cattle, camels, and horses are particularly sensitive. Natural infections with *Trypanosoma congolense, T. vivax, T. brucei*, and *T. evansi* have been described in goats. Trypanosomosis in goats produces acute, subacute, chronic, or subclinical forms, being *T. vivax, T. congolense,* and *T. evansi,* the most invasive trypanosomes for goats. However, the role of goats in the epidemiology of trypanosomosis is largely discussed and not well understood. Thus, it has commonly been assumed that trypanosomosis presents a subclinical course and that goats do not play an important role in the epidemiology of the disease. This can partially be due to parasitemia caused by trypanosomes which has been considered low in goats. However, this assumption is currently undergoing a critical reappraisal because of goats may also serve as a reservoir of trypanosome infection for other species, including the human beings in the case of *T. brucei rhodesiense*. The present article describes the current status of trypanosomosis in goats in Africa, Asia, and South America. Pathogenesis, clinical features, diagnosis, and treatment of the different trypanosomes are also described. The possible role in the epidemiology of the disease in the different areas is also discussed.

KEYWORDS: *Trypanosoma* spp.; trypanosomosis; goats; current status

INTRODUCTION

Trypanosomosis is a major constraint on ruminant livestock production in many areas of Africa, Asia, and South America. Many animal species can be

Address for correspondence: Carlos Gutierrez, Veterinary Faculty, University of Las Palmas, Arucas, Las Palmas, 35416 Canary Islands, Spain. Voice: 34-928451115; fax: 34-928451142.
e-mail: cgutierrez@dpat.ulpgc.es

Ann. N.Y. Acad. Sci. 1081: 300–310 (2006). © 2006 New York Academy of Sciences.
doi: 10.1196/annals.1373.040

affected by the different trypanosomes, thus severely impairing the economic efficiency in endemic areas.

Trypanosoma are classically divided into Stercoraria and Salivaria sections, according to their life cycle in the insect vector. Within the Salivaria section, some species (e.g., *T. congolense* and *T. brucei*) are transmitted only by tsetse flies (*Glossina* spp.) and are called the tsetse-transmitted trypanosomes. Others may be either cyclically transmitted by tsetse flies, or mechanically transmitted by other hematophagous insects (e.g., *T. vivax*). Still others are only mechanically (*T. evansi*) or sexually (*T. equiperdum*) transmitted (TABLE 1).

Tsetse-transmitted trypanosomosis is a disease complex caused by several species of *Trypanosoma*. The many species of tsetse infest 10 million square kilometers and affect 37 countries in Africa. The disease affects both humans and livestock. It is currently estimated that about 50 million people[1] and 48 million cattle[2] are at risk of contracting trypanosomosis. From an economic point of view, the disease is particularly important in cattle, although other mammals can also be affected. The livestock-carrying capacity of such areas in West and Central Africa could be increased five- to sevenfold by eliminating or controlling animal trypanosomosis.[3]

Trypanosomosis caused by *T. evansi* (surra) is the most widely distributed of the pathogenic animal trypanosomes affecting livestock in South America, Africa, and Asia. The most affected animal species are buffalo, horses, camels, and cattle, although geographical differences are observed. Other hosts, including small ruminants, can be affected.

There are approximately 228 million goats in Africa[4] (data on Somalia are not available) with as many as 173 million in the tsetse-infested regions of the continent.

It is commonly believed that goats are highly resistant to infection, that caprine trypanosomosis is only sporadic, and that the disease in goats is of little economic consequence.[3] However, current epidemiological information indicates that goats can play an important role in the dissemination of the disease. Thus, goats naturally infected with *T. congolense*, *T. vivax*, or *T. brucei* and presenting clinical disease are regularly observed in Africa. Regional differences in the prevalence of caprine trypanosomosis exist, but can be high in some areas.[5,6] In general, caprine trypanosomosis is more common in East than in West Africa. This has been attributed to differences in feeding preferences between riverine and savannah species of *Glossina*; the latter being more inclined to feed on goats.[7]

Trypanotolerance has clearly been established in cattle, particularly in the breeds N'dama of West Africa and West African Shorthorn. The existence of trypanotolerance in certain goat and sheep breeds is under study. Dwarf goats are known to be more resistant to trypanosomosis than exotic breeds or breeds living in tsetse-free areas.[5,8] Studies carried out by Goossens *et al.*[9] seem to demonstrate that African Dwarf goats are less trypanotolerant than Djallonke

TABLE 1. Trypanosomosis in goats

Species	Major species affected	Geographic distribution	Vectors involved	Natural infection in goats	Experimental infection in goats	Clinical manifestation
T. vivax	Domestic ruminants, camels, horses, antelope	Widespread in tropical Africa and South America	*Glossina* spp., various biting flies	Common	Readily	Acute and chronic forms, mild to fatal
T. uniforme	Domestic ruminants, antelope	Zaire, Uganda	*Glossina* spp.	Yes	Not reported	Nonpathogenic or subclinical infection
T. congolense	All domestic animals, wild game	Widespread in tropical Africa	*Glossina* spp.	Common	Yes	Acute, subacute, and chronic forms, mild to fatal outcome
T. simiae	Domestic pigs, camels, wild warthogs	Widespread in tropical Africa	*Glossina* spp. and *Stomoxys*, *Tabanus* flies	Uncommon	Not reported	Mainly subclinical or mild clinical disease
T. brucei	Domestic ruminants, horses, dogs and cats	Widespread in tropical Africa	*Glossina* spp.	Common but with strain variation	Yes, with strain variation	Noninfective to fatal outcomes
T. b. gambiense (West African sleeping sickness)	Humans	Tropical West and Central Africa	*Glossina* spp. and various biting flies	Uncommon	Yes	Noninfective or a chronic form leading to death or spontaneous recovery
T. b. rhodesiense (East African sleeping sickness)	Humans	East and Southern Africa	*Glossina* spp.	Uncommon	Yes	Experimental infections subacute and fatal
T. evansi	Camels, equines, dogs, water buffaloes	India, Far East, Near East, Philippines, North Africa, Central and South America	Various biting flies	Yes	Yes	Subclinical, moderate or acute disease.
T. equiperdum	Horses	Northern and South Africa, Central and South America, Mexico, Middle East, Italy, former USSR	Venereal reported	Not reported	Not reported	Not reported
T. cruzi (Chagas disease)	Humans	South and Central America, sporadic in USA	Reduvid blood-sucking bugs	Yes	Yes	Not reported

Source: Adapted from Reference 7.

sheep. The trypanotolerance in cattle has been defined as their ability to control parasitemia and anemia.[10] However, small ruminant are less able to control parasitemia and drop in packed cell volume (PCV) following trypanosome infection.[11] On the other hand, Murray *et al.*[12] described that *Glossina* flies may select other livestock over goats when mixed animal populations are present, which can contribute to survival in tsetse areas. The studies carried out in goats seem to be insufficient to understand the true mechanism of trypanotolerance in this species.

Regarding treatment, drug resistance has become a significant problem because no new drugs have been marketed for quite some time. In general, curative doses used in cattle are also appropriate for goats and sheep.[13] Diminazene aceturate is given intramuscularly as a 7% water solution at a dose of 3.5 mg/kg; quinapyramine dimethyl sulfate given intramuscularly as a 10% water solution at a dose of 10.0 mg/kg. Both are considered as very effective. Relapse of infection has been reported in goats treated with diminazene aceturate, presumably because of re-emergence of trypanosomes from the central nervous system where they were inaccessible to the drug during earlier treatment.[8]

Homidium chloride or homidium bromide are given in a 2% water solution at a dose of 1.0 mg/kg intramuscularly, both are effective against *T. vivax* and *T. congolense*. Isometamidium chloride is also effective against the trypanosomes in the blood when given at a dose of 0.25–0.75 mg/kg intramuscularly as a 1% or 2% water solution. This drug was shown to produce signs of shock or death in goats if given intravenously at doses greater than or equal to 0.5 mg/kg.[14] Goats experimentally infected with *T. evansi* were cured after a single inoculation of 0.3 mg/kg of an arsenal compound (Cymelarsan®; Merial, Lyon, France).[15]

In many areas in the world, goats are reared near or in contact to highly susceptible species (particularly cattle, dromedaries, and horses). However, their role as possible reservoirs and carriers of the trypanosomes is largely discussed. In this article, we expose the current knowledge of trypanosomosis in goats.

T. EVANSI

T. evansi is the causative agent of surra, a disease of camel and horses that produces important economic losses in endemic areas (FIGS. 1–3). The disease has been described in small ruminants causing subclinical infection,[16–18] moderate infection,[19] and severe infection.[19,20] Ngeranwa *et al.*[19] described erratic parasitemia, weight loss, and significant drop in PCV in an experimental inoculation using a *T. evansi* strain isolated in Kenya and inoculating small East African bucks. Natural infection has been described in goats by serology[21,22] in a survey carried out in Sudan. However, goats kept in contact with parasitemic camels and horses were found aparasitemic in Jordan.[23] To

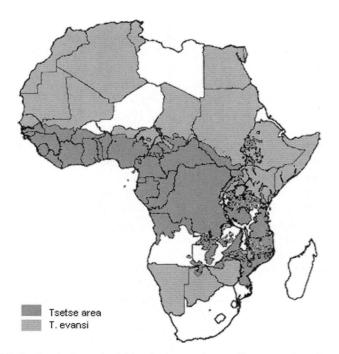

FIGURE 1. Tropical area in Africa (tsetse area) as well as countries where *T. evansi* has been reported.

isolate *T. evansi* from affected goats is very difficult due to low parasitemia. Ngeranwa *et al.*[19] observed a predominant presence of *T. evansi* in extravascular locations (synovial, peritoneal and cerebrospinal fluids, and lymph nodes). *T. evansi* can pass to blood from these extravascular locations in febrile or advances stages in goats. Common parasitological detection tests for *Trypanosoma* spp. employed in other animal species are also valid for goats, including the mini anion exchange centrifugation technique.[24]

The small size of the caprine erythrocytes (3.2 μm; for comparison: 6.5 μm for camels, 5.5 μm for horses, and 5.8 μm for cattle) must be taken into consideration for obtain a valid PCV (Woo technique[25]). A mean cell hemoglobin concentration (MCHC) around 30–36% is considered a proper centrifugation for normal goat blood.[26]

Indirect methods seem to be more appropriate to detect *T. evansi* infections in goats. An enzyme-linked immunosorbent assay (ELISA) for the detection of *T. evansi* in goat sera using a monoclonal antibody has been reported.[27] Indirect immunofluorescence (IFI) has also been used to detect *T. evansi* antibodies in goats.[28] A direct card agglutination test (CATT/*T. evansi*) and an indirect latex agglutination test (LATEX/*T. evansi*) have been shown adequate to detect *T. evansi* antibodies in goat sera.[29]

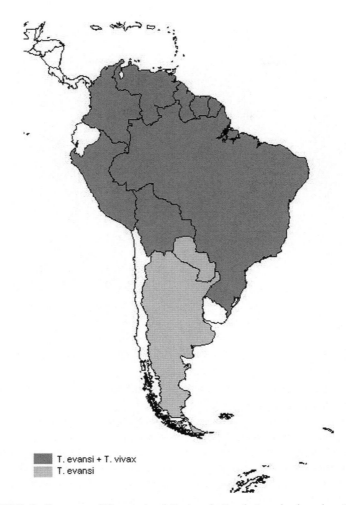

FIGURE 2. Presence of *T. evansi* and *T. vivax* in South America based on Dávila and Silva.[41]

T. CONGOLENSE

T. congolense is the most common trypanosome of goats in Africa. Goats can also act as a reservoir of *T. congolense* for other species. In the Sudan, goats infected with *T. congolense* developed a chronic form of disease from which many spontaneously recovered. When the organism was passaged from goats into calves, however, acute fatal bovine trypanosomosis occurred.[18]

The trypanotolerance to *T. congolense* of West African Dwarf goats is similar to its F1 crosses with the Sahelian breed (trypanosusceptible).[30] Similar results have also been reported by Dhollander *et al.*[31] studying West African Dwarf goats and its F1 crosses with Saanen goats (trypanosusceptible). The African

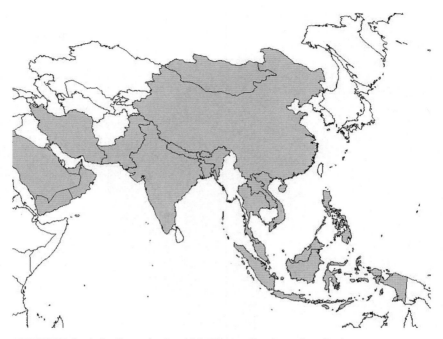

FIGURE 3. Asia. Countries in which *T. evansi* has been described.

gray duiker (*Sylvicapra grimmia*) is also considered as trypanotolerant, even much more than sheep and goats.[32]

T. congolense produces immunosuppressive effects in West African Dwarf goats infected simultaneously with *Haemonchus contortus*.[30] Experimental *T. congolense* infection in the same breed affected reproductive performance with abortions, premature births, and perinatal losses. Transplacental transmission of the parasite or lesions in placenta could not be demonstrated.[33] In another experimental inoculation of *T. congolense* in goats, Witola and Lovelace[34] indicated that erythrophagocytosis by mononuclear cells is a mechanism of anemia pathogenesis.

From the diagnosis point of view, detection of *T. congolense* DNA by polymerase chain reaction (PCR) using GOL as primer set was 100% concordant with buffy coat examination.[22] Also, an indirect ELISA to detect *T. congolense* antibodies in goats has been described by Lejon *et al*.[35]

T. BRUCEI

Natural infection of goats with *T. brucei* is sporadically reported. A survey carried out in Gambia showed that *T. brucei* was present in West African Dwarf goats but only in a few cases.[36] From the experimental viewpoint,

T. brucei infection has been reproduced in Nigerian West African Dwarf goats using a local virulent strain.[37] In an immunity study, infection of goats with *T. brucei* resulted in depressed responses to mitogen stimulation of lymphocyte transformation.[38]

Goats and other domestic animals are relatively resistant to *T. brucei gambiense*, which is the cause of West African human sleeping sickness; however, goats have been suggested as reservoir host of the parasite.[39] When infection does occur, the clinical course is chronic. *T. brucei rhodesiense* is an uncommon cause of caprine disease.[7] Goats also have been implicated as a reservoir of *T. brucei rhodesiense*, transmissible to man.[40]

T. VIVAX

T. vivax is the second most common trypanosome of goats in Africa. *T. vivax* can be transmitted to domestic livestock by tsetse flies (*Glossina* spp., cyclical transmission) as well as directly (mechanical transmission) by other bloodsucking insects thus allowing *T. vivax* to extend its distribution beyond tropical Africa. *T. vivax* was introduced in South America in 1830 by a shipment of zebu cattle from Senegal.[41] Today, goats are recognized as reservoir host for *T. vivax* in many countries in South America.[42]

T. vivax produces immunosuppression, which has also been demonstrated in goats.[43] Thrombocytopenia, microthrombus formation and hemorrhage suggestive of disseminated intravascular coagulation (DIC) have been observed in goats infected with *T. vivax*.[44,45]

T. CRUZI

Natural infection of *T. cruzi* in goats has been detected by Herrera *et al.*[46] using indirect fluorescent antibody test. Clinical manifestation of the disease has not been reported. Kids experimentally infected with *T. cruzi* showed no clinical signs of disease and carried the infection for 38 days.[47] Regarding the epidemiology of the disease in a Brazilian endemic area of Chagas' disease, Herrera *et al.*[46] described that goats did not play an apparent role.

OTHER TRYPANOSOMES

Goats are susceptible to *T. uniforme*, in Uganda and Zaire, but only mild infections occur. *T. simiae*, a trypanosome of swine and camels is transmissible to goats by either *Glossina* spp. or by biting flies but causes mostly mild or subclinical disease.[7]

A nonpathogenic trypanosome, *T. theodori*, was found incidentally in goats in Israel.[7] It is transmitted by a hippoboscid fly, *Lipoptena caprina*. This organism is morphologically similar to the common, nonpathogenic sheep trypanosome, *T. melophagium.*

In conclusion, goats are highly susceptible to pathogenic trypanosomes, although the disease follows commonly a subclinical course. Parasitemia is usually low but persistent, and therefore, goats can be considered as an important reservoir for the majority of trypanosomes of other animals and humans. In those areas of the world where the presence of goats is important (in desert or semi-desert zones), caprine trypanosomosis should be taken into consideration in all programs to control the disease.

REFERENCES

1. KUZOE, F.A.S. 1991. Perspectives in research on control of African trypanosomiasis. Ann. Trop. Med. Parasitol. **85:** 33–41.
2. KRISTJANSON, P.M., B.M. SWALLOW, G.J. ROWLANDS, et al. 1999. Measuring the costs of African animal trypanosomosis, the potential benefits to control and returns to research. Agr. System **59:** 79–98.
3. GRIFFIN, L. 1978. African trypanosomosis in sheep and goats: a review. Vet. Bull. **48:** 819–825.
4. FAO (FOOD AND AGRICULTURE ORGANIZATION). 2004. FAOSTAT. www.fao.org.
5. GRIFFIN, L. & E.W. ALLONBY. 1979. Studies on the epidemiology of trypanosomiasis in sheep and goats in Kenya. Trop. Anim. Health Prod. **11:** 133–142.
6. KRAMER, J.W. 1966. Incidence of trypanosomes in the West African Dwarf sheep and goat in Nsukka, eastern Nigeria. Bull. Epizoot. Dis. Afr. **14:** 423–428.
7. SMITH, M.C. & D.M. SHERMAN. 1994. Blood, lymph, and immune system. *In* Goat Medicine. M.C. Smith & D.M. Sherman, Eds.:193–230. Lea & Febiger. Philadelphia.
8. WHITELAW, D.D., J.E. MOULTON, W.I. MORRISON, et al. 1985. Central nervous system involvement in goats undergoing primary infections with *Trypanosoma brucei* and relapse infections after chemotherapy. Parasitology **90:** 255–268.
9. GOOSSENS, B., S. OSAER & S. KORA. 1997. Long-term effects of an experimental infection with *Trypanosoma congolense* on reproductive performance of trypanotolerant Djallonké ewes and West African Dwarf does. Res. Vet. Sci. **63:** 169–173.
10. MURRAY, M., W.I. MORRISON & D.D. WHITELAW. 1982. Host susceptibility to African trypanosomiasis: trypanotolerance. Adv. Parasitol. **21:** 1–68.
11. OSAER, S., B. GOOSSENS, D.J. CLIFFORD, et al. 1994. A comparison of the susceptibility of Djallonke sheep and West African Dwarf goats to experimental infection with two different strains of *Trypanosoma congolense*. Vet. Parasitol. **51:** 191–204.
12. MURRAY, M., J.C.M. TRAIL, C.E. DAVIS, et al. 1984. Genetic resistance to African trypanosomosis. J. Infect. Dis. **149:** 311–319.
13. ILEMOBADE, A.A. 1986. Tripanosomiasis (nagana, samore, tsetse fly disease). *In* Current Veterinary Therapy, Food Animal Practice, 2nd ed. J. Howard, Ed.: 642–645. WB Saunders. Philadelphia.
14. SCHILLINGER, D., S.H. MALOO & D. ROTTCHER. 1985. The toxic effect of intravenous application of the trypanocide isometamidium (samorin). Zbl. Vet. Med. A **32:** 234–239.

15. ZWEYGARTH, E., J. NGERANWA & R. KAMINSKY. 1992. Preliminary observations on the efficacy of mel Cy (Cymelarsan) in domestic animals infected with stocks of *Trypanosoma brucei brucei* and *T. b. evansi*. Trop. Med. Parasitol. **43:** 226–228.

16. KHASANOV, L. & E.D. IVANITSKAYA. 1974. Experimental trypanosomiasis (*T. ninaekolhjakimovi*) infection in sheep and goats. Trudy Uzbekskogo Nauchoissledovatelskogo Veterinarnogo Instituta **22:** 98–100.

17. OTIENO, P.S. & J.W. GACHANJA. 1976. Studies of experimental *Trypanosoma evansi* infection in goats. Bull. Anim. Health Prod. Afr. **24:** 295–297.

18. MAHMOUD, M.M. & K.H. ELMALIK. 1977. Trypanosomiasis: goats as a possible reservoir of *Trypanosoma congolense* in the Republic of the Sudan. Trop. Anim. Health Prod. **9:** 167–170.

19. NGERANWA, J.J., P.K. GATHUMBI, E.R. MUTIGA, *et al.* 1993. Pathogenesis of *Trypanosoma (brucei) evansi* in small east African goats. Res. Vet. Sci. **54:** 283–289.

20. ANTAO, S., D. STEEL & G.M. WARUI. 1968. The infectivity of *Trypanosoma evansi* to some East African mammals. 12th Meeting of the International Scientific Council for Trypanosomiasis. Banjul, The Gambia. Publication number 102, 123–124.

21. BOID, R., E.A. EL-AMIN, M.M. MAHMOUD, *et al.* 1981. *Trypanosoma evansi* infections and antibodies in goats, sheep and camels in the Sudan. Trop. Anim. Health Prod. **13:** 141–146.

22. PEREIRA DE ALMEIDA, P.J., M. NDAO, B. GOOSSENS, *et al.* 1998. PCR primer evaluation for the detection of trypanosome DNA in naturally infected goats. Vet. Parasitol. **80:** 111–116.

23. ABO-SHEHADA, M.N., H. ANSHASSI, G. MUSTAFA, *et al.* 1999. Prevalence of surra among camels and horses in Jordan. Prev. Vet. Med. **38:** 289–293.

24. GUTIERREZ, C., J.A. CORBERA, F. DORESTE, *et al.* 2004. Use of miniature anion exchange centrifugation technique to isolate *Trypanosoma evansi* from goats. Ann. N. Y. Acad. Sci. **1026:** 149–151.

25. WOO, P.T.K. 1969. The haematocrit centrifuge for the detection of trypanosomes in blood. Can. J. Zool. **47:** 921–923.

26. JAIN, N.C. 1986. Schalm's Veterinary Hematology, 4th Ed. Lea & Febiger. Philadelphia.

27. OLAHO-MUKANI, W., W.K. MUNYUA & A.R. NJOGU. 1992. An enzyme-linked immunosorbent assay (ELISA) for the detection of trypanosomal antigens in oat serum using a monoclonal antibody. J. Immunoassay **13:** 217–229.

28. JACQUIET, P., D. CHEIKH, A. THIAM, *et al.* 1993. La trypanosomose à *Trypanosoma evansi* (Steel 1885), Balbiani 1888 chez les petits ruminants de Mauritanie: résultats d'inoculation expérimentale et d'enquetes sur le terrain. Rev. Elev. Méd. Vét. Pays Trop. **46:** 574–578.

29. GUTIERREZ, C., J.A. CORBERA, M. MORALES, *et al.* 2004. Performance of serological tests for *Trypanosoma evansi* in experimentally inoculated goats. Ann N. Y. Acad. Sci. **1026:** 152–153.

30. FAYE, D., S. OSAER, B. GOOSSENS, *et al.* 2002. Susceptibility of trypanotolerant West African Dwarf goats and F1 crosses with the susceptible Sahelian breed to experimental *Trypanosoma congolense* infection and interactions with helminth infections and different levels of diet. Vet. Parasitol. **108:** 117–136.

31. DHOLLANDER, S., J. BOS, S. KORA, *et al.* 2005. Susceptibility of West African Dwarf goats and WAD x Saanen crosses to experimental infection with *Trypanosoma congolense*. Vet. Parasitol. **130:** 1–8.

32. OGUNSANMI, A.O. & V.O. TAIWO. 2001. Pathobiochemical mechanisms involved in the control of the disease caused by *Trypanosoma congolense* in African grey duiker (*Sylvicapra grimmia*). Vet. Parasitol. **96:** 51–63.

33. FAYE, D., J. SULON, Y. KANE, *et al.* 2004. Effects of an experimental *Trypanosoma congolense* infection on the reproductive performance of West African Dwarf goats. Theriogenology **62:** 1438–1451.

34. WITOLA, W.H. & C.E.A. LOVELACE. 2001. Demonstration of erythrophagocytosis in *Trypanosoma congolense*-infected goats. Vet. Parasitol. **96:** 115–126.

35. LEJON, V., D.E. REBESKI, M. NDAO, *et al.* 2003. Performance of enzyme-linked immunosorbent assays for detection of antibodies against *T. congolense* and *T. vivax* in goats. Vet. Parasitol. **116:** 87–95.

36. OSAER, S., B. GOOSSENS, S. KORA, *et al.* 1999. Health and productivity of traditionally managed Djallonke sheep and West African dwarf goats under high and moderate trypanosomosis risk. Vet. Parasitol. **82:** 101–119.

37. CHIEJINA, S.N., G.A. MUSONGONG, B.B. FAKAE, *et al.* 2005. The modulatory influence of Trypanosoma brucei on challenge infection with Haemonchus contortus in Nigerian West African Dwarf goats segregated into weak and strong responders to the nematode. Vet. Parasitol. **128:** 29–40.

38. DIESING, L., J.S. AHMED, E. ZWEYGARTH, *et al.* 1983. *Trypanosoma brucei brucei* infection in goats. Response in peripheral blood lymphocytes to mitogen stimulation. Tropenmed. Parasitol. **34:** 79–83.

39. MAKUMYAVIRI, A.M. 1991. Epidemiological importance of the experimental host and of the animal reservoir of *Trypanosoma brucei gambiense*. Rev. Med. Vet. **141:** 873–875.

40. ROBSON, J. & L.R. RICKMAN. 1973. Blood incubation infectivity test results for *Trypanosoma brucei* subgroup isolated in the Lambwe Valley, South Nyanza, Kenya. Trop. Anim. Health Prod. **5:** 187–191.

41. DAVILA, A.M.R. & R.A.M.S. SILVA. 2000. Animal trypanosomiasis in South America. Current status, Partnership, and information technology. Ann. N. Y. Acad. Sci. **916:** 199–212.

42. GARDINER, P.R. & M.M. MAHMOUD. 1992. Salivarian trypanosomes causing disease in livestock outside Sub-Saharan Africa. *In* Parasitic Protozoa. J.P. Kreier & J.R. Baker, Eds.: Vol. **2:** 277–314. Academic Press. San Diego, California.

43. VAN DAM, R.H. *et al.* 1981. Trypanosome mediated suppression of humoral and cell-mediated immunity in goats. Vet. Parasitol. **8:** 1–11.

44. VAN DEN INGH, T.S.G.A.M., D. ZWART, A.J. SCHOTMAN, *et al.* 1976. The pathology and pathogenesis of *Tripanosoma vivax* in the goat. Res. Vet. Sci. **21:** 264–270.

45. VEENENDAAL, G.H., A.S. VAN MIERT, T.S. VAN DEN INGH, *et al.* 1976. A comparison of the role of kinins and serotonin in endotoxin induced fever and *Trypanosoma vivax* infections in the goat. Res. Vet. Sci. **21:** 271–279.

46. HERRERA, L., P.S. DE´ANDREA, S.C.C. XAVIER, *et al. Trypanosoma cruzi* infection in wild mammals of the National Park "Serra da Capibara" and its surroundings (Piauí, Brazil), an area endemic for Chagas disease. Trans. Royal Soc. Trop. Med. Hyg. **99:** 379–388.

47. DIAMOND, L.S. & R. RUBIN. 1958. Experimental infection of certain farm animals with a North American strain of *Trypanosoma cruzi* from the raccoon. Exp. Parasitol. **7:** 383–390.

Detection of *T.b. rhodesiense* Trypanosomes in Humans and Domestic Animals in South East Uganda by Amplification of Serum Resistance-Associated Gene

JOHN CHARLES K. ENYARU, ENOCK MATOVU, BARBRA NERIMA, MARGARET AKOL, AND CHARLES SEBIKALI

Livestock Health Research Institute, 96, Tororo, Uganda

ABSTRACT: The human serum resistance-associated (SRA) gene was identified in 28 (80%) of the 35 *T.b. rhodesiense* trypanosomes from parasitologically confirmed sleeping sickness cases, using the primers designed by Radwanska and in 27 (77.1%) of the same 35 *T.b. rhodesiense* trypanosomes using the primers designed by Gibson. However, about 20% of the 35 *T.b. rhodesiense* trypanosomes could not be detected by SRA—polymerase chain reaction (PCR) even when an aliquot of the first PCR was used in the second PCR, indicating that the gene may be absent in those trypanosomes or the trypanosomes could be having another variant of SRA not detectable by these primers since three variants of SRA genes have so far been identified or the amount of trypanosomal DNA extracted from infected blood was too low to be detected. The trypanosome isolates that are SRA gene negative may indicate the presence of some *T.b. rhodesiense* trypanosomes with modified or lack SRA genes or simple loss of the SRA gene from the expression site in which it resides during antigenic variation. Analysis of trypanosomes derived from domestic animals showed that 79 (90.8%) of the 87 trypanosomes isolated from cattle were positive by *Trypanosoma brucei* (TBR)–PCR, indicating that they were *Trypanozoon* while 8 (9.2%) of the trypanosome isolates which were negative by TBR–PCR could be *T. vivax, T. congolense,* or *T. theileri.* When subjected to SRA–PCR, 10 (11.5%) of the 87 trypanosomes isolates derived from cattle were positive, indicating that there could be *T.b. rhodesiense* circulating in cattle, which is similar to the percentage of *T.b. rhodesiense* previously obtained in cattle in Serere, Soroti district.

KEYWORDS: *Trypanosoma brucei rhodesiense*; detection; humans; domestic animals; amplification; serum resistance-associated gene

Address for correspondence: J.C.K. Enyaru, Livestock Health Research Institute, 96, Tororo, Uganda.Voice: +256-772220007; fax: +256-4545520.
e-mail: johnenyaru@yahoo.com

Ann. N.Y. Acad. Sci. 1081: 311–319 (2006). © 2006 New York Academy of Sciences.
doi: 10.1196/annals.1373.041

INTRODUCTION

The ability of only certain subspecies of *Trypanosoma brucei (T. brucei)* trypanosomes to infect humans has been one of the most important problems in the epidemiology of sleeping sickness in tropical Africa. This is a zoonotic disease with a wide variety of wild and domestic animals, which act as reservoir hosts, especially in rhodesiense sleeping sickness. Human pathogenic trypanosomes of the subspecies *T. brucei* are morphologically indistinguishable from those found only in other animals; and this has greatly hampered research on animal reservoirs. However, with the advent of biochemical and molecular markers some trypanosome stocks circulating in animals were shown to be similar to those found in man.[1–5] The importance of both wild and domestic animals in the epidemiology of *T.b. rhodesiense* sleeping sickness in East Africa was recognized early by Heisch, *et al.*,[6] but it was not until when Onyango *et al.*[7] conclusively showed that domestic cattle were reservoirs of *rhodesiense* sleeping sickness by direct human inoculation with cattle-derived trypanosomes. Since then, the role played by domestic animals in the transmission of *T.b. rhodesiense* has been the subject of several investigations and is well documented.[4,8–10]

However, the demonstration that human serum resistance-associated (SRA) gene from a Ugandan *T.b. rhodesiense* isolate is expressed only in serum resistant associated variants of *T.b. rhodesiense*[11] opened the way to find out the trypanolytic factor in human serum. This gene, which is related to variant surface glycoprotein (VSG) genes, was able to sufficiently confer human serum resistance on *T.b. brucei* by transfection.[12,13] It is now known that resistance to normal human serum (NHS) is conferred by SRA gene that encodes a truncated form of the variant surface glycoprotein called serum resistance-associated protein whose amino-terminal α–helix is responsible for resistance to NHS.[14] The study therefore aimed at evaluating the SRA gene for the detection of *T.b. rhodesiense* trypanosomes in humans and in domestic animals as well as to identify domestic animals that act as animal reservoirs of *T.b. rhodesiense* sleeping sickness in south eastern Uganda.

MATERIALS AND METHODS

Trypanosome Stocks

Selection of villages in the districts was based on high prevalence of human and animal trypanosomosis as per the respective district records of sleeping sickness cases in the health centers/hospitals. Villages with about 10% prevalence of animal trypanosomosis were selected and domestic animals screened for the presence of trypanosomes.

A cross-sectional study of *T. brucei* infections in domestic animals was conducted in the *T.b. rhodeisense* endemic districts of Kaberamaido, Soroti, and

Tororo; and nonendemic district of Sembabule. A team screened domestic animals in the selected areas using hematocrit centrifugation technique (HCT). Each blood sample from parasitologically confirmed case was divided into two portions. One portion was inoculated intraperitoneally into *Mastomys nantalensis* rat for *T.b. rhodesiense* isolation or was stabilated using 10% glycerol in phosphate-buffered saline glucose, pH 8.0, and preserved in liquid nitrogen. The second portion of the blood sample was used for DNA extraction for polymerase chain reaction (PCR) technique for detecting *T.b. rhodesiense*.

Animal Trypanosomosis

A total of 87 trypanosomal DNA samples from parasitologically positive cattle with trypanosomes were prepared and analyzed by *Trypanosoma brucei* (TBR)–PCR and SRA–PCR. All the positive cattle were treated with samorin free of charge.

Human Trypanosomosis (Sleeping Sickness)

Two of 1672 persons examined by the HCT were positive for trypanosomes in Kaberamaido district. The two diagnosed sleeping sickness cases were referred to Serere Health Centre for treatment since Kaberamaido district did not have a sleeping sickness treatment center at that time. All positive blood samples were divided into two portions; one portion stabilated using 10% glycerol in phosphate-buffered saline glucose, pH 8.0, and preserved in liquid nitrogen. The second portion of the blood sample was inoculated into one mouse for propagation and isolation of trypanosomes. Blood samples from previously diagnosed sleeping sickness cases in Soroti and Tororo districts were included in the analysis for the presence of SRA gene.

Extraction of DNA

Total DNA was extracted using Qiamp (Qiagen, GmbH, Hilden, Germany) blood DNA extraction protocol from all the 87 infected blood samples from cattle and 35 infected blood samples from humans as described by Radwanska *et al.*[15] The DNA in the eluent was precipitated using 20 μL of 3 M sodium acetate (pH 5.2) and 400 μL of prechilled 100% ethanol, mixed and centrifuged at 8000 *g* for 5 min. The pellet was washed once with 70% ethanol, centrifuged at 8000 *g* for 5 min and the DNA pellet resuspended in 20 μL of double distilled water.

PCR for T. brucei Subspecies

The DNAs from trypanosome isolates from domestic animals were amplified by TBR1-2 primers (TBR1 5′-CGA ATG AAT ATT AAA CAA TGC GCA GT-3′ and TBR2 5′AGA ACC ATT TAT TAG CTT TGT TGC-3′) for *T. brucei* subspecies in order to ascertain whether the trypanosomes derived from domestic animals were, indeed, *T. brucei* subgroup trypanosomes before PCR involving TgsGP primers specific for *T.b. gambiense* was done. It also served as a way of estimating the amount of DNA in the solution and hence what volume to use in the PCR. The PCR amplification was carried out as described by Penchenier *et al.*[16] in 25 μL reaction mixture containing final concentrations of 10 mM Tris-HCl, pH 8.3, 50 mM KCl, 1.5 mM $MgCl_2$, 0.1% (v/v) Triton X-100, 200 μmol each of dATP, dCTP, dGTP, and dTTP, 0.1 μmol each of the 5′ and 3′ primers, 50 ng DNA template or 2 μL crude DNA preparation, and 1 unit of Taq DNA polymerase. The amplification started with the initial denaturation step at 94°C for 3 min and subjected to 35 cycles involving denaturation for 1 min at 94°C, annealing at 56°C for 1 min, and extension at 72°C for 1 min and final elongation of 5 min at 72°C. The absence of contaminants was routinely checked by inclusion of negative control samples in which the DNA sample was replaced with sterile water. Fifteen microliters of each sample alongside control and marker DNA were electrophoresed in 2.0% w/v agarose gel containing 0.5 μg/mL ethidium bromide. The amplified products were observed by Ultraviolet (UV) transillumination.

PCR Using T.b. rhodesiense-Specific Primers

PCR assay using primers (SRA-R 5′ ATA GTG ACA AGA TGC GTA CTC AAC GC 3′ and SRA-F 5′ AAT GTG TTC GAG TAC TTC GGT CAC GCT 3′) specific for *T.b. rhodesiense* (SRA) gene was conducted to identify *T.b. rhodesiense* as described by Radwanska *et al.*[15] PCR amplification was performed using 50 ng of DNA extracted from purified *T.b. rhodesiense* trypanosomes as control DNA, or 10 μL of DNA extracted from domestic animal blood. The DNA amplifications were carried out in 25 μL reaction mixture containing final concentrations of 20 mM Tris-HCl, pH 8.7, 100 mM KCl, 50 mM $(NH_4)_2SO_4$, 1.5 mM $MgCl_2$, 200 uM each of dATP, dCTP, dGTP, and dTTP, 0.5 uM each primers and 2.5 units of HotStar Taq DNA polymerase (Qiagen). SRA–PCR was performed using a GeneAmp PCR System 9700 from Applied Biosystems (Foster City, CA) with the initial incubation for 15 min at 95°C, followed by 45 cycles involving denaturation for 1 min at 94°C, annealing at 68°C for 1min, extension at 72°C for 1 min, and a final extension for 10 min at 72°C. The absence of contaminants was routinely checked by inclusion of negative control samples in which the DNA sample was replaced with sterile water. All samples were subjected to an initial PCR, followed by a second

TABLE 1. Results of PCR amplification of trypanosomal DNA isolated from infected humans from three different areas

			Primers used in PCR					
Origin	Host	No. of isolates examined	TBR 1&2 +	−	SRA (Radwanska) +	−	SRA (Gibson) +	−
Serere	Humans	11	11	0	7	4	8	3
Tororo	Humans	22	22	0	20	2	18	4
Kaberamaido	Humans	2	2	0	1	1	1	1
Total (%)		35	35 (100)	0 (0)	28(80.0)	7 (20.0)	27(77.2)	8(22.8)

PCR using 1 μL of the first PCR product in order to increase sensitivity. Twenty microliters of each sample were electrophoresed in a 2% agarose containing 1 μg/mL ethidium bromide. The amplified products were observed by UV transillumination.

RESULTS

The human SRA gene was identified in 28(80%) of the 35 *T.b. rhodesiense* trypanosomes from parasitologically confirmed sleeping sickness cases, using the primers designed by Radwanska *et al.*[15] and in 27 (77.1%) of the same 35 *T.b. rhodesiense* trypanosomes using the primers designed by Gibson *et al.*[17] (TABLE 1). In Serere area, 4 of the 11 *T.b. rhodesiense* isolates were SRA–PCR negative using Radwanska *et al.*[15] primers and 3 of the same isolates were again SRA–PCR negative using Gibson *et al.*[17] primers (TABLE 1). Similarly in Tororo area, 2 of the 22 *T.b. rhodesiense* isolates were SRA–PCR negative using Radwanska *et al.*[15] primers and 4 including the 2 of the same isolates were again SRA–PCR negative using Gibson *et al.*[17] primers (TABLE 1). However, about 20% of the 35 *T.b. rhodesiense* trypanosomes could not be detected by SRA–PCR even when an aliquot of the first PCR (TABLE 2) was used in the second PCR, indicating that the SRA gene may be absent in those trypanosomes or the trypanosomes could be having another variant of SRA not detectable by these primers since three variants of SRA genes have so far been identified or the amount of trypanosomal DNA extracted from infected blood was too low to be detected. The trypanosome isolates that are SRA negative may indicate the presence of some *T.b. rhodesiense* trypanosomes with a modified SRA or lack SRA gene of simple loss of SRA gene from the expression site in which it resides. The number of *T.b. rhodesiense* isolates, which are SRA gene negative are too many to be accounted for as misidentification, but could be explained by simple loss of the SRA gene from the expression site in which it resides during antigenic variation.

TABLE 2. Molecular differentiation of *T.b. rhodesiense* trypanosomes from infected cattle blood samples from Kaberamaido, new focus on sleeping sickness

Serial No.	Code No.	Inoculum	Origin	Tryp species	TBR	SRA (Radwanska) 1st	2nd	SRA (Gibson) 1st	2nd
1	Cow110	Blood	Kaberamaido	*T. brucei*	+++	−	−	−	−
2	326	Blood	Kaberamaido	*T. brucei*	+++	−	−	−	−
3	327	Blood	Kaberamaido	*T. brucei*	+++	−	+	−	+
4	328	Blood	Kaberamaido	*T. brucei*	+++	−	−	−	−
5	329	Blood	Kaberamaido	*T. brucei*	+++	−	−	−	−
6	330	Blood	Kaberamaido	*T .brucei*	+	−	−	−	−
7	334	Blood	Kaberamaido	*T. brucei*	+++	−	−	−	−
8	336	Blood	Kaberamaido	*T. brucei*	+++	−	−	−	−
9	337	Blood	Kaberamaido	*T.brucei*	+	−	−	−	−
10	338	Blood	Kaberamaido	*T.brucei*	+++	−	−	−	−
11	339	Blood	Kaberamaido	*T.brucei*	+++	−	−	−	−
12	340	Blood	Kaberamaido	*T.brucei*	++	−	−	−	−
13	341	Blood	Kaberamaido	*T.brucei*	++	−	−	−	−
14	342	Blood	Kaberamaido	*T .brucei*	+	−	−	−	−
15	343	Blood	Kaberamaido	*T. brucei*	+++	−	−	−	−
16	344	Blood	Kaberamaido	others	−	−	−	−	−
17	347	Blood	Kaberamaido	*T. brucei*	++	−	−	−	−
18	348	Blood	Kaberamaido	*T. brucei*	++	−	−	−	−
19	352	Blood	Kaberamaido	*T. brucei*	+	−	−	−	−
20	353	Blood	Kaberamaido	*T .brucei*	+	−	−	−	−
21	354	Blood	Kaberamaido	*T. brucei*	+	−	−	−	−
22	356	Blood	Kaberamaido	*T. brucei*	+++	−	−	−	−
23	377	Blood	Kaberamaido	*T. brucei*	++	−	−	−	−
24	378	Blood	Kaberamaido	*T. brucei*	++	−	−	−	−
25	380	Blood	Kaberamaido	*T. brucei*	+++	−	−	−	−
26	381	Blood	Kaberamaido	*T. brucei*	++	−	−	−	−
27	382	Blood	Kaberamaido	*T. brucei*	++	−	−	−	−
28	383	Blood	Kaberamaido	*T. brucei*	+++	−	−	−	−
29	384	Blood	Kaberamaido	*T. brucei*	+++	−	−	−	−
30	385	Blood	Kaberamaido	*T. brucei*	+++	−	−	−	−

−=negative;+=positive;++=strong positive;+++=very strong positive.

Analysis of trypanosomes derived from domestic animals showed that, 79 (90.8%) of the 87 trypanosomes isolated from cattle (TABLE 3) were positive by TBR–PCR, indicating that they are *Trypanozoon* while 8 (9.2%) were negative, suggesting that they could be *T. vivax, T. congolense,* or *T. theileri.* When subjected to SRA–PCR, 10 (11.5%) of the 87 trypanosomes isolates derived from cattle were positive, indicating that there could be *T.b. rhodesiense* circulating in cattle, which is similar to the percentage of *T.b. rhodesiense* previously obtained in cattle in Serere, Soroti district by Welburn *et al.*[18] Some of the SRA–PCR negatives could as well be *T.b. rhodesiense* since this

TABLE 3. Results of PCR amplification of trypanosomal DNA isolated from infected domestic animals from four different areas

Origin	Host	No. of isolates tested	Primers used in PCR					
			TBR 1&2		SRA (Radwanska)		SRA (Gibson)	
			+	−	+	−	+	−
Serere, N. E. Uganda	Domestic animals	46	39	7	6	40	7	39
Kaberamaido N.E. Uganda	Domestic animals	30	29	1	1	29	1	29
Sembabule in south Uganda	Domestic animals	5	5	0	0	5	0	5
Tororo in S.E Uganda	Domestic animals	6	6	0	3	3	2	4
Total (%)		87	79 (90.8)	8 (9.2)	10(11.5)	77(88.5)	10(11.5)	77(88.5)

technique appears to miss some of the parasitologically confirmed cases of *T.b. rhodesiense* sleeping sickness, which could be due to modified SRA genes or loss of the SRA genes from the expression sites in which they reside during the gene rearrangements associated with antigenic variation.

DISCUSSION

Radwanska *et al.*[15] analyzed 25 different *T.b. rhodesiense* strains from Uganda, Kenya, and Rwanda and found out that 24 strains were SRA–PCR positive, but one strain STIB 884 was negative and was thought to be a misidentification of the strain. In the present study 8 (20.0%) of the 35 *T.b. rhodesiense* from parasitologically confirmed sleeping sickness cases were SRA–PCR negative, indicating that there may be more than one factor involved in resistance to lysis by NHS. Furthermore, Radwanska *et al.*[15] also showed that strain TREU 927/4 used as the reference *T. brucei* strain for the trypanosome genome sequencing project (TIGR database) was both SRA gene and SRA transcript negative, but resistant to lysis by NHS, again indicating that resistance to NHS may be conferred by other factors not yet identified besides the SRA gene. Similar analysis using the same 35 *T.b. rhodesiense* strains and primers developed by Gibson *et al.*[17] showed that 7 (22.8%) were SRA–PCR negative (TABLE 1). Since SRA gene resembles VSG gene, it may be that these *T.b. rhodesiense* isolates, which are SRA gene negative, are true *T.b. rhodesiense* with modified SRA gene or lack SRA gene. The number of *T.b. rhodesiense* isolates, which are SRA gene negative are too many to be accounted for as misidentification of the isolates, but the SRA–PCR negativity could be explained by simple loss of the SRA gene from the expression site in which it resides in the Ugandan *T.b. rhodesiense*[13] during the gene rearrangements involved in antigenic variation. It is intended that DNA hybridization will be done on some of the *T.b. rhodesiense* isolates that are SRA gene negatives to confirm their status.

Analysis of trypanosomes derived from domestic animals showed that 79 (90.8%) of the 87 trypanosomes isolated from cattle (TABLE 3) were positive by TBR–PCR, indicating that they were *Trypanozoon* while 8 (9.2%) were negative, suggesting that they could be *T. vivax, T. congolense,* or *T. theileri.* When subjected to SRA–PCR, 10 (11.5%) of the 87 trypanosomes isolates derived from cattle were positive, indicating that there could be *T.b. rhodesiense* circulating in cattle, which is similar to the percentage of *T.b. rhodesiense* previously obtained in cattle in Serere, Soroti district by Welburn *et al.*[18]

On the other hand, some of the SRA–PCR negatives could as well be *T.b. rhodesiense* since this technique appears to miss some of the parasitologically confirmed cases of *T.b. rhodesiense* sleeping sickness, which could be due to modified SRA gene or loss of the SRA genes from the expression sites in which they reside during gene rearrangements, associated with antigenic variation. Alternatively, SRA gene-negative trypanosome isolates could represent a group truly *T.b. brucei,* which are nonpathogenic to humans; and is similar to what Gibson *et al.,*[17] had found—that SRA gene was absent from West African *T.b. brucei.*

ACKNOWLEDGMENTS

We are thankful to the Director of LIRI, Uganda, for logistic support and for allowing me to attend this meeting. We also thank all district and field staff and local council members for assistance in the research activities. This investigation was supported by the International Atomic Energy Agency (IAEA).

REFERENCES

1. GIBSON, W.C. *et al.* 1980. Numerical analysis of enzyme polymorphism: a new approach to the epidemiology and taxonomy of trypanosomes of the subgenus *Trypanozoon*. Advances Parasitol. **18:** 175–246.
2. MEHLITZ, D. *et al.* 1982. Epidemiological studies on the animal reservoir of Gambian sleeping sickness part III. Characterization of *Trypanozoon* stocks by isoenzymes and sensitivity to human serum. Tropenmedizin und Parasitologie **33:** 113–118.
3. MIHOK, S. *et al.* 1990. Population genetics of *Trypanosoma brucei* and the epidemiology of human sleeping sickness in the Lambwe Valley, Kenya. Parasitology **100:** 219–233.
4. ENYARU, J.C.K. *et al.* 1992. Characterization by isoenzyme electrophoresis of *Trypanozoon* stocks from sleeping sickness endemic areas of South East Uganda. Bull. WHO **70:** 631–638.
5. ENYARU, J.C.K. *et al.* 1993. The isolation and genetic heterogeneity in *Trypanosoma brucei gambiense* from north west Uganda. Acta Tropica **54:** 31–39.

6. HEISCH, R.B. *et al.* 1958. The isolation of *Trypansosoma rhodesiense* from a bushbuck. Br. Med. J. **2:** 1203–1204.

7. ONYANGO, R.J. *et al.* 1966. The epidemiology of *Trypanosoma rhodesiense* sleeping sickness in Alego location, Central Nyanza, Kenya. I. Evidence that cattle may act as reservoir hosts of trypanosomiasis infective to man. Trans. Royal Soc. Trop. Med. Hygiene **60:** 175–182.

8. HIDE, G. *et al.* 1991. *Trypanosoma brucei rhodesiense*:characterisation of stocks from Zambia, Kenya and Uganda using repetitive DNA probes. Exp. Parasitol. **72:** 430–439.

9. BITEAU, N. *et al.* 2000. Characterisation of *Trypanosoma brucei* isolates using genetic microsatellite and minisatellite markers. Mol. Biochem. Parasitol. **105:** 185–201.

10. MACLEOD, A. *et al.* 2001. Evidence for multiple origins of human infectivity in *Trypanosoma brucei* revealed by minisatellite variant repeat mapping. J. Mol. Evol. **52:** 290–301.

11. DE GREEF, C. & R. HAMERS. 1994. The serum resistance associated (SRA) gene of *Trypanosome brucei rhodesiense* encodes a VSG like protein. Mol. Biochem. Parasitol. **68:** 277–284.

12. DE GREEF, C. *et al.* 1998. A gene expressed only in serum resistant variants of *Trypanosome brucei rhodesiense*. Mol. Biochem. Parasitol. **36:** 169–176.

13. XONG, H. *et al.* 1998. A VSG expression site-associated gene confers resistance to human serum in *Trypanosome rhodesiense*. Cell **95:** 839–846.

14. VANHAMME, L. *et al.* 2003. Apolipoprotein L-1 is the trypanosome lytic factor of human serum. Nature **422:** 83–67.

15. RADWANSKA, M. *et al.* 2002. The serum resistance associated gene as a diagnostic tool for the detection of *Trypanosoma brucei rhodesiense*. Am. J. Trop. Med. Hygiene **67:** 684–690.

16. PENCHENIER, L. *et al.* 1996. Improvement of blood and fly gut processing for PCR diagnosis of trypanosomiasis. Parasite **4:** 387–389.

17. GIBSON, W.C. *et al.* 2002. The human serum resistance associated gene is ubiquitous and conserved in *Trypanosoma brucei rhodesiense* throughout East Africa. Infect. Genet. Evol. **25:** 1–8.

18. WELBURN, S.C. *et al.* 2001. Identification of human infective trypanosomes in animal reservoirs of sleeping sickness in Uganda by means of serum-resistance-associated (SRA) gene. Lancet **358:** 2017–2019.

Trypanosomiasis in Domestic Animals of Makwanpur District, Nepal

MAHENDRA MAHARJAN AND DINESH R. MISHRA

Central Department of Zoology, T.U. Kirtipur, Kathmandu, Nepal

ABSTRACT: **Trypanosomiasis is an infectious emerging hemoprotozoan parasitic disease in domestical animals of Nepal. The prevalence of disease was found in 16 of 240 (6.67%) in domestic animals of Makawanpur district, out of which 9 of 105 were (8.57%) cattle; 5 of 75 (6.67%) buffalos, and 2 of 15 (13.3%) dogs, while none of the goats and pigs acquired infection. The disease was found maximum during rainy season 9 of 82 (10.98%) with higher prevalence among cross breeds than that of local breeds.**

KEYWORDS: *Trypanosoma*; blood parasite; domestic animals; Geimsa

INTRODUCTION

Nepal, a sovereign independent kingdom, is located in between the latitude 26°22′N to 30°27′N and longitude 80°4′E to 88°12′E with elevation ranges from 60 to 8848 meters. Makawanpur, a hilly district of the central development region is geographically located into central hill and inner Terai. The climate here is tropical, subtropical, and temperate, respectively from south to north—with scorching heat to snowfall in winter.[1] According to the district livestock service office, the total number of livestock is 336,439. Among them, cattle comprise 30.5%, buffalos 20.3%, goats 47.4%, sheep 0.2%, and pigs 1.4% with the majority of animals being indigenous varieties.[2,3] Cattle contribute 33.19% of total milk production whereas buffales provide 68.81%. Infectious hemoprotozoan diseases caused by *Babesia*, *Theileria*, *Trypanosoma*, *Leishmania*, and *Toxoplasma* constitute the greatest hindrance to the growth of animal production in this area.

METHODS

Out of the 43 village development committees (VDCs) in the district, four major VDCs (Hatiya, Padampokhari, Basamadi, and Handikhola) and Hetauda

Address for correspondence: Mahendra Maharjan, Central Department of Zoology, Tribhuvan University Kirtipur, P.O. Box 23414, Kathmandu, Nepal. Voice: +977-1-4312314; fax: +977-1-4331896.
e-mail: mahendra_maharjan@yahoo.ca

Ann. N.Y. Acad. Sci. 1081: 320–321 (2006). © 2006 New York Academy of Sciences.
doi: 10.1196/annals.1373.042

Municipality were randomly selected for the present study. A total of 240 blood samples comprising 105 blood smears of cattle, 75 buffalos, 30 goats, 15 pigs, and 15 dogs were collected from four selected VDCs and Hetauda Municipality during three different seasons. The thick and thin smear blood samples were collected in the morning from peripheral blood by pricking ear lobes with a sterilized needle. The collected blood smears were stained with Giemsa and examined microscopically.

RESULTS AND DISCUSSION

Out of 240 suspected animal examined, 16 (6.67%) animals were found to be infected with *Trypanosoma* spp. The distribution of the organism among cattle was 9/105 (8.57%), among buffalos 5/75 (6.67%), and in dogs 2/15 (13.3%), while none of the goats and pigs acquired infection. The study was conducted in three consecutive seasons of the country. Trypanosomiasis was found in 6/80 (7.50%) during the dry season, 9/82 (110.98%) during the rainy season, and 1/78 (1.28%) during the winter season. Vector dynamics and activities increased during the rainy season, which show a positive correlation with the disease prevalence. Out of a total of 16 positive cases in different domestic animals, maximum disease prevalence was observed among cross breeds than that of the local breeds (12 and 4 cases, respectively). The degree of resistance to disease exhibited by local animals resulted in decreased clinical trypanosomiasis but they may remain carriers and thus a constant source of reinfection to the susceptible exotic animals in enzootic area. The overall distribution of *Trypanosoma* infection indicated a maximum in Hatiya VDC with a total of seven domestic animals infected (with five cases in cattle). Hetauda municipality had five cases of trypanosomiasis while one case each was reported in Handi Khola and Padampokhari. The present study indicated that hemoparasitic diseases, particularly trypanosomiasis, are solely related to the economic loss of the farming communities. Neither control measures nor preventive strategies have been developed through related sectors and are still a low priority. In order to raise the economic standard, strategy for vector (ticks/biting flies) control programs should be encouraged as well as regular animal health camps. Diagnostic treatment modalities and effective quarantine law must be regularly organized among farming communities.

REFERENCES

1. DISTRICT AGRICULTURE DEVELOPMENT. 2002. Annual Progress Report. HMG/N, Hetaunda, Makawanpur.
2. DISTRICT LIVESTOCK SERVICE. 2002. Annual Progress Report. HMG/N, Hetaunda, Makwanpur.
3. VETERINARY LABORATORY AND ANIMAL DISEASE CONTROL SECTION. 2000. Annual Report. Central Veterinary Laboratory, Veterinary Complex, Tripureshor.

Prevalence of *Trypanosoma evansi* Infection in Equines and Camels in the Punjab Region, Pakistan

MURTAZ UL HASAN,[a] GHULAM MUHAMMAD,[a]
CARLOS GUTIERREZ,[b] ZAFAR IQBAL,[a]
ABDUL SHAKOOR,[a] AND ABDUL JABBAR[a]

[a]*Faculty of Veterinary Sciences, University of Agriculture,
38040 Faisalabad, Pakistan*

[b]*Veterinary Faculty, University of Las Palmas, 35416 Canary Islands, Spain*

ABSTRACT: A cross-sectional study has been carried out in order to determine the prevalence of *Trypanosoma evansi* infection in susceptible hosts in the Punjab region (Pakistan). A total of 170 equines and 150 dromedary camels were examined. Five (3.3%) and 6 (4%) camels were positive at parasitological and serological examination, respectively. None of the equines tested positive at any method. These results seem to indicate that *T. evansi* infection has a relatively low prevalence in the Punjab region. However, efforts must be done in order to establish control measures in affected herds and avoid dissemination of the disease.

KEYWORDS: *Trypanosoma evansi*; surra; prevalence; camels; horses; Pakistan

INTRODUCTION

Animal trypanosomosis caused by *Trypanosoma evansi (T. evansi)*, commonly known as "surra," is a frequent health problem of equines and camels in a wide range of climate and vegetation zones in the world. Thus, the prevalence of the disease can vary greatly between the different geographical areas due to different reasons. In Pakistan, previous studies on surra prevalence using different diagnostic methods have been carried out in Gujranwala,[1] Faisalabad,[2,3] and in the North West Frontier Province (NWFP).[4] The purpose of this study was to investigate the prevalence of *T. evansi* infection in horses and camels in different areas of Punjab using different serological and parasitological methods.

Address for correspondence: Carlos Gutierrez, Veterinary Faculty, University of Las Palmas, 35416, Arucas, Las Palmas, Canary Islands, Spain. Voice: 34-928451115; fax: 34-928451142.
  e-mail: cgutierrez@dpat.ulpgc.es

Ann. N.Y. Acad. Sci. 1081: 322–324 (2006). © 2006 New York Academy of Sciences.
doi: 10.1196/annals.1373.043

MATERIALS AND METHODS

A total of 320 animals (170 equines and 150 dromedary camels) were randomly selected for this study. The animals belonged to several herds located at various areas of the Punjab region and they had not previously been introduced from other regions. Blood samples were collected from the jugular vein using tubes containing EDTA (2 mg/mL) and without anticoagulant for serum extraction. Trypanosomes were searched using microhematocrit centrifugation technique (m-HCT), as well as examination of wet blood film and stained thin smears (Giemsa). Antigens were detected using Suratex® (AccuPharma, Inc., NY, NY). Suratex detects trypanosome-circulating antigens using a monoclonal antibody against a *T. evansi* internal antigen. Biochemical tests included formol-gel test, mercuric chloride precipitation, and thymol turbidity test, and were performed following procedures described in the *Manual for Diagnostic Tests and Vaccines* (OIE).

RESULTS AND DISCUSSION

The presence of *T. evansi* was only demonstrated in dromedary camels (5/150 animals, 3.3%). Serum antigens detection was also evident in dromedaries, with a prevalence of 4%. No horses were found positive at any diagnostic method. All seropositive camels also tested parasitemic except one of them, in which *T. evansi* was not discovered. On the other hand, all parasitemic and seropositive camels were also positive to biochemical tests. In contrast, 7 positive cases at formol-gel test, 10 at mercuric chloride test, and 6 at thymol turbidity test were negative to *T. evansi* diagnostic specific methods. Given that only visualization of the trypanosomes by microscopy could confirm the disease, those positive cases at biochemical tests but negative at parasitological tests would be considered as false positive. The prevalence of surra in camels observed in the Punjab region ranged between 3.3% and 4% and can be considered as low compared with other endemic regions (56% in Somalia,[5] or 48% in Kenya.)[6] Previous surveys carried out in several areas of Pakistan reported surra prevalence in Faisalabad of 5.18% and 9.09% in horses and donkeys, respectively[2] and 3% in camels,[3] 7.41% in horses in NWFP,[4] and 3.35% in Gujranwala.[1] Further studies are necessary in order to establish control measures in the affected herds, detect possible reservoirs, and avoid dissemination of the disease controlling animal movements in the country.

REFERENCES

1. WAHEED, M.A., G.H. QURESHI & J.L. GONDAL. 2003. A report on Surra in Gujranwala. Pakistan Vet. J. **23:** 170–172.

2. KHAN, M.Q., B. HAYAT & C.S. HAYAT. 1987. Prevalence of blood parasites in equines in and around Faisalabad. Pakistan Vet. J. **7:** 113–116.
3. BUTT, A.A., N.I. CHAUNDHRY, G. MUHAMMAD, *et al.* 1996. Prevalence of haemoparasites among dromedary in and around Faisalabad (Punjab). J. Camel Pract. Res. **3:** 103–106.
4. BANO, L. & A.H. JAN. 1986. Natural occurrence of Trypanosomiasis in ungulates of N.W.F.P. (Pakistan). Pakistan Vet. J. **6:** 137–139.
5. BAUMANN, M.P.O. & K.H. ZESSIN. 1992. Productivity and health of camels (*Camelus dromedarius*) in Somalia. Association with Trypanosomosis and Brucellosis. Trop. Anim. Health Prod. **24:** 145–156.
6. OLAHO, W. & A.J. WILSON. 1983. The prevalence of camel trypanosomiasis in selected areas of Kenia. 17th Meeting of the International Scientific Council for Trypanosomiasis Research and Control. Arusha, Tanzania. 246–253.

Clinical, Hematological, and Biochemical Findings in an Outbreak of Abortion and Neonatal Mortality Associated with *Trypanosoma evansi* Infection in Dromedary Camels

CARLOS GUTIERREZ, JUAN A. CORBERA, MARIA C. JUSTE, FRANCISCO DORESTE, AND INMACULADA MORALES

Department of Animal Medicine and Surgery, Veterinary Faculty, University of Las Palmas, Las Palmas, 35416 Canary Islands, Spain

ABSTRACT: This article presents the clinical and laboratorial findings in an outbreak of abortions and high neonatal mortality attributable to *Trypanosoma evansi* infection in camels. A total of 16 females were diagnosed, 2 of which showed moderate signs of chronic form, particularly hyporexia and intolerance to exercise. The main laboratory findings were regenerative anemia (hemolytic anemia), lymphocytic and monocytic leukocytosis, hyperproteinemia, hyperglobulinemia, hypoglycemia, serum urea increased, and serum iron decreased. The most characteristic finding in the examined females would be the uremia, probably due to the higher protein metabolism.

KEYWORDS: Camel; *Trypanosoma evansi*; laboratory findings; abortion; neonatal mortality

INTRODUCTION

Trypanosomosis due to *Trypanosoma evansi* is a major enzootic disease of the dromedary camel. From the clinical viewpoint, camels affected of trypanosomosis usually show anemia, emaciation, recurrent fever, atrophy of the thigh muscles, edema of the dependent parts, corneal opacity, and diarrhea.[1] In pregnant female camels abortions can occur,[2] although the mechanisms responsible for the reproductive disturbances in trypanosomosis are not fully understood. There is only little information on clinical assessment in pregnant or just-delivered females in the available literature. This article presents the relevant clinical, hematological, and biochemical findings in an outbreak of

Address for correspondence: Carlos Gutierrez, Veterinary Faculty, University of Las Palmas, Arucas, Las Palmas, 35416 Canary Islands, Spain. Voice: 34-928451115; fax: 34-928451142.
e-mail: cgutierrez@dpat.ulpgc.es

Ann. N.Y. Acad. Sci. 1081: 325–327 (2006). © 2006 New York Academy of Sciences.
doi: 10.1196/annals.1373.044

abortion and high neonatal mortality associated with *T. evansi* in a camel herd in the Canary Islands.

MATERIALS AND METHODS

A total of 16 pregnant or just-delivered dromedary females, aged 6–12 years, were diagnosed to suffer *T. evansi* infection, using wet blood film, microhematocrit technique, and stained blood smear. The affected animals were assessed by means of clinical examination and laboratorial analysis. The "positive" animals were consequently treated with trypanocidal drug (Cymelarsan®; Merial, Lyon, France). Blood samples were taken from the jugular vein using EDTA (for hematology), heparin (for parasitology), and without anticoagulant for serum collection. For comparison, 16 female camels belonging to another camel farm, with similar management conditions and negative to parasite detection tests and serological tests, were used as controls.

RESULTS AND DISCUSSION

At clinical examination, 2 out of 16 affected animals showed moderate signs of chronic form, particularly hyporexia and intolerance to exercise. The remaining 14 animals did not show any clinical evidence of the disease. The aborted fetuses (five) were aged 6–8 months of gestation, approximately. Of the eight premature and weak calves born from the affected females, only one survived. At stained smear examination, anisocytosis and immature erythrocytes were observed in four animals from the outbreak group. The hematological data would indicate anemia and leukocytosis in the examined animals. Both findings are common in trypanosomosis in camels.[3,4] Clinical biochemistry showed significant variations in total proteins, A/G ration, glucose, urea, and iron. Laboratory parameters in all affected camels returned to normal ranges within 3 weeks after trypanocidal treatment. The hypoproteinemia is common in trypanosomosis due to hypergammaglobulinemia that the patients suffer as a response to infection.[5] The hypoglycemia is also common in trypanosomosis. Jaktar and Singh (1974)[6] described that parasite count is inversely proportional to glucose concentration. Uremia showed a significant increase in the outbreak group. The fact that creatinine did not suffer significant variations with respect to the control group suggests that there were no renal failures but an increased catabolism of body proteins. Uremia is not a common finding in trypanosomosis, but it could appear in pregnant or just-delivered females related to disease due to the higher metabolic requirements. Serum iron levels showed a significant decrease in the outbreak group. These findings have also previously been reported and would be due to a decrease in iron-transporting protein.[7]

REFERENCES

1. BOID, R., T.W. JONES & A.G. LUCKINS. 1986. Protozoal diseases of camels. *In* The Camel in Health and Disease. A. Higgins, Ed: 41–59. Baillière Tindall. London.
2. DONALD, V. & G.V. JUDITH. 1990. Biochemistry. Viley. New York, p. 263.
3. WERNERY, U. & O.R. KAADEN. 2002. Infectious Diseases in Camelids. Blackwell Science, Berlin.
4. WOO, P.T.K. 1969. The haematocrit centrifuge technique for the detection of trypanosomes in blood. Can. J. Zool. **47:** 921–923.
5. YAGIL, R. 1982. FAO Animal Production and Health paper No 26. Camels and Camel Milk. Food and Agriculture Organization of the United Nations, Rome, p. 41.
6. JAKTAR, P.R., M. SINGH. 1974. Pathogenesis of anaemia in *Trypanosoma evansi* infection. IV. Blood glucose studies. Indian Vet. J. **51:** 710–714.
7. YAGOUB, I.A. 1989. Haematological studies in dromedary camels with single or concurrent natural infection of *Trypanosoma evansi* and *Haemonchus longistipes*. Acta Vet. (Beogr.) **39:** 109–119.

Prevalence of *Cryptosporidium* among Dairy Cows in Thailand

SATHAPORN JITTAPALAPONG,[a] NONGNUCH PINYOPANUWAT,[a]
WISSANUWAT CHIMNOI,[a] CHUTATIP SIRIPANTH,[b]
AND ROGER W. STICH[c]

[a]*Department of Parasitology, Faculty of Veterinary Medicine, Kasetsart
University, Bangkok 10900, Thailand*

[b]*Department of Protozoology, Faculty of Tropical Medicine, Mahidol University,
Bangkok 10400, Thailand*

[c]*Department of Veterinary Pathobiology, University of Missouri, Columbia,
Missouri 65211, USA*

ABSTRACT: *Cryptosporidium* species are frequently associated with diarrhea among AIDS patients in Thailand, and dairy herds are a possible
source of some of these infections. A cross-sectional study was performed
to determine if *Cryptosporidium* is present among dairy cows in Thailand.
Fecal samples were randomly collected from 363 Holstein-Friesian dairy
cows from 108 of 860 farms in the Nong Pho region of central Thailand.
The average prevalence of *Cryptosporidium* among dairy cows was 9.4%,
according to an assay for *Cryptosporidium*-specific antigen (CSA) and
0.6% by microscopic examination of acid-fast stained feces. CSA was
detected in all host age categories tested, but was most prevalent among
calves (15.1%). Overall, 31.5% of farms were contaminated with *Cryptosporidium* infections. Fifty percent of poorly managed farms had CSA-
positive cows, which were more likely to contaminate water and raw
milk, while 12.9% of farms with acceptable management practices had
CSA-positive cows. There was no association between the detection of
Cryptosporidium and other gastrointestinal parasites. These results indicate that *Cryptosporidium* is enzootic among Thai dairy cattle, and
suggest that cattle could have a role in zoonotic cryptosporidiosis in
Thailand.

KEYWORDS: *Cryptosporidium*; gastrointestinal parasites; dairy cows;
CSA assay; Thailand

Address for correspondence: Sathaporn Jittapalapong, DVM, Ph.D., Department of Parasitology,
Faculty of Veterinary Medicine, Kasetsart University, Bangkok 10900, Thailand. Voice: 662-942-
8438; fax: 662-942-8438.
e-mail: fvetspj@ku.ac.th

Ann. N.Y. Acad. Sci. 1081: 328–335 (2006). © 2006 New York Academy of Sciences.
doi: 10.1196/annals.1373.045

INTRODUCTION

Cryptosporidium is a unique genus of apicomplexan parasites that infect a broad range of vertebrates and that can cause severe enteritis in naïve hosts.[1] *Cryptosporidium* oocysts, which are shed with four sporozoites, are small (approximately 5 μm in diameter) and colorless, thus difficult to observe in fecal specimens with conventional light microscopy. More recent investigations suggested that there are more *Cryptosporidium* species and genotypes than originally thought, and that human hosts are affected by both anthroponotic and zoonotic transmission cycles of different parasite genotypes. For example, some investigations suggested that *Cryptosporidium parvum* consists of an anthroponotic "human" genotype and a zoonotic "bovine" genotype, and that the anthroponotic genotype is a more common agent of cryptosporidiosis outbreaks among immunocompetent human populations.[2]

In recent years, the public has become aware of severe cryptosporidiosis because of its incidence in AIDS patients and because of outbreaks of cryptosporidial enteritis worldwide. The prevalence of *C. parvum* infections among immunocompetent human patients with diarrhea was estimated at 2%, while the average prevalence was estimated at approximately 22% among AIDS patients in developing countries.[3] Water-borne *C. parvum* has become a global concern due to the resistant nature of the oocysts and their widespread environmental contamination.

Cryptosporidium species are also considered important agents of diarrhea among AIDS patients in Thailand. Surveys in this country revealed up to 12.8% prevalence of *Cryptosporidium* infection among HIV-infected patients,[4–8] while the infection rate among immunocompetent Thai human hosts appears to be no more than that reported for immunocompetent human hosts in other countries.[3,7–9] Prevalence of these parasites among AIDS patients with diarrhea is even higher at approximately 20%.[4,8,10,11] Additionally, a broad range of zoonotic *Cryptosporidium* species was associated with diarrheic AIDS patients in Thailand, including the *C. parvum* "bovine" genotype.[12]

Cattle could be an important source of zoonotic *Cryptosporidium*.[13] Cattle in Canada and the United States, particularly calves, are commonly infected with *Cryptosporidium* species,[14] and cattle are believed to be a major source of water-borne *Cryptosporidium*.[15] The purpose of this article was to determine if *Cryptosporidium* is present among dairy herds in a major dairy production region of Thailand. Fecal shedding of *Cryptosporidium* oocysts and *Cryptosporidium*-specific antigen (CSA) were examined by microscopy and CSA assay, respectively; and parasite detection was evaluated in the context of host age, farm management practices, and the prevalence of other gastrointestinal parasitic infections.

MATERIALS AND METHODS

Farms and Cows

Holstein-Friesian cows at ages from 6 months to over 5 years were randomly selected from 108 of 860 farms in Nong Pho dairy area of central Thailand. Animals from each farm belonged to one of three age groups (<1 year, 1–5 years, and > 5 years; $n = 36$ farms per age group), and farms were chosen with poor ($n = 54$) or acceptable ($n = 54$) management practices. Farm management conditions were defined as poor or acceptable based on the presence of cement floors and bedding, water quality, and cleaning and storage of silage, grain, and hay.

Sample Collection

Previous investigations indicated that the rate of parasitic infection in dairy cows at Nong Pho was highest during the rainy season.[16] Thus, samples were collected during the 2001 rainy season from June to October. One fecal specimen was obtained from each animal tested. Each sample was collected directly from the rectum and put into a plastic carton that was then sealed with a plastic snap-on lid. The cartons were placed in an insulated portable cooler and transported to the laboratory within a few hours of collection, stored at 4°C, and examined the same day.

Parasite Detection

Fecal samples were prepared by maceration with a stick in the presence of a small quantity of sugar solution; and the sugar solution was continuously added with stirring until a volume of 15 mL was reached. This was strained through gauze into a centrifuge tube, and the sugar solution was added to form a positive meniscus. A coverslip was placed over the tube and the preparation centrifuged at $500g$ for 10 min before the coverslip was removed and the sample smeared onto a microscope slide. Smears were air dried and immersed in 100% methanol for 10 min to fix the sample. Fixed smears were rinsed with tap water, and stained with basic fuchsin dye (Carbol Fuchsin stain; Life Science Dynamic Division, Arnaparn, Thailand) for 2 min, rinsed with water followed by acid–alcohol solution (5% Sulfuric acid, 95% Ethanol) until destained, rinsed again with water, and stained with Methylene Blue background stain (Counter stain; Life Science Dynamic Division) for 2 min. After a final rinse with water, the slides were allowed to air dry, and permount and a coverslip were applied prior to examination by light microscopy with the 100X objective lens. Other parasites were identified by diagnostic stage morphology and size.

CSA Assay

The ProSpectT® *Cryptosporidium* Rapid Assay (Alexon-Trend, Inc., Alexon-Trend, Ramsey, MN, lot no. 9906243) was used for detection of CSA in aqueous extracts of all fecal specimens. Fresh stool specimens were processed according to the manufacturer's instructions. All reagents and samples were brought to room temperature, and reagents diluted with washing buffer. Stool specimens were immersed in specimen dilution buffer and emulsified thoroughly by vigorously shaking to assure uniform distribution of antigen. Diluted stool specimens were applied to membranes containing immobilized anti-CSA antibodies. After incubation, membranes were washed to remove unbound material, incubated with biotinylated anti-CSA antibody, and washed again. Membranes were then incubated with Horseradish Peroxidase (HRP) conjugated to streptavidin, washed again, and developed with a colorimetric HRP substrate provided with the kit. CSA-positive specimens were identified by visual detection of blue color associated with the HRP product.

Statistical Analysis

Overall and individual dairy cow test concordance between the microscopic and CSA detection methods were compared with the McNemar's χ^2 test. Infection rates between different age groups and between poor and acceptable dairy management were compared with the χ^2 or Fisher's exact test, according to the number of samples per group tested. Significance was determined at $P < 0.05$.

RESULTS

Fecal samples were collected from a total of 363 animals on 108 farms with an average of 3 animals per farm. There were 119 animals less than 1 year of age, 129 animals between 1 and 5 years of age, and 115 animals more than 5 years of age. *Cryptosporidium* oocysts were detected in 2 of 363 cows (0.6%) by microscopic examination of acid-fast stained feces. CSA was detected in feces from 34 cows (9.4%). Eighteen calves less than 1 year old (15.1%) were CSA-positive, and oocysts were observed in feces from 2 of these calves (1.7%). No oocysts were found by acid-fast stain in dairy cows more than 1 year old (TABLE 1). The χ^2 test showed that the difference between the numbers of CSA- and oocyst-positive samples was significant ($P < 0.001$). In addition, infection rates were significantly higher in dairy cows less than 1 year old than the remaining age groups ($P < 0.05$).

Cryptosporidium was the only parasite detected in 6.1% of cattle tested, while co-infections with other protozoan and gastrointestinal parasites were observed in 3.3% of the samples tested (TABLE 1). Analysis of infection rates in

TABLE 1. Number and percentage of *Cryptosporidium* and other parasite infections classified by host ages and parasites in Nong Pho, Thailand

| Parasites detected | Host age | | | |
	<1 year ($n = 119$)	1–5 years ($n = 129$)	>5 years ($n = 115$)	Total ($n = 363$)
Cryptosporidium				
Oocysts	2 (1.7)*	0 (0)	0 (0)	2 (0.6)
CSA	18 (15.1)	10 (7.8)	6 (5.2)	34 (9.4)
CSA only	12 (10.1)	6 (4.7)	4 (3.5)	22 (6.1)
Co-infections	6 (5.0)	4 (3.1)	2 (1.7)	12 (3.3)
Other parasites				
Strongyloides	51 (42.9)	46 (35.7)	35 (30.4)	132 (36.4)
Strongyles	39 (32.8)	46 (35.7)	34 (29.6)	119 (32.8)
Coccidia	55 (46.2)	35 (27.1)	7 (6.1)	97 (26.7)
Trichuris	32 (26.9)	7 (5.4)	0 (0)	39 (10.7)
Moniezia	15 (12.6)	6 (4.7)	1 (0.9)	22 (6.1)
Capillaria	6 (5.0)	6 (4.7)	2 (1.7)	14 (3.9)
Giardia	0 (0)	2 (1.6)	1 (0.9)	3 (0.8)
Trematode	1 (0.8)	1 (0.8)	0 (0)	2 (0.6)

*% positive for corresponding column indicated in parentheses.

the youngest age group showed that 10.1% were CSA-positive, and that 5.0% were CSA-positive and co-infected with other gastrointestinal parasites.

The number of farms with one or more infected hosts was also analyzed (TABLE 2). Of the 108 dairy farms tested, 50% of those with poor management conditions were CSA-positive, while 12.9% of those with acceptable management practices were CSA-positive. There was a significant association between the infection rate of *Cryptosporidium* species and the quality of farm management ($P < 0.01$). Gastrointestinal parasites were detected in 78.7% of the farms surveyed. Other parasites detected among these cattle, with their corresponding prevalence in parentheses, were *Strongyloides* (36.4%), strongyles (32.8%), coccidia (26.7%), *Trichuris* (10.7%), *Moniezia* (6.1%), *Capillaria* (3.9%), *Giardia* (0.8%), and trematodes (0.6%). There was no association between detection of CSA and co-infection with other gastrointestinal parasites.

DISCUSSION

Cryptosporidium infections appear to be present among dairy herds in Thailand. In our hands, the CSA assay was more sensitive than the traditional parasitological procedure. In addition, host age and poor management practices were the primary factors associated with the prevalence of *Cryptosporidium* infection among these cattle. Diagnosis of cryptosporidiosis is

TABLE 2. Number and percentage of *Cryptosporidium*-specific antigen (CSA) positive farms classified by host ages and farm conditions in Nong Pho, Thailand

Host age ($n = 36$ per group)	Farm condition ($n = 54$ per group)		Total
	Poor	Acceptable	
<1 year	12 (22.2)*	4 (7.4)	16 (44.4)
1–5 years	8 (14.8)	2 (3.7)	10 (27.8)
>5 year	7 (12.9)	1 (1.9)	8 (2.8)
Total	27 (50)	7 (12.9)	34 (31.5)

*% positive for corresponding column indicated in parentheses.

often dependent on observation of *Cryptosporidium* oocysts in fecal smears. One widely used technique includes Sheather's sugar floatation,[17] which, when combined with an acid-fast stain, can give similar results as those obtained with sedimentation methods.[18] This method is thought to be sufficient for clinical purposes, because the number of oocysts excreted by symptomatic animals is thought to be high. However, in our hands, this technique did not appear to be sensitive enough to detect carriers that would shed small numbers of oocysts. In addition, the combined sugar flotation and acid-fast staining procedure is laborious, time-consuming, and often fails to detect infections.[19]

To our knowledge, this work represents the first survey for *Cryptosporidium* in dairy cows of Thailand with a CSA assay. A number of immunoassays are commercially available for rapid screening of large numbers of stool samples for *Cryptosporidium*.[20] Overall, the sensitivities of these assays are considered superior to traditional microscopy and similar to those based on immunofluorescence microscopy or the polymerase chain reaction.[20,21] Although commonly used for examination of human feces, the CSA assay was previously adapted for detection of *Cryptosporidium* in bovine feces.[22]

Our results indicated that 9.4% of cattle and 15.1% of calves less than 1 year of age were CSA-positive. This result was in agreement with those from other countries.[14,23–25] An infection rate of 25% was reported in calves 8 to 14 days old, which apparently decreased to less than 10% when the calves were more than 1 month old.[26] This work also confirmed *Cryptosporidium* infections of dairy animals in Asia. For example, 11% and 15% of calves in Japan and Korea, respectively, were *Cryptosporidium*-positive by microscopic examination of feces,[27,28] and 4.7% of adult cattle surveyed in slaughterhouses were positive for *Cryptosporidium* oocysts in Japan.[29] Interestingly, 33.6% of goats tested were reported to shed *Cryptosporidium* oocysts in Sri Lanka.[30] In Thailand, cattle could be an important factor in the epidemiology of cryptosporidiosis as asymptomatic carriers that intermittently shed oocysts, possibly transmitting the parasite to humans through contamination of water or food products.

In summary, this investigation indicates that the prevalence of *Cryptosporidium* species among dairy cattle in Thailand is similar to that described for other parts of the world. Thus, there is potential for zoonotic cryptosporidiosis in Thailand, and further work is warranted to investigate the risk of human infection through environmental contamination and contaminated dairy products.

ACKNOWLEDGMENTS

This study was supported by a grant (K.I.P. 9.43) from Kasetsart University Research and Development Institute (KURDI), Thailand. We appreciate the excellent assistance of the Nong Pho Teaching Hospital staff.

REFERENCES

1. XIAO, L., R. FAYER, U. RYAN, *et al.* 2004. *Cryptosporidium* taxonomy: recent advances and implications for public health. Clin. Microbiol. Rev. **17:** 72–97.
2. PENG, M.M., L. XIAO, A.R. FREEMAN, *et al.* 1997. Genetic polymorphism among *Cryptosporidium parvum* isolates: evidence of two distinct human transmission cycles. Emerg. Infect. Dis. **3:** 567–573.
3. ADAL, K.A. 1994. From Wisconsisn to Nepal—*Cryptosporidium, Cyclospora,* and *Microsporidia.* Curr. Opin. Infect. Dis. **7:** 609–615.
4. MOOLASART, P., B. EAMPOKALAP, M. RATANASRITHONG, *et al.* 1995. Cryptosporidiosis in HIV infected patients in Thailand. Southeast Asian J. Trop. Med. Public Health **26:** 335–338.
5. PUNPOOWONG, B., P. VIRIYAVEJAKUL, M. RIGANTI, *et al.* 1998. Opportunistic protozoa in stool samples from HIV-infected patients. Southeast Asian J. Trop. Med. Public Health **29:** 31–34.
6. SAKSIRISAMPANT, W., B. EAMPOKALAP, M. RATTANASRITHONG, *et al.* 2002. A prevalence of *Cryptosporidium* infections among Thai HIV-infected patients. J. Med. Assoc. Thai. **85**(Suppl 1): S424–S428.
7. UGA, S., N. KUNARUK, S.K. RAI, *et al.* 1998. *Cryptosporidium* infection in HIV-seropositive and seronegative populations in southern Thailand. Southeast Asian J. Trop. Med. Public Health **29:** 100–104.
8. WIWANITKIT, V. 2001. Intestinal parasitic infections in Thai HIV-infected patients with different immunity status. BMC Gastroenterol. **1:** 3.
9. JANTANAVIVAT, C., P. SUCHARIT, S. HARIKUL, *et al.* 1991. *Cryptosporidium* oocysts in stool specimens submitted to routine ova & parasite examination: 38 months survey. J. Med. Assoc. Thai. **74:** 259–264.
10. MANATSATHIT, S., S. TANSUPASAWASDIKUL, D. WANACHIWANAWIN, *et al.* 1996. Causes of chronic diarrhea in patients with AIDS in Thailand: a prospective clinical and microbiological study. J. Gastroenterol. **31:** 533–537.
11. WAYWA, D., S. KONGKRIENGDAJ, S. CHAIDATCH, *et al.* 2001. Protozoan enteric infection in AIDS related diarrhea in Thailand. Southeast Asian J. Trop. Med. Public Health **32**(Suppl 2): 151–155.
12. GATEI, W., Y. SUPUTTAMONGKOL, D. WAYWA, *et al.* 2002. Zoonotic species of *Cryptosporidium* are as prevalent as the anthroponotic in HIV-infected patients in Thailand. Ann. Trop. Med. Parasitol. **96:** 797–802.

13. BEDNARSKA, M., A. BAJER & E. SINSKI. 1998. Calves as a potential reservoir of *Cryptosporidium parvum* and *Giardia* sp. Ann. Agric. Environ. Med. **5:** 135–138.
14. MANN, E.D., L.H. SEKLA, G.P. NAYAR, *et al.* 1986. Infection with *Cryptosporidium* spp. in humans and cattle in Manitoba. Can. J. Vet. Res. **50:** 174–178.
15. FAYER, R. 2004. *Cryptosporidium*: a water-borne zoonotic parasite. Vet. Parasitol. **126:** 37–56.
16. JITTAPALAPONG, S., J.W. & P.T. 1987. Survey of internal parasites of dairy cows in Nong Pho. Kasetsart Veterinarians **8:** 124–132.
17. ANDERSON, B.C. & M.S. BULGIN. 1981. Enteritis caused by *Cryptosporidium* in calves. Vet. Med. Small Anim. Clin. **76:** 865–868.
18. MCNABB, S.J., D.M. HENSEL, D.F. WELCH, *et al.* 1985. Comparison of sedimentation and flotation techniques for identification of *Cryptosporidium* sp. oocysts in a large outbreak of human diarrhea. J. Clin. Microbiol. **22:** 587–589.
19. ALLES, A.J., M.A. WALDRON, L.S. SIERRA, *et al.* 1995. Prospective comparison of direct immunofluorescence and conventional staining methods for detection of *Giardia* and *Cryptosporidium* spp. in human fecal specimens. J. Clin. Microbiol. **33:** 1632–1634.
20. GARCIA, L.S. & R.Y. SHIMIZU. 1997. Evaluation of nine immunoassay kits (enzyme immunoassay and direct fluorescence) for detection of *Giardia lamblia* and *Cryptosporidium parvum* in human fecal specimens. J. Clin. Microbiol. **35:** 1526–1529.
21. BIALEK, R., N. BINDER, K. DIETZ, *et al.* 2002. Comparison of fluorescence, antigen and PCR assays to detect *Cryptosporidium parvum* in fecal specimens. Diagn. Microbiol. Infect. Dis. **43:** 283–288.
22. MCCLUSKEY, B.J., E.C. GREINER & G.A. DONOVAN. 1995. Patterns of *Cryptosporidium* oocyst shedding in calves and a comparison of two diagnostic methods. Vet. Parasitol. **60:** 185–190.
23. NACIRI, M., M.P. LEFAY, R. MANCASSOLA, *et al.* 1999. Role of *Cryptosporidium parvum* as a pathogen in neonatal diarrhoea complex in suckling and dairy calves in France. Vet. Parasitol. **85:** 245–257.
24. SCOTT, C.A., H.V. SMITH & H.A. GIBBS. 1994. Excretion of *Cryptosporidium parvum* oocysts by a herd of beef suckler cows. Vet. Rec. **134:** 172.
25. VILLACORTA, I., E. ARES-MAZAS & M.J. LORENZO. 1991. *Cryptosporidium parvum* in cattle, sheep and pigs in Galicia (N.W. Spain). Vet. Parasitol. **38:** 249–252.
26. HENRIKSEN, S.A. & H.V. KROGH. 1985. Bovine cryptosporidiosis in Denmark. 1. Prevalence, age distribution, and seasonal variation. Nord. Vet. Med. **37:** 34–41.
27. MIYAJI, S., Y. SAKANASHI, H. ASAMI & J. SHIKATA. 1990. Cryptosporidial infections in calves in Kanto District, Japan, and experimental infections in mice. Nippon Juigaku Zasshi **52:** 435–437.
28. WEE, S.H., H.D. JOO & Y.B. KANG. 1996. Evaluation for detection of *Cryptosporidium* oocysts in diarrheal feces of calves. Korean J. Parasitol. **34:** 121–126.
29. KANETA, Y. & Y. NAKAI. 1998. Survey of *Cryptosporidium* oocysts from adult cattle in a slaughter house. J. Vet. Med. Sci. **60:** 585–588.
30. NOORDEEN, F., R.P. RAJAPAKSE, A.C. FAIZAL, *et al.* 2000. Prevalence of *Cryptosporidium* infection in goats in selected locations in three agroclimatic zones of Sri Lanka. Vet. Parasitol. **93:** 95–101.

Toxoplasmosis in Piglets

ANYARAT THIPTARA, WANDEE KONGKAEW, UMAI BILMAD,
TEERAPHUN BHUMIBHAMON, AND SOMSAK ANAN

*Southern Veterinary Research and Development Center, Nakhonsithammarat
80110, Thailand*

ABSTRACT: Seventeen-day-old piglets in a small holding farm in southern Thailand manifested signs of convulsion, fever, and death. The morbidity and mortality rate were approximately 26.09% (6/23) and 4.35%
(1/23), respectively. Impression smear from lungs demonstrated tachyzoite stage of *Toxoplasma gondii*. Histopathological investigation revealed
interstitial pneumonia. Further investigation, blood collection, educating
the farmer, and prescribed affected herd with sulfa-trimethoprim were
performed soon after *Toxoplasma* infection was demonstrated. A serological detection of *T. gondii* infection among affected herds using latex
agglutination test was conducted on 14 serum samples. The overall seroprevalence was 71.43% (10/14). The titers were 1:64 in 3 pigs (21.43%),
1:128 in 4 (28.57%), 1:256 in 2 (14.29%), and 1:512 in 1 (7.14%). A cat
in this farm showed antibody titer 1:32 while a dog was seronegative.
Data derived from this case indicated two possible routes of transmission: transplacental infection and ingested food or water contaminated
with oocysts shed by cat in this farm. However, rodents can not exclude as
a role of toxoplasmosis transmission. Serological monitoring at slaughter
houses combine with good sanitary practices, rodent and cat control in
the farm are important measures to prevent toxoplasma infection and
improve human health in the future.

KEYWORDS: piglets; *Toxoplasma gondii*; seroprevalence

INTRODUCTION

Toxoplasmosis, caused by infection with *Toxoplasma gondii*, is a contagious
disease of warm-blooded animals worldwide and is one of the major zoonoses.
Infection occurs either by ingesting or drinking contaminated food with sporu-
lated oocysts. Ingestion of oocysts shed by cats is the main route of infection on
pig farms. Pork is considered to be the most important meat source of human

Address for correspondence: Anyarat Thiptara, DVM (2nd Class Honors), Veterinary epidemiologist,
Epidemiology section, Southern Veterinary Research and Development Center (SVRDC), Tee-wang,
Thungsong, Nakhonsithammarat 80110 Voice: 6675-538035-6; fax: 6675-538035-6, 6675-363423-4,
ext. 102.
e-mail: thiptara9@yahoo.com

Ann. N.Y. Acad. Sci. 1081: 336–338 (2006). © 2006 New York Academy of Sciences.
doi: 10.1196/annals.1373.047

infection. Most infections in swine are generally asymptomatic. Infection during pregnancy causes abortion, mummified fetuses, and congenitally infected piglets. The purpose of this article is to describe epidemiological observations and clinical signs of toxoplasmosis in piglets.

METHODS AND RESULTS

A small holding swine farm has a population of 48 pigs including 4 sows, a boar, 20 growing pigs, and 23 suckling piglets (17–28 days). In August 2001, two piglets were submitted at SVRDC. These piglets were born in the same parity of nine pigs in which three were reported stillborn. They manifested signs of convulsion, fever, dyspnea, anorexia, diarrhea, and death. The morbidity rate and mortality rate were nearly 26.09% (6/23) and 4.35% (1/23), respectively. Gloss lesions only showed multiple white spot foci on the lung, while lung impression smears demonstrated tachyzoite stage of *T. gondii*. Internal organs were processed for histopathological examination and were collected for bacterial culture. Swine fever virus (SFV) and Aujeszky's disease virus (ADV) antigens were determined by Fluorescent antibody (FA) assay. Once the histopathology result confirmed toxoplasmosis, follow-up procedures on this farm included farmer interviewing, farmer education, and animal medication with sulfa-trimethoprim. Serum samples were collected from pigs, a cat, and a dog to detect antibody titer against *T. gondii* by using Latex Agglutination test kits (Eiken Chemical Co., Tokyo, Japan). The overall, 71.43% (10/14) of pigs from the affected farm had antibody against *T. gondii* (titer ≥ 1:64). The cat was suspicious (1:32), while a dog was negative. After 1 month, case follow-up was arranged in order to monitor the outcome. All affected pigs appeared healthy and had no evidence of abnormal signs relating to toxoplasmosis.

DISCUSSION

In most species, toxoplasmosis develops in young animals. Clinical signs in pigs vary depending on age, strain, and immune status. In this case, toxoplasmosis was established by suggestive clinical signs and confirmed by laboratory tests. Clinical signs and lesions observed in these piglets were similar to those described by Ito *et al.*[1] Multifocal of necrosis area on lungs was similar to those explained by Dubey *et al.*[2] Moreover, the manifested sign of stillbirth in dam and the developing sing in surviving piglets at 1–3 weeks of age were supported the odds of toxoplasmosis that was similarly described by Basil.[3] It is not clear how the piglets in our report became infected. However, the data derived from this case might indicate two sources. The first way is transplacental transmission. The supporting events were that the sow of infected piglets gave birth to nine piglets which included three stillbirths; and the members of the same litter showed high antibody titer. Moreover, only this sow gave a seropositive result. The second way is the piglets acquired infection by ingestion with *T. gondii* oocysts from infected cat. This event was supported by seropositivity in the cat and additional observations of seropositivity distributed among all pig groups. Strategies to prevent and control *T. gondii* infection on swine farms must focus on control measures for cats and rodents. Serological monitoring at slaughter houses, combined with good sanitary practices to control rodent and cat populations, should lead to the implementation of strategies to prevent infection in pigs.

REFERENCES

1. ITO, S., K. TSUNODA, H. NISHIKOWA & T. MADSUI. 1997. Pathogenicity for piglets of Toxoplasma oocysts originated from naturally infected cat. Nat. Inst. Anim. Health **14**(4): 182–187.
2. DUBEY, J.P., S.E. WEISBRODE, S.P. SHARMA, *et al.* 1979. Porcine toxoplasmosis in Indiana. J. Am. Vet. Med. Assoc. **174**(6): 604–609.
3. BASIL, O. 1994. Diseases caused by protozoa; Toxoplasmosis. *In* Veterinary Medicine, 8th ed. O.M. Radostits, D.C. Blood & C.C. Gay, Eds.: 1201–1206. The Bath Press. Avon.

Cysticercosis of Slaughter Cattle in Southeastern Nigeria

MAXWELL N. OPARA,[a] UKEME MICHAEL UKPONG,[a]
IFEANYI CHARLES OKOLI,[a] AND JUDE CHUKS ANOSIKE[b]

[a]*Tropical Animal Health and Production Research Laboratory, Department Of Animal Science and Technology, Federal University of Technology P.M.B 1526, Owerri, Imo State Nigeria*

[b]*Department of Biological Sciences, Faculty of Science Imo State University, P.M.B. 2000 Owerri Nigeria*

ABSTRACT: The incidence of cysticercosis due to *Taenia saginata* in both local and exotic breeds of cattle slaughtered for meat in southeastern Nigeria between November 1999 and April 2002 is reported. The examination of various organs of 25,800 cattle in 10 major abattoirs of this region showed that 6750 (26.2%) were infected with *Cysticercus (C.) bovis*. The prevalence rates varied from one abattoir to another while the rates of cysticercosis in local and exotic breeds varied significantly ($P >$ 0.05). Sixty percent of all the infected animals had cysts. The tongue, cardiac, and masseter muscles were the main predilection sites of the cysts. Out of 11,720 male cattle, examined, 3215 (27.4%) had cysts of *C. bovis* while 160 (13.6%) of the 1180 female animals investigated were infected. There was an inverse relationship between the ages of the animals and prevalence of infection with *C. bovis* ($r = -0.8743, P < 0.05$). Monthly occurrence of the cysts in the animals revealed an upsurge of infected animals during the dry season. The epidemiology and epizootiology of *Taenia saginata* and *C. bovis* in relation to the veterinary service agencies and public health planners in southeastern Nigeria are highlighted.

KEYWORDS: cysticercosis; cattle; southeastern Nigeria

INTRODUCTION

Cysticercus (C.) bovis, the larval stage of the beef tapeworm *Taenia saginata* is found in the striated muscles of cattle. When cattle are infected with this parasite, it leads to a condition referred to as "beef measles" or cysticercosis. *C. bovis* has a cosmopolitan distribution and is really very common in

Address for correspondence: Dr. M. N. Opara, Tropical Animal Health and Production Research Laboratory, Department Of Animal Science and Technology, Federal University Of Technology P.M.B 1526, Owerri, Imo State Nigeria. Voice: +234 8035373748.
e-mail: oparamax@yahoo. com

Ann. N.Y. Acad. Sci. 1081: 339–346 (2006). © 2006 New York Academy of Sciences.
doi: 10.1196/annals.1373.048

Africa. In some endemic areas of Africa over 80% of cattle are believed to be infected.[1,2] Cysticercosis has little effect on the health of the animals, but it is socially, and economically important as a zoonosis. Affected meat is very often condemned and control measures are usually expensive. The preferred hosts of *Taenia saginata* cysticerci are cattle, especially young animals, since the older ones are known to be more resistant to the infection.[3] Cysticerci are sometimes observed in other ruminants (sheep, goats, buffalo, gazelles, some antelopes, and dromedaries) but their development is unlikely.[4,5] Some researchers comprehensively reviewed the epidemiology and epizootiology of *T. saginate* and *C. bovis* as well as the factors that control their transmission.[6] A WHO memorandum in outlining some research needs equally recommended the establishment of centers in endemic foci to deal with the problems of taeniasis and cysticercosis.[7]

Incidence rates of cysticercosis in several endemic areas of Africa vary from 0% to 40%.[3] In Sierra Leone, 34.8% of cattle slaughtered in that country were infected, while an incidence rate of 17.5% was reported in Kenya.[8] The incidence of this disease in tropical Africa is based on reports from routine meat inspection of the abattoirs. Consequently, there are no data collected on the incidence of cysticercosis among several cattle slaughtered and consumed in the rural areas. In addition, meat inspection facilities in most of our abattoirs are highly inadequate, while the procedures in meat inspection are not uniform or standardized. In places where abattoir practice is reasonably developed, for example, Kenya,[1] incision is restricted to certain muscles.[3]

Available literature tend to presume that cysticercosis is mainly prevalent in northern Nigeria.[9–11] The only isolated reports of this disorder in southeastern Nigeria are those from Imo,[3] Anambra,[12] and Ebonyi States.[13]

Presently, there is no documented record on the incidence of *C. bovis* in the other two states of this region or a comprehensive report of the disorder in the entire region as a whole. This research work was therefore carried out to highlight the incidence of this parasite in both local and exotic breeds of cattle slaughtered for meat in the entire southeastern region. The study therefore, provides information in the epizootiology of cysticercosis in southeastern Nigeria.

MATERIALS AND METHODS

Postmortem investigations were carried out in a total of 10 abattoirs comprising of two, randomly selected from each of the five states that make up southeastern Nigeria, between November 1999 and April 2002. This was very necessary as there are no rapid and accurate antemortem diagnostic tests available for bovine cysticercosis in any of these states. The abattoirs visited were selected such that one from each state was located in the rural area where only local breeds of cattle are slaughtered. The other was located in the urban

TABLE 1. Incidence of *C. bovis* in cattle slaughtered in southeastern states of Nigeria

	Local breeds in rural areas		Exotic breeds in urban areas		
State (Abattoirs)	No. Examined.	No (%) infected	(Abattoirs)	No. Exam.	No (%) infected
Abia (Ohafia)	1,050	340 (32.4)	Umuahia	3,290	960 (29.2)
Anambra (Oba)	1,260	360 (28.6)	Awka	5,120	1,060 (20.7)
Ebonyi (Ogbala)	1,320	390 (29.5)	Abakaliki	4,420	1,100 (24.9)
Enugu (Awgu)	1,030	270 (26.2)	Enugu	4,610	1,210 (26.2)
Imo (Obinze)	900	250 (27.8)	Owerri	2,800	810 (28.9)
Total	5,560	1,610 (29.0)	Total	20,240	5,140 (25.4)

or semiurban center where only exotic breeds of cattle are slaughtered. Each abattoir was visited twice monthly and was such that the butchers were met while slaughtering in the morning. This was also necessary so as to determine the age and sex of each animal slaughtered. The diaphragm, triceps, masseter, heart, and intercostal muscles as well as lungs, liver, tongue, and spleen of 12,900 cattle (consisting of 2786 local and 10,114 exotic breeds of cattle) slaughtered during the period of this investigation were examined for tapeworm cysts following the methods earlier described.[1,3] The cysts observed were categorized into live and calcified cysts. Thereafter, they were carefully dissected from the tissues and the number in each organ recorded for each animal. At the end of the examination, the cysts collected were taken to the laboratory for further diagnosis following the procedures already reported.[14] The cysts were released by enzymatic excystation. If they did not excyst, they were then transferred to a hatching solution. Hatching usually occurred within 30 to 60 min. The cysts were then identified as *C. bovis* if there were no hooks on the envaginated scolex.[3]

RESULT

Out of 25,800 cattle carcasses examined, 6750 (26.2%) were infected with *C. bovis*. The prevalence was highly variable between abattoirs (TABLE 1). There was no significant variation in the prevalence rates of cysticercosis in local and exotic breeds ($P > 0.05$) of the cattle examined.

The distribution of cysts in slaughtered cattle in southeastern Nigeria, shows that 66.8% of the animals that harbored calcified cysts had between 1–2 cysts while among animals with live cysts, majority had between 4–10 cysts (TABLE 2).

However, 61.8% of all the infected animals with cysts had live cysts. Intensity of the infection revealed that there were light-to-moderate live infections. On enzymatic digestion, all the calcified cysts did not yield live parasites. Our observations showed that more cysts were isolated during the dry season months of November to March.

TABLE 2. Distribution of cysts in slaughtered cattle in southeastern state of Nigeria

Calcified cysts		Live cysts	
No. of cysts/animal	No. of animals	No. of cysts/animal	No. of animals
1	1,250	1	650
2	420	2	420
3	–	3	640
4—10	340	4—10	740
11—15	60	11—15	410
16—20	120	16—20	400
21—30	70	21—30	420
Above 30	240	Above 30	370
Total	2,500	Total	4,050

On the predilection sites of the cysts (TABLE 3), 29.9%, 21.9%, 15.6%, 8.7%, 5.5%, 3.1%, and 1.6% of the cysts were collected from the tongue, heart muscles, masseter muscles, thigh muscles, liver, diaphragm, and kidney as well as triceps muscles, respectively. Cysts were not found in the lungs, spleen, intercostal muscles, and intestinal mucosa.

The sex distribution of *C. bovis* infection of cattle is shown in TABLE 4. Of the 25, 800 cattle examined, 90.9% were males. Of the 23,452 male animals examined, 6426 (27.4%) had cysts of *C. bovis,* while 324 (13.8%) of the 2348 female animals examined were infected. Although more males than females were examined, the prevalence of infections did not show any significant difference ($P > 0.05$).

The infection of cattle with *C. bovis* was more prevalent in younger animals than older ones irrespective of the breed (FIG. 1). Analysis of the actual data showed that there was a significant inverse relationship between the ages of the animals with regard to the prevalence of *C. bovis* infection ($r = 0.8743$, $P < 0.05$). Investigation into the monthly occurrence of the cysts in the animals revealed that the infection was recorded in all the months of the study. However,

TABLE 3. Predilection sites of the cysts in slaughtered cattle in southeastern states

Predilection sites	No. infected	% Prevalence
Kidney	210	3.1
Tongue	2,020	29.9
Heart muscles	1,480	21.9
Diaphragm	370	5.5
Intercostal muscle	–	–
Triceps	110	1.6
Thigh muscles	810	12.0
Masseter muscles	1,050	15.6

Over total No. of cattle infected (6750).

TABLE 4. Sex distribution of *C. bovis* infection of cattle slaughtered in southeastern Nigeria

State (Abattoirs)	No. of males examined	No. (%) infected	No. of females examined	No. (%) infected
Abia	4,000	1,300 (32.5)	340	64 (18.8)
Anambra	6,200	1,110 (17.9)	180	48 (26.7)
Ebonyi	5,000	1,220 (24.4)	740	75 (10.1)
Enugu	5,400	2,250 (41.7)	240	70 (29.7)
Imo	2,852	546 (19.1)	848	67 (7.3)
Total	23452 (90.9%)	6,426 (27.4%)	2,348 (9.1%)	324 (13.8)

there was a drop in live cysts infection as the rainy season months set in (FIG. 2). The pattern of infection following the months showed that most of the local breeds were more infected than the exotic cattle. More so, there was an upsurge of infection during the dry season months.

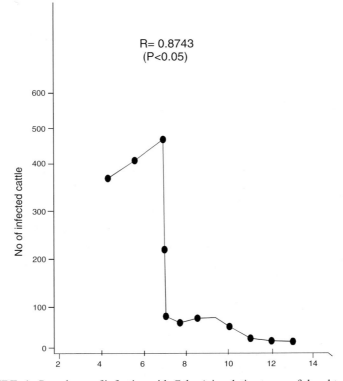

FIGURE 1. Prevalence of infection with *C. bovis* in relation to age of slaughtered cattle.

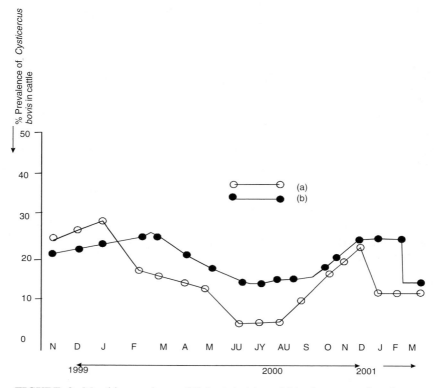

FIGURE 2. Monthly prevalence of *C. bovis* in (a) rural (b) urban areas of southeastern Nigeria.

DISCUSSION

This work documents the incidence and distribution of *C. bovis* infections among slaughtered cattle in southeastern Nigeria. With an overall prevalence rate of 26.2%, *C. bovis* infection is indeed high in southeastern Nigeria. The incidence in the local breeds as well as the exotic breeds of cattle is also high. The pattern of infection in the study area is not analogous to what was observed in the southwestern and northeastern parts of the country.[11,15] The high rate is equally not surprising compared with the results from Chad Republic and Cameroon of prevalence rates varying from 3.0% to 40%, as most of the exotic cattle slaughtered here are imported from those countries.[16] The variation in prevalence rates recorded in the different abattoirs could be attributed to the different modes of transportation of these animals. It has been recorded,[1] that in the past when nomads walked their animals to the southern parts of the country, infected animals got sick enroute and were sold off on the way, accounting for the differences recorded in Bauchi[9] or in Kano,[11] all in the northeastern and northcentral parts of the country, respectively. On the other hand, nowadays lorries are used to transport these animals to southeastern Nigeria. Consequently, the improvement in the mode of transportation of the cattle has undoubtedly introduced distortions in the epizootiology and increased prevalence of *C. bovis* in southern Nigeria.[3] Furthermore, animals grazed by nomads who are always on the move have fewer but more intense infection than sedentary cattle, which have lighter infection, but show higher incidence of cysticercosis.[17] This could also explain the high prevalence rate of *C. bovis* among local breeds of cattle reared and grazed in the rural areas. Our observations showed that the tongue, heart muscles, and masseter muscles as well as thigh muscles among others were the preferred organs (predilection sites) for the cysts of *C. bovis* similar to earlier reports in various endemic areas.[3,6,9,18] It appears that several factors, such as breed of cattle, activity of the muscles, age, and the geographical area concerned determine largely the predilection sites in slaughtered cattle.[14,19,20]

It is interesting to observe that some live cysts were isolated from the kidneys but not from the intercostal muscles, lungs, spleen, and intestinal mucosa.

Sex-related distribution of *C. bovis* infection of the slaughtered cattle in this study showed that sex of the animals and infection are independent. Though more males than females were infected, it could be related to the sample size and not sex. This is in agreement with the observations in Anambra State of Nigeria.[3] There was an inverse relationship of prevalence with the ages of the animals similar to documented records.[21]

Slaughtering of cattle continued throughout the study period. However, there was increase in the number of slaughter during the dry season months, perhaps due to festivities. Infection was recorded in all the months of study. This could be attributed to the long period of the development of the parasite, which takes 3–5 months for the infection to be established in the muscles of the animals and also the ability of the cysts to survive long periods for about 1 year once established.[4] From our observations on the epidemiology and epizootiology of *T. saginata* and *C. bovis* in southeastern Nigeria, the present study has brought to focus some public health implications:

1. The habit of buying and slaughtering cattle especially in the rural areas without proper meat inspections may result in serious health risks.
2. There is a potential outbreak of epidemics of tapeworm infections in the region if proper preventive measures are not taken urgently.
3. The widespread practice of eating spiced roasted beef (called *suya*), which is heated over open fire at 45°C for 15 min, is enough to destroy the cysticerci.[16] Eating of *suya* is a common practice in all the states of southeastern Nigeria.

The present observations should therefore be of interest not only to the veterinary service agencies but also to the public health planners in the states of southeastern Nigeria.

REFERENCES

1. ANOSIKE, J.C. 1985. A survey of gastrointestinal parasites of some ruminants in Etiti Local Government Area of Imo State, Nigeria. Thesis, Imo State University. 96 p. Etiti, Nigeria.
2. TESFA-YOHANNES, T.M. 1990. Effectiveness of Praziquantel against *Taenia saginata* infections in Ethiopia. Ann. Trop. Med. Parasitol. **84:** 581–585.
3. OKAFOR, F.C. 1988. Epizootiology of Cysticercus bovis in Imo State, Nigeria. Angew. Parasitol. **29:** 25–30.
4. TRONCY, P.M. 1981. Helminths of livestock and poultry in tropical Africa. *In* Manual of Tropical Veterinary Parasitology. 99 p. C.A.B. International. Wallingford, UK.
5. HARRISON, L.J.S. & M.M.H. SEWEL. 1991. The zoonotic *Taenia* of Africa. *In* Parasitic Helminths Zoonoses in Africa C.N.L. Macpherson & P.S. Craig, Ed.: 54–82. Unwin Hyman. London.
6. PAWLOWSKI, Z.S. & M.G. SCHULTZ. 1992. Taeniasis and Cysticercosis (*Taenia saginata*). Adv. Parasitol. **10:** 269–273.
7. ABDUSSALAM, M., M.A. GEMMELL, R.B. GRIFFINS, *et al*. 1975. Research needs in taeniasis-cysticercosis {Memorandum}. Bull. World Health Org. **53:** 67–73.
8. FROYD, G. 1960. Cysticercosis and hydatid diseases of cattle in Kenya. J. Parasitol. **46:** 491–496.
9. BELLINO, E.E. 1975. Some observations on *Taenia saginata* cysticercosis in slaughter cattle in Nigeria. Int. J. Zoonoses **2:** 92–99.
10. DADA, B.J.O. 1977. Prevalence of taeniids encountered at meat inspection in Nigeria Vet. Rec. **101:** 347.
11. DADA, B.J.O. & E.D. BELLINO 1978. Prevalence of hydatidosis and cysticercosis in slaughtered livestock in Nigeria. Vet. Rec. **103:** 311–312.
12. ONAH, D.N. & S.N. CHIEJINA 1983. Bovine cysticercosis in Anambra State, Nigeria. A paper presented at the 7th annual conference of Nigerian Society for Parasitology. University of Calabar, Nigeria.
13. ANOSIKE, J.C. 2001. Some observations on *Taenia saginata* cysticercosis in slaughter cattle in Nigeria. Int. J. Zoonoses **2:** 82–89.
14. PETROVIC, A.P. 1976. On the incidence of *Cysticercus bovis* in Tanzania. Vet. Glesnik. **30:** 709–713.
15. ATSANDA, N.N. & S.A. AGBEDE. 1999. A survey for brucellosis, tuberculosis and cysticercosis in cattle slaughtered in Ibadan and Maiduguri abattoirs. Nig. Vet. J. **20:** 61–66.
16. UKOLI, F.M.A.. 1984. Introduction to Parasitology in Tropical Africa. 464 pp. John Wiley and Sons. New York.
17. GRABER, M., R. TABO. 1968. La cysticercose bovine en milien sedemarie et en million nomade. Rev. Elev. Med. Vet. Pays. Trop. **21:** 29–33.
18. PAWLOWSKI, Z.S.. 1990. Perpectus and control of Taenia saginata. Parasitol. Today **6:** 371–372.
19. SCHILLHORN VAN VEEN, T.W. 1976. The occurrence of *Cysticercus bovis* in cattle livers. Vet. Rec. **101:** 370.
20. MITCHELL, J.R.. 1978. Bovine cysticercosis. Vet. Rec. **102:** 469.
21. SOULSBY, E.J.L.. 1975. Taeniasis and cysticercosis: the problem of the old world. Scientific Publications No. 295, 127–132.

Use of *Bacillus thuringiensis* Toxin as an Alternative Method of Control against *Haemonchus contortus*

MARIA E. LÓPEZ,[a] JAIME FLORES,[a] PEDRO MENDOZA,[a]
VICTOR VÁZQUEZ,[a] ENRIQUE LIÉBANO,[a] ALEJANDRA BRAVO,[b]
DAVID HERRERA,[a] ELENA GODÍNES,[a] PATRICIA VARGAS,[a]
AND FABIAN ZAMUDIO[a]

[a]*Centro Nacional de Investigación Disciplinaria en Parasitología Veterinaria,
INIFAP, Jiutepec, Morelos, México C.P. 62550*

[b]*Instituto de Biotecnología, Universidad Nacional Autónoma de México,
Circuito Universitario Chamilpa, Cuernavaca, Morelos, México C.P. 62209*

ABSTRACT: The biocide activity of *Bacillus thuringiensis* (*B. thuringiensis*) IB-16 strain was evaluated against the blood-feeding nematode *Haemonchus contortus* (*H. contortus) in vitro* and *in vivo* assays. Twenty experimental jirds (*Meriones unguiculatus*) and 32 sheep were infected with *H. contortus* by oral route. Fourteen days post infection 10 jirds were treated with 0.2 mg per mL of IB-16 soluble toxin by intraperitoneal (i.p.) route and 8 sheep were treated with 0.5 mg of toxin per kg of body weight by intramuscular route 35 days after *H. contortus* infection. Same number of treated jirds and sheep were used as control. Fecal and blood samples were analyzed from experimental sheep to estimate the number of parasitic eggs, percentage of eosinophils, packed cell volume (PCV), and IgG title. All experimental jirds and 16 sheep (8 treated and 8 controls) were sacrificed at days 5, 7, and 30 after *B. thuringiensis* treatment. The percentage of nematode reduction was estimated from L_4 and *H. contortus* adults. The percentage of protection was 80.0 to jirds and 73.8 and 53.3 to sheep, sacrificed at days 7 and 30, respectively. Moreover, nonsignificant difference ($P \geq 0.05$) was detected from parasitic eggs, eosinophils, and PCV parameters. Significance level of IgG was observed only before *H. contortus* treatment with *B. thuringiensis* soluble toxin ($P \leq 0.05$) but nonsignificant difference was observed after treatment. These results showed that *B. thuringiensis* activity was similar to those observed by anthelmintic treatment and it could be used as an alternative biological method.

KEYWORDS: *Bacillus thuringiensis*; *Haemonchus contortus*; adults and L_4; biological control; sheep; jirds

Address for correspondence: María López, Centro Nacional de Investigacion Disciplinaria en Parasitologia Veterinaria, INIFAP. Apdo. Postal 206 CIVAC, Jiutepec, Morelos, Mexico C.P. 62550. Voice: 0052-777-3-19-28-50; fax: 0052-777-320-55-44.
e-mail: lopez.mariaeugenia@inifap.gob.mx

Ann. N.Y. Acad. Sci. 1081: 347–354 (2006). © 2006 New York Academy of Sciences.
doi: 10.1196/annals.1373.049

INTRODUCTION

Bacillus thuringiensis (*B. thuringiensis*) is a Gram (+) bacterium that has been isolated from soil, stored grains, insect cadavers, and plant surface.[1] *B. thuringiensis* is a endospore-forming bacterium, which synthesizes an inclusion body with different molecules during sporulation.[2,3] Some of these molecules are called "crystal" proteins and they have shown high toxicity against a wide range of insects.[4] Currently, some commercial products are available containing *B. thuringiensis* crystal (Cry) proteins against agriculture pests and some strains are used to control insects like human pathogenic vectors.[5] Moreover, a few studies have also shown the lethal effect of *B. thuringiensis* against parasitic and free-living nematodes.[6,7] These reports open new expectations in the new alternatives of control against parasitic nematodes. Recently, IB-16 strain of *B. thuringiensis* showed more than 98% of lethal effect against *Haemonchus contortus* (*H. contortus*) eggs and free-larvae *in vitro* assays.[8] This nematode is recognized as the most important pathogen to ruminants from tropical and temperate regions. The availability of broad spectrum anthelmintics has helped to reduce the incidence of *H. contortus* infection. However, the extensive use and improper dosage of anthelmintics have resulted in drug resistance to *H. contortus*.[9] The soluble toxin of *B. thuringiensis* IB-16 strain might be considered as an alternative control against *H. contortus*. Therefore, this article shows preliminary observations of *B. thuringiensis* against the fourth larvae (L_4) and the adult of *H. contortus*.

MATERIALS AND METHODS

Production of IB-16 Soluble Toxin

B. thuringiensis IB-16 strain was generously provided by Dr. Alejandra Bravo from the Institute of Biotechnology, Universidad Nacional Autonoma de Mexico. The IB-16 strain was cultured in petridishes containing SP media (0.15 g agar, 0.5 M $CaCl_2$, 1N Fe [SO_4], 0.5 M $MnCl_2$) and incubated at 30°C for 5 days. Then, free-crystal proteins were harvested by centrifugation in phosphate-buffered saline (PBS) pH 10.5 and 1 μM phenil-methyl-sulphoxide. Crystal proteins were solubilized with 10 mM 2-mercapto-ethanol at 37°C for 4 h and centrifuged at 1280 g and 10,000 g. Soluble toxin was dialyzed in PBS buffer pH 8.0 for 24 h and protein concentration was estimated by the method of Bradford.[10] The soluble toxin was examined by SDS-PAGE at 4% and 12%.[11]

Identification of IB-16 Cry Genes

Three general primers were used to detect *cry*1, *cry*3, and *cry*5 genes selected from highly conserved regions by using a simultaneous alignment of previously described sequences.[12,13] IB-16 strain was cultured at 30°C on Luria-Bertani media. One single colony was transferred to 100 μL of H_2O water (Milli-Q.; Millipore, Mexico) and frozen at –70°C and at 95°C to lyses the cell. Samples were centrifuged at 10,000 g and 20 μL of supernatant was used in polymerase chain reactior (PCR) assays (Thermal Cycler Omniogene HB-TRB; Techne, Princeton, NJ). Amplification was performed by using a single step of denaturalization at 72°C for 2 min, followed by a step cycle program set for 30 cycles. Each cycle of this program consists of denaturalization step at 95°C for 2 min, annealing at 50°C for 1 min, extension at 72°C for min, and extra step of extension at 72°C for 5 min. Then, PCR samples were analyzed in electrophoresis agarose gel at 3% for 35 min at 250 V.

H. contortus L_3 and L_4 Stages

H. contortus-infective larvae (L_3) susceptible isolate to bencimidazole was obtained from an infective donor sheep. Fecal culture was made by Curticelli technique and L_3 were obtained by migration technique. The fourth stage (L_4) of *H. contortus* was obtained from unsheathed L_3 with 0.368% sodium hypochloride and maintained in sterile media with 0.1% sucrose, 0.02% bovine sera albumin, 5 μL of erythrocytes, PBS pH 4.0, antibiotiotic and antimicotic (Amersham Pharmacia Stockholm, Sweden) at 39°C in 5% of Co_2 atmosphere. Interaction between *H. contortus* L_4 with soluble toxin was carried to estimate the lethal effect of IB-16.

Experimental Design

Two experimental trials were carried out at the National Centre of Disciplinary Research in Veterinary Parasitology (CENID-PAVET), INIFAP in Morelos District of Mexico.

Trial I: Forty jirds of 30–35 g were treated with anthelmintic (Piperazine; Columbia Labs, Tolvca, Mexico) and corticosteroids (Schering-Plough, Mexico City, Mexico) previous to *H. contortus* infection. Jirds were infected with 7000 L_3 *per os* and 13 days after infection they were divided in two groups: (*a*) treated with 0.2 mg of soluble toxin and (*b*) treated with PBS pH 8 by intraperitoneal (i.p.) route per animal. Then, jirds were sacrificed with anesthesia 9 days after *B. thuringiensis* treatment. Stomachs were removed and longitudinally opened and put in vials containing distilled water and placed in a water bath at 37°C for 6 h. L_4 stages were preserved in 2% formaldehyde solution and then counted.

Trial II: Sixteen 8- to 10-month-old native sheep were fed with hay, concentrate and water *ad libitum* and kept indoors. Fifteen days before infections, sheep were orally treated with albendazole (Valbazen, Pfizer, San Juan del Rio, Mexico). Animals were infected with 350 L_3 of *H. contortus* per kg of body weight by oral route at day 0. After 35 days all sheep were positive to *H. contortus* infection. Then, sheep were assigned in 4 groups with 4 sheep in each one: groups A and C were treated with 0.5 mg per kg of body weight of soluble toxin and groups B and D received PBS pH 8 by intramuscular (i.m.) route. In order to determine the activity of IB-16 toxin on adults, experimental sheep were slaughtered at days 7 (A and B) and 30 (C and D) after treatment. The biocide activity of the IB-16 soluble toxin was estimated using the following formula[8]:

$$\text{Percentage of efficacy} = \frac{XA - XB}{XA} \times 100$$

Where XA = mean of recovered adult nematodes in treated group with *B. thuringiensis* and XB = mean of recovered adult nematodes in control group with PBS.

Fecal, Hematological, and Immunological Examination

Fecal egg samples were analyzed by McMaster technique. Blood samples were taken to determine the packed cell volume percentage (PCV %), peripheral eosinophil percentage (Eo %), and IgG kinetics by enzyme-linked immunosorbent assay (ELISA) from sacrificed groups at day 30 after *B. thuringiensis* treatment (C and D). ELISA technique was carried out using L_3 crude-extract antigen, anti-IgG of rabbit anti-sheep polyclonal antibody with peroxidase (1:1000), and ABTS as substrate (Sigma-Aldrich, St. Louis, MO).

Statistical Analyses

Hematological, fecal, and immunological parameters were analyzed using ANOVA analysis ($P \leq 0.05$).[14]

RESULTS

Gene and Protein Pattern

The *cry* gene of IB-16 of *B. thuringiensis* strain did not match using general oligonucleotide primers to *cry1*, *cry3*, and *cry5*. On the other hand, protein pattern of IB-16 of *B. thuringiensis* soluble toxin showed five groups of proteins with molecular weight around 100, 62, 40, 30, and 22 kDa.

Experimental Animals

Trial 1: Careful examination of experimental jirds stomachs was carried out to determine external damage. Light red color of epithelial mucus and edema was observed on the surface from control group. In contrast, treated group with *B. thuringiensis* did not show damage on the stomach tissue. The number of L_4 recovered after necropsy was 6 and 38 from A and B groups, respectively, then the percentage of protection was 80.2.

Trial II: At necropsy, treated groups (A and C) showed a yellow-pale mucus color with a few microhemorrhages on the abomasal tissue. In contrast, control groups (B and D) showed severe damage on the abomasal tissue as hyperemic mucus, microhemorrhages, and edema. The biocide activity of *B. thuringiensis* on A and C groups was 73.87% and 53.3% on *H. contortus* adult reductions, at days 7 and 30 after treatment. The number of parasites, percentage of protection, and the ANOVA analyses of *H. contortus* recovered per group are showed in TABLE 1.

Hematological, Fecal, and Immunological Analysis

The number of PCVs and Eo % cells was counted before and after treatment and nonsignificant difference was observed ($P \geq 0.05$). Although, the percentage of eosinophils corresponding to group C (sacrificed 30 day after treatment) suddenly felt 1 week after treatment, indicating that *H. contortus* circulated antigens had decreased because of the nematode reduction. The number of *H. contortus* eggs and IgG title between control and treated sheep for groups C and D was not significant ($P \geq 0.05$) after *B. thuringiensis* treatment. However, it is an important observation that infected hosts treated with *B. thuringiensis* consistently increased the level of IgG anti-*H.contortus* after treatment. In contrast, control group showed variable response against *H. contortus* (FIG. 1).

DISCUSSION

Different alternatives of biological control are currently explored against *H. contortus*. The biocide activity of IB-16 soluble toxin could be used as a new method of control against *H. contortus*. The percentage of protection against *H. contortus* was not so high (80.2%, 73.8%, and 53.3%) when they

TABLE 1. Percentage of protection and ANOVA analysis of infected sheep treated with IB-16 soluble toxin of *B. thuringiensis*

Group	Adult nematodes	Mean (X)	Standard deviation (sd±)	P value	% of protection
A	580	145	65	$P \leq 0.05$	73.87
B	2220	555	120		
C	2180	545	390	$P \geq 0.05$	53.3
D	3070	1023	633		
Total	8050	2268			

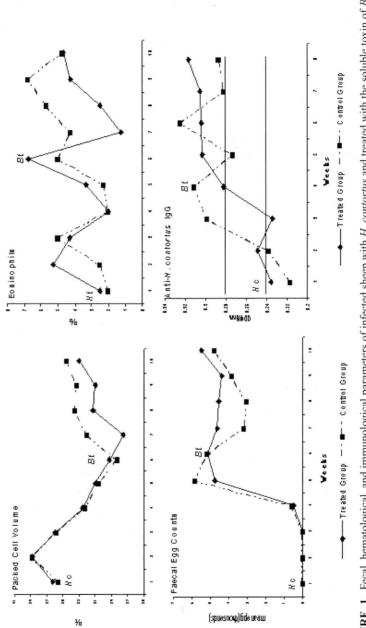

FIGURE 1. Fecal, hematological, and immunological parameters of infected sheep with *H. contortus* and treated with the soluble toxin of *B. thuringiensis* IB-16. Hc = *H. contortus* infection; Bt = treatment of IB-16 soluble toxin; % = percentage.

are compared with the nematicide effect of macrocyclic-lactones and benz-imidazole, whose effectiveness is close to 100%. However, it is important to consider that IB-16 toxin is only a crude extract. It is important to consider that IB-16 toxin is a crude extract. It is likely that after purification, such toxins might increase their nematicide activity as it has been observed with other recombinant *B. thuringiensis* products.[7] The advantage of IB-16 toxin by i.m. injection was that it did not cause damage to treated hosts as hyper-sensitivity. These results are similar to other experimental observations, such as mouse and humans treated with different species of *Bacillus*.[5,15] Moreover, the number of parasitic eggs, percentage of eosinophils, and PCV were only indicative of *H. contortus* infection as other studies have been notified[16] and they were not related to the treatment with *B. thuringiensis*. Although, the level of peripheral Eo % suddenly fell 7 day after *B. thuringiensis* treatment, this result was related with the reduction of *H. contortus* antigen, therefore less quantity of eosinophils were detected. Meeusen and Balic[17] have mentioned the importance of eosinophils against *H. contortus* endoparasitic larvae and we observed that eosinophils and IgG antibodies were also important parameters to determine the host immune response against *H. contortus* before and after *B. thuringiensis* treatment. The mode of action of IB-16 against this nematode is not clear; it might presumably cause a cytological damage on the mid-gut cells of endoparasitic stages (L_4 and adults), similar to other free-living nema-todes (i.e., *Ceanorhabiditis elegans*) whose feeding is by oral route.[7] Besides Cry proteins some *B. thuringiensis* strains have other kinds of virulent factors, including exotoxins (α,β), chitinase, and phospolipases. The L_3 and L_4 stages of *H. contortus* have an external cuticule, which could have been affected by these enzymes. On the other hand, IB-16 strain was not matched with some notified *cry*-gene with nematicide genes; furthermore, this strain is a candidate for harboring putative novel *cry* gene with nematicide action. The nematicide action of IB-16 needs to be clarified. The identification and purification of the components of the toxin might help to increase the percentage of protection against *H. contortus* and to understand the mechanisms of action of IB-16 on parasitic nematodes.

ACKNOWLEDGMENTS

This project received a grant by Consejo Nacional de Ciencias y Tecnología, Mexico, Num. 28803-B. Elena Godínez and Fabian Zamudio received a schol-arship from CONACYT-Mexico.

REFERENCES

1. SCHNEPF, E., N. CRICKMORE, J. VAN RIE, *et al.* 1998. *Bacillus thuringiensis* and its pesticidal crystal proteins. Microbiol. Mol. Biol. Rev. **62:** 775–806.

2. FEITELSON, S.J., J. PAYNE & L. KIM. 1992. *Bacillus thuringiensis*: insects and Beyond. Biotechnology **10**: 271–275.
3. DE-MAAGD, R.A., A. BRAVO, B. COLIN, *et al.* 1998. Structure, diversity and evolution of protein toxins from spore-forming entomopathogenic bacteria. Annu. Rev. Genet. **37**: 409–433.
4. DE-MAAGD, R., A. BRAVO & N. CRICKMORE. 2001. How *Bacillus thuringiensis* has evolved specific toxins to colonize the insect world. Trend Genet. **17**: 193–199.
5. SANDERS, M.E., L. MORELLI & T.A. TOMPKINS. 2003. Sporoformes as human probiotics: *Bacillus*, *Sporolactobacillus* and *Brevibacillus*. Compr. Rev. Food Sci. Food Safety **2**: 101–110
6. BOTTJER, P.K. & W.L. BONE. 1987. Changes in morphology of *Trichostrongylus colubriformis* eggs and juveniles caused by *Bacillus thuringiensis israelensis*. J. Nematol. **3**: 282–286.
7. WEI, J.-Z., K. HALE, L. CARTA, *et al.* 2003. *Bacillus thuringiensis* crystal proteins that target nematodes. Microbiology **100**: 2760–2765.
8. LÓPEZ-ARELLANO, M.E., J. FLORES-CRESPO, P. MENDOZA-DE-GIVES, *et al.* 2002. *In vitro* lethal activity of *Bacillus thuringiensis* toxins against *Haemonchus contortus* eggs and infective larvae. Int. J. Nematol. **12**: 66–72.
9. VAN WYK, J.A. 2001. Refugia. Overlooked as perhaps the most potent factor concerning the development of anthelmintic resistance. Onderstepoort J. Vet. Res. **68**: 55–67
10. BRADFORD, M.M. 1976. A rapid and sensitive method for the quantitation of microgram quantities of protein utilizing the principle of protein-dye binding. Anales de Bioquimica **72**: 248–254.
11. LAEMMLI, U.K. 1970. Cleavage of structural proteins during the assembly of the head of bacteriophage T4. Nature **227**: 680–685.
12. CERON, J., A. ORTIZ, R.L. QUINTERO, *et al.* 1995. Specific PCR primers directed to identify *cryI* and *cryIII* genes within a *Bacillus thuringiensis* strain collection. Appl. Environ. Microbiol. **61**: 3826–3831.
13. BRAVO, A., S. SARABIA, L. LOPEZ, *et al.* 1998. Characterization of *cry* genes in a Mexican *Bacillus thuringiensis* strain collection. Appl. Environ. Microbiol. **64**: 4965–4972.
14. MENDELHALL, W. 1982. Introducción a la probabilidad y la estadística. Wadsworth Internacional/Iberoamérica, USA.
15. MAYERS, M.E., G.A.C. HELD, J.C. LAU, *et al.* 1989. Characterization of the mammalian toxicity of the crystal polypeptides of *Bacillus thuringiensis* subesp *israelensis*. Fund. Appl. Toxicol. **13**: 310–316.
16. HOODA, V., C.L. YADAV, S.S. CHAUDHRI, *et al.* 1999. Variation in resistance to haemonchosis: selection of female sheep resistant to *Haemonchus contortus*. J. Helminthol. **73**: 137–142.
17. MEEUSEN, E.N.T. & A. BALIC. 2000. Do eosinophils have a role in the killing of Helminto Parasites? Parasitol. Today **16**: 95–101.

Biological Control of Gastrointestinal Parasitic Nematodes Using *Duddingtonia flagrans* in Sheep under Natural Conditions in Mexico

PEDRO MENDOZA-DE GIVES,[a] CLAUDIA ZAPATA NIETO,[a] ENRIQUE LIÉBANO HERNÁNDEZ,[a] MARÍA EUGENIA LÓPEZ ARELLANO,[a] DAVID HERRERA RODRÍGUEZ,[a] AND ROBERTO GONZÁLEZ GARDUÑO [b]

[a]*CENID-Parasitología Veterinaria, INIFAP, Jiutepec, Morelos México CP 62550*

[b]*Universidad Autónoma Chapingo, Centro Regional Universitario del Sureste, Teapa, Tabasco, México 86800*

ABSTRACT: This investigation was aimed to evaluate the use of an oral bio-preparation containing *Duddingtonia flagrans* chlamydospores for the control of sheep gastrointestinal parasitic nematodes under the Mexican cold high plateau conditions. Two groups of gastrointestinal parasitic nematode naturally infected sheep, were randomly selected and located into two free-gastrointestinal nematode larvae paddocks. Group 1 received once a week a supplement containing *D. flagrans* chlamydospores mixed with oats and molasses. Group 2 received a similar supplement without any fungal material. After 5 months grazing animals were discarded from the experiment and two groups of free-nematode "tracer" sheep were located into the same paddocks to collect larvae from the contaminated pastures. Animals were slaughtered and necropsied and the nematodes were obtained and counted. A screening of the number of gastrointestinal nematode larvae present on the grass was performed and compared between the two grazing areas. The results showed 56% reduction in the *Ostertagia (Teladorsagia) circumcincta* and 94% reduction in the *Nematodirus* sp. population of the "tracer" sheep who grazed on the *D. flagrans*-treated sheep area, compared to the nematode population in animals grazed on the non-treated area. The results of the number of larvae on the grazing pastures showed a 51.1% reduction for *H. contortus*, and 100% for *Cooperia* sp. in the area with fungi. In the case of *Trichostrongylus* sp. no reduction was observed, when compared to the control group.

Address for correspondence: Pedro Mendoza de Gives, CENID-Parasitología Veterinaria, INIFAP, A.P. 206, CIVAC, Morelos, México, 62550. Voice: 01777-3192850; ext.: 124; fax: 01777-3192850; ext.: 129.

e-mail: pedromdgives@yahoo.com

Ann. N.Y. Acad. Sci. 1081: 355–359 (2006). © 2006 New York Academy of Sciences.
doi: 10.1196/annals.1373.050

KEYWORDS: *Duddingtonia flagrans*; gastrointestinal parasitic nematodes; sheep

INTRODUCTION

Anthelmintic efficacy of some commercial chemical products is sometimes seriously reduced, because of the presence of anthelmintic resistance in the parasites.[1,2] In addition, some anthelmintic products can be harmful for beneficial fauna from soil.[3] Alternatives of control (different than chemotherapy) have being intensively explored; for instance, the use of nematode-natural enemies. *Duddingtonia flagrans* is a nematode-trapping fungus, which develops traps to capture nematodes from mycelia. Such fungus produces a large quantity of chlamydospores which are able to resist the passage through the gastrointestinal tract of ruminants, once they are orally administered into animals.[4] Once chlamydospores are expelled with faeces to the environment, they colonize faecal material and due to a recognition of chemical signals produced by the nematode cuticle, fungi detect the presence of nematodes and in this way a mycelia-differentiation process is triggered, leading to a heavy trap production, where finally nematodes are trapped and destroyed by the fungi[5] reducing either the infectivity of surrounding grass by larvae and the re-infections in sheep.[6–8] In the National Centre of Disciplinary Research in Animal Parasitology (Mexico), an autochthonous strain of *D. flagrans* (FTHO-8) has being isolated from sheep feces[4] and it has displayed an enormous potential in the control of animal parasitic nematodes in different controlled trials[7,9]; however, there is still no investigation about the use of such technology under field conditions in Mexico. This paper evaluates the use of *D. flagrans* chlamydospores in the control of gastrointestinal parasitic nematodes in Mexican sheep farming in a cold high plateau.

METHODS

The use of D. flagrans for the control of gastrointestinal nematodes in Mexican sheep farming in a cold high plateau was evaluated. Two groups of five sheep were considered as treated (group 1) and control (group 2), respectively. Group 1 received 1×10^6 *D. flagrans* chlamydospores per kg of live weight mixed with oat grains and molasses, once a week for 5 months. Group 2 received the same nutritional regime but without fungi. A $1000 \, m^2$ nematode-free grazing area was divided in two equal parts. Each group was located in the corresponding individual grazing area along the experiment. Sheep are thought to spread either larvae (group 1) or larvae plus chlamydospores (group 2). Following the grazing period, sheep from both groups were discarded from the experiment. In order to screen the parasitic conditions of both areas, 2 groups of 4 nematode-free sheep, (1 and 2 "tracer" groups) were assigned to graze and collect larvae from the nonprotected and protected area, respectively for 4 weeks. After this period, "tracer" sheep were slaughtered and recovered nematodes were counted and identified.[7] The larval reduction on grass was evaluated by a random sampling of grass taking 20 circle-shape samples of 15 cm diameter each from the soil surface of every area that was at a height of 10 cm. The total grass samples were weighted and the larval migration technique was applied for 24 h to obtain the total larvae present in the samples.[10] The results were expressed as the total number of larvae per kg of grass, and compared between both grazing areas. Reduction percentage was estimated based on the following formula:

Percentage of larval reduction on grass $= LT - LC/LT \times (100)$

From which LT = total number of larvae recovered from treated area and LC = total number of larvae recovered from control area.

The variable "number of adult nematodes" was N_{log} transformed to obtain an approximation to the normal distribution.[11] The General Linear Model (GLM) (SAS) procedure was used.[12]

RESULTS

The nematodes recovered from abomasums of both "tracer" sheep groups were identified as *Teladorsagia circumcincta (T. circumcincta)*. A total of 820 nematodes [mean = 205 ($\pm$139.1) and 360, mean = 90 ($\pm$88.3)] were recorded from sheep that corresponded to the nonfungal and fungal areas, respectively. Fifty-six reduction percentage was recorded when means in both groups were compared. All the specimens collected from small intestine corresponded to *Nematodirus* sp. The total number of worms of this genus was 13,110 (mean = 3277.5 $\pm$ 3250.9) in the animals corresponding to the "nonfungal protected area." In contrast, only 790 worms (mean = 197.5 $\pm$ 155.2), were obtained from the "fungal protected area." The reduction percentage of this nematode was 94%. Regarding the results obtained from large intestine, a large variability in both groups was observed and no effect of the fungi was observed against nematodes from this compartment. The total number of infective larvae recovered from grass in the fungi-free area was 18, 292. In contrast, 8928.4 larvae were recovered from the "fungi protected area." The results showed 51.1% reduction for *H. contortus*, and 100% for *Cooperia* sp. in the area with fungi. In the case of *Trichostrongylus* sp. no reduction was observed.

DISCUSSION

The results showed evidence of a reduced parasitic burden in the "tracer" sheep group grazing in the area previously grazed by *D. flagrans-* treated sheep.

A clear reduction in the parasitic burden of *T. circumcincta* and *Nematodirus* sp. was observed at necropsy. On the other hand, the number of larvae obtained from the grass screening in both grazing areas, showed clear evidence of the effect of the *D. flagrans* treatment in the reduction in the populations of *H. contortus* and *Cooperia* sp. Additional control measures must be considered to integrate an antiparasitic control program focused to control either adult and free-living nematode stages, minimizing the effects of the gastrointestinal parasitic nematodes and reducing the alarming threat of anthelmintic resistance.

ACKNOWLEDGMENTS

This work received financial support from the *International Foundation for Science* Agreement B/3022-1. This research was part of the M.Sc. thesis work of Miss Claudia Zapata at the Autonomous University of Morelos State, Mexico.

REFERENCES

1. CHARLESTON, T. 1994. Control of gastrointestinal parasites in beef production systems. Veterinary Continuing Education, Massey University **159:** 157–174.
2. SAUER, S. 1996. Epidemiologie und klinische auswirkungen von infektionen in Koppelhaltung. 151 pp. Inaugural Dissertation, Fechbereich Veterinarmedizin, Justus Liebig-Universität, Giessen, Germany.
3. BULMAN, G.M., M.E. MUÑOZ-COBENAS, & R.R. AMBRUSTOL. 1996. The environmental impact of the macrocyclic lactones (endectocides): a comprehensive and comparative update. Veterinaria Argentina **13:** 490–504.
4. LLERANDI-JUAREZ, R.D. & P. MENDOZA DE GIVES, 1998. Resistance of chlamydospores of nematophagous fungi to the digestive processes of sheep. *J. Helminthol.* **72:** 209–213.
5. PRYADKO, E.I., & P.P OSIPOV. 1996. Trials of nematophagous fungi in field conditions. *Biologycheskaya* **1:** 30–33.
6. FAEDO, M., E.H. BARNES, R.J. DOBSON, *et al.* 1998. The potential of nematophagous fungi to control the free-living stages of nematode parasites of sheep: pasture plot study with *Duddingtonia flagrans*. *Veterinary Parasitology* **72:** 129–135.
7. MENDOZA DE GIVES, P., C.J. FLORES, R.D. HERRERA, *et al.* 1998. Biological control of *Haemonchus contortus* infective larvae in ovine faeces by administering an oral suspension of *Duddingtonia flagrans* chlamydospores to sheep. *J. Helminthol* **72:** 343–347.
8. PEÑA, M.T., J.E. MILLER, M.E. FONTENOT, *et al.* 2002. Evaluation of *Duddingtonia flagrans* in reducing infective larvae of *Haemonchus contortus* in faeces of sheep. *Vet. Parasitol.* **103:** 259–265.
9. ARROYO-BALÁN, L.F. 2006. Evaluation of a combined method of control of the ovine Haemonchosis under controlled conditions (*Original title in Spanish: Evaluación de un método combinado de control de la hemoncosis ovina bajo*

condiciones controladas). M.Sc. Degree Thesis. Universidad Juárez Autónoma de Tabasco.

10. LIÉBANO HERNÁNDEZ, E. & J. FLORES-CRESPO. 2002. Identificación morfométrica de larvas infectantes de nematodos gastrointestinales y pulmonares en rumiantes domésticos. *En: Primer curso de Diagnóstico y control de las nematodiasis gastrointestinales y pulmonares de los rumiantes*. Huamantla, Tlaxcala, México, 18 -19 de Noviembre del 2002. págs 1–21.

11. BOUIX, J.J., R. KRUPINSKI, B. RZEPECKI, *et al*. 1998. Genetic resistance to gastro-intestinal nematode parasites in Polish Ion-wool sheep. *Int. J. Parasitol*. **28:** 1797–1804.

12. SAS. 1998. The SAS System for Windows, Release 7.00 SAS Institute Inc., Cary, NC. USA.

New Findings on Anaplasmosis Caused by Infection with *Anaplasma phagocytophilum*

EUGENIO LILLINI, GLADIA MACRÌ, GABRIELLA PROIETTI, AND MANUELA SCARPULLA

Istituto Zooprofilattico Sperimentale delle Regioni Lazio e Toscana, 00187 Rome, Italy

ABSTRACT: *Ixodes ricinus (I. ricinus)* is one of the vectors of *Anaplasma phagocytophilum (A. phagocytophilum)* in Europe, in which rates of infection range from 1.9% to 34%. In 1998, human granulocytic ehrlichiosis-like (HGE-like) *Ehrlichia* DNA was detected in Italy, by PCR technique in one *I. ricinus* nymph out of 55 ticks that were examined. In 1996, 6.3% of 310 human sera in high-risk subjects from Italy were found positive for antibodies to *Ehrlichia phagocytophila (E. phagocytophila)*. In the same year, the authors reported the first case of equine granulocytic ehrlichiosis. In 1997, only 2 out of 563 equine blood samples examined were found positive for antibodies to *E. phagocytophila* in the Latium region. In 1998, serological positivity was not observed in 14 symptomatic race horses. In 2002, a symptomatic horse living in Rome was found positive for *Ehrlichia equi (E. equi)* antibodies, as confirmed by PCR. *E. equi* was also demonstrated in horses by detection of specific antibodies from two asymptomatic ponies. We tested 128 sera from sheep in different flocks, and antibodies to *E. phagocytophila* were detected in 17 sera (13.3%) of these sheep. From 2000 to 2004, 147 dog sera were tested for antibodies against *A. phagocytophilum,* and 7 of these sera were positive (4.8%). These data confirm the presence of the infection in human, domestic animals, and pets in Italy. Studies are under way to correlate the distributions of the disease and tick vector, *I. ricinus.*

KEYWORDS: anaplasmosis; *Anaplasma phagocytophilum*; human; horse; sheep; dog

INTRODUCTION

Anaplasma phagocytophilum (A. phagocytophilum), classified in the genus *Anaplasma,* family *Anaplasmataceae,* order *Rickettsiales,* is an obligate intracellular Gram-negative bacterium, that is the causative agent of granulocytic

Address for correspondence: Dr. Eugenio Lillini, Istituto Zooprofilattico Sperimentale delle Regioni Lazio e Toscana, Via Appia Nuova 1411, 00187 Roma, Italy. Voice: 39-06-79099451; fax: 39-06-79340724.

e-mail: elillini@rm.izs.it

Ann. N.Y. Acad. Sci. 1081: 360–370 (2006). © 2006 New York Academy of Sciences.
doi: 10.1196/annals.1373.053

ehrlichiosis in humans, horses, dogs, cattle, and sheep. On the basis of genetic analysis (16 S rRNA gene), the unification of *Ehrlichia equi (E. equi), Ehrlichia phagocytophila (E. phagocytophila),* and human granulocytic ehrl agent (HGE) in the single species *A. phagocytophilum* was published.[1] Analysis of the 16 S rRNA gene has shown a very low grade of genetic variability, also supported by similar *groESL clades,* and biological and antigenic characteristics.[1,2] These micro-organisms can be frequently found in microcolonies, called *morulae,* in the cell cytoplasm of host cells, mainly neutrophil granulocytes. Enclosed bodies are frequently pleomorphic and more than one *morula* can be present in the same cell.[3-5]

At present, the family *Anaplasmataceae* includes six genera: *Ehrlichia, Anaplasma, Neorickettsia, Wolbachia, Aegyptianella,* and "*Candidatus* Neoehrlichia." These bacteria infect cells of hematopoietic origin and the bone marrow except *Wolbachia.* Generally, wild animals are reservoirs of *Anaplasma* infection and humans are generally infected by the bite of infected ticks.

Mechanisms of Pathogenesis during A. phagocytophilum *Infection*

Organisms of the family *Anaplasmataceae* have evolved remarkable ways to survive inside host leukocytes. It has been recently demonstrated that these bacteria lack all genes for biosynthesis of lipid A and most genes for biosynthesis of peptidoglycan.[6] Deletion of these genes in *Anaplasma* sp. eliminated a means of triggering these microbicidal activities in leukocytes, thus increasing their chance for intraleukocytic survival. The bacteria have developed the ability to take up cholesterol from the environment to acquire significant levels of membrane cholesterol, required for their survival, to compensate the loss of mechanical strength due to the lack of these genes and of their products as well as to the lack of genes for cholesterol biosynthesis or modification. Furthermore *A. phagocytophilum* cell entry and intracellular infection involve membrane phagosomes that bypass lysosomes.[7] These bacteria actively suppress host cells to survive inside leukocytes. Superoxide (O_2^-) generated by activated NADPH oxidase is one of major antimicrobial mechanisms. *A. phagocytophilum* actively inhibits NADPH oxidase activation. In addition, *A. phagocytophilum* prolongs the life span of human peripheral blood neutrophils *in vitro,* inhibiting human neutrophil spontaneous apoptosis, thus enabling the establishment of infection and transmission of this pathogen to new host cells.[8,9]

A. phagocytophilum *in the Tick Vector,* I. ricinus

I. ricinus is the tick vector of *A. phagocytophilum* and other several pathogens to human and animals in Europe. This tick species can feed on greater than

200 host species, primarily wild rodents and ruminants.[2,10] The prevalence of *A. phagocytophilum* infection is usually higher in adult ticks than in nymphs and ranging from zero or very low to greater than 30%.[11]

Infection of ticks has been studied in many European countries. *A. phagocytophila* DNA has been detected in 5.1% of 235 investigated *I. ricinus* adult ticks using PCR targeting 16 S rRNA in Austria.[12] In northeastern Poland, among 559 examined ticks (adults and nymphs), 8.7% were found positive (PCR).[13] *E. phagocytophila* group DNA were detected in 6 of 141 adult *I. ricinus* examined in Slovakia.[14] In Bulgaria and Slovenia the infection rate of ticks were found to be 34% and 3.2%, respectively.[15,16] In Germany 4.1% of 1022 adult and nymph *I. ricinus* investigated were found infected.[17] In Switzerland 1.4% of 417 *I. ricinus* ticks (adult and nymphs), collected by flagging vegetation, included ehrlichial DNA.[18] In Hungary 452 ticks collected from 100 different foxes were tested and some of them turned out to be infected.[19] In Portugal (Madeira Island), 4% out of 142 collected nymphs tested positive for *A. phagocytophilum* DNA.[20] It is likely that technical and methodological differences account for at least part of the different prevalence of the infection found in various studies.

In our study, a total of 55 *I. ricinus* nymphs were collected from mid-October to mid-November 1998 in four localities of the Feltre area, in Italy. The ticks, preserved in ethanol 70%, were grouped in 11 pools and examined by PCR technique to screen the presence of both *Borrelia burgdorferi (B. burgdorferi)* and *Ehrlichia* species DNA. The PCR screening was positive for *B. burgdorferi* in 45% of samples and also positive for *Ehrlichia* DNA in 9% of them. At a further characterization, the *Ehrlichia* ribosomal fragment sequence showed identity with HGE-like *Ehrlichia*. The pool proved positive for both pathogens was used to develop a multiplex PCR assay and the different molecular size of the two amplified fragments allowed an easy identification of both pathogens after electrophoretic run in agarose gel.[10]

A. phagocytophilum *in Humans*

The first documented HGE case in Europe caused by granulocytic ehrlichia species was reported by Petrovec *et al.*[21] in 1997 in Slovenia. The patient, reporting a history of a tick bite, presented a self-limited but moderately severe illness mainly characterized by fever, up to 40°C, malaise, thrombocytopenia, and high C-reactive protein concentration. The diagnosis was established by seroconversion to HGE agent and by PCR with sequence analysis of the gene encoding the HGE agent 16 S rRNA and the etiological agent was isolated in HL60 cell culture.[21] After the first description, details of other human patients with confirmed HGE and several patients fulfilling criteria for probable HGE had been reported in Europe (up to early 2003 about 65 human patients).[11] The majority of these patients live in Central Europe (Slovenia)[22–24] and Scandinavia (Sweden)[25] and there are few reports from other countries, the Netherlands,[26] Norway,[27] Poland,[28] Spain,[29] Austria,[30] Estonia,[31] France,[32] and Italy.[33]

In 1996, in Italy, 310 sera were obtained from 220 high-risk human subjects living in Belluno and Feltre areas (Veneto region). We tested these sera for detection of antibodies to *E. phagocytophila* and *Borrelia*. Antibodies positivity rate for *E. phagocytophila,* by indirect fluorescent antibody test (IFAT), was 6.3% compared to a value of 1.1% of controls. The subgroup of forestry workers showed the highest rates of positivity and 4 of the 12 sera (33.3%) tested positive for anti-*Ehrlichia* antibody showed concomitant positivity to *Borrelia.*[34]

A. phagocytophilum *in Horses*

In Europe, EGE cases were reported in Great Britain,[35,36] Denmark,[37] Sweden,[38,39] Switzerland,[40] France,[41,42] Germany,[43–45] and Italy.[46,47] The first case of EGE in Italy was reported from the authors in 1996 in a symptomatic 6-year-old saddle horse from East Europe on the basis of positivity to anti-*E. equi* antibodies by IFAT, the presence of characteristic *morulae* in neutrophils and the recovery from the infection by the use of oxytetracycline therapy.[46] In 1997 only 0.3% out of 563 equine blood samples examined by IFAT in the Latium region, were found serologically positive to *E. phagocytophila.*[46] In 1998 no serological positivity was observed in 14 symptomatic race horses.[46]

In 2002, five horses (2–18 years old) coming from the Latium and Tuscany areas, with symptoms of the disease, were investigated. Several blood tests of each subject were examined by enzyme-linked immunosorbent assay (ELISA) and/or by IFAT to detect antibodies against *A. phagocytophilum* (*E. equi* Equine ELISA KIT, Vita Research, catalog N° VRCEEE96G; *E. equi* IFA Equine 120 test IgG Kit, Fuller Laboratories, Fullerton, CA). The samples were considered positive from 1:80 dilution by IFAT and from OD 0,3 for ELISA. For microscope detection of the bacterium in leukocytes, smears were prepared from buffy coat, stained with Hemacolor® (Merck, Darmstadt, Germany, catalog N° 1.11661) and examined in a light microscope.

The buffy coat, added 1:1 with DMSO 10% in fetal calf serum, were frozen at −80°C to further perform PCR and culture. The extraction of DNA was carried out starting from 200 μL of buffy coat according to the protocol Blood and Body Fluid Spin, QIAamp® DNA Mini Kit (Qiagen, Inc., Valencia, CA). A PCR was carried out with the Kit ADIAVET® Ehrlichia-test (Adiagene, Saint-Brieuc, France) to detect *E. phagocytophila* DNA. The samples were considered as positive when a 900-bp band was observed after electrophoresis on agarose gel.

Out of the 5 horse samples examined, 4 were positive by ELISA and/or IFAT and PCR, and one of these revealed the presence of *morulae*. One sample

TABLE 1. Laboratory tests results

S	ELISA	IFAT	PCR	ME	L	PLT	I
1	+	n.t.	+	−	N	N	
2	+	n.t.	−	−	N	↓	Be
3	+	+	+	n.t.	↑	↓	Be−Bc
4	+	n.t.	+	+	n.t.	n.t.	Bc
7	+	+	+	−	n.t.	n.t.	Lb

S = samples; ME = microscopic examination; L = leucocytes; PLT = platelets; I = intercourrant infections with *B.equi* (Be), *B.caballi* (Bc), and *Leptospira bratislava* (Lb); n.t. = not tested; (+) = positive; (−) = negative; N = normal; (↑) =augmentation; (↓): reduction

was positive by test ELISA and negative by PCR. Hematological findings on two horses showed thrombocytopenia in two seropositive subjects. One animal positive by PCR showed leukocytosis. The biochemistry carried out did not reveal relevant changes (TABLE 1 and FIG. 1). The infectious agent was not isolated by propagation in the HL-60 cell line.

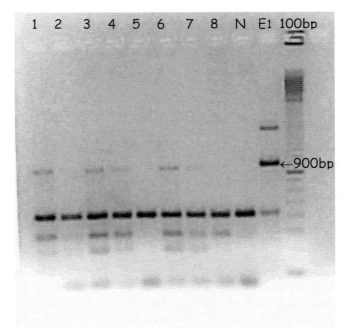

FIGURE 1. PCR to detect *A. phagocytophilum* DNA. Lines 1 to 8: samples tested. Line N: negative control. Line E1: marker of size ADIAGENE. Line 100 bp: marker of size 100 bp ladder. Samples 1, 3, 4, 6, and 7 were positive.

A. phagocytophilum *in Sheep*

In domestic ruminants *A. phagocytophilum* causes a disease known as tick-borne fever (TBF). *A. phagocytophilum* in sheep causes very high fever, reduced milk yield and abortion in pregnant animals. Main laboratory findings are severe neutropenia and cytoplasmatic inclusions with more than 95% of the neutrophils infected. Besides, it is known that TBF has profound effects on the immune system and can increase the susceptibility to disease. TBF is seldom fatal unless complicated by other infections.[48] The disease is common in Spain, Norway, United Kingdom, Scandinavia, and in other areas of mainland Europe.[49–51]

Our personal experience on sheep was limited on the investigation of 73 sera from aborted ewes collected during 1997 from different flocks in the Pordenone province, in northeastern Italy. Antibodies to *E. phagocytophila* were detected in 12.3% of sera from different flocks. The IFAT, using *E. phagocytophila* infected ovine granulocytes as antigen and anti sheep IgG FITC (Sigma-Aldrich, St. Louis, MO) Sigma at 1:100 dilution as conjugate, was performed. The infected cells were fixed on multispot slides, made in UK by the Royal School of Veterinary Sciences (University of Edinburgh). Sera were considered positive at 1:80 dilution.

In 2002 the investigation was carried out on 55 sheep sera coming from 7 flocks in Parco Nazionale d'Abruzzo, in Central Italy, during the transhumance period. Antibodies against *E. phagocytophila* were detected in 14.5% of sera from different flocks using commercial IFAT (Fuller Laboratories Slides) and anti-sheep IgG FITC by Sigma at 1:100 dilution as conjugate.

A. phagocytophilum *in Dogs*

A. phagocytophilum that frequently causes chronic disease in dogs with non-specific clinical and hematological findings of fever, anorexia, and thrombocytopenia are often observed. The frequent occurrence of polyarthritis, involving joint swelling and pain, lameness of one or multiple limbs, and stiffness, with a reluctance to rise, often with neutrophilic inflammation, is recorded.[52] Cases of canine granulocytic ehrlichiosis (CGE) in Europe has been reported in Sweden, Greece, Italy, Slovenia, Austria, Poland, and Switzerland.[53–61]

In 2000, 40 sera from dogs living in the Latium Region, in Central Italy, were investigated by IFAT (Fuller Laboratories Slides) using anti-dog IgG FITC by Sigma at 1:100 dilution as conjugate, to detect antibodies against *A. phagocytophilum*. The cut-off titer for positive serological assay was 1:80. Positivity was found in 5 of them (12.5%). In 2004, 107 stray dogs living in Rome were examined, and only 2 of them (1.87%) were found to be positive. In some of these dogs a concomitant high title seropositivity to *E. canis* was evidenced.

DISCUSSION

The results analyzed thus far confirm the perpetuation of *A. phagocytophilum* in northeastern Italy, the identification of *I. ricinus* as the vector of the infection and forestry employment as a risk factor for HGE seropositivity. A mixed infection of *A. phagocytophilum* and *E. canis* in ticks suggests that dogs may acquire both infections as a consequence of a multiple tick bite. The coexistence of antibodies against *A. phagocytophilum* and *E. canis* in dogs occurs rarely and only in hyperimmunized sera.[62,63] These cross-reactions, generally observed at very low titers, are taken into consideration to represent nonspecific reactions to highly conserved antigens among the members of the *Ehrlichia* genus.[64]

Thorough intensive surveillance is needed, including its reservoir hosts, vector, and tick-exposed populations, to clarify the epidemiology of human anaplasmosis in Europe. Studies carried out in Switzerland and in Israel on small rodents and jackals demonstrated the role of wild animals as reservoirs.[65,66] Further studies are also required to verify the existence of a wild cycle of circulation of the agent, the supposed sentinel role of horse, dog, and sheep on human anaplasmosis and to study the disproportion between the high percentage of infection in ticks and the low numbers of clinical signs in humans and animals.

REFERENCES

1. DUMLER, J.S., A.F. BARBET, C.P. BEKKER, *et al*. 2001. Reorganization of genera in the families *Rickettsiaceae* and *Anaplasmataceae* in the order *Rickettsiales*: unification of some species of *Ehrlichia* with *Anaplasma*, *Cowdria* with *Ehrlichia* and *Ehrlichia* with *Neorickettsia*, descriptions of six new species combinations and designation of *Ehrlichia equi* and 'HGE agent' as subjective synonyms of *Ehrlichia phagocytophila*. Int. J. Syst. Evol. Microbiol. **51**(Pt 6): 2145–2165.
2. MADIGAN, J.E. & N. PUSTERLA. 2000. Ehrlichial diseases. Vet. Clin. North Am. Equine Pract. **16**: 487–499.
3. REUBEL, G.H. *et al*. 1998. Experimental transmission of *Ehrlichia equi* to horses through naturally infected ticks (*Ixodes pacificus*) from northern California. J. Clin. Microbiol. **36**: 2131–2134.
4. MUNDERLOH, U.G. *et al*. 1996. Isolation of the equine granulocytic ehrlichiosis agent, *Ehrlichia equi*, in tick cell culture. J. Clin. Microbiol. **34**: 664–670.
5. MADIGAN, J.E. 1993. *Equine ehrlichoisis*. Vet. Clin. North Am. Equine Pract. **9**: 423–428.
6. LIN, M. & Y. RIKIHISA. 2003. *Ehrlichia chaffeensis* and *Anaplasma phagocytophilum* lack genes for lipid A biosynthesis and incorporate cholesterol for their survival. Infect. Immun. **71**: 5324–5331.
7. LIN M. Y. RIKIHISA. 2003. Obligatory intracellular parasitism by *Ehrlichia chaffeensis* and *Anaplasma phagocytophilum* involves caveolae and glycosyl-phosphatidyilinositol-anchored proteins. Cell. Microbiol. **5**: 809–820.

8. MOTT, J., Y. RIKIHISA & S. TSUNAWAKI. 2002. Effect of *Anaplasma phagocytophila* on NADPH oxidase components in human neutrophils and HL-60 cells. Infect. Immun. **70:** 1359–1366.

9. LIN, Q., Y. RIKIHISA, N. OHASHI & N. ZHI. 2003. Mechanism of variable p44 expression by *Anaplasma phacytophilum*. Infect. Immun. **71:** 5650–5661.

10. FAVIA, G., G. CANCRINI, A. CARFI', *et al.* 2001. Molecular identification of *Borrelia valaisiana* and HGE-like *Ehrlichia* in *Ixodes ricinus* ticks sampled in north-east Italy: first report in Veneto region. Parassitologia **43:** 143–146.

11. STRLE, F. 2004. Human granulocytic ehrlichiosis in Europe. Int. J. Med. Microbiol. **293**(Suppl 37): 27–35.

12. SIXL, W. *et al.* 2003. Investigation of *Anaplasma phagocytophila* infections in *Ixodes ricinus* and *Dermacentor reticulatus* ticks in Austria. Ann. N. Y. Acad. Sci. **990:** 94–97.

13. GRZESZCZUK, A. *et al.* 2004. Human anaplasmosis in north-eastern Poland: sero-prevalence in humans and prevalence in *Ixodes ricinus* ticks. Ann. Agric. Environ. Med. **11:** 99–103.

14. SPITALSKA, E. & E. KOCIANOVA. 2003. Tick-borne microorganisms in southwestern Slovakia. Ann. N. Y. Acad. Sci. **990:** 196–200.

15. CHRISTOVA, I. *et al.* 2001. High prevalence of granulocytic *Ehrlichiae* and *Borrelia burgdorferi sensu lato* in *Ixodes ricinus* ticks from Bulgaria. J. Clin. Microbiol. **39:** 4172–4174.

16. PETROVEC, M., J.W. SUMNER, W.L. NICHOLSON, *et al.* 1999. Identity of ehrlichial DNA sequences derived from *Ixodes ricinus* ticks with those obtained from patients with human granulocytic ehrlichiosis in Slovenia. J. Clin. Microbiol. **37:** 209–210.

17. VON LOEWENICH, F. D. *et al.* 2003. High diversity of *ankA* sequences of *Anaplasma phagocytophilum* among *Ixodes ricinus* ticks in Germany. J. Clin. Microbiol. **41:** 5033–5040.

18. LIZ, G. *et al.* 2000. PCR detection of granulocytic ehrlichiae in *Ixodes ricinus* ticks and wild small mammals in western Switzerland. J. Clin. Microbiol. **38:** 1002–1007.

19. SRETER, T. *et al.* 2004. *Anaplasma phagocytophilum*: an emerging tick-borne pathogen in Hungary and Central Eastern Europe. Ann. Trop. Med. Parasitol. **98:** 401–405.

20. SANTOS, A.S. *et al.* 2004. Detection of *Anaplasma phagocytophilum* DNA in *Ixodes* ticks (Acari: *Ixodidae*) from Madeira Island and Setubal District, mainland Portugal. Emerg. Infect. Dis. **10:** 1643–1648.

21. PETROVEC, M., S. LOTRIC FURLAN, T.A. ZUPANAC, *et al.* 1997. Human disease in Europe caused by a granulocitic *Ehrlichia* species. J. Clin.Microbiol. **35:** 1556–1559.

22. LOTRIC-FURLAN, S. *et al.* 1998. Human ehrlichiosis in Central Europe. Wien Klin Wochenschr. **110:** 894–897.

23. LOTRIC-FURLAN, S. *et al.* 2001. Prospective assessment of the etiology of acute febrile illness after a tick bite in Slovenia. Clin. Infect. Dis. **33:** 503–510.

24. LOTRIC-FURLAN, S. *et al.* 2003. Human granulocytic ehrlichiosis in Slovenia. Ann. N. Y. Acad. Sci. **990:** 279–284.

25. KARLSSON, U. *et al.* 2001. Human granulocytic ehrlichosis—a clinical case in Scandinavia. Scand. J. Infect. Dis. **33:** 73–74.

26. VAN DOBBENBURGH, A *et al.* 1999. Human granulocytic ehrlichiosis in western Europe. N. Engl. J. Med. **340:** 1214–1216.

27. KRISTIANSEN, B.E. *et al.* 2001. Human granulocytic ehrlichiosis in Norway. Tidsskr Nor Laegeforen. **121:** 805–806.
28. TYLEWSKA-WIERZBANOWSKA, S., T. CHMIELEWSKI, M. KONDRUSIK, *et al.* 2001. First cases of acute human granulocytic ehrlichiosis in Poland. Eur. J. Clin. Microbiol. Infect. Dis. **20:** 196–198.
29. OTEO, J.A., J.R. BLANCO, V. MARTINEZ DE ARTOLA & V. IBARRA. 2000. First report of human granulocytic ehrlichiosis from southern Europe (Spain). Emerg. Infect. Dis. **6:** 430–432.
30. WALDER, G., B. FALKENSAMMER, J. AIGNER, *et al.* 2003. First documented case of human granulocytic ehrlichiosis in Austria. Wien Klin Wochenschr. **115:** 263–266.
31. PRUKK, T., K. AINSALU, E. LAJA & A. AIGRO. 2003. Human granulocytic ehrlichiosis in Estonia. Emerg. Infect. Dis. **9:** 1499–1500.
32. REMY, V., Y. HANSMANN, S. DE MARTINO, *et al.* 2003. Human anaplasmosis presenting as atypical pneumonitis in France. Clin. Infect. Dis. **37:** 846–848.
33. RUSCIO, M. & M. CINCO. 2003. Human granulocytic ehrlichiosis in Italy: first report on two confirmed cases. Ann. N. Y. Acad. Sci. **990:** 350–352.
34. NUTI, M., F. RUSSINO, D. GRAZIOLI, *et al.* 1996. Anticorpi anti-*Ehrlichia in soggetti a rischio di zone pedemontane del Veneto. Microbiologia Medica. **11:** 492–495.
35. KORBUTIAK, E. & D.H. SNEIDERS. 1994. First confirmed case of equine ehrlichiosis in Great Britain. Equine Vet. Edu. **6:** 303–304.
36. SHAW, S. *et al.* 2001. Equine granulocytic ehrlichiosis in the UK. Vet. Rec. **28:** 127–128.
37. MADIGAN, J.E. & N. PUSTERLA. 2000. Ehrlichial diseases. Vet. Clin. North Am. Equine Pract. **16:** 487–499.
38. BJOERSDORFF, A. 1990. *Ehrlichia equi* infection diagnosed in horses. Svensk Vet. Tid. **42:** 357–360.
39. BJOERSDORFF, A., B. BAGERT, R.F. MASSUNG, *et al.* 2002. Isolation and characterization of two European strains of *Ehrlichia phagocytophila* of equine origin. Clin. Diagn. Lab. Immunol. **9:** 341–343.
40. BUSCHER, G., R. GRANDRAS, G. APEL, K.T. FRIEDHOFF. 1984 Der erste Fall von Ehrlichiosis beim Pferd in Deutschland. Dtsch tierarztl.Wschr. **91:** 408–409.
41. DAVOUST, B. *et al.* 1999. Survey of horses from southeast France for antibodies reactives with the agent of human granulocytic ehrlichiosis. International Conference on Rickettsiae and Rickettsiology 14th Sesquiannual Joint Meeting, 12–16 June 1999(Marseille).
42. BERMANN, F. *et al.* 2002. *Ehrlichia equi* (*Anaplasma phagocytophila*) infection in an adult horse in France. Vet. Rec. **150:** 787–788.
43. HERMANN, M. 1985. Colitis X in the horse: 9 cases. Schweiz Arch Tierheilkd. **127:** 385–396.
44. VON LOEWENICH, F.D., G. STUMPF, B.U. BAUMGARTEN, *et al.* 2003. Human granulocytic ehrlichiosis in Germany: evidence from serological studies, tick analyses, and a case of equine ehrlichiosis. Ann. N. Y. Acad. Sci. **990:** 116–117.
45. VON LOEWENICH, F.D., G. STUMPF, B.U. BAUMGARTEN, *et al.* 2003. A case of equine granulocytic ehrlichiosis provides molecular evidence for the presence of pathogenic *Anaplasma phagocytophilum* (HGE agent) in Germany. Eur. J. Clin. Microbiol. Infect. Dis. **22:** 303–305.
46. SCARPULLA, M., M.E. CARISTO, G. MACRÌ & E. LILLINI. 2003. Equine ehrlichiosis in Italy. Ann. N. Y. Acad. Sci. **990:** 259–263.

47. CUBEDDU, G.M. *et al.* 2001. Equine ehrlichiosis in Asinara's Island—Clinical signs. *In* Proceeding of "7th World Congress of World Equine Veterinary Association." 5–7 October 2001. Sorrento (Naples) – Italy. Ed.: 317.

48. GARCIA-PEREZ, A.L., J. BARANDIKA, B. OPORTO, *et al.* 2003. *Anaplasma phagocytophila* as an abortifacient agent in sheep farms from northern Spain. Ann. N. Y. Acad. Sci. **990:** 429–432.

49. JUSTE, R.A., A.L. GARCIA-PEREZ & I. POVEDANO-FERNANDEZ. 1986. Estudio experimental de algunos agentes patogenos transimitdos por garrapatas (*Babesia*, *Theileria*, *Cytoecetes* y *Anaplasma*) en ovejas del Pais Vasco. Med. Vet. **3:** 431–439.

50. STUEN, S., S. NEVLAND & T. MOUM. 2003. Fatal cases of tick-borne fever (TBF) in sheep caused by several 16 S rRNA gene variants of *Anaplasma phagocytophilum*. Ann. N. Y. Acad. Sci. **990:** 433–434.

51. WOLDEHIWET, Z., B.K. HORROCKS, H. SCAIFE, *et al.* 2002. Cultivation of an ovine strain of *Ehrlichia phagocytophila* in tick cell cultures. J. Comp. Pathol. **127:** 142–149.

52. BREITSCHWERDT, E.B. 2000. The rickettsioses. *In* Ettinger S.J., E.C. Feldman. Eds.: 400–408. Textbook of Veterinary Internal Medicine. W.B. Saunders. Philadelphia.

53. PUSTERLA, N., J.B. PUSTERLA, P. DEPLAZES, *et al.* 1998. Seroprevalence of *Ehrlichia canis* and of canine granulocytic *Ehrlichia* infection in dogs in Switzerland. J. Clin. Microbiol. **36:** 3460–3462.

54. SKOTARCZAK, M., M. ADAMSKA & M. SUPRON. 2004. Blood DNA analysis for *Ehrlichia* (*Anaplasma*) *phagocytophila* and *Babesia* spp of dogs from Northern Poland. Acta Vet. Brno. **73:** 347–351.

55. STADTBAUMER, K., M.W. LESCHNIK & B. NELL. 2004. Tick-borne encephalitis virus as a possible cause of optic neuritis in a dog. Vet. Ophthalmol. **7:** 271–277.

56. TOZON, N., M. PETROVEC & T. AVSIC-ZUPANC. 2003. Clinical and laboratory features of the first detected cases of *A. phagocytophila* infections in dogs from Slovenia. Ann. N. Y. Acad. Sci. **990:** 424–428.

57. MANNA, L., A. ALBERTI, L.M. PAVONE, *et al.* 2004. First molecular characterization of a granulocytic *Ehrlichia* strain isolated from a dog in South Italy. Vet. J. **167:** 224–227.

58. GRAVINO, A.E., D. DE CAPRARIIS, L. MANNA, *et al.* 1997. Preliminary report of infection in dogs related to *Ehrlichia equi*: description of three cases. New Microbiol. **20:** 361–363.

59. EGENVALL, A.E., A.A. HEDHAMMAR & A.I. BJOERSDORFF. 1997. Clinical features and serology of 14 dogs affected by granulocytic ehrlichiosis in Sweden. Vet. Rec. **140:** 222–226.

60. MYLONAKIS, M.E., A.F. KOUTINAS, G. BANETH, *et al.* 2004. Mixed *Ehrlichia canis*, *Hepatozoon canis*, and presumptive *Anaplasma phagocytophilum* infection in a dog. Vet. Clin. Pathol. **33:** 249–251.

61. JOHANSSON, K.E., B. PETTERSSON, M. UHLEN, *et al.* 1995. Identification of the causative agent of granulocytic ehrlichiosis in Swedish dogs and horses by direct solid phase sequencing of PCR products from the 16 S rRNA gene. Res Vet Sci. **58:** 109–112.

62. DUMLER, J.S., K.M. ASANOVICH, J.S. BAKKEN, *et al.* 1995. Serologic cross-reactions among *Ehrlichia equi*, *Ehrlichia phagocytophila* and human granulocytic *Ehrlichia*. J. Clin. Microbiol. **33:** 1098–1103.

63. NICHOLSON, W.L., J.A. COMER, J.W. SUMMER, *et al.* 1997. An indirect immunofluorescence assay using a cell culture-derived antigen for detection of antibodies to the agent of human granulocytic ehrlichiosis. J. Clin. Microbiol. **35:** 1510–1516.

64. WANER, T., S. HARRUS, F. JONGEJAN, *et al.* 2001. Significance of serological testing for ehrlichial disease in dogs with special emphasis on diagnosis of canine monocytic ehrlichiosis caused by *Ehrlichia canis*. Vet. Parass. **95:** 1–15.

65. LIZ, J.S., L. ANDERES, J.W. SUMNER, *et al.* 2000. PCR detection of granulocytic ehrlichiae in *Ixodes ricinus* ticks and small mammals in western Switzerland. J. Clin. Microbiol. **38:** 1002–1007.

66. WANER, T., G. BANETH, C. STRENGER, *et al.* 1999. Antibodies reactive with *Ehrlichia canis*, *Ehrlichia phagocytophila* genogroup antigens and the spotted fever group rickettsial antigens, in free-ranging jackals (*Canis aureus syriacus*) from Israel.Vet. Parasitol. **82:** 121–128.

Molecular Diagnosis of Granulocytic Anaplasmosis and Infectious Cyclic Thrombocytopenia by PCR-RFLP

ALBERTO ALBERTI[a] AND OLIVIER A.E. SPARAGANO[b]

[a]Istituto di Patologia Speciale e Clinica Medicina Veterinaria, and Center for Biotechnology Development and Biodiversity Research, University of Sassari, 07100, Italy

[b]Newcastle University, School of Agriculture, Food and Rural Development, Newcastle upon Tyne NE1 7RU, United Kingdom

ABSTRACT: *Anaplasma phagocytophilum* (*A. phagocytophilum*, formerly *Ehrlichia phagocytophila*) is a tick-borne pathogen responsible for tick-borne fever in ruminants, equine granulocytic ehrlichiosis (EGE) in horses, canine granulocytic ehrlichiosis (CGE) in dogs, and for human granulocytic ehrlichiosis (HGE). Human cases have been registered in many countries with a broad range of symptoms and pathogenicity. This article focused on Sardinia as the prevalence in humans was almost seven times higher than in the rest of Italy. To evaluate the risk, blood samples were collected from dogs and horses on the island. Genomic DNA was extracted from the buffy coat and amplified by heminested polymerase chain reaction (PCR) using the *groEL* gene primers. The first PCR reaction amplified a 624-bp fragment for both *A. phagocytophilum* and *A. platys* while the second PCR reaction amplified 573-bp and 515-bp fragments for the above two pathogens, respectively. Six *A. phagocytophilum* samples were PCR positive (3 dogs and 3 horses) while another dog was *A. platys* PCR positive. A phylogenetic analysis was conducted with *A. phagocytophilum* sequences in GenBank from the United States, Slovenia, Switzerland, Germany, UK, Austria, and Czech Republic. Surprisingly, the related phylogenetic tree showed that the Sardinian isolates were closer to the American isolates, which were showing highest mortality rates than from the other two European lineages.

KEYWORDS: Italy; anaplasmosis; ehrlichiosis; dog; horse; PCR

Address for correspondence: Dr. Olivier A.E. Sparagano, School of Agriculture, Food and Rural Development, Newcastle University, Agriculture Building, Newcastle upon Tyne NE1 7RU, UK. Voice: 44-191-2225071; fax: 44-191-2226720.
  e-mail: Olivier.sparagano@ncl.ac.uk

Ann. N.Y. Acad. Sci. 1081: 371–378 (2006). © 2006 New York Academy of Sciences.
doi: 10.1196/annals.1373.055

INTRODUCTION

Human granulocytic ehrlichiosis (HGE) due to *Anaplasma phagocytophilum* (*A. phagocytophilum)* is in fact a multihost pathogen also known as *Ehrlichia equi* in horses, *Ehrlichia phagocytophila* in cattle, and small ruminants. The new taxonomy is now regrouping all these names under the *A. phagocytophilum* cluster.[1] The HGE agent has been found in small ruminants,[2] according to the same colleagues,[3] tick density on sheep can change the transmission pattern of the pathogen. Wildlife animals have also been linked with HGE.[4–6]

A study on forest workers in the region of mideastern Poland found that 45.7%, 4.5%, and 0.9% of the female, male, and nymph ticks were PCR positive for *A. phagocytophilum* with 20.6% of the forest workers showing a seroprevalence for this disease (furthermore, 84.6% of this seroprevalent group was also showing seroprevalence for anti-*Borrelia burgdorferi* antibodies).[7] Prevalence of HGE is currently 6.4 times higher in Sardinia compared to mainland Italy.

This article investigated the prevalence of *A. phagocytophilum* in dogs and horses and the phylogenetic links with already sequenced isolates from worldwide origin.

METHODS

Samples were collected on the west coast of Sardinia (Latitude 40° 00′ N; Longitude 9° 00′ E). Four groups were followed, two groups of dogs (one showing symptoms of TBD and one asymptomatic) and two groups of horses (as for the dogs). DNA was extracted from the buffy coat and *A. phagocytophilum* and *A. platys* were detected by two heminested polymerase chain reactions (PCRs) targeting the *groEL* gene (see FIG. 1). DNAs were also sequenced and compared with existing sequences available in the GeneBank database. Phylogenetic trees were also produced and edited as previously published.[8,9]

Plasmids pAphgroEL and pAplgroEL were generated by cloning two first round PCR products into pCR2.1-TOPO (Invitrogen, Paisley, UK), obtained from field samples of *A. phagocytophilum* and *A. platys*, respectively, and were diluted to 50,000 copies/µL. The limit of detection for the two heminested assays was evaluated with samples for which the number of plasmids containing alternatively *A. phagocytophilum* and *A. platys* amplification products obtained from the first PCR round was previously determined. Twofold dilutions of the two plasmids (pAphgroEL and pAplgroEL) were produced until the concentration of 3 copies/µL was reached. One microliter of each tube of the two dilution series was coupled to 100 ng of calf thymus DNA (Sigma, Poole, UK), and tested by heminested PCR, performed as described above. For each of the two heminested PCR assays, three replicates of

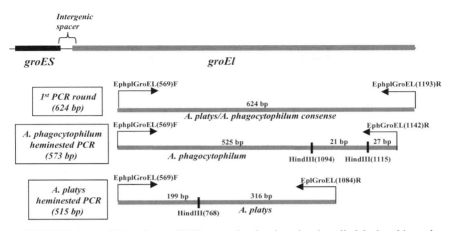

FIGURE 1. *groEL* heminested PCR strategies developed and applied during this study. Numbers in parentheses indicate positions of primers and Hind III restriction sites calculated using the sequence of the *A. phagocytophilum* NCH-1 strain as a consensus.

experiments were independently performed with both GoTaq DNA polymerase (Promega, Southampton, UK) and HotMaster Taq DNA polymerase (Eppendorf, Cambridge, UK), starting from three different twofold series of plasmid dilutions.

In order to evaluate the potential interference determined by the presence of *A. platys* DNA during *A. phagocytophilum* amplifications, all the twofold dilutions of pAphgroEL (from 50,000 copies to 3 copies) were coupled to fixed amounts of pAplgroEL (100, 1000, and 10000 copies) and tested by *A. phagocytophilum*-specific heminested PCR. Similar experiments were performed in order to establish the interference level determined by the presence of *A. phagocytophilum* DNA when testing samples with the heminested PCR specific for *A. platys*. Specificity experiments were repeated independently three times.

The ABI PRISM Big Dye Terminator Cycle Sequencing Ready Reaction Kit (Applied Biosystems, Foster City, CA) was used for direct cycle sequencing of the PCR products obtained, according to the protocol supplied by the manufacturer. To assure that polymorphisms did not represent PCR errors, all the amplicons obtained were cloned into the pCR2.1-TOPO vector (Invitrogen), and three clones/samples were sequenced using universal M13 primers. The generated sequences were edited with CHROMAS (Technelysium Pty. Ltd., Tewantin, Australia) and checked against the GenBank database using BLASTn (European Bioinformatics Institute, Cambridge, UK). After submission, GenBank accession numbers for *A. phagocytophilum* (TABLE 1) and *A. platys* (AY848753) were obtained. In order to confirm the identity of the *groEL* sequences as gene regions peculiar of Sardinian *A. phagocytophilum*

TABLE 1. Variable nucleotide positions of the six new *groEL* sequence type identified in Sardinian horses and dogs and alignment to pathogenic U.S. and European strains

groEL sequence type	Position[a]																		
	5	27	72	74	86	112	120	138	252	261	345	351	381	384	391	408	434	510	525
1-HGESlovSwissGer	A	A	T	T	A	C	A	T	C	G	C	T	A	C	A	G	A	T	A
39-HorseSWEDEN	•[b]	•	•	•	•	•	•	•	T	•	T	•	•	•	•	•	•	•	•
2-HGE USA	•	•	C[c]	•	•	•	•	•	•	A	•	•	G	A	•	T	•	•	G
29-IxodesCalifornia	•	•	C	•	•	•	G	•	•	A	•	•	G	A	•	T	•	•	G
7-ITHorseQuada	•	G	C	•	T	T	G	•	•	A	•	•	G	A	•	T	•	•	G
8-ITHorseDollaro	•	•	C	•	•	•	•	•	•	A	•	•	G	A	G	T	•	•	G
9-ITDogStechi	•	•	C	•	•	•	•	•	•	A	•	A	G	A	•	T	•	•	G
6-ITDogPippo	•	•	C	C	•	•	C	•	•	A	•	•	G	A	•	T	•	C	G
10-ITHorseSogno	T	•	C	•	•	•	•	•	•	A	•	•	G	A	•	T	•	•	G
3-ITDogPerla	•	•	C	•	•	•	•	•	•	A	•	•	G	A	•	T	G	•	G
IT-USA consense	W[d]	R	C	Y	W	Y	R	Y	Y	A	Y	Y	G	A	R	T	R	Y	G

[a] numbering according to the *groEL* partial sequence of *A. phagocytophilum* considered in this study.

[b] a dot indicates a nucleotide identical to the HGE European type sequence.

[c] italic lettering indicates nucleotides are shared by the USA HGE strains and by the strains isolated during this study.

[d] polymorphisms nomenclature according to the International Union of Biochemistry.

and *A. platys* isolates, the edited sequences were aligned to the corresponding region of other species belonging to the genera *Anaplasma* and *Ehrlichia*, using CLUSTALX (IGBMC, Strasbourg, France).

Based on the alignment of all the *A. phagocytophilum groEL* sequences available in the GenBank database with the sequences of *A. phagocytophilum* generated during this study (573 bp), 39 type sequences were identified. The 39 *groEL* type sequences were used as operational taxonomic units (OTUs) for phylogenetic analyses, performed with MEGA version 3.0.[10] Genetic distances among the OTUs were computed as a percentage of total nucleotide differences or by the Kimura two-parameters method and were used to construct neighbor-joining (NJ) trees. Statistical support for internal branches of the trees was evaluated by bootstrapping. Maximum parsimony (MP) trees and consensus values were also generated.

RESULTS AND DISCUSSION

Four percent of the dogs and 8% of the horses from their respective symptomatic groups were PCR positive for *A. phagocytophilum* showing the correct fragment of 573 bp, while samples from the asymptomatic group did not show any positive results.

The six *groEL A. phagocytophilum* amplicons obtained in this study generated a pattern identical to the Hind III digestion pattern obtained from the *A. phagocytophilum* NCH-1 amplification, and to the Hind III pattern predicted for *A. phagocytophilum*.[11]

The limit of detection of the heminested PCR specific for amplification of *A. phagocytophilum* DNA (FIG. 2 A, C, and D), evaluated by testing the twofold dilution series of the plasmid pAphgroEL, was different depending on the polymerase used (3 plasmid copies when using the GoTaq DNA polymerase and 6 plasmid copies with the HotMaster Taq DNA polymerase). Furthermore, the use of the GoTaq DNA polymerase resulted in bands of stronger intensity even at the highest plasmid dilutions. Similar results were obtained with the twofold dilution series of pAplgroEL when testing the limit of detection of the heminested PCR specific for amplification of *A. platys* DNA (FIG. 2 B, E, and F). No interference determined by the presence of *A. platys* DNA during *A. phagocytophilum* amplifications (and *vice versa*) was observed in specificity experiments, conducted as described above.

As recently observed by Massung and Slater[12] when comparing different PCR assays for *A. phagocytophilum* detection, each laboratory should determine the efficacy of any PCR assay within their local environment, including positive and negative controls, the use of replicates, and specificity evaluation. We satisfied the requirements of Massung and Slater,[12] and developed a PCR method able to detect at least three copies of the *groEL* gene of *A. phagocytophilum* or *A. platys*, in the presence of calf DNA. Coinfection

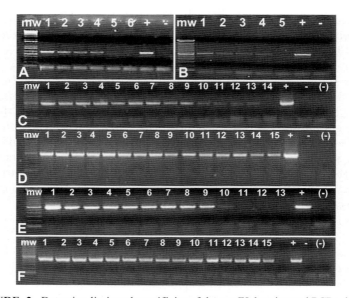

FIGURE 2. Detection limit and specificity of the *groEL*-heminested PCRs developed during this study. (**A**) PCR results obtained from twofold dilutions of plasmid pAph-groEL with primers EphplgroEL(569)F and EphplgroEL(1193)R. (**B**) PCR results obtained from twofold dilutions of plasmid pAplgroEL with primers EphplgroEL(569)F and EphplgroEL(1193)R. (**C**) Heminested PCR results obtained from twofold dilutions of plasmid pAphgroEL with primers EphplgroEL(569)F and EphgroEL(1142)R using HotMaster Taq DNA polymerase. (**D**) Heminested PCR results obtained from twofold dilutions of plasmid pAphgroEL with primers EphplgroEL(569)F and EphgroEL(1142)R using GoTaq DNA polymerase. (**E**) Heminested PCR results obtained from twofold dilutions of plasmid pAplgroEL with primers EphplgroEL(569)F and EplgroEL(1084)R using HotMaster Taq DNA polymerase. (**F**) Heminested PCR results obtained from twofold dilutions of plasmid pAplgroEL with primers EphplgroEL(569)F and EplgroEL(1084)R using HotMaster Taq DNA polymerase. + indicates a PCR positive control, – indicates a PCR negative control (water), (–) indicates a PCR negative control of the first PCR round used as negative control in heminested PCR. Numbers indicate twofold plasmid DNA dilutions, starting from 50,000 copies (1), to 3 copies (15).

with multiple tick-borne pathogens has been extensively described in dogs and other species.[13,14] Our experiments of interference/specificity demonstrated that the presence of different concentrations of *A. platys* DNA during *A. phagocytophilum* amplifications (and *vice versa*) does not affect the PCR limit of detection, thus making the method suitable for amplification from clinical samples even when mixed infections are suspected. Furthermore, when two recombinant Taq polymerases were tested, GoTaq resulted in more evident bands even at the lower DNA target concentrations in twofold dilution experiments.

Sequencing results showed some variability between isolates (see TABLE 1). Surprisingly, the six *A. phagocytophilum* isolates from Sardinia did not link with one of the two European lineages for this pathogen but were closely related to American strains.[15,16] However, considering that the first HGE case on the island of Sardinia was coming from U.S. military based on a U.S. Navy base there are some epidemiological grounds for the origin of the American strains circulating in Sardinia. Work from colleagues for other vector-borne diseases, such as *Theileria annulata* in Sicily[17] or Blue Tongue viruses in Corsica[18] showed that Mediterranean islands sometimes have a different epidemiological situation than the nearest mainland. However, it is important to consider that migratory birds could also have brought *A. phagocytophilum*-infected ticks on the island and more epidemiological studies mainly from North Africa would help to trace similar strains in different countries in the region.

Concluding, molecular analyses are required in order to characterize the *A. phagocytophilum* strains circulating in hosts (especially human) and vectors in the Mediterranean area, and to confirm our observations. For instance, this could be accomplished by using additional highly discriminating phylogenetic probes, such as the *ank* gene, already successfully applied for *A. phagocytophilum* phylogenetic studies at the species and strain levels.[19,20]

REFERENCES

1. DUMLER, J.S., A.F. BARBET, C.P.J. BEKKER, *et al*. 2001. Reorganization of genera in the families Rickettsiaceae and Anaplasmataceae in the order Rickettsiales: unification of some species of Ehrlichia with Anaplasma, Cowdria with Ehrlichia, and Ehrlichia with Neorickettsia, descriptions of six new species combinations and designation of *Ehrlichia equi* and 'HGE agent' as subjective synonyms of Ehrlichia phagocytophila. Int. J. Syst. Evol. Microbiol. **51:** 2145–2165.
2. OGDEN, N.H., A.N.J. CASEY, N.P. FRENCH, *et al*. 2002b. Field evidence for density-dependent facilitation amongst *Ixodes ricinus* ticks feeding on sheep. Parasitology **124:** 117–125.
3. OGDEN, N.H., A.N.J. CASEY, C.H. LAWRIE, *et al*. 2002a. IgG responses to salivary gland extract of *Ixodes ricinus* ticks vary inversely with resistance in naturally exposed sheep. Med. Vet. Entomol. **16:** 186–192.
4. PICHON, B., D. EGAN, M. ROGERS & J. GRAY. 2003. Detection and identification of pathogens and host DNA in unfed host-seeking *Ixodes ricinus* L. (Acari: Ixodidae). J. Med. Entomol. **40:** 723–731.
5. SRETER, T., Z. SRETER-LANCZ, Z. SZELL & D. KALMAN. 2004. *Anaplasma phagocytophilum*: an emerging tick-borne pathogen in Hungary and central Eastern Europe. Ann. Trop. Med. Parasitol. **98:** 401–405.
6. De La FUENTE, J., V. NARANJO, F. RUIZ-FONS, *et al*. 2004. Prevalence of tick-borne pathogens in Ixodid ticks (Acari: Ixodidae) collected from European wild boar (*Sus scrofa*) and Iberian red deer (*Cervus elaphus hispanicus*) in central Spain. Eur. J. Wild. Res. **50:** 187–196.

7. TOMASIEWICZ, K., R. MODRZEWSKA, A. BUCZEK, *et al.* 2004. The risk exposure to *Anaplasma phagocytophilum* infection in Mid-Eastern Poland. Ann. Agr. Envir. Med. **11:** 261–264.
8. MAGNARELLI, L.A., J.S. DUMLER, J.F. ANDERSON, *et al.* 1995. Co-existence of antibodies to tick-borne pathogens of Babesiosis, Ehrlichiosis, and Lyme Borelliosis in human sera. J. Clin. Microbiol. **33:** 3054–3057.
9. MANNA, L., A. ALBERTI, L.M. PAVONE, *et al.* 2004. First molecular characterisation of a granulocytic *Ehrlichia* strain isolated from a dog in South Italy. Vet. J. **167:** 224–227.
10. KUMAR, S., K. TAMURA & M. NEI. 2004. MEGA3: integrated software for molecular evolutionary genetics analysis and sequence alignment. Brief. Bioinform. **5:** 150–163.
11. ALBERTI, A., R. ZOBBA, B. CHESSA, *et al.* 2005. Equine and canine *Anaplasma phagocytophilum* strains isolated on the island of Sardinia (Italy) are phylogenetically closely related to USA pathogenic strains. Appl. Environ. Microbiol. **71:** 6418–6422.
12. MASSUNG, R.F. & K.G. SLATER. 2003. Comparison of PCR assays for detection of the agent of human granulocytic ehrlichiosis, *Anaplasma phagocytophilum*. J. Clin. Microbiol. **41:** 717–722.
13. KORDICK, S.K., E.B. BREITSCHWERDT, K.L. SOUTHWICK, *et al.* 1999. Co-infection with multiple tick-borne pathogens in a Walker Hound kennel in North Carolina. J. Clin. Microbiol. **37:** 2631–2638.
14. SUKSAWAT, J., C. PITULLE, C. ARRAGA-ALVARADO, *et al.* 2001. Co-infection with three *Ehrlichia* species in dogs from Thailand and Venezuela with emphasis on consideration of 16S ribosomal DNA secondary structure. J. Clin. Microbiol. **39:** 90–93.
15. PETROVEC, M.M., J. BIDOVEC, W.L. SUMNER, *et al.* 2002. Infection with *Anaplasma phagocytophila* in cervids from Slovenia: evidence of two genotypic lineages. Wien. Klin. Wochenschr. **114:** 641–647.
16. VON LOEWENICH, F.D., B.U. BAUMGARTEN, K. SCHROPPEL, *et al.* 2003. High diversity of *ankA* sequences of *Anaplasma phagocytophilum* among *Ixodes ricinus* ticks in Germany. J. Clin. Microbiol. **41:** 5033–5040.
17. GEORGES, K., G.R. LORIA, S. RIILI, *et al.* 2001. Detection of haemoparasites in cattle by reverse line blot hybridization with a note on the distribution of ticks in Sicily. Vet. Parasitol. **99:** 273–286.
18. BREARD, E., C. HAMBLIN, C. SAILLEAU, *et al.* 2004. The epidemiology and diagnosis of bluetongue with particular reference to Corsica. Res. Vet. Sc. **77:** 1–8.
19. CHAE, J.S., J.E. FOLEY, J.S. DUMLER & J.E. MADIGAN. 2000. Comparison of the nucleotide sequence of 16S rRNA, 444*Ep-ank*, and groESL heat shock operon genes in natural occurring *Ehrlichia equi* and human granulocytic ehrlichiosis agent isolates from northern California. J. Clin. Microbiol. **38:** 1364–1369.
20. MASSUNG, R.F., J.H. OWENS, D. ROSS, *et al.* 2000. Sequence analysis of the *ank* gene of granulocytic ehrlichiae. J. Clin. Microbiol. **38:** 2917–2922.

Development of an Immunosensor for the Diagnosis of Bovine Anaplasmosis

MARTA SILVA,[a] SILVINA WILKOWSKY,[b]
SUSANA TORIONI DE ECHAIDE,[c] MARISA FARBER,[b]
AND ABEL OLIVA[a]

[a] Instituto de Biologia Experimental e Tecnológica (IBET)/Instituto de Tecnologia Química e Biológica (ITQB), 2781-901 Oeiras, Portugal

[b] Instituto de Biotecnología, Instituto Nacional de Tecnología Agropecuaria (INTA), 1712 Castelar, Argentina

[c] Estacion Experimental Agropecuaria Rafaela, (INTA), 2300 Rafaela, Argentina

ABSTRACT: An optical immunosensor based in major surface protein 5 (MSP5) of *Anaplasma marginale* was developed towards detection of anti-*Anaplasma* sp. antibodies in acute infection as well as in vaccinated cattle. This study was performed using recombinant MSP5 covalently immobilised in controlled pore glass (CPG) beads to detect anti-MSP5 antibodies in serum samples. The quantification is based on the measurement of the Cy5 fluorescence of the detection antibody, anti bovine IgG, after reaction with serum. Sera were collected in enzootic and tick-free regions of Argentina. The immunosensor showed a detection range of 1.2 g/ml to 48 g/ml of antibody in sera, with a sensitivity of 93% and a specificity of 70%. The optical immunosensor developed is suitable for quantification of antibodies in sera of naturally or experimentally infected animals.

KEYWORDS: optical immunosensor; *Anaplasma*; MSP5; veterinary diagnostic

INTRODUCTION

Anaplasmosis, caused by the intraerythrocytic rickettsial pathogen *Anaplasma (A.) marginale,* is the most prevalent tick-borne infection in cattle worldwide, causing significant morbidity and mortality in tropical and subtropical regions.[1,2] In Argentina, anaplasmosis is becoming a more relevant sanitary problem as it is widespread exceeding the limit of tick- infected area. Outbreaks of anaplasmosis in dairy herds outside the known anaplasmosis endemic area in

Address for correspondence: Abel Oliva, Biosensors/Biomolecular Diagnostics Laboratory, Instituto de Biologia Experimental e Tecnológica (IBET)/Instituto de Tecnologia Química e Biológica (ITQB), Apartado 12, P-2781-901 Oeiras, Portugal. Voice: +351-214469427; fax: +351-214421161.
e-mail: oliva@itqb.unl.pt

Ann. N.Y. Acad. Sci. 1081: 379–381 (2006). © 2006 New York Academy of Sciences.
doi: 10.1196/annals.1373.056

the temperate region of the country had already been detected.[3] This situation is a consequence of mechanical transmission via blood-contaminated fomites, being the carriers for *A. marginale,* the introduced animals from enzootic areas.

An immunosensor is generally defined as a sensor combining immuno-compounds with a transducer element. The system takes advantage of the high specificity and sensitivity of antigen–antibody interaction, which is detected by the transduction of a parameter (electron transfer, fluorescence, mass change, thermal variation) into an electrical signal.[4]

Previous work demonstrated that major surface protein 5 (MSP5) is present not only in *A. marginale* but also in *A. centrale,* the low virulence nontick-transmitted vaccine strain, and *A. ovis.* Remarkably, MSP5 protein is broadly conserved among *A. marginale* isolates. We tested the hypothesis that an MSP5-based immunosensor would detect anti-*Anaplasma* sp. antibodies in acute infection as well as in vaccinated and experimentally infected cattle.

MATERIALS AND METHODS

The study was performed using recombinant MSP5 covalently immobilized in controlled pore glass (CPG) beads to detect anti-MSP5 antibodies in serum samples. The immunosensor system was configured as a distal-phase optode. A multimode optical fiber guides the excitation radiation into the flow cell, where the immunoreaction takes place. Fluorescence quantification was achieved using anti-bovine IgG-Cy5(ABIgG-Cy5) and HeNe laser as a light source. Sera were collected in enzootic and tick-free regions of Argentina. The samples were simultaneously tested using competitive ELISA (cELISA)[5] and direct agglutination test (card test) as reference techniques.

RESULTS

First of all, the detection range of the immunosensor was determined with a reference positive antiserum. The immunosensor detection range was 1.2 μg/mL to 48 μg/mL. A total of 32 sera were analyzed. The samples tested were the following: (*a*) 10 sera from an outbreak of *Anaplasma* from a nonen-zootic area, (*b*) 9 sera from vaccinated bovines from a tick-free zone; (*c*) 10 negative sera from a nonenzootic area, and (*d*) 3 sera from vaccinated bovines from an enzootic area. All sera were also analyzed with an indirect ELISA using the same MSP5. The results showed a good concordance with standard serological methods. The sensor had a relative sensitivity of 93% and a rel-ative specificity of 70% when compared with cELISA using ROC analysis. The specificity could be increased if a larger number of negative samples were tested. A good advantage of the immunosensor is that the recombinant MSP5 covalently immobilized in CPG beads can be reused up to 10 times with a loss of fluorescence of 30%.

CONCLUSION

The optical immunosensor developed is sensitive enough for detection of anti-MSP5 antibodies in sera of naturally or experimentally infected animals but its specificity should be improved. Finally, it presents advantages to the standard immunoassay techniques like simplicity, rapidity, and reproducibility

ACKNOWLEDGMENTS

This work was financially supported by Secretaría de Ciencia y Tecnología (SECyT), Argentina and Gabinete de Relações Internacionais da Ciência e do Ensino Superior (GRICES), Portugal, as an international cooperation grant.

REFERENCES

1. WYATT, W.C. *et al*. 1996. Effect on intraerythrocytic Anaplasma marginale of soluble factors from infected calf blood mononuclear cells. Infect. Immun. **64:** 4846–4849.
2. DE LA FUENTE, J. *et al*. 2004. *Anaplasma* infection in free-ranging Iberian red deer in the region of Castilla-LA Mancha, Spain. Vet. Microbiol. **100:** 163–173.
3. GUGLIELMONE, A.A. *et al*. 1997. Different seasonal occurrence of anaplasmosis outbreaks in beef and dairy cattle of an area of Argentina free of *Rhipicephalus microplus*. Vet. Q. **19:** 32–33.
4. CANH, T.M. 1993. General principles. *In* Biosensors. Sensors Physics and Technology Series. Chapman & Hall, London, UK.
5. TORIONI DE ECHAIDE, S. *et al*. 2005. Detection of antibodies against *Anaplasma marginale* in milk using recombinant MSP5 indirect ELISA. Vet. Microbiol. **106:** 287–292.

Identification of Common Antigens in *Babesia bovis*, *B. bigemina*, and *B. divergens*

JULIO V. FIGUEROA,[a] ERIC PRECIGOUT,[b†] BERNARD CARCY,[b]
AND ANDRÉ GORENFLOT[b]

[a]*CENID-PAVET, INIFAP, Jiutepec, Morelos, 62550, Mexico*

[b]*Laboratoire Biologie Cellulaire et Moléculaire, Fac de Pharmacie,
Université Montpellier I, Montpellier, 34000, France*

[†]*Deceased.*

ABSTRACT: Bovine babesiosis, caused by *Babesia bovis*, *B. bigemina*, and
B. divergens, is a significant impediment to livestock production in countries with tropical/subtropical and temperate climates. Previous studies
conducted on the immunoprophylaxis against the disease and diagnosis of these parasites has demonstrated the presence of similar antigens.
The objective of this article was to identify and partially characterize
antigens conserved among these three species. Immunochemical analysis using sera from cattle immunized individually with antigens from
these three *Babesia* species revealed a number of antigens recognized by
heterologous antisera. Cross-reactions were more evident in sera from
cattle immunized with *B. bovis*/*B. bigemina* which recognized several
antigens (15 kDa to >200 kDa) in *B. divergens*. Immunoscreening of a
B. divergens cDNA library with bovine serum to *B. bigemina* allowed the
isolation of five clones and DNA sequencing of plasmid BdJF5 showed
a 680 bp cDNA insert. Basic Local Alignment Search Tool (BLAST)
analysis of the predicted amino acid sequence revealed 47% identity
with a protein identified as α NAC. Serum from mice immunized with a
recombinant Glutathione S-Transferase-BdJF5 fusion protein immunoprecipitated a 20 kDa *B. bovis* antigen. However, 30 kDa and 18 kDa
antigens were immunoprecipitated from *B. divergens* and immunoblotting analysis revealed the recognition of a 35 kDa *B. bigemina* antigen. An
indirect fluorescence antibody assay on merozoites showed strong reaction with *B. divergens* and weak recognition of *B. bovis* and *B. bigemina*.
Despite the existent antigenic polymorphism among the *Babesia* spp.,

Address for correspondence: Dr. Julio V. Figueroa, CENID-PAVET, INIFAP, Apartado Postal 206,
CIVAC, Morelos, 62550 Mexico. Voice: +52-777-3-192850; ext.: 139; fax: +52-777-3-192850; ext.:
129.

e-mail: figueroa.julio@inifap.gob.mx

Ann. N.Y. Acad. Sci. 1081: 382–396 (2006). © 2006 New York Academy of Sciences.
doi: 10.1196/annals.1373.057

these results demonstrated that common antigens occur between European *B. divergens* and Mexican *B. bovis/B. bigemina.*

KEYWORDS: *Babesia bovis*; *b. bigemina*; *b. divergens*; common antigens; αNAC protein

INTRODUCTION

Babesiosis is a tick-transmitted disease of mammalian hosts, caused by the intraerythrocytic protozoan parasites of the genus *Babesia*, and manifested by anemia, fever, occasional hemoglobinuria, and death.[1] More than 70 species of *Babesia* have been listed in the phylum apicomplexa,[2] and several species of *Babesia* of cattle have been reported in the literature: *B. divergens*, *B. bovis*, *B. bigemina*, *B. major*, *B. ovata*, *B. jakimovi*, *B. beliceri*, and *B. occultans*.[3,4] These species are distributed worldwide, and on a global basis bovine babesiosis is considered one of the most important tick vector-borne infections of ruminants.[4-6] Babesiosis persists in tropical and semitropical regions of the world between the 32nd parallel south and the 40th parallel north of the equator.[4,7] With its wide geographic distribution, it exerts an important economic impact on livestock industries, especially in developing countries. Approximately one-half billion cattle throughout the world may be endangered by the disease caused by species of *Babesia*.[7] The economic impact of the disease includes losses due to death or production loss in terms of milk or meat production.[1,4,5] It has been found that due to vector distribution, concomitant or multiple infections in the host can occur in endemic areas. Consequently, two or more *Babesia* species of cattle may be microscopically found in clinical cases.[8] Most common, however, is the case in which there is serological cross-reactivity among the babesial antigens, particularly when the indirect fluorescent antibody test (IFAT) is used in trying to differentiate the *Babesia* species involved in the infection of cattle.[9,10] The latter has motivated researchers to develop more sensitive and specific assays by identifying the species-specific antigens recognized by antibodies in the serum of infected animals with a particular species.[10,11] In this attempt, the presence of several cross-reactive antigenic components has been described,[12,13] including immunogenic material that induces protection in cattle against a challenge with the heterologous *Babesia* species.[13]

In search of this type of antigenic components that could potentially be used as a multi-purpose *Babesia* immunogen, we report on the identification of cross-reactive epitopes existing in *B. bovis*, *B. bigemina*, and *B. divergens* by use of immunochemical assays. The isolation of a cDNA clone from a *B. divergens* gene library is also reported, the sequence of which encodes a deduced amino acid sequence with homology to the protein denominated αNAC (Nascent-polypeptide Associated Complex, α chain).

MATERIALS AND METHODS

Source of Parasite Antigen

B. bovis and *B. bigemina* parasites from Mexico were cultivated *in vitro* under standard culture conditions.[14,15] *B. divergens* was cultured in human O[+] erythrocytes essentially as described previously.[16]

Source of Bovine Immune Serum

Samples from four cattle immunized with a *B. bovis* culture-derived population,[17] four serum samples from cattle immunized with a *B. bigemina* culture-derived population,[17] and one sample from a bovine immunized and challenged with *B. divergens*[18] were used in the immunochemical assays.

Biosynthetic Labeling of Parasite

B. bovis and *B. divergens* cultures were expanded to 25 cm^2 culture flasks, and [^{35}S]methionine metabolic labeling of parasite polypeptides was accomplished as follows: At 24-h postinitiation of cultures, the culture supernatant was replaced with complete culture medium supplemented with [^{35}S]L-methionine to a final concentration of 50 μCi/mL of culture (specific activity $(3.7 \times 10^4$ GBq/mmol^{-1}, Amersham, Buckinghamshire, England). Cultures were returned to the incubator and incubated at 37°C for 12 hours.[19]

Antigen Solubilization

For immunoprecipitation and/or immunoblotting analysis of parasite components, cultured *Babesia* parasites were extracted for 1 h at 0–4°C in nine volumes of extraction buffer [2% Triton X-100, 0.6 M KCl, 0.15 M NaCl, 5 mM EDTA, 0.01 M Tris-HCl, pH 7.8, 1 mM phenylmethylsulfonyl fluoride (PMSF), and 0.1 mM N-tosyl-L-lysine chloromethyl ketone (TLCK)]. The extract was then centrifuged at 15,600g for 15 min 4°C to remove the insoluble material. The supernatant was removed and kept at −70°C. Preparations of normal bovine erythrocytes cultures were solubilized, and the components extracted in a similar manner.[19]

Immunoprecipitation

The assay included the overnight incubation of 1 × 10^6 cpm of radiolabeled antigen incubated overnight at 4°C with 5 μL of bovine immune serum (BIS) or mouse serum samples. The antigen/antibody complex was precipitated by adding 75 μL of Protein G-Sepharose (Pharmacia Biotech, Uppsala, Sweden) during 1 h at room temperature. Reaction tubes were then washed twice by centrifugation (13,600g, for 2 min at 4°C) with washing buffer A [20 mM Tris HCl, pH 7.5, 5 mM EDTA, 100 mM NaCl (TEN), 1% Nonidet-P40, 1% BSA]; four times with washing buffer B (TEN, 1% NP-40, 2 mM NaCl); and twice with washing buffer C (TEN, 1% NP-40). Bound [35S]methionine-labeled antigens were eluted with sodium dodecyl sulphate (SDS) sample buffer for electrophoretic analysis.

SDS-PAGE

The [35S]methionine-labeled parasite antigens immunoprecipitated by the procedure described above were boiled for 5 min in sample buffer containing 62.5 mM tris-HCl, pH 6.8, 3% SDS, 20% glycerol, and 5% 2-mercaptoethanol. Samples were analyzed by separation of components in 10 cm × 16 cm slab gels using a 12% discontinuous gel system.[20] The separating gel from the immunoprecipitation experiment was processed for fluorography, before drying for exposure to X-OMAT XAR5 film (Eastman Kodak, Rochester, NY).

Immunoblotting

The electrophoresed proteins from unlabeled material were transferred from the gel onto a sheet of nitrocellulose as described before.[21] The electrophoretic transfer of polypeptide bands was performed at room temperature at 100 mA for 1 h using a semi-dry transfer unit (Transfor, Biorad, Marnes-la-Coquette, France). Blocking of the nitrocellulose sheets, incubation with primary and secondary antibodies and substrate color development were carried out essentially as described previously.[19]

B. divergens cDNA Clones

Six clones containing recombinant pBK-CMV plasmids (pBDJF1 to pBdJF6) derived from a screening performed with BIS to *B. bigemina* on a *B. divergens* cDNA library[22] constructed in the λZAP II vector (Stratagene, Amsterdam, The Netherlands) were originally isolated. Clones were subjected to the *in vivo* excision of plasmids as recommended by the manufacturer and processed by the alkaline lysis method for plasmid purification.[23]

Restriction Enzyme Digestion of pBdJF Clones and Sequencing

Babesia divergens cDNA present on pBdJF clones was double-digested with *Eco*RI/*Xho*I, restriction enzymes as recommended by the manufacturer

(Life Technologies, Paisley, UK). Digested DNA was separated by agarose gel electrophoresis and visualized by ultraviolet light exposure.[23] An aliquot of purified plasmid pBdJF5 was sent out for sequencing to Genome Express S.A. (Meylan, France). The sequencing reaction was performed by the dideoxychain-termination method[24] on both strands of the cDNA insert.

Expression of Glutathione S-Transferase-BdJF5 Fusion Protein

The *Eco*RI/*Xho*I fragment of the encoding amino acid sequence of the *B. divergens* cDNA was excised from the pBdJF5 recombinant plasmid and subcloned into the *Eco*RI/*Xho*I-digested, phosphatase-treated pGEX-4T3 expression vector (Pharmacia Biotech). Positive clones were selected from transformed *Escherichia coli* (Sure strain) by using *Eco*RI/*Xho*I restriction enzyme digestion analysis. Glutathione *S*-transferase (GST)-BdJF5 fusion protein was overexpressed in BL 21 cells transformed with the recombinant plasmid according to the manufacturer's protocols (Pharmacia Biotech). Culture of transformed *E. coli* BL 21 cells, induction of expression and purification of the recombinant protein was performed as described before.[19]

Production of Polyclonal Antibodies to GST-BdJF5 Fusion Protein

The production of polyclonal antibodies to the GST-BdJF5 fusion protein was carried out by immunizing mice three times, 3 weeks apart, with 10 μg of fusion protein emulsified with complete Freund's adjuvant (first immunization) and incomplete Freund's adjuvant (second and third immunizations).

Indirect Fluorescent Antibody Test

The IFAT on acetone-fixed, parasite-infected erythrocytes was carried out as described before.[19] Infected erythrocytes smears made out of *in vitro*-cultured parasites were reacted with 1:50 dilution of serum collected from the mice immunized with GST fusion protein. Pre-immune mouse serum diluted 1:50 in phosphate-buffered saline was used as a negative control. In addition, a polyclonal antibody developed in gerbils against *B. divergens*[16] was included in the test as positive control. The antigen slides were allowed to incubate at 37°C for 30 min and washed with phosphate buffered saline (PBS) three times for 5 min. The antigen slides were reacted with sheep anti-mouse IgG-FITC conjugate (Sigma-Aldrich Chimie, Lyon, France), and incubated for a further 30 min. After three washes in PBS, smears were examined on an epifluorescent light microscope.

RESULTS

The immunoblot analysis showed that besides revealing a number of antigenic components recognized by antibodies present in the homologous system, the BIS to *B. bigemina* recognized cross-reactive epitopes present on three well-defined bands in the *B. bovis*-infected erythrocyte extract (50 kDa, 70 kDa, and 95 kDa) in addition to a smear of antigenically minor components (FIG. 1 A, lane 7). The 95 kDa and 70 kDa bands were also reacted within the *B. divergens*-infected erythrocyte extract (FIG. 1 A, lane 6). Moreover, the 95 kDa cross-reactive antigen present in *B. divergens* was also detected in the culture supernatant of this species (FIG. 1, lane 5). By comparison, when similar blots were reacted with BIS to *B. bovis*, although weakly, the 95 kDa band was cross-reactive in the *B. divergens* and *B. bigemina* corpuscular antigen extracts (FIG. 1 A, lanes 2 and 4, respectively). Immunoblot analysis of parasite culture supernatants revealed again the 95 kDa band present in *B. divergens* (FIG. 1 C, lane 6). However, two major components of >130 kDa were detected in culture supernatants of *B. bovis* and *B. bigemina* (FIG. 1 C, lanes 7 and 8). Conversely, even though the BIS to *B. divergens* reacted strongly with several major antigenic components of *B. divergens*, apparently it did not recognize corpuscular *B. bovis* or *B. bigemina* antigens (FIG. 1 B, lanes 3 and 4). However, and rather weakly, a 95-kDa component was reactive in the culture supernatant of *B. bovis* antigen (FIG. 1 B, lane 7), whereas a band of approximately 40 kDa was recognized in the *B. bigemina* culture supernatant (FIG. 1 C, lane 8). The 95 kDa *B. divergens* soluble antigen was also detected with the BIS to *B. divergens*, in addition to two other minor components of 40 kDa and 15 kDa (FIG. 1 B, lane 6). Contrary to what was observed on the immunoblots, FIGURE 2 shows a more defined and higher number of parasite polypeptides immunoprecipitated either with the species-homologous or -heterologous BIS. Out of the more than

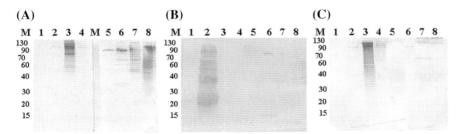

FIGURE 1. Immunoblot analysis of *Babesia* antigens. Panel **A**: lanes 1 and 5, *B. divergens* culture supernatant; lanes 2 and 6, *B. divergens*-infected erythrocytes (IE); lanes 3 and 7, *B. bovis* IE; lanes 4 and 8, *B. bigemina* IE; lanes 1–4, reacted with BIS to *B. bovis*; lanes 5–8, reacted with BIS to *B. bigemina*. Panels **B** and **C**: lane 1, uninfected erythrocytes; lane 2; *B. divergens*-IE; lane 3, *B. bovis*-IE; lane 4, *B. bigemina*-IE; lanes 5–8; culture supernatants, same identification as in lanes 1–4. Panel **B**: reacted with BIS to *B. divergens*. Panel **C**: reacted with BIS to *B. bovis*.

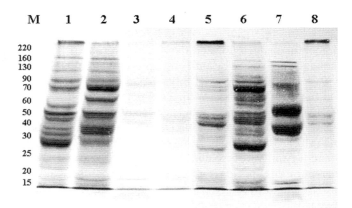

FIGURE 2. Immunoprecipitation assay of [^{35}S]methionine-labeled *Babesia* parasites reacted with BIS to *Babesia* sp. Lanes 1–4: *B. bovis* protein extract reacted with BIS to *B. bovis* (1); BIS to *B. bigemina* (2); BIS to *B. divergens* (3); and uninfected bovine serum (4). Lanes 5–8: *B. divergens* protein extract reacted with BIS to *B. bovis* (5); BIS to *B. bigemina* (6); BIS to *B. divergens* (7); and uninfected bovine serum (8).

20 *B. bovis* antigens immunoprecipitated with the homologous BIS to *B. bovis* (relative sizes from 15 kDa to >220 kDa), cross-reactivity was demonstrated for most, if not all, the *B. bovis* polypeptides when immunoprecipitated with BIS to *B. bigemina*. The major antigenic bands precipitated were those with relative sizes of 70 kDa, 60 kDa, 50kDa, 40 kDa, and 35 kDa (FIG. 2, lane 2). The heterologous BIS to *B. divergens* immunoprecipitated, albeit very weakly, the 70 kDa, 60 kDa, and 50 kDa polypeptides present in *B. bovis* (FIG. 2, lane 3). Immunoprecipitation assays carried out with *B. divergens* as antigen showed that up to 15 *B. divergens* antigenic bands were clearly immunoprecipitated with anti-*B. bigemina* serum (FIG. 2, lane 6), highlighting the 90 kDa, 70 kDa, 60 kDa, 50 kDa, and 30 kDa bands as the more abundant in the precipitates. Although less strongly, these *B. divergens* polypeptides were also immunoprecipitated with the BIS to *B. bovis* (FIG. 2, lane 5). The *B. divergens* polypeptides with relative sizes of 45 kDa and 40 kDa immunoprecipitated with both the BIS to *B. bigemina* and to *B. bovis* were considered nonspecific, as they were also immunoprecipitated with normal bovine serum (FIG. 2, lane 8). To confirm these results four species-heterologous BIS to *B. bigemina* were utilized. As it can be observed in FIGURE 3, lanes 1–4, out of the more than 20 *B. bovis* antigens immunoprecipitated with four different species-homologous BIS to *B. bovis,* up to 16 *B. bovis* polypeptides were also immunoprecipitated with four different species-heterologous BIS to *B. bigemina* (FIG. 3, lanes 5–9). The immunoprecipitated bands were considered *bona fide* and specific as demonstrated by the reaction provided by the immunoprecipitation of *B. bovis* antigen with normal bovine serum (FIG. 3, lane 9). Similar results were observed when

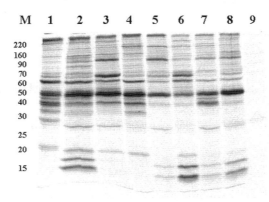

FIGURE 3. Immunoprecipitation assay of [^{35}S]Methionine-labeled *B. bovis* parasites reacted with BIS from cattle infected with *B. bovis* and *B. bigemina*. Lanes 1–4, *B. bovis* protein extract reacted with BIS to *B. bovis*. Lanes 5–8, *B. bovis* protein extract reacted with BIS to *B. bigemina*. Lane 9, *B. bovis* protein extract reacted with uninfected bovine serum.

the four different species-heterologous BIS to *B. bovis* and to *B. bigemina* were tested by immunoprecipitation against *B. divergens* radiolabeled antigen, that is, up to 15 *B. divergens* bands were precipitated with the species-heterologous sera (not shown, but see FIG. 2, lanes 5 and 6), having higher cross-reactivity for those polypeptides with relative sizes of 90 kDa, 70 kDa, 60 kDa, 50 kDa, and 30 kDa.

Six clones were originally isolated from the *B. divergens* cDNA library and plasmids from five clones were identified to contain cDNA inserts of approximately 600 bp as demonstrated by restriction enzyme analysis (*Eco*RI/*Xho*I double digestion) and agarose gel electrophoresis (not shown). Sequence analysis of the cDNA insert of *B. divergens* carried by pBdJF5 revealed a nucleotide stretch of 684 residues in length (nucleotide sequence deposited in the GenBank database under accession number DQ138321). FIGURE 4 shows that the cDNA insert contained a 593 bp long open-reading frame, between nucleotide position numbers 25 (corresponding to a initiation codon ATG) and 618 (corresponding to a stop codon TAA). This unique open-reading frame would code for a 197 translated amino acid sequence of a protein with a predicted size of 21,151 Daltons and an isoelectric point of 4.98 (Protean module, Lasergene software, DNAStar, Madison, WI). The nucleotide sequence was translated using Editseq (Lasergene Package, DNAStar) and the deduced amino acid sequence was submitted to PSI-BLAST at the NCBI website (http://www.ncbi.nlm.nih.gov/BLAST). The search revealed sequences with significant alignments (47% and 45% protein sequence identity) with a putative αNAC-like protein of the protozoan parasites *Theileria annulata* (Accession No. CAI76866) and *T. parva* (Accession No. EAN32216), respectively. The IFAT was utilized to determine the distribution of the BdJF5 protein. As

```
GCA CGA GAA AAA GTT GAG GGC ACT ATG GCC GAG CCT GTG GAG GAC AGC GTT GAC GAG ATC    60
                                M   A   E   P   V   E   D   S   V   D   E   I    12
TCC AGT GAA GGT GAT TCA GAC GTT GAA GAA TCC AAG GGT CCG GAG GGA AGC GCG CCC AAA   120
 S   S   E   G   D   S   D   V   E   E   S   K   G   P   E   G   S   A   P   K    32
AAC CGG CAG GAC AAG AAC GAG CGC AAA TCA CGC AAA CTT CTT GGG AAG CTT GGT ATG AAA   180
 N   R   Q   D   K   N   E   R   K   S   R   K   L   L   G   K   L   G   M   K    52
CCT GTT GAT GGT GTA ACC AAG GTC TGC ATC AAG AAG TCC AAG CAG ATT TAC TTC GTT GTC   240
 P   V   D   G   V   T   K   V   C   I   K   K   S   K   Q   I   Y   F   V   V    72
AAC AAG CCC GAC GTG TAC AAG TTG CCC AAC TCG GAC ACC TAT GTG ATC TTC GGA GAG GCT   300
 N   K   P   D   V   Y   K   L   P   N   S   D   T   Y   V   I   F   G   E   A    92
AAG GTT GAG GAC ATG AGC CAA AAC AGC GCG CTG GAG GCG GCT CAG AGG TTG TCT CAG CTG   360
 K   V   E   D   M   S   Q   N   S   A   L   E   A   A   Q   R   L   S   Q   L   112
TCA TCT GCG CTG CAG GCT GTG GGT GCT GAC CGC GGC ACT GAT TCC TCC GCT GCA GCT CAC   420
 S   S   A   L   Q   A   V   G   A   D   R   G   T   D   S   S   A   A   A   H   132
GCC TCT GGC CAT GAC CAT GCA CAT GAT CAC GAT CAC TCA CAT GGC GAT TGT GCA TCA AAG   480
 A   S   G   H   D   H   A   H   D   H   D   H   S   H   G   D   C   A   S   K   152
GCA GAC GAG TCT TCA GTC AAC CAA AGT GAC ATT GAC CTG GTA GTT AGC CAG GTT GGG TGT   540
 A   D   E   S   S   V   N   Q   S   D   I   D   L   V   V   S   Q   V   G   C   172
ACC CGT GAA CAG GCT GTA GAG GCG CTG ATT AAG AAC AAG GGT GAC ATA GTG GAG ACC ATA   600
 T   R   E   Q   A   V   E   A   L   I   K   N   K   G   D   I   V   E   T   I   192
ATG CAG CTT TCA ACC TAA CTG TAA AAA CCG TAC TAA TTT TGG TAT GAA TTA GCT TAA AAA   660
 M   Q   L   S   T                                                               197
AAAAAAAAAAACTCGGTCATAGCT                                                         684
```

FIGURE 4. DNA sequence of *Babesia divergens* cDNA insert from clone pBdJF5 and deduced amino acid sequence. The ATG start initiation site and TAA stop site are underlined. The stretch of amino acid residues identified as the NAC domain (60 residues) from position 37 (K) to 96 (H) is bold underlined.

demonstrated in FIGURE 5 D, the serum from a mouse immunized with the GST-BdJF5 fusion protein and tested against acetone-fixed *B. divergens*-infected erythrocytes contained antibodies that reacted primarily, in a diffuse pattern, with merozoite-stage parasite bodies. The mouse pre-immune serum did not contain antibodies that would bind to the parasite or red cell ghosts (FIG. 5 C). The control sera used in the assay, Gerbil immune serum to *B. divergens* (FIG. 5 A), and uninfected gerbil serum (FIG. 5 B), showed that the fluorescent staining of *B. divergens* merozoites is an authentic and specific reaction. Importantly, the expression of a parasite component similar to BdJF5 protein was identified in the other two species of *Babesia* tested, that is, *B. bigemina* (FIG. 5 E) and *B. bovis* (FIG. 5 F). To confirm the parasite expression of the BdJF5 protein (or its homolog) in the *Babesia* species analyzed in this study, immunoprecipitation assays with ^{35}S-methionine-labeled parasite extracts showed that the polyclonal mouse anti-GST-BdJF5 antibodies prepared by inoculating mice with the recombinant protein, reacted primarily with a 20 kDa *B. bovis* antigen, and only weakly with a doublet of approximately 30 kDa (FIG. 6 A, lane 3). The specificity of the reaction was demonstrated when reacting the same antigen with mouse pre-immune serum (FIG. 6 A,

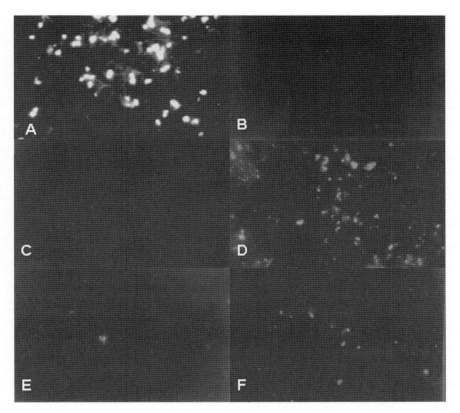

FIGURE 5. Indirect fluorescent antibody test. *B. divergens* infected erythrocytes (IE) (**A**), (**B**), (**C**), and (**D**); *B. bigemina*-IE (**E**) and *B. bovis*-IE (**F**) were reacted with anti-*B. divergens* gerbil immune serum (**A**), uninfected gerbil serum (**B**), pre-immune mouse serum (**C**), and immune mouse serum anti-recombinant protein GST-BdJF5 (**D**), (**E**), and (**F**). All reactions were revealed with rabbit anti-mouse IgG-FITC conjugate.

lanes 1 and 2). The 30 kDa doublet and an 18 kDa protein were strongly immunoprecipitated from extracts containing *B. divergens* antigens (FIG. 6 A, lane 4). When comparing the mouse immunoprecipitation reactions with the bovine immunoprecipitation reactions side by side, it became evident that even though bands with similar relative mobility were weakly immunoprecipitated with the bovine sera, seemingly these parasite antigens are not naturally highly immunogenic as demonstrated by the immunoprecipitation assays carried out with BIS to *B. bovis* (FIG. 6 A, lane 5) and BIS to *B. divergens* (FIG. 6 A, lane 8).

As *B. bigemina* radioactive material was not available, electrophoresed *Babesia* proteins were transferred to nitrocellulose, and the membrane reacted with the mouse immune serum to the GST-BdJF5 recombinant protein. Two components were recognized (approximate calculated molecular mass of

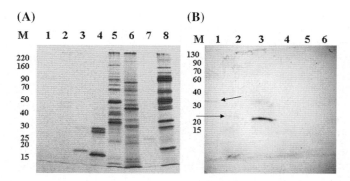

FIGURE 6. (**A**) Immunoprecipitation assay of [^{35}S]methionine-labeled *Babesia* parasites reacted with mouse or BIS to *Babesia* sp. Lanes 1, 3, 5, and 7, *B. bovis* protein extracts. Lanes 2, 4, 5, and 6, *B. divergens* protein extracts. Lanes 1 and 2, immunoprecipitation (IP) with mouse pre-immune serum; lanes 3 and 4, IP with mouse immune serum to GST-BdJF5; lanes 5 and 6, IP with BIS to *B. bovis*; and lanes 7 and 8, IP with BIS to *B. divergens*. (**B**) Immunoblot analysis with mouse immune serum to recombinant protein GST-BdJF5. Lane 1, *B. bigemina*-infected erythrocytes (IE); lane 2, *B. bovis*-IE; lane 3, *B. divergens*-IE; and lanes 4–6, culture supernatants of *B. bigemina*, *B. bovis,* and *B. divergens,* respectively.

30 kDa and ≈20 kDa) by the immunized mouse serum in the *B. divergens* sample (FIG. 6 B lane 3); only one component (≈35 kDa) was weakly detected in the *B. bigemina* antigen extract (FIG. 6 B, lane 1), and the only antigen weakly recognized in the *B. bovis* antigen extract had an estimated size of 20 kDa (FIG. 6 B, lane 2). None of these *Babesia* sp. components was recognized in the culture supernatant (FIG. 6 B, lanes 4–6).

DISCUSSION

In order to identify the cross-reactive epitopes existing in *B. bovis*, *B. bigemina,* and *B. divergens*, immunoblotting analysis of parasite-infected red blood cell extracts reacted with species-specific BIS was initially carried out. That antigens being common to *B. bovis* and *B. bigemina* exist has been previously demonstrated by immunoblotting analysis, in which bovine antiserum to *B. bigemina* or to *B. bovis* avidly stained the homologous and heterologous antigens, revealing a two-way cross-reactivity.[13] More importantly, a protective immune response was induced in 75% of the calves immunized with an enriched *B. bigemina* antigenic fraction (containing the cross-reactive components) against an heterologous *B. bovis* challenge.[13] Recently, studies conducted by Western blot analysis of *B. bovis* antigen tested with BIS to *B. divergens*, showed cross-reactivity with a band of 183 kDa.[10] However, no cross-reactivity was demonstrated for *B. bigemina* antigens when *B. bovis*, *B. divergens,* and *B. major* heterologous immune sera were tested, whereas antigenic preparations of these parasite species displayed considerable cross-reactivity when tested against the heterologous immune sera.[10]

To precisely define and confirm that the cross-reactive components detected in the immunoblots were derived from the Babesia parasites, [35S]methionine-labeled polypeptides were immunoprecipitated with homologous and heterologous BIS and separated by SDS-PAGE. The major cross-reactive *B. bovis* antigens immunoprecipitated with BIS to *B. bigemina* were those with relative sizes of 70 kDa, 60, kDa, 50kDa, 40 kDa, and 35 kDa; and components with relative sizes of 90 kDa, 70 kDa, 60 kDa, 50 kDa, and 30 kDa were more abundant in the immunoprecipitates using *B. divergens* as antigen. Other researchers have previously reported on the identification of 16 *B. bigemina* and eight *B. bovis* merozoite proteins containing species cross-reactive epitopes, when species-heterologous immunoprecipitation studies were conducted.[12] In general, based on the immunoprecipitation results, it appears that the BIS serum to *B. bigemina* contains antibodies which more avidly react with both *B. bovis* and *B. divergens* antigenic components. That this is not a haphazard result based on the use of only one serum sample can be demonstrated by the immunoprecipitation results obtained when four other BIS samples to *B. bigemina* were used. As for the cross-reactive immunoprecipitation studies with the *B. bigemina* antigen, an insufficient number of live parasites precluded the appropriate [35S]methionine-labeling of *B. bigemina* merozoites. Nonetheless, and based on the results of previous studies in which a two-way cross-reaction between *B. bovis* and *B. bigemina* antigens has been demonstrated,[11,12] a different scenario would not be expected. This, however, would perhaps not be the case for the *B. bigemina*/*B. divergens* species-heterologous antigen system, in which the cross-reactive antigen analysis has only been conducted by Western blots.[10] As it has been shown in this study, even though the immunoblotting is highly specific, it appears that it lacks analytical sensitivity as compared to the immunoprecipitation technique, at least with the antigens prepared and utilized here. Analysis of the pBdJF5 cDNA sequence using the PSI-BLAST application program[25] revealed sequences with significant alignments (47% and 45% protein sequence identity) with a putative αNAC-like protein of the protozoan parasites *T. annulata* (Accession No. CAI76866) and *T. parva* (Accession No. EAN32216), respectively. The BLAST search showed that the BdJF5 cDNA-encoded protein also shared similarities and identities with αNAC proteins from a large number of organisms including those from the apicomplexan parasites *Plasmodium falciparum*, *P. berghei*, *P. chabaudi*, *P. yoelii*, *Cryptosporidium parvum*, and *C. hominis*. To identify the possible conserved domains present in the BdJF5 deduced sequence, a Conserved Domain Database[26] search was conducted by submitting the sequence to http://www.ncbi.nlm.nih.gov/Structure/cdd/cdd.shtml. In effect, the search produced significant alignments with pfam01849, NAC (αNAC domain sequences) and COG1308, EGD2 (a domain present in a transcription factor homologous to αNAC). Moreover, by using the

Conserved Domain Architecture Retrieval Tool (CDART),[27] also available at NCBI (http://www.ncbi.nlm.nih.gov/Structure/lexington/lexington.cgi), the search showed significant alignments with a family of 201 protein sequences associated with basic transcription functions of the Eukaryota which contained a NAC single domain. The search results included the putative Transcription factor B3 of *T. parva* (Accession No. EAN32376), the putative Nascent-polypeptide Associated Complex, α subunit of *T. parva* (Accession no. EAN32216) and a putative Transcription factor Btf3 homolog of *T. annulata* (Accession no. CA174885). The CDART search showed that the deduced BdJF5 sequence had protein architecture similarities with three sequences having both, the NAC and the EGD2 domains: a putative NAC of *P. berghei* (Accession no. XP-673748); a putative NAC of *P. chabaudi* (Accession No. CAH79122); and putative transcription factor homologous to αNAC from *P. yoelii* (Accesion No. EAA20799). Moreover, 23 protein sequences having exclusively the EGD2 domain resulted from the CDART search. This group of sequences included that from the *T. annulata* putative NAC, α chain (Accession No. CA176866). The stretch of amino acid residues covered by the NAC domain in the BdJF5 deduced amino acid sequence (60 residues) starts on position 37 (K) up to position 96 (H), whereas the putative EGD2 domain present in the BdJF5 sequence encompassed residues 38 to 196. It has been reported that αNAC prevents short ribosome-associated nascent polypeptides from inappropriate interactions with proteins in the cytosol[28] and purified NAC from bovine brain consists of two polypeptides with apparent molecular masses of 33 and 22 kDa[28] when resolved by SDS-PAGE. However, under nondenaturing conditions on PAGE purified NAC migrated as a single moiety. Furthermore, when NAC is analyzed by mass spectrometry, three peaks are obtained that correspond to the predicted molecular masses of αNAC (22,492 Da), βNAC (17,352 Da) and the heterodimeric complex (40,864 Da).[29] As noted by the authors, the differences in the calculated and apparent molecular masses deduced by SDS-PAGE are not the result of modifications but of an unusual running behavior in SDS-PAGE.[29] Based on the predicted size of the molecule (21,151 Da) and on the homology search results, the protein encoded by the cDNA present in BdJF5 most probably is the α chain of the NAC complex. There seemed to be a particular compartmentalization or accumulation of BdJF5 protein in the interior of the merozoite as evidenced by the dotted staining pattern observed after incubation with the mouse immune serum. However, the specific site for accumulation of the BdJF5 protein cannot be resolved at this time. Immunolocalization with confocal or electron microscopy studies will have to be carried out to determine the compartment localization of αNAC-like protein. In conclusion, despite the existent antigenic polymorphism present among the *Babesia* spp. of cattle analyzed in this study, we were able to identify common antigens that are shared between geographically and biologically different species, i.e., the European *B. divergens* and the Mexican *B. bovis*/*B. bigemina* transmitted by *Ixodes* and *Boophilus* ticks, respectively. Moreover, an immunogenically minor parasite component was identified in the three *Babesia* spp. studied. The parasite protein may be considered as a novel αNAC-like protein. Future immunization studies in cattle will have to be conducted to define the protective potential, if any, of the babesial αNAC.

ACKNOWLEDGMENTS

Financial support for this study was received in part from the Ministére d'Education Nationale et la Researche, France, and SAGARPA-CONACyT, Mexico, Project No. 2003-C01-139. The Mexican *Babesia* parasites and the bovine serum samples were kindly provided by Dr. J. Antonio Alvarez at the Hemoparasite Research Unit, CENID-PAVET, INIFAP.

REFERENCES

1. McCosker, P.J. 1981. The global importance of babesiosis. *In* Babesiosis. M. Ristic & J.P. Kreier, Eds.: 1–24. Academic Press. New York, NY.
2. Levine, N.D. *et al.* 1980. A newly revised classification of the protozoa. J. Protozool. **27:** 37–58.
3. Morel, P.C. 2000. Maladies à tiques du bétail en Afrique. *In* Précis De Parasitologie Véterinaire Tropicale. Éditions Médicales Nationales, Éds: 519–574. Tec & Doc Lavoisier. Paris.
4. Bock, R. *et al.* 2004. Babesiosis of cattle. Parasitology **129**(Suppl l): 247–269.
5. Zintl, A. *et al.* 2003. *Babesia divergens*, a bovine blood parasite of veterinary and zoonotic importance. Clin. Microbiol. Rev. **16:** 622–636.
6. Uilenberg, G. 1980. Ticks and tick-borne diseases of veterinary interest in Europe and Africa: prospects for control and eradication. *In* Ticks and Tick-Borne Diseases: Proceedings of the 56th Annual Conference of the Australian Veterinary Association. L.A.Y. Johnston & M.G. Cooper, Eds.: 1–3. Townsville. Queensland, Australia.
7. Ristic, M. 1984. Research on babesiosis vaccines. *In* Malaria and Babesiosis: Research Findings and Control Measures. M. Ristic, P. Ambroise-Thomas & J.P. Kreier, Eds.: 103–122. Martinus Nijhoff. Boston, MA.
8. Figueroa, J.V. & G.M. Buening. 1995. Nucleic acid probes as a diagnostic method for tick-borne hemoparasites of veterinary importance. Vet. Parasitol. **75:** 75–92.
9. Leeflang, P. & M.M. Perie. 1972. Comparative immunofluorescent studies on 4 *Babesia*-species of cattle. Res. Vet. Sci. **13:** 342–346.
10. Edelhofer, R. *et al.* 2004. Differentiation of *Babesia bigemina*, *B. bovis*, *B. divergens* and *B. major* by Western blotting—First report of *B. bovis* in Austrian cattle. Parasitol. Res. **92:** 433–435.
11. Passos, L.M.F., L. Bell-Sakyi & C.G.D. Brown. 1998. Immunochemical characterization of in vitro culture-derived antigens of *Babesia bovis* and *Babesia bigemina*. Vet. Parasitol. **76:** 239–249.
12. McElwain, T.F. *et al.* 1988. Identification of *Babesia bigemina* and *Babesia bovis* merozoite proteins with isolate- and species-common epitopes recognized by antibodies in bovine immune sera. Infect. Immun. **56:** 1658–1660.

13. WRIGHT, I.G. *et al*. 1987. Protection of *Babesia bigemina*-immune animals against subsequent challenge with virulent *Babesia bovis*. Infect. Immun. **55:** 364–368.
14. PALMER, D.A., G.M. BUENING & C.A. CARSON. 1982. Cryopreservation of *Babesia bovis* for in vitro cultivation. Parasitology **84:** 567–572.
15. VEGA, C.A. *et al*. 1985. In vitro cultivation of *Babesia bigemina*. Am. J. Vet. Res. **46:** 416–420.
16. GORENFLOT, A. *et al*. 1991. Cytological and immunological responses to *Babesia divergens* in different hosts: ox, gerbil, man. Parasitol. Res. **77:** 3–12.
17. VEGA, C.A. *et al*. 1999. Insuficiente inmunidad cruzada en bovinos por *Babesia bigemina* y/o *Babesia bovis* derivadas de cultivo in vitro. Tec. Pecu. Mex. **37:** 13–22.
18. VALENTIN, A. *et al*. 1993. Cellular and humoral immune responses induced in cattle by vaccination with *Babesia divergens* culture-derived exoantigens correlate with protection. Infect. Immun. **61:** 734–741.
19. FIGUEROA, J.V. *et al*. 2004. Identification of a coronin-like protein in *Babesia* species. Ann. N.Y. Acad. Sci. **1026:** 125–138.
20. LAEMMLI, U.K. 1972. Cleavage of structural proteins during the assembly of the head of bacteriophage T4. Nature **227:** 680–685.
21. TOWBIN, H., T. STAEHELIN & J. GORDON. 1979. Electrophoretic transfer of proteins from polyacrylamide gels to nitrocellulose sheets: procedures and some applications. Proc. Natl. Acad. Sci. USA **76:** 4350–4354.
22. DELBECQ, S. *et al*. 2002. *Babesia divergens*: cloning and biochemical characterization of Bd37. Parasitology **125:** 305–312.
23. SAMBROCK, J. & D.W. RUSSELL. 2001. Molecular Cloning: a Laboratory Manual, 3rd ed. Cold Spring Harbor Laboratory Press. Cold Spring Harbor, NY.
24. SANGER, F., S. NICKLEN & A.R. COULSON. 1977. DNA sequencing with chain-terminating inhibitors. Proc. Natl. Acad. Sci. USA **74:** 5463–5467.
25. ALTSCHUL, S.F. *et al*. 1997. Gapped BLAST and PSI-BLAST: a new generation of protein database search programs. Nucleic Acids Res. **25:** 3389–3402.
26. MARCHLER-BAUER, A. *et al*. 2005. CDD: A conserved domain database for protein classification. Nucleic Acids Res. **33:** D192–D196.
27. GEER, L.Y. *et al*. 2002. CDART: protein homology by domain architecture. Genome Res. **12:** 1619–1623.
28. WEIDMANN, B. *et al*. 1994. A protein complex required for signal-sequence-specific sorting and translocation. Nature **370:** 434–440.
29. BEATRIX, B., S. HIDEAKI & M. WEIDMANN. 2000. The α and β subunit of the nascent polypeptide-associated complex have distinct functions. J. Biol. Chem. **275:** 37838–37845.

Evaluation of Cattle Inoculated with *Babesia bovis* Clones Adhesive *In Vitro* to Bovine Brain Endothelial Cells

GERMINAL J. CANTO,[a] JULIO V. FIGUEROA,[b] JUAN A. RAMOS,[b]
EDMUNDO E. ROJAS,[b] DAVID GARCIA-TAPIA,[b,c]
J. ANTONIO ALVAREZ,[b] DAVID R. ALLRED,[d]
AND CHARLES A. CARSON[c]

[a]*CENID–Fisiologia Animal, INIFAP, Ajuchitlan, Qro., 76280 Mexico*

[b]*CENID–Parasitologia Veterinaria, INIFAP, Jiutepec, Morelos, 62550 Mexico*

[c]*Department of Veterinary Pathobiology, University of Missouri, Columbia, Missouri 65211, USA*

[d]*Department of Pathobiology, College of Veterinary Medicine, University of Florida, Gainesville, Florida 32611-0880, USA*

ABSTRACT: A comparative assessment of the virulence of *Babesia bovis* clones that adhere or not to bovine brain endothelial cells was done using two clones of *B. bovis*: (1) a clone phenotypically characterized as virulent (2F8) and (2) a clone of reduced virulence (RAD). Of these subpopulations, we selected those that had adhesive characteristics (a) or nonadhesive characteristics (na) in cultured endothelial cells. Twenty Holstein cattle, 12 months of age or older, were used in this study, and these cattle were randomly assigned to five groups of four animals each. The clones and their respective subpopulations were inoculated via intramuscular injection at a 0.5×10^7 infected erythrocyte dosage. Group A was inoculated with aRAD, group B with naRAD, group C with a2F8, group D with na2F8, and group E remained as a control. All inoculated animals showed a decrease in the packed cell volume (PCV), with group D showing the largest decrease (39.53%) and longest time (7 days) with rectal temperature above 39.5°C. *Babesia* was observed in stained blood smears from only six cattle. While the four parasite subpopulations were pathogenic, significant differences were not noted among them, despite that the subpopulations considered to be virulent caused the greatest reduction in PCV per individual.

KEYWORDS: *Babesia bovis*; *in vitro* adhesive clones; *in vivo* assessment

Address for correspondence: Dr. Julio V. Figueroa, CENID-PAVET, INIFAP, Apartado Postal 206, CIVAC, Morelos, 62550 Mexico. Voice: +52-777-3-192850; ext.: 139; fax: +52-777-3-192850; ext.: 129.

e-mail: figueroa.julio@inifap.gob.mx

Ann. N.Y. Acad. Sci. 1081: 397–404 (2006). © 2006 New York Academy of Sciences.
doi: 10.1196/annals.1373.058

INTRODUCTION

Babesiosis, caused by intra-erythrocytic *Babesia* protozoans, is a disease transmitted by ticks to mammalian hosts. The disease is characterized by pale mucosa and jaundice, hemoglobinuria, fever, hemolytic anemia, depression, decreased appetite, ruminal stasis, prostration, lachrymation, increased salivation, and in severe cases, death.[1] Of the six *Babesia* species that infect cattle, *B. bovis* is considered to be the most pathogenic. *Babesia* sp. can cause a wide range of clinical manifestations due to the differences in virulence and pathogenicity of the strains within each species. Infections with *B. bovis* always cause an acute syndrome, although the severity of the disease can vary.[2] This disease persists in tropical and subtropical regions of the world between parallel 35 South and parallel 40 North of the equator, and has economic impact on livestock production, especially in developing countries. The presence of babesiosis restricts translocation and establishment of new livestock production in these regions. *B. bovis* and *B. bigemina* have a wide distribution corresponding to the distribution of *Boophilus microplus*, *B. decoloratus*, and *B. annulatus* ticks.[1]

Infection with *B. bovis* stimulates a controlling immune response but it does not eliminate the parasite, resulting in persistent chronic infection.[2-4] The parasite remains hidden from the immune response of cattle when erythrocytes infected with mature parasites are sequestered in capillaries,[2,3,5] thus possibly avoiding elimination by the spleen.[6] Nevertheless, the mechanisms used by *B. bovis* to achieve sequestering of the erythrocytes into capillaries have not been described. Infected erythrocytes may be sequestered in the capillaries through receptor-type interactions between the infected erythrocytes and the endothelium, such as in human infections caused by *Plasmodium falciparum*.[4,7] In many aspects, these parasites have similar interactions with their host cells. Each parasite induces the formation of protrusions on the infected erythrocyte cell surface, which then allows adhesion to the endothelium.[2,4,7] Antigens derived from the parasite and associated to the surface of the erythrocyte, and potentially involved in cell adhesiveness, are subject to a rapid antigenic variation.[6,8] Both in human malaria and bovine babesiosis, parasites are sequestered in the capillaries of several organs in the host, an activity hypothesized to contribute to their pathology, particularly in cerebral complications that are present in both diseases.[2-5] In malaria, most of this interaction has been determined with an *in vitro* model, through adhesion studies of infected erythrocytes to umbilical chord endothelial cells.[7,9] For bovine babesiosis, recently published data suggested that adhesiveness of bovine endothelial cells for erythrocytes infected with *B. bovis* represents an acceptable model for the study of interactions that occur between infected erythrocytes and endothelial cells during the *in vivo* sequestering of the parasite.[4,7,8] In this article, we report the results of a study in cattle in which we compared the virulence of subpopulations of *B. bovis* repeatedly selected for adhesiveness to cultured bovine brain endothelial cells against their nonadhesive homologous subpopulations.

MATERIALS AND METHODS

Two clones of *B. bovis*, previously characterized as virulent (2F8) and attenuated (RAD) were used in this study.[3] In order to select subpopulations with positive or negative cell adhesion characteristics, the clones were subjected to cell culture in the presence of bovine brain endothelial cells through procedures that included four rounds of enrichment-depletion, essentially as it has previously been described.[4,8] The subpopulations were maintained *in vitro* using culture conditions for *Babesia* sp.[10] and amplified to prepare fresh inocula kept in refrigeration until their final use in Rancho GB, Queretaro, Mexico. For the experiment, 20 susceptible male *Bos taurus* Holstein breed cattle, 12 months of age or older, which were obtained from a *Boophilus* sp. tick-free area, were used. These cattle were confirmed free of antibodies against anaplasmosis (enzyme-linked immunosorbent assay, ELISA), babesiosis (Indirect Fluorescence Antibody Test), and negative to IBR, brucellosis, and tuberculosis. The animals were randomly assigned into five groups of four animals each and were separated into different enclosures located in the Rancho GB. The two clones (2F8 and RAD) and their corresponding subpopulations, adhesive (a) and nonadhesive (na), were inoculated by intramuscular injection (IM) with a dose of 0.5×10^7 *B. bovis* infected erythrocytes. The experimental groups were as follows: group A: aRAD; group B: naRAD; group C: a2F8; group D: na2F8, and group E: uninoculated control group. The study was carried out under a double-blind arrangement. A clinical and hematological follow-up was carried out in all animals. Starting from day 4 post-inoculation (PI), rectal temperature and blood samples were obtained daily in order to determine the packed cell volume (PCV) by using the microhematocrit technique. The blood samples were obtained by puncture of the coccygeal vein. The prepatent period, days PI when infected erythrocytes appear in smears made from peripheral blood, was expressed as an average in days. Blood from all animals was collected every other day during the week prior to inoculation and daily during the following weeks. On the same dates, body temperatures were recorded for each animal and the whole blood samples were processed to determine the presence of parasitized erythrocytes in Giemsa-stained blood smears. The average rectal temperatures (T) and PCV values from the five groups were compared through generalized linear models (GLM procedure of the SAS statistical package software; SAS Institute, SA de CV, Mexico), using a fully random model for classification and the mean temperature and PCV values as co-variables.

RESULTS

All inoculated animals, regardless of type of inoculum, showed a decrease in the percentage of PCV as well as temperature above 39.5°C, which indicates that the infecting material originating from *in vitro* culture, was viable.

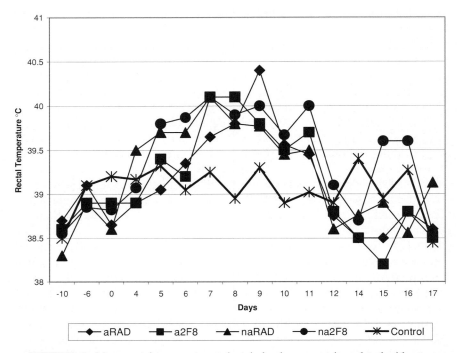

FIGURE 1. Mean rectal temperature values in bovine groups inoculated with attenuated (RAD) and virulent (2F8) *Babesia bovis* clones adhesive (a) and nonadhesive (na) to brain endothelial cells *in vitro*.

Overall, there were no differences in the clinical signs among the groups inoculated with the *B. bovis* clones. The average rectal temperature values for each group are shown in FIGURE 1. The maximum temperature reached (40.4°C) was observed in the group inoculated with the endothelial cell-adhering clone aRAD (FIG. 1, TABLE 1) at day 9 PI. Furthermore, cattle in the other inoculated groups showed the maximum temperature (40.1°C) at day 7 PI (FIG. 1, TABLE 1). As for the PCV in animals inoculated with the RAD clone, the group inoculated with aRAD had an average PCV value of 17 on day 10 PI, whereas the group inoculated with naRAD showed a mean PCV value of 20 on day 9 PI (FIG. 2). Animals inoculated with a2F8 and na2F8 had a minimum average PCV of 18.2 and 17.2, respectively, on day 10 PI. When determining the maximum average reduction in PCV per individual (i.e., calculated from the PCV values determined in each individual pre- and post-inoculation) values of 28.74%, 30.89%, 35.33%, and 39.53% were obtained for the cattle groups inoculated with the aRAD, naRAD, a2F8, and na2F8 clones, respectively (TABLE 1). Out of the 20 animals inoculated with *B. bovis*, only six animals showed parasites in smears stained with Giemsa, corresponding to two each for groups aRAD

TABLE 1. Temperature and PCV in cattle inoculated with attenuated (RAD) and virulent (2F8) *Babesia bovis* clones adhesive (a) and nonadhesive (na) to bovine brain endothelial cells *in vitro*

Variables	Groups				
	aRAD	naRAD	a2F8	na2F8	Control
Temperature >40°C (No. of days)	1	1	2	3	–
Mean maximum temperature (C)	40.4	40.1	40.1	40.1	39.3
Mean lowest PCV (%)	17	20	18.2	17.2	24.7
Lowest PCV per animal (%)	16	16	15	14	24
Mean maximum reduction of PCV (%) per individual	28.74	30.89	35.33	39.53	5.4
Positive animals in Giemsa-stained smears	2	1	1	2	–
Number of animals with a PCV decrement >30%	2	2	3	3	–

and na2F8, whereas only one from the naRAD and the a2F8 groups (TABLE 1) showed parasites. During the experiment, two animals died: one belonging to group aRAD died during the night of day 9 PI and the cause of death could not be determined. Nevertheless, on the previous day it had not shown any signs characteristic of babesiosis, such as fever, decrease in PCV, or parasites in the blood. Therefore, death of the animal caused by the protozoan parasite was ruled out. The second animal death belonged to group na2F8 and died of classical bovine babesiosis.

DISCUSSION

The main objective of the study was to assess if cattle inoculated with two clonal *B. bovis* populations, with or without *in vitro* endothelial cell adhesion phenotype, could be differentiated, by following the clinical manifestations of the disease in susceptible cattle. The four parasite subpopulations inoculated into cattle were pathogenic and significant differences were not noted among them, despite that the subpopulations considered to be virulent caused the greatest reduction in PCV per individual. Furthermore, regardless of the *B. bovis* clone used for inoculation, no significant differences were noted in rectal temperature values between the groups of animals inoculated with the adhesive and nonadhesive populations of parasites. Taken together, this could mean that the virulence mechanisms of the parasites are other and that the cell adhesiveness is only a protection mechanism for the parasite,[4,7] and that all populations of *B. bovis*, regardless their origin, have the capability to produce it without causing severe damage in the host. Several researchers have observed this fact from a different perspective. For example, it has been pointed out that the endothelial cell adhesiveness would provide *B. bovis* with the capacity for establishing very long-term chronic infections,[11,12] while others report

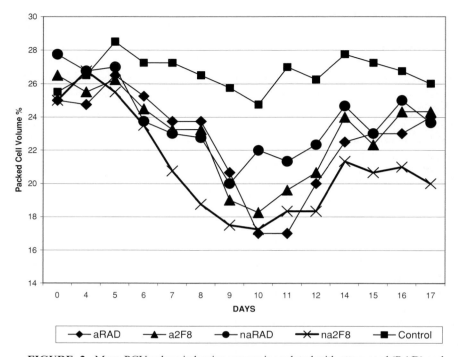

FIGURE 2. Mean PCV values in bovine groups inoculated with attenuated (RAD) and virulent (2F8) *Babesia bovis* clones adhesive (a) and nonadhesive (na) to brain endothelial cells *in vitro.*

that in spite of the immune response mounted by the bovine host, the parasite continues proliferating in the blood flow and that the parasitemia appears below the microscopic detection level.[7] The pathology associated with the most severe forms of the acute disease has been attributed to the sequestration of infected erythrocytes, particularly in the brain endothelial cells.[5] However, in this study, acute severe disease was not seen in cattle inoculated with the adhesive or nonadhesive populations. Therefore, the concentration of erythrocytes infected with trophozoite or merozoite forms of *B. bovis* in endothelial cells of the host may only be a mechanism to avoid destruction of the parasites when passing through the spleen. Moreover, by sequestering in the capillaries, parasites are made inaccessible to other types of immune responses such as antibody-dependent cytotoxicity, or opsonization and phagocytosis,[2] and that this process induces the chronic phase of the infection in babesiosis and other hemoparasite diseases.[6,7] As mentioned above, the objective of the study was fulfilled when the virulence of the strains was assessed; nevertheless, the hypothesis originally established could not be tested as all clones studied showed a similar virulence regardless of their adhesive or nonadhesive phenotype. In this sense, similar results were recently reported in that animals inoculated with erythrocytes infected with *B. bovis* adherent *in vitro* to endothelial cells from bovine umbilical chord did not show an exacerbation of clinical signs when compared to animals inoculated with the nonadhesive mother strain.[9] In conclusion, through *in vitro* selection and enrichment, it is possible to obtain endothelial cell-adhesive and nonadhesive populations from originally pathogenic and nonpathogenic populations of *B. bovis*. However, at this point in time, it is not clear if the variations in these properties could explain the differences in the degree of virulence that is observed in the various *B. bovis* isolates, and if the loss of this adhesiveness explains the attenuation of the protozoan[4] or if this is only a feature for preserving the parasite within the host by evading the immune protection mechanisms.[8]

ACKNOWLEDGMENTS

This research was supported in part by the USDA-FAS Grant 58-3148-8-042; PAIEPEME, A. C., and SAGARPA-CONACYT, Mexico, Project No. 2003-C02-139.

REFERENCES

1. McCosker, P.J. 1981. The global importance of babesiosis. *In* Babesiosis M. Ristic & J P. Kreier, Eds.: 1–24. Academic Press. New York.
2. Wright, I.G., B.V. Goodger & I.A. Clark. 1988. Immunopathophysiology of *Babesia bovis* and *Plasmodium falciparum* infections. Parasitol. Today **4:** 214–218.
3. Nevils, M.A., J.V. Figueroa, G.J. Canto, *et al.* 2000. Cloned lines of *Babesia bovis* differ in their ability to induce cerebral babesiosis in cattle. Parasitol. Res. **86:** 437–443.
4. O'Connor, R.M., J.A. Long & D.R. Allred. 1999. Cytoadherence of *Babesia bovis*-infected erythrocytes to bovine brain capillary endothelial cells provides an in vitro model for sequestration. Infect. Immun. **67:** 3921–3928.
5. Callow, L.L. & M. McGavin. 1963. Cerebral babesiosis due to *Babesia argentina*. Aust. Vet. J. **39:** 15–21.
6. Allred, D.R. 1995. Immune evasion by *Babesia bovis* and *Plasmodium falciparum*: cliff-dwellers of the parasite world. Parasitol. Today **11:** 100–105.
7. Allred, D.R. 2003. Babesiosis: persistence in the face of adversity. Trends Parasitol. **19:** 51–55.
8. O'Connor, R.M. & D.R. Allred. 2000. Selection of *Babesia bovis*-infected erythrocytes for adhesion to endothelial cells co-selects for altered variant erythrocyte surface antigen isoforms. J. Immunol. **164:** 2031–2045.
9. Molloy, J.B., P.M. Bowles, W.K. Jorgensen, *et al.* 2003. *Babesia bovis:* adhesion of parasitized red blood cells to bovine umbilical vein endothelial cells *in vitro* does not select for virulence. Exp. Parasitol. **103:** 182–184.

10. PALMER, D.A., G.M. BUENING & C.A. CARSON. 1982. Cryopreservation of *Babesia bovis* for in vitro cultivation. Parasitology **84:** 567–572.

11. MAHONEY, D.F., I. WRIGHT & G. MIRRE. 1973. Bovine babesiasis: the persistence of immunity to *Babesia argentina* and *B. bigemina* in calves (*Bos taurus*) after naturally acquired infection. Ann. Trop. Med. Parasitol. **67:** 197–203.

12. CALDER, J.A., G.R. REDDY, L. CHIEVES, *et al*. 1996. Monitoring *Babesia bovis* infections in cattle by using PCR-based tests. J. Clin. Microbiol. **34:** 2748–2755.

Bovine Babesiosis Live Vaccine Production

Use of Gamma Irradiation on the Substrate

CARMEN ROJAS,[a] JULIO V. FIGUEROA,[a] ARCELIA ALVARADO,[b]
PEDRO MEJIA,[b] JUAN J. MOSQUEDA,[a] ALFONSO FALCON,[a]
CARLOS A. VEGA,[a] AND ANTONIO ALVAREZ[a]

[a]CENID Parasitología Veterinaria, INIFAP, Morelos, C.P. 62500, México

[b]CENID-Microbiología INIFAP, Morelos, C.P. 62500, México

ABSTRACT: Gamma irradiation on bovine serum and red blood cells (RBC) allows proliferation and growth of *in vitro*-cultured *Babesia* sp., and has potential application to inactivate contaminating viruses and bacteria from the substrate. Gamma irradiation with 25 kGy in a source of ^{60}Co was able to inactivate infectious bovine rinotracheitis (IBR) and bovine viral diarrhea (BVD) viruses in artificially contaminated serum; besides, bacteria were also eliminated. *In vitro* culture of *Babesia bovis* (*B. bovis*) in modified substrate, by adding irradiated serum with ^{60}Co at 25 kGy was propagated from 24-well culture plates to 225 cm^2 tissue culture flasks, and percentages of parasitized erythrocytes (PPE) from 2.4% to 8.8% were obtained. Infected RBC adapted to Irrad S were transferred to the irradiated substrate *in vitro* culture system, by using serum irradiated at 25 kGy and RBC from 10 to 70 Gy. The PPE ranged from 3.1 to 11. Culture of *Babesia bigemina* (*B. bigemina*) was established with Irrad S (25 kGy); its propagation was achieved in tissue culture flasks reaching PPE from 0.5 to 4.3 with no statistical difference ($P >$ 0.05) when compared to the nonirradiated control culture (1.2–4.8). *B. bigemina*-infected RBCs were transferred to the modified culture system by adding irradiated serum and RBC (25 kGy and 70 Gy, respectively). PPE obtained in culture flasks were from 0.8 to 4.2. The results indicate that gamma irradiation is a suitable method to inactivate potential viral contamination and eliminate bacteria from bovine serum, to produce a live attenuated vaccine through the *in vitro* culture.

KEYWORDS: bovine babesiosis; live attenuated vaccine; cattle

Address for correspondence: Antonio Alvarez, CENID-PAVET, INIFAP, Apartado Postal 206, CIVAC, Morelos, C.P. 62500. Mexico. Voice: +52-777-3192850; fax: 52-777-3192850; ext.: 129. e-mail: alvarez.jesus@inifap.gob.mx

Ann. N.Y. Acad. Sci. 1081: 405–416 (2006). © 2006 New York Academy of Sciences.
doi: 10.1196/annals.1373.059

INTRODUCTION

Bovine babesiosis is one of the most important diseases in tropical and sub-tropical areas of Mexico. It is caused by the protozoa *Babesia (B.) bovis* and *Babesia bigemina*, transmitted by the one host tick *Boophilus* spp.[1,2] Immunization is considered to be the method that offers the best perspectives for the prevention and/or control of bovine babesiosis outbreaks. In Mexico, several studies on vaccination have been carried out; starting up with *in vitro* culture-derived parasites.[3,4] Previously in Australia, an attenuated live vaccine was obtained through multiple passages of the *Babesia* parasites in splenectomized[5] or intact calves.[6] This procedure allows the production of large number of vaccine doses. However, the risk of contamination with adventitious pathogens has been documented to occur after several passages carried out in bovines.[7] To allow growth of the *Babesia* parasites by the *in vitro* culture method, animals are required as donors to provide for red blood cells (RBCs) and serum as part of the culture substrate, thus the risk for contamination is also latent. Furthermore, bovine blood donor selection is a complicating factor because it has been stated that many different viruses and bacteria are present in many cattle farms in Mexico.

Therefore, the implementation of procedures to remove or inactivate such potential disease agents is a high priority for the bovine babesiosis vaccine production. Gamma irradiation has been used successfully for sterilization of medical devices and to inactivate bacteria and viruses in animal sera and biotherapeutics.[8] In the present article we used increasing gamma irradiation doses ranging from 10 to 25 kGy on bovine serum, and from 10 to 70 Gy to treat bovine RBCs. We measured the reduction of infectivity of two viruses, bovine herpes virus 1 (IBR) and bovine viral diarrhea (BVD) virus, as well as the elimination of some bacteria species. The *in vitro* proliferation of *B. bovis* and *B. bigemina* maintained in cultures was monitored microscopically to evaluate the effect of gamma irradiation on the substrate–bovine serum and RBCs.

MATERIALS AND METHODS

Animal Donors

Two selected 12-month-old *Bos taurus* type bulls, were used as donors of normal erythrocytes and fresh serum substrate to be included in the *Babesia in vitro* culture medium. These bovines came from a tick-free area in Mexico and were free of bovine brucellosis, tuberculosis, leucosis, IBR, BDV, *Anaplasma marginale*, and *Babesia* sp.

Babesia *Parasites*

B. bovis BOR, a biological clone derived from the KBb strain by the critical dilution method[9] and irradiated with a source of Cobalt-60 (^{60}Co),[10] has been maintained by alternate *in vitro* culture and cryopreservation. *B. bigemina* BIS, is a culture strain that was originally obtained from a field isolate in Mexico, and kept in the laboratory by alternate freezing and continuous propagation by *in vitro* culture.[4]

In vitro *Culture System*

Media: Consisted of Medium M199 (Sigma Chemical Co., St. Louis, MO) buffered with 30 mM N-Tris (hydroxymethyl)-methyl-2-aminoethanesulfonic acid (TES) (Sigma) and 26 mM $NaHCO_3$ (Sigma) and supplemented with 40% (v/v) normal bovine serum. The media was added 100 IU/mL penicillin, and 100 μg/mL streptomycin, and then sterilized by using a 0.22 μm pore size filter.

Substrate

Normal bovine erythrocytes (nRBC) were collected into sterile flasks with defibrinating glass beads, washed twice with VYM's solution,[4] and after removing the buffy coat and uppermost erythrocyte layer, were resuspended at 25% (v/v) concentration in VYM's solution. Obtained defibrinated serum and the processed erythrocytes were stored at 4°C, until used.

Initiation of Culture

Thawed *B. bovis* and *B. bigemina* cryostabilates were added to VYM's solution and centrifuged at 1000g for 10 min. After centrifugation, 0.1 mL of the RBCs pellet was added to 1000 μL of complete culture media containing 5% fresh, uninfected bovine RBCs, and were added to a well of a 24-well tissue culture plate. Plates were incubated at 37°C in an atmosphere of 5% O_2, 5% CO_2, and 90% N_2. Culture medium was replaced every 24 h, and subcultures were initiated every 72 h, by reducing the percentage of parasitized erythrocytes (PPE) to 1% with the addition of normal RBC. The PPE were determined for each well by microscopic observation of Giemsa-stained smears. The PPE were estimated by counting at least 1000 cells.

Expansion to Large Volumes of in Vitro–*Cultured* Babesia *sp.*

To produce a continuous supply of larger volumes of parasites, the latter were scaled up using 25, 75, and 225 cm^2 tissue culture flasks, which were kept as the culture plates at 37°C in an atmosphere of 5% O_2, 5% CO_2, and 90% N_2.

Cryopreservation Procedure

The cryoprotectant solution was 20% (v/v) poly vinyl pirrolidone (PVP-40, Sigma) in VYM's solution. Cultures were centrifuged at 1000g for 10 min, the medium was discarded, the packed RBC mixed with an equal volume of 20% PVP, dispensed in 2 mL cryotubes, placed in a container with isopropyl-alcohol at −70°C for 2 h, and finally transferred to the liquid N_2 storage.

Gamma Irradiation Procedure

Bovine serum, with or without artificial viral contamination, dispensed as 500 mL aliquots in plastic containers. Bovine erythrocytes were packed as 25 mL aliquots in 50 mL plastic tubes. Samples were irradiated in a ^{60}Co irradiator. Virus-spiked samples (serum and erythrocytes), and virus-free controls were both irradiated at the National Institute of Nuclear Research (Salazar, Mexico) in an MDS Nordion (Ottowa, Canada) Gamma-cell 220.

Measurement of Virus Inactivation

Stock suspensions of IBR virus (strain IBR758) with a titer of $10^{5.6}$ 50% tissue culture infective dose ($TCID_{50}$)/mL, and BVD virus (strain NADL) at 10^3 $TCID_{50}$/mL were used. Virus-spiked samples and controls without virus were prepared in triplicate. After irradiation, viruses were assayed by standard $TCID_{50}$ assays. IBR virus was assayed using MDBK cells, whereas BVD virus was assayed with TB cells. MDBK and TB cells were grown in MEM's medium, containing 10% fetal bovine serum (FBS), to reach complete confluence. Before carrying out each viral assay, cell suspensions were seeded in 96-well microtiter plates (Corning Costar, Corning, NY). Plates were incubated in 5% CO_2 at 37°C for 48 h. IBR and BVD viral titers were calculated by the Reed and Muench method[11] and cell layers were analyzed for cytopathic effect (CPE).[12] Immunoenzymatic assay (ELISA) (Bommeli Diagnostics, Intervet, Liebefeld-Bern, Switzerland) was used for BVD detection and titration.

Measurement of Bacteria Elimination

The bacterial contamination was evaluated as a vaccine sterility test approach. Thus, seven different bacteria-spiked serum samples and negative controls without bacteria were prepared in duplicate. The bacteria included in this test were; *Bacillus cereus* (ATCC 11778), *Escherichia coli* (ATCC 4350), *Listeria monocytogenes* (ATCC 7644), *Klebsiella peumoniae* (ATCC 10031), *Proteus mirabilis, Staphylococcus aureus* 6835P, and *Salmonella senftenberg*. After gamma irradiation, each sample was incubated at 25°C for 14 days in tryptone-casein soy broth and at 35°C for 14 days in thioglycolate broth and saboraud broth tubes. Bacterial growth, if any, was detected by turbidity test in the medium, and samples were then seeded on baby heart infusion agar (BHI) at 35°C for 24 h in order to verify the presence of bacteria colonies.

Statistical Analysis

Percentages of erythrocytes parasitized were analyzed as hypothesis test for proportions by using the mean for each treatment and a t-test was applied.[13]

Experimental Procedures

Experiment 1. Five 1 mL aliquots of bovine serum with two replicates were contaminated with 500–1000 $TCID_{50}$ of IBR virus. Similarly, bovine serum samples were added with 300–500 $TCID_{50}$ of the BVD virus. Each sample was irradiated with a different radiation dose, 0, 10, 15, 20, and 25 kGy, and three replicates were performed per radiation dose. After gamma irradiation virus-spiked samples were assayed as described above.

Experiment 2. Similar to experiment 1, aliquots of bovine serum were individually contaminated with seven different bacteria. The tubes containing the contaminated bovine serum were irradiated at 25 kGy. After gamma irradiation bacteria-spiked samples were inoculated into culture broth as indicated above.

Experiment 3. Uninfected bovine RBCs resuspended in VYM's solution were irradiated at 10, 20, 40, 60, and 70 Gy as low doses range, and at 10, 15, 20, and 25 kGy as high radiation doses, in a ^{60}Co irradiator.

Experiment 4. *B. bovis*- and *B. bigemina*-infected RBCs from a cryostabilate were incorporated to the *in vitro* culture system. The culture medium included normal bovine serum and normal RBCs as substrate. A short period of time was allowed in culture to reactivate infectivity of the parasites *in vitro*.

Experiment 5. *B. bovis*-infected RBCs derived from experiment 4 were maintained in the *in vitro* system. Nonradiated RBCs (N-Irrad/RBC) and 25 kGy irradiated-serum (25 kGy Irrad/S) were incorporated as substrate. Since the PPE were 2%, expansion was performed from 24-well plates to 225 cm² flasks. One culture flask without any irradiated substrate was the control. PPE were determined every 24 h after culture initiation.

Experiment 6. The *B. bovis*-infected RBCs from the N-Irrad/RBC, 25 kGy-Irrad/S substrate were used, keeping as fixed factor the 25 kGy Irrad/S, but adding increased irradiation doses of 10, 20, 40, 60, and 70 Gy for the RBCs substrate. One control treatment with normal RBC was included.

Experiment 7. *B. bigemina*-infected RBCs derived from experiment 4 were maintained in the *in vitro* system; N-Irrad/RBC and 25 kGy Irrad/S were incorporated as substrate. When PPE were above 2%, expansion was performed to 225 cm^2 flasks. One treatment without any irradiated substrate served as the control culture.

Experiment 8. *B. bigemina*-infected RBCs from experiment 7 were used modifying the substrate composition to 25 kGy Irrad/S and 70 Gy Irrad/RBCs.

RESULTS

The results of experiment 1 indicated that ^{60}Co irradiation was an appropriate method to achieve virus inactivation of artificially contaminated bovine serum. Serum aliquots contaminated with IBR virus, ^{60}Co irradiated from 10 to 25 kGy, were negative to the antigen detection assay as compared to the nonirradiated sample. Cell monolayers were confluent even at 1:128, the highest dilution tested. The viral titer determined was 10^4 TCID$_{50}$, showing a one log$_{10}$ reduction of the original titer. BVD virus-contaminated and irradiated samples showed also negative antigen detection in the cultures assayed. The values detected were lower than 20% positive in an ELISA test (Bommeli Diagnostics, Intervet). In contrast, nonirradiated samples were, albeit weak, positives (30%). The selected dose to irradiate serum was 25 kGy to conduct the subsequent experiments.

In experiment 2, the seven bacteria included (*Bacillus cereus, Escherichia coli, Listeria monocytogenes, Klebsiella peumoniae, Proteus mirabilis, Staphylococcus aureus,* and *Salmonella senftenberg)* were effectively eliminated by the irradiation procedure. Bacteria growth measured by the turbidity test showed that 25 kGy irradiation caused its elimination. In contrast, all nonirradiated samples showed turbidity in three different media. Similarly, nonirradiated samples showed the presence of colonies on BHI agar, which were not seen on the 25 kGy ^{60}Co-irradiated samples.

Experiment 3 was designed to verify the endurance of RBC to gamma irradiation exposure at different doses. RBCs irradiated with doses ranging from 10 to 25 kGy in a ^{60}Co source (Irrad/RBC), were completely damaged, with 100% hemolysis observed. Consequently, these irradiation levels were discarded for treating RBC as substrate for the *in vitro* culture of *Babesia.* Lower irradiation doses from 10 to 70 Gy did not cause lysis of the RBC. The selected dose for the subsequent experiments was the highest tested in this experiment (70 Gy).

Experiment 4. *In vitro* culture recovery to propagate *B. bovis* and *B. bigemina* was successfully initiated from frozen stages. The substrate con-

TABLE 1. *In vitro* culture of *B. bovis*

Treatment	Container type			
	24-well plate	6-well plate	75 cm flask	225 cm flask
Control	5.8[a]	5.6[b]	4.0[c]	6.2[d]
Irradiated serum-nonirradiated RBC	5.3[a]	5.9[b]	5.1[c]	5.3[d]

Values represent PPE determined by Geimsa-stained smears counting 1000 cells. PPE means followed by same letters in a column are not significantly different ($P > 0.05$). Control = nonirradiated substrate. Irradiated serum with 25 kGy: [a,b,c,d] same letters in same column indicates no significant difference.

sisted of nonirradiated bovine RBC and normal serum. Three days after removal from the liquid N_2 stage, PPE above 2% were obtained. As a result, these *Babesia*-infected RBCs were used in the next experiments.

Experiment 5 was carried out to adapt the *B. bovis*-infected RBC to the substrate containing 25 kGy-Irrad/Ser. Nonirradiated serum (N-irrad/S) was included as the control culture. Cultures were expanded to larger volumes by sequentially transferring the parasites from 24-well to 6-well plates, then to 75 cm² and finally to 225 cm² tissue culture flasks. PPE observed at different volumes of culture were not statistically different ($P > 0.05$) (5.8 versus 5.3; 5.6 versus 5.9; 4.0 versus 5.1; 6.2 versus 5.3) (TABLE 1). *B. bovis* iRBCs from this experiment were included in experiment 6.

Experiment 6 evaluated the *B. bovis* proliferation when both components of the substrate were irradiated 25 kGy-Irrad/S remained as fixed factor and 10 to 70 Gy- Irrad/RBC were considered as the variable factor. PPE determined were similar in cultures tested with Irrad/RBC at different irradiation doses. The highest PPE mean was estimated in cultures containing RBC irradiated at 70 kGy (7.7), whereas the lowest PPE were estimated for the nonirradiated RBC substrate (4.1) (see TABLE 2).

Experiment 7 included the adaptation of *B. bigemina* parasites maintained *in vitro* with normal RBC and serum to a substrate containing 25 kGy-Irrad/Ser. *In vitro* cultures were expanded to larger volumes by transferring sequentially from 24-well to 6-well plates, then to 75 cm² and finally to 225 cm² flasks (see TABLE 3). PPE values were higher for the control treatment PPE estimated

TABLE 2. *In vitro* culture of *B. bovis* with increasing irradiation doses for RBCs

RBC irradiation dose	0 Gy	10 Gy	20 Gy	40 Gy	60 Gy	70 Gy
PPE (mean)	4.1	5.3	6.3	7.1	6.3	7.7

In vitro culture of *B. bovis* with 25 kGy Irrad/S kept as fixed variable and increasing irradiation doses for RBC (0, 10,20, 40, 60, and 70 Gy). PPE determined by Giemsa-stained smears counting 1000 cells.

TABLE 3. *In vitro* culture of *B. bigemina*

Treatment	Container type			
	24-well plate	6-well plate	75 cm flask	225 cm flask
Control	5.9[a]	6.1[a]	4.3[a]	6.0[a]
Irradiated serum nonirradiated RBC	2.4[b]	2.3[b]	2.9[a]	2.6[b]
Irradiated substrate	nd	nd	nd	2.8[b]

Values represent PPE determined by Geimsa-stained smears counting 1000 cells. PPE means followed by different letters in a column are significantly different ($P < 0.05$). Control = nonirradiated substrate. Irradiated serum with 25 kGy. Irradiated substrate is composed by serum with 25 kGy, and RBCs with 70 G. [a], [b]: same letter in same column indicates no significant difference; nd: nodetermined.

for *B. bigemina* parasites cultivated in 225 cm^2 flasks, specifically comparing irradiated serum/nonirradiated RBC to the irradiated substrate (serum with 25 kGy and RBC with 70 Gy) showed no significant difference ($P > 0.05$) (2.6 versus 2.8). Control treatment by using nonirradiated substrate showed higher PPE and was significantly different ($P < 0.05$) to the irradiated substrate treatment, (6.0 versus 2.8).

DISCUSSION

This study describes the gamma irradiation of the substrate (bovine serum and RBCs) of the culture media, used for the *in vitro* cultivation of *B. bovis* and *B. bigemina*. An effort to inactivate BVD and IBR viruses and eliminate potential bacterial contamination from parasite cultures would benefit the culture system, particularly by reducing the risk for pathogen transmission when used as an attenuated live vaccine. Fetal serum providers usually agree to that cattle are infected with viruses, and it is therefore important to ensure that the blood products do not contain such pathogens.[14,15] The viral inactivation observed in this study by using ^{60}Co at 25 kGy in bovine serum was similar to studies describing that a similar dose of gamma irradiation inactivated 6 logs TCID$_{50}$ of BVD virus when spiked serum was irradiated in bottles.[16,17] Moreover, viral inactivation properties have been described for different methods, such as the use of dyes and irradiation.[18] It has been suggested that a polymeric compound, poly 1,4-dimethyl-6-vynilnaphthalene-1,4-endoperoxide (PVNE) may be useful to mediate virus inactivation for biological fluids.[19] Another kind of irradiation, by UV light, has also been studied.[20] There are some principles for determination of the virus inactivating or removal capacity, and some additional substances, such as antioxidants and freeze-drying of the irradiated biological products can minimize the potential for generating free radicals, maintaining the ability to inactivate greater than 5 logs of porcine parvovirus infectivity, as well as the functional activity for monoclonal antibody preparations infected with the virus.[21]

In this study the highest dose used to irradiate RBCs was 70 Gy, which was not detrimental to the cells. However, it has been reported that 400 Gy caused less than 5% hemolysis 24 h after irradiation.[22] It is important to assess if any alteration on the RBC can be unfavorable for the *in vitro* culture system for *Babesia* spp. Thus, a gamma irradiation dose that avoids bacterial contamination but causes no RBC hemolysis is a requisite to allow the babesial multiplication within the *in vitro* culture system. One study reported that different bacteria (*Brucella abortus, Campylobacter fetus* subsp. *fetus, Campylobacter jejuni, Campylobacter coli, Campylobacter laridis, Mycobacterium fortuitum, Aspergillus fumigatus, Salmonella muenster, Candida albicans, Clostridium difficile,* and *Streptococcus faecalis*) were successfully eliminated after gamma irradiation.[23] Surviving of bacteria was quantitatively determined by selective and enrichment techniques. The irradiating dose required to reduce the population by 90% ranged from 13.4 kRad for *Campylobacter fetus* to 156.6 kRad for *Streptococcus faecalis.*[23]

The *in vitro* culture system that we have initiated in this study without any irradiated component perfectly adapted to the irradiated substrate for *B. bovis* and *B. bigemina,* achieving acceptable PPE in culture flasks. Other studies have used different irradiation systems, such as UV on sera, and maintained their growth-promoting activities for various cell types (MRC-5, Vero, CHO) indicating the lack of significant damage during UVC exposure.[24] Similarly, gamma irradiation has proved to inactivate viral and prion pathogens without excessive damage to albumin structure and good quality of diagnostic reagents.[8,25]

The ideal condition to use bovine blood to be included in the *Babesia-in vitro* culture process, is the absence of pathogens that cause disease in cattle, such as: IBR, BVD virus, bovine leucosis virus, *Mycobacterium bovis, Brucella abortus,* etc., as *B. bovis* and *B. bigemina* vaccine strains still require the bovine components to grow in the *in vitro* culture system.[1,2,26] The use of the gamma irradiation approach has reduced protein damage in substrate to acceptable levels to sustain cultivation of parasites. Various methods have been described for the inactivation of viruses in bovine blood. However, a disadvantage of most inactivation approaches is that they affect the growth-promoting properties of bovine sera.

The safety, purity, and efficacy of viral vaccines might in turn be questioned, as the use of contaminated cells for vaccine production may result in contaminated vaccines, which may lead to seroconversion or disease in the vaccinated animal, and may also interfere with the diagnosis of viral infections.[14,15,27]

To regularly produce an attenuated live vaccine against babesiosis and in order to minimize the risk of viruses being introduced into an animal or animal population directly by the vaccination procedure, it would be advisable to use gamma irradiation of the substrate. However, it is important to recall that some viruses may become activated, such as that reported for human cytomegalovirus (HCV) after gamma irradiation.[28] Another study describes the difficulty for using radiation on HIV sterilization, and concluded that gamma irradiation should be disregarded as a significant virus inactivation method for bone allograft, as the irradiation dose required to achieve a sterility assurance level is 89 kGy, which exceeds current recommendations.[29]

We observed negative antigen detection and one log titer reduction in IBR virus-spiked substrate by using 25 kGy. It has been reported that larger irradiation doses are required for virus inactivation. By using pseudorabies virus (PRV) as a model for human herpesviruses; bovine viral diarrhea virus (BVDV) for HCV; and bovine parvovirus (BPV) for parvovirus B19, it was shown, for example, that for BPV, a dose of 34 kGy was required to reduce by 4 log the infectivity titers.[30] Another study described the comparison of gamma irradiation, moist heat, and chemical sterilization on enveloped viruses (human immunodeficiency virus type 2, HIV-2), PRV, BVDV, and nonenveloped viruses (hepatitis A virus (HAV), poliovirus (PV-1), porcine/bovine parvovirus (PPV, BPV). The three methods achieved 4–7 log reduction of virus titers.[31] However, it has also been demonstrated that the viruses have different susceptibility to gamma irradiation, which means that different doses are required to inactivate different virus families.[32]

Gamma irradiation of RBCs and sera appears advantageous to currently recommended inactivation procedures, for at least: (*a*) it possesses a high inactivation capacity for BVD virus, IBR virus, and bacteria, such as *Bacillus cereus, Escherichia coli, Listeria monocytogenes, Klebsiella peumoniae, Proteus mirabilis, Staphylococcus aureus,* and *Salmonella senftenberg*; (*b*) it causes no noticeable impairment in *B. bovis* and *B. bigemina* growth, and (*c*) it can be performed in a controlled manner at the production site.

Thus, the procedure followed in this study using ^{60}Co at 70 Gy as an irradiating dose for bovine RBC, it is probably not the optimal to reduce bacterial load. However, we found that higher doses pose an additional obstacle to avoid RBC damage so that irradiated RBC can be used as substrate for *in vitro* culture of Babesial parasites. Nonetheless, it was important to notice the apparent absence of damage induced to serum proteins by irradiating it with 25 kGy, so that the substrate could still promote and maintain the *Babesia* parasites *in vitro*.

In conclusion, the gamma irradiation method tested with ^{60}Co is recommended for viral inactivation and bacteria elimination from substrate (RBC and serum) for the *in vitro* culture of cattle *Babesia*. However, additional safety measures, such as full clinical history of cattle, negative serological and polymerase chain reaction (PCR) assay results must be taken into consideration for the selection of multiple bovine blood donors.

REFERENCES

1. ALVAREZ, J.A., J.A. RAMOS, E.E. ROJAS, *et al.* 2004. Field challenge of cattle vaccinated with a combined *Babesia bovis* and *Babesia bigemina* frozen immunogen. Ann. N. Y. Acad. Sci. **1026:** 277–283.
2. CANTO, G.J., J.V. FIGUEROA, J.A. RAMOS, *et al.* 1999. Evaluacion de la patogenicidad y capacidad protectora de un inmunogeno fresco combinado de *Babesia bigemina* y *Babesia bovis*. Vet. Mex. **30:** 215–220.
3. ERP, E.E., S.M. GRAVELY, R.D. SMITH, *et al.* 1978. Growth of *Babesia bovis* in bovine erythrocyte cultures. Am. J. Trop. Med. Hyg. **27:** 1061–1064.
4. VEGA, C.A., G.M. BUENING, S.D. ROIGUEZDR, *et al.* 1986. Cloning of *in vitro* propagated *Babesia* bigemina. Vet. Parasitol. **22:** 223–233.
5. CALLOW, L.L. & L.T. MELLORS. 1966. A new vaccine for *Babesia argentina* infection prepared in splenectomised calves. Aust. Vet. J. **42:** 464–467.
6. DALGLIESH, R.J., L.L. CALLOW, L.T. MELLORS, *et al.* 1981. Development of a highly infective *Babesia bigemina* vaccine of reduced virulence. Aust. Vet. J. **57:** 8–11
7. ROGERS, R.J., C.K. DIMMOCK, A.J. DE VOS, *et al.* 1988. Bovine leucosis virus contamination of a vaccine produced *in vivo* against bovine babesiosis and anaplasmosis. Aust. Vet. J. **65:** 285–287.
8. MIEKKA, S.I., R.Y. FORNG, R.G. ROHWER, *et al.* 2003. Inactivation of viral and prion pathogens by g-irradiation under conditions that maintain the integrity of human albumin. Vox Sanguinis. **84:** 36–44.
9. RODRIGUEZ, S.D., G.M. BUENING, T.J. GREEN, *et al.* 1983. Cloning of *Babesia bovis* by *in vitro* cultivation. Infect. Immun. **42:** 15–18.
10. RODRIGUEZ, S.D., G.M. BUENING & C.A. CARSON. 1993. Caracterizacion bioquimica preliminar de clonas de *Babesia bovis* irradiadas con cobalto 60. Tec. Pecu. Mex. **31:** 16–22.
11. ROSSI, C.H., G.K. KIESEL & P.F. RUMPH. 1982. Association between route of inoculation with infectious bovine rhinotracheitis virus and site of recrudescence after dexamethasone treatment. Am. J. Vet. Res. **43:**1440–1453.
12. JENNEY, E.W., S.J. WESSMAN & F.L. SPINKA. 1978. Microtitration serology methods for bovine virology. U.S. Department of Agriculture. Animal and Plant Health Inspection Service. Ames, Iowa.
13. GLANTZ, S.A. 1997. How to analyze rate and proportions. *In* Primer of Biostatistics, 4th ed. M. Wonsiewicz & P. McCordy, Eds.:pp. 108–150. McGraw-Hill. New York.
14. LEVINGS, R.L. & S.J. WESSMAN. 1991. Bovine viral diarrhea virus contamination of nutrient serum, cell cultures and vaccines. Dev. Biol. Stand. **75:** 177–181.
15. STURDE, E., G. BERTONI & U. CANDRIAN. 2002. Detection and characterization of pestivirus contaminations in human live viral vaccines. Biologicals **30:** 289–296.
16. HANSON, G. & L. FOSTER. 1997. Viral safety in serum for cell culture use. Art Sci. **16:** 1–7. Newsletter
17. DALEY, J.P., D.J. WEPPER & M.Z. PLAVSIC. 1998. Virus inactivation by gamma irradiation of fetal bovine serum. Focus. **20:** 86–88. Newsletter.
18. PREUSS, T., S. KAMSTRUP, N.C. KYVSGAARD, *et al.* 1997. Comparison of two different methods for inactivation of viruses in serum. Clin. Diagn. Lab. Immunol. **4:**504–508.

19. KASSERMANN, F. & C.H. KEMF. 1998. Inactivation of enveloped viruses by singlet oxygen thermally generated from a polymeric naphthalene derivative. Antiviral Res. **38:** 55–62.
20. DE RODA, H.A., P. BIJKERK, W. LODDER, et al. 2004. Calicivirus inactivation by nonionizing (253.7-nanometer-wavelength [UV]) and ionizing (gamma) radiation. Appl. Environ. Microbiol. **70:** 5089–5093.
21. GRIEB, T., R.Y. FORNG, R. BROWN, et al. 2002. Effective use of gamma irradiation for pathogen inactivation of monoclonal antibody preparations. Biologicals **30:** 207–216.
22. CHATTERJEE, S., S. PREMACHANDRAN, R.S. BAGEWADIKAR, et al. 2005. The use of ELISA to monitor amplified hemolysis by the combined action of osmotic stress and radiation: potential applications. Radiat. Res. **163:** 351–355.
23. GARCIA, M.M., B.W. BROOKS, R.B. STEWART, et al. 1987. Evaluation of gamma radiation levels for reducing pathogenic bacteria and fungi in animal sewage and laboratory effluents. Can. J. Vet. Res. **51:** 285–289.
24. KURTH, J., R. WALDMANN, J. HEITH, et al. 1999. Efficient inactivation of viruses and mycoplasma in animal sera using UVC irradiation. Dev. Biol. Stand. **99:** 111–118.
25. WHITE, L.A., C.Y. FREEMAN, H.E. HALL, et al. 1990. Inactivation and stability of viral diagnostic reagents treated by gamma radiation. Biologicals **18:** 271–280.
26. FIGUEROA, J.V., G.J. CANTO, J.A. ALVAREZ, et al. 1998. Capacidad protectora en bovinos de una cepa de *Babesia bigemina* derivada del cultivo *in vitro*. Tec. Pecu. Mex. **36** 95–107.
27. WESSMAN, S.J. & R.L. LEVINGS. 1999. Benefits and risks due to animal serum used in cell culture production. Dev. Biol. Stand. **99:** 3–8.
28. OHAGEN, A., V. GIBAJA, J. HORRIGAN, et al. 2004. Induction of latent human cytomegalovirus by conventional gamma irradiation and prevention by treatment with INACTINE PEN110. Vox Sang. **87:** 1–9.
29. CAMPBELL, D.G. & P. LI. 1999. Sterilization of HIV with irradiation: relevance to infected bone allografts. Aust. N. Z. J. Surg. **69:** 517–521.
30. PRUSS, A., M. KAO, U. GOHS, et al. 2002. Effect of gamma irradiation on human cortical bone transplants contaminated with enveloped and non-enveloped viruses. Biologicals **30:** 125–133.
31. PRUSS, A., A. HANSEN, M. KAO, et al. 2001. Comparison of the efficacy of virus inactivation methods in allogeneic vital bone tissue transplants. Cell Tissue Bank. **2:** 201–215.
32. HOUSE, C., J.A. HOUSE & R.J. YEDLOUTSCHNIG. 1990. Inactivation of viral agents in bovine serum by gamma irradiation. Can. J. Microbiol. **36:** 737–740.

Comparative Genomics of Three Strains of *Ehrlichia ruminantium*

A Review

ROGER FRUTOS,[a] ALAIN VIARI,[b] CONCHITA FERRAZ,[c]
ALBERT BENSAID,[a,d] ANNE MORGAT,[b,e] FREDERIC BOYER,[b]
ERIC COISSAC,[b] NATHALIE VACHIÉRY,[a]JACQUES DEMAILLE,[c]
AND DOMINIQUE MARTINEZ[a]

[a]*Cirad, Emvt Department, TA30/G, Campus International de Baillarguet, 34398,
Montpellier Cedex 05, France*

[b]*Inria Rhône-Alpes-Projet HELIX, 655, Av. de l'Europe, 38330
Montbonnot-Saint Martin, France*

[c]*Centre de Séquençage Génomique, IGH-CNRS-UPR 1142, 141 rue de la
Cardonille, 34396 Montpellier Cedex 05, France*

[d]*Centre de Recerca en Sanitat Animal, Campus de Belleterra, Edifici V, 08193
Bellaterra, Barcelona, Spain*

[e]*Swiss Institute of Bioinformatics, Swiss-Prot Group, 1 rue Michel, Servet,
CH-1211 Geneva 4, Switzerland*

ABSTRACT: The tick-borne *Rickettsiale Ehrlichia ruminantium (E. ruminantium)* is the causative agent of heartwater in Africa and the
Caribbean. Heartwater, responsible for major losses on livestock in
Africa represents also a threat for the American mainland. Three complete genomes corresponding to two different groups of differing phe-
notypes, Gardel and Welgevonden, have been recently described. One
genome (Erga) represents the Gardel group from Guadeloupe Island
and two genomes (Erwo and Erwe) belong to the Welgevonden group.
Erwo, isolated in South Africa, is the parental strain of Erwe, which was
maintained for 18 years in Guadeloupe under different culture conditions than Erwo. The three strains display genomes of differing sizes with
1,499,920 bp, 1,512,977 bp, and 1,516,355 bp for Erga, Erwe, and Erwo,
respectively. Gene sequences and order are highly conserved between
the three strains, although several gene truncations could be pinpointed,
most of them occurring within three regions of accumulated differences
(RAD). *E. ruminantium* displays a strong leading/lagging compositional
bias inducing a strand-specific codon usage. Finally, a striking feature
of *E. ruminantium* is the presence of long intergenic regions containing

Address for correspondence: Roger Frutos, CIRAD TA30/G, Campus International de Baillarguet,
34398 Montpellier Cedex 5, France. Voice: +33-4-67-59-39-62; fax: +33-4-67-59-39-60.
e-mail: roger.frutos@cirad.fr

Ann. N.Y. Acad. Sci. 1081: 417–433 (2006). © 2006 New York Academy of Sciences.
doi: 10.1196/annals.1373.061

tandem repeats. **These repeats are at the origin of an active process, specific to** *E. ruminantium*, **of genome expansion/contraction based on the addition or removal of tandem units.**

KEYWORDS: *Ehrlichia ruminantium;* heartwater; comparative genomics; complete genome

INTRODUCTION

The rickettsia, *Ehrlichia ruminantium (E. ruminantium)* is an obligate intracellular pathogen of endothelial cells of ruminants responsible for heartwater or cowdriosis in Africa where it causes major economic losses[1,2] and the Caribbean from where it threatens the American mainland due to the presence of potentially transmitting ticks.[3,4] The control of current strategy for controlling heartwater is based on a combination of vector control and immunization to achieve endemic stability. Vector eradication can only be envisaged in islands where the incoming flow of ticks is highly limited[5] and vaccine development, therefore, remains critical. However, the only commercial vaccine available is 50 years old and relies on the high-risk method of infection of cattle with infected blood followed by treatment with antibiotics.[6] Good attenuated and DNA vaccines were developed,[7–9] but their use in the field was limited by the occurrence of strain combinations.[7,10–13] Strain-specific diagnostics are thus crucial to efficient vaccine development and management. Serodiagnosis of heartwater is hampered by a lack of specificity and sensitivity of the various tests available.[14] The use of MAP1-related proteins in ELISA tests[15,16] has greatly improved the specificity but cross-reactions remain with other *Ehrlichia* spp.[17] In addition, MAP1 bears polymorphic epitopes, which could interfere with the sensitivity of the test depending on strains circulating in the field. Furthermore, sensitivity for bovine sera is poor.[18] PCR-based methods are widely used[19–21] and confirm the presence of various *E. ruminantium* genotypes simultaneously circulating in limited geographic areas.[22] Additional diagnostic targets, protective proteins, and potential drug targets are, therefore, still needed. A better global understanding of the variability is a prerequisite to any step toward improvement of diagnostic tools and vaccines. We thus report here the differential analysis of the genome of three phenotypically different strains of *E. ruminantium.*

MATERIALS AND METHODS

Origin of Bacterial Strains and Sequencing

The strain Gardel of *E. ruminantium* (Erga) was isolated on Guadeloupe Island in 1982 from a goat injected with a homogenate of a female tick of

A. variegatum collected on cows.[23] The strain Welgevonden of *E. ruminantium* (Erwe/Erwo) was isolated in South Africa in 1985 from mice injected with individually homogenized infected field-collected *A. hebraeum* ticks.[24] A sample of this Welgevonden strain, received in Guadeloupe Island in 1988, was immediately injected to a naïve goat. A blood sample was used to inoculate a cell culture and total of 13 additional successive passages were done. Passages 11 to 14 were used to provide DNA for cloning and sequencing. This strain was denominated Erwe. The original field-isolated Welgevonden strain was maintained in South Africa where its genome was recently sequenced.[25] This Welgevonden strain is further referred to as Erwo. The strain Welgevonden (Erwe/Erwo) is infective and pathogenic to mice whereas the strain Gardel (Erga) is not. Strains Erga, Erwe on one hand and Erwo on the other were sequenced, assembled, and annotated completely independently. More details about DNA extraction, cloning, and sequencing are found in the respective publications on Erwo[25] and Erga/Erwe.[26]

Gene Prediction and Annotation

The Erga and Erwe genomes were both annotated as previously described[26] using the integrated computer environment GenoStar (www.genostar.com).[27] A five-order periodic Markov Model was used for detecting coding sequences (CDS), with a 120-bp cut-off value for CDS length and a probability threshold $P = 0.80$ for CDS of length less than 360 bp. All of these CDS were subsequently manually checked by using the GenoStar graphic display capabilities.[27] Similarity search of the products deduced from these CDS was performed using BlastP[28] against a database resulting from the nonredundant concatenation of SwissProt (Release 41) (www.expasy.org) and the proteomes of two completely sequenced *Rickettsiae*: *R. conorii*[29] and *R. prowazekii*[30] because of their close phylogenetic relationship to *Ehrlichiae*. Clusters of Orthologous Groups of proteins (COGs) were assigned using the same procedure by comparison with a database of annotated proteins displaying references to COG numbers and categories.[31] Cross-genomes comparisons were performed using BlastP.[28] A pair of CDS exhibiting more than 70% of identity and whose length was not differing for more than 20% was considered as a pair of homologous genes. Moreover, thanks to the high conservation of gene order, homologous genes with same relative position in Erga, Erwe, or Erwo were considered as orthologs. The sequence conservation between pairs of orthologs has been measured by pairwise alignment, using the "gap free end" variant of dynamic programming (i.e., gaps at 3′ and 5′ ends are ignored). Genome GC-skew analysis was performed with the procedure described by Grigoriev[32] and an arbitrary origin of coordinates was assigned at the putative origin of replication (no clear DNA-box could be located). Codon usage was analyzed by correspondence analysis[33] using the GenoBool module embedded in GenoStar.

The Erwo genome was independently annotated by Collins *et al.*[25] based on slightly differing parameters. The annotations of Erwo were kept as it is. Other genomes discussed in this study were extracted from genome reviews database (http://www.ebi.ac.uk/GenomeReviews/) and annotations were kept as it is.

RESULTS

General Genome Features

The general genome features are summarized in TABLE 1. The genome of Erga, Erwe, and Erwo are 1,499,920, 1,512,977, and 1,516,355 bp long, respectively with a G+C content of 27.5%. The genome of Erga comprises 950 CDS of an average size of 1007 bp. The genome of Erwe bears 958 CDS of an average size of 998 bp (TABLE 1). The Erwo genome bears 920 CDS out of which 32 are considered as pseudogenes.[28] The differences in the number of CDS between Erwe and Erwo (38 CDS) are due to slightly different annotation strategies. One reason is the minimum CDS length threshold (120 bp with probability 0.8 for Erga and Erwe). Another reason is the presence of pseudogenes that were split into two CDS for Erga and Erwe,[26] whereas they have been annotated as a single entity (with a frameshift) in Erwo.[25]

A striking feature of the three *E. ruminantium* genomes is their very low coding ratio (number of bp involved in CDS/total number of bp) of 64% (TABLE 1). As compared to all annotated bacterial and archebacterial genomes available from databanks, *E. ruminantium* exhibits the lowest coding ratio observed so far (FIG. 1) with the exception of *Mycobacterium leprae.*[34] However, in the latter case, the low coding ratio is due to the very high number of pseudogenes.[34] Since the average gene length in *E. ruminantium* is the same as usually observed in bacteria (TABLE 1), this lower ratio is actually due to longer intergenic regions.[26]

TABLE 1. General features of Erga, Erwe, and Erwo genomes

Features	Genome		
	Erga	Erwe	Erwo[a]
Genome size (bp)	1,499,920	1,512,977	1,516,355
G+C content	27.51%	27.48%	27.5%
Number of predicted CDS	950	958	920
Coding ratio[b]	64.4%	63.8%	63.1%
Mean CDS size (bp)	1,007	998	1,032
Number tRNA	36	36	36
Number of rRNA	3	3	3

[a] = As described by Collins *et al.*[25]
[b] = number of bp in CDS / total number of bp.

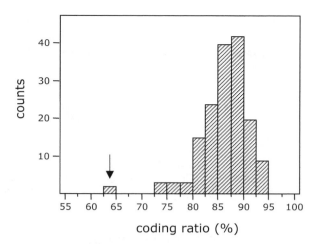

FIGURE 1. Coding ratio of bacterial and archaeabacterial genomes. Distribution of the coding ratio (number of bp involved in CDS/ total number of bp) observed in 160 bacterial and archebacterial genomes. The arrow denotes the position of *E. ruminantium*.

Comparative Analysis of the Genomes and Genome Size Plasticity

Erga and Erwe display 903 pairs of orthologs (95.0% of the genes) (see "Materials and Methods" section) and Erwe an Erwo display 873 pairs of orthologs (94.8%). FIGURE 2 A displays the differences of the CDS length of Erga/Erwe and Erwe/Erwo orthologs, showing that most of them actually have exactly the same length. FIGURE 2 B displays the percentage of identity between

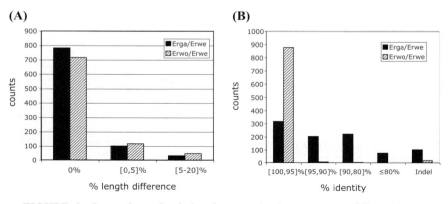

FIGURE 2. Comparison of orthologs between the three genomes of *E. ruminantium*. (**A**) Differences of the CDS length between Erga/Erwe (*black*) and Erwe/Erwo (*gray*) orthologs. (**B**) Percentage of identity at the nucleotidic level between Erga/Erwe (*black*) and Erwe/Erwo (*gray*) orthologs.

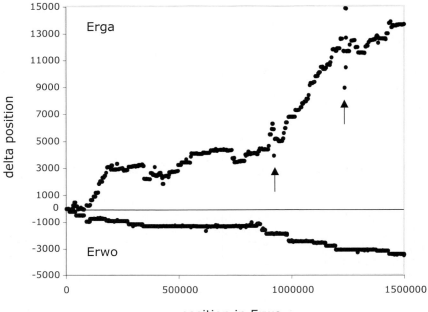

FIGURE 3. Repartition of size differences between the three genomes of *E. ruminantium.*Each dot corresponds to a pair of orthologs between Erga/Erwe (top curve) and Erwo/Erwe (*bottom curve*). The x axis represents the absolute position (in bp) in Erwe. The y axis represents the variation of the position of the corresponding ortholog in Erga (*top curve*) and Erwo (*bottom curve*). The total genome size difference is 13 kb between Erga and Erwe and 3 kb between Erwo and Erwe. The arrows denote the positions of the two small inversions between Erga and Erwe/Erwo. Note that, for the sake of comparison the origin of the Erwo chromosome has been shifted by 19 kb.

Erga/Erwe and Erwe/Erwo orthologs (see "Materials and Methods" section). This shows that despite the fact that Erwe and Erwo have been sequenced independently, their CDS are highly similar. In spite of their slight difference in length Erga, Erwe, and Erwo exhibit a highly conserved gene order and the perfect colinearity is only affected by two small inversions involving 2 and 3 CDS, respectively, between Erga and Erwe/Erwo. Full genome alignments, using the orthologs as anchor points, indicate that the differences in genome size between Erwe and Erwo (3 kb) and between Erga and Erwe (13 kb) are not due to specific large deletions but due to small size increments/decrements scattered almost uniformly along the genomes (FIG. 3). FIGURE 3 displays the variations of position in Erga (y-axis top curve) and Erwo (y-axis bottom curve) versus the absolute position in Erwe (x axis). The region between 250 kb and 800 kb is slightly more stable. Since gene length is very well conserved between the three strains, these increments/decrements are actually due to intergenic regions of varying size. A striking trait of *E. ruminantium* is the presence of a high number of tandem repeats making up to 8.3% of the chromosome[25] and mostly located in noncoding regions. Moreover, Frutos *et al.*[26] reported that these intergenic regions exhibit important size plasticity related to the presence of the tandem repeats. More precisely, the genome expansion/contraction in noncoding regions occurs by loss/gain of tandem repeat units of about 150 bp, that is, by varying the number of copies rather than by insertion or deletion of fragments of differing size.

Comparative Analysis of Unique and Truncated Genes

Fifty-seven unique CDS, defined as sequences for which no predicted orthologs are found in the other genome, are observed within the three genomes. Careful examination of sequence alignments shows that the same sequences are actually found in Erwe and Erwo and that the differences between Erwe and Erwo are only due to different annotation strategies (see above). Altogether, 34 CDS are specific to the Erwe/Erwo group when compared to Erga, whereas 22 are found only in Erga. Only 7 out of these 57 unique CDS correspond to major rearrangements, such as complete or partial deletions or extensive mutations. The remaining 49 CDS are unique CDS because of decay of the corresponding sequence in the other strain, making it too short to reach the minimal ORF size set for prediction. Beside these unique genes, several other CDS display full-length orthologs in two strains and a truncated version in the third one. More precisely, 18 such CDS truncations differentiate the genome of Erga from that of Erwe/Erwo, out of which 8 are specific to Erga and 10 are found only in Erwe/Erwo. Out of these 18 truncations, only 2 affect known genes, that is, *map1–2* (truncated in Erga) and *ftsA* (truncated in Erwe/Erwo). Finally, an additional set of 7 truncations affect the three genomes but differently depending upon the strain. Only one CDS out of these has a known function (putative type IV secreted protein). Most of the unique and truncated CDS are affected by a single (STOP codon) or very few point mutations and thus are not suited for differential diagnostics since most of the homologous sequence is still present in the other strains. However, 12 genes bear large deletions or extensive mutations and thus represent targets of choice for the development of differential diagnostics. These target CDS are listed in TABLE 2. Finally, although the mutated CDS are evenly distributed in the genome of *E. ruminantium*, we identified three regions of accumulated differences (RAD) where contiguous CDS were affected by different kinds of truncations or genomic rearrangements. These RAD are displayed in FIGURE 4.

Functional Annotation of the E. ruminantium Genome

Out of the 950 CDS described in the chromosome of Erga, 340 (36%) do not correspond to any COG category and no function could be attributed.

TABLE 2. Target genes for differential diagnostic of Erga and Erwe/Erwo

Target gene in Erga	Status	Target gene in Erwe	Status
ERGA_CDS_05600	Unique gene	None	Sequence absent (full deletion)
ERGA_CDS_07600	Unique gene	None	Sequence absent (full deletion)
ERGA_CDS_04990	Unique gene	None	Partial deletion
ERGA_CDS_05610	Unique gene	None	Extensive mutations
None	Partial deletion	ERWE_CDS_08340	Unique gene
ERGA_CDS_04350	Unique gene	None	Extensive mutations
ERGA_CDS_00120	Full length gene	ERWE_CDS_00120	Truncated gene (partial deletion)
ERGA_CDS_01350	Full length gene	ERWE_CDS_01390	Truncated gene (partial deletion)
ERGA_CDS_07340	Truncated gene partial deletion	ERWE_CDS_07420	Full length gene
ERGA_CDS_05750	Full length gene	ERWE_CDS_05840	Truncated gene (partial deletion)
ERGA_CDS_04510	Full length gene	ERWE_CDS_04590	Frameshift (partial deletion)
		ERWE_CDS_04600	Frameshift (partial deletion)
ERGA_CDS_05360	Full length gene	ERWE_CDS_05460	Frameshift (partial deletion)
		ERWE_CDS_05470	Frameshift (partial deletion)

For the remaining CDS (64%), some COG functional categories are underrepresented in *E. ruminantium* when compared to the overall COG database (FIG. 5): carbohydrate transport and metabolism (G), transcription (K), cell wall/membrane/envelope biogenesis (M), signal transduction mechanisms (T), and defense mechanisms (V). The latter category is also underrepresented when compared to the phylogenetically related *Rickettsia* (*R. conorii* and *R. prowazekii*). Interestingly, groups H (coenzyme transport and metabolism) and F (nucleotide transport and metabolism) are overrepresented when compared to both the overall COG database and the *Rickettsia* (FIG. 5). Some groups are under- or overrepresented with respect to the overall COG database but are present at a similar ratio in *Rickettsia*: cell motility (N), lipid transport and metabolism (I), intracellular trafficking, secretion and vesicular transport (U), amino acid transport and metabolism (E), and posttranslational modification, protein turnover, and chaperones (L). The same results were observed for the genomes of Erwe and Erwo and no significant differences were observed in terms of metabolic capabilities between the three strains.

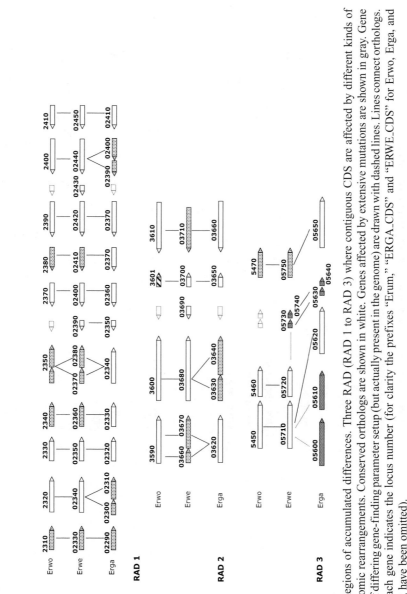

FIGURE 4. Regions of accumulated differences. Three RAD (RAD 1 to RAD 3) where contiguous CDS are affected by different kinds of truncations or genomic rearrangements. Conserved orthologs are shown in white. Genes affected by extensive mutations are shown in gray. Gene missing because of differing gene-finding parameter setup (but actually present in the genome) are drawn with dashed lines. Lines connect orthologs. The label above each gene indicates the locus number (for clarity the prefixes "Erum," "ERGA_CDS" and "ERWE_CDS," for Erwo, Erga, and Erwe, respectively, have been omitted).

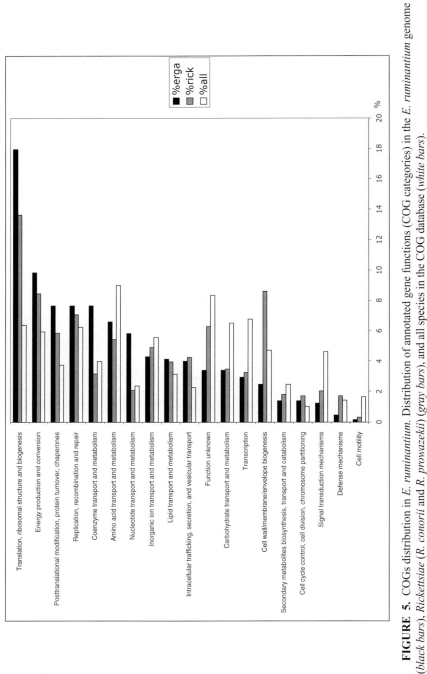

FIGURE 5. COGs distribution in *E. ruminantium*. Distribution of annotated gene functions (COG categories) in the *E. ruminantium* genome (*black bars*), Rickettsiae (*R. conorii* and *R. prowazekii*) (*gray bars*), and all species in the COG database (*white bars*).

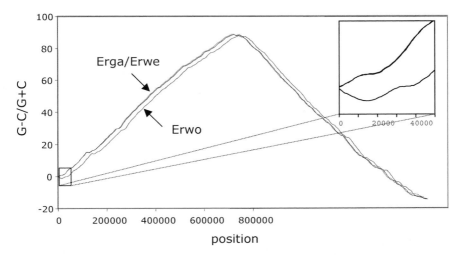

FIGURE 6. GC-skew of the *E. ruminantium* genomes. The y axis represents the GC-skew (G-C/G+C) versus the position (in bp) along the three genomes. In the absence of clear DNA box, this curve is used to assign a putative location of the origin of replication ORI (minimum of the curve). The slight difference observed between Erga/Erwe and Erwo is due to a shift of 19 kb in ORI location between authors. The inset is a zoom over the first 50 kb.

Compositional Biases

As shown in FIGURE 6, *E. ruminantium* exhibits a strong GC-skew.[35] The slight difference observed between Erga/Erwe and Erwo on the figure arise from a shift of 19 kb in the origin of replication assigned in Erwo. In the absence of clear DNA box, the precise location of the origin of replication is difficult to ascertain. However, the position indicated in Erga/Erwe[26] fits better to the GC-skew than the one proposed for Erwo.[25] The leading/lagging compositional bias is strong enough to influence drastically the codon usage of *E. ruminantium*, a phenomenon already observed in spirochetes.[36] Correspondence analysis of codon usage clearly shows two separated gene clusters (FIG. 7) associated with the leading and lagging strands. FIGURE 7 also shows the presence of an additional cluster when looking on the lower part of axis 2. Genes present in this cluster are localized indifferently on both strands and have an amino acid composition biased toward the enrichment of large, hydrophobic amino acids: phenylalanine and tryptophan.[26] One hundred sixteen CDS are present in this cluster out of which 47 have been assigned to known proteins, all of them being membrane proteins.[26] The unknown proteins from this cluster might, therefore, also be membrane proteins specific to *E. ruminantium*.

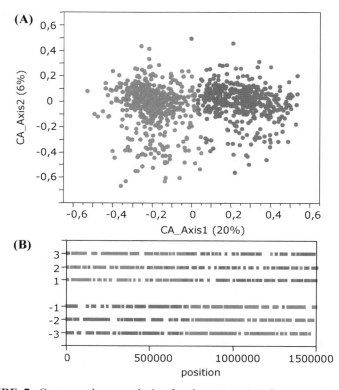

FIGURE 7. Correspondence analysis of codon usage. (**A**) Correspondence analysis (CA) of codon usage of all CDS in Erga (same results are observed for Erwe and Erwo). Each dot corresponds to a CDS. The axis represents respectively 20% and 6% of the total inertia. (**B**) Location of the red and green CDS in (**A**) along the chromosome. Red dots correspond to genes mostly on the leading strand whereas green dots correspond to genes mostly on the lagging strand.

DISCUSSION

Developing efficient vaccines remains a key issue in the control of heartwater since the efficacy of the current vaccines is limited in the field.[7,8,10–13] An attenuated vaccine, recently derived from the Welgevonden strain, is protective against several strains, including Gardel, under laboratory conditions.[9] However, it is not known yet whether this strain will, like other vaccines, be limited in field efficiency. The simultaneous presence of various *E. ruminantium* genotypes in limited geographic areas[22] provides an explanation for the limited field efficacy of single-strain vaccines. Owing to this diversity, vaccine management is therefore a key issue and comparative genomics makes an efficient approach for tackling this issue and understanding the phenomena potentially involved.

The first interesting feature, well in phase with this observed variability, is the high level of genome plasticity in *E. ruminantium*. Genome plasticity is an ongoing process in *E. ruminantium* and is characterized by a permanent deletion insertion of tandem repeats and occurrence of gene disruptions. This differentiates *E. ruminantium* from other intracellular bacteria for which genome stability following initial size reduction is usually a key feature.[35,37–40] *E. ruminantium* seems to be capable of rapidly undergoing genomic rearrangements upon exposure to a novel environment, which may well explain for a large part the poor field efficacy of vaccines. Another trait is the apparent ability of *E. ruminantium* to undergo gene disruptions following environmental changes. This is exemplified by the mutations observed in Erwe, but also by the recombination the *map1–2* and *map 1–3* genes of CTVM Gardel isolate, a subset strain of Erga, which led to the lack of production of Map1-2.[41] The development of an attenuated phenotype of the Welgevonden strain by propagation in an unusual cell environment, that is, a canine macrophage–monocyte cell line[9] also illustrates this phenomenon. In addition to its ability to accumulate gene truncations, *E. ruminantium* is also characterized by the presence of a specific mechanism of genomic plasticity based on the insertion/deletion of tandem repeat units of about 150 bp[26] compatible with RecA-independent recombination.[42,43] Interestingly, although *E. ruminantium* bears the *recA* gene as well as other genes involved in DNA repair, the RecA-independent mechanism seems to be favored. This suggests that selection pressure is still active or that some elements of the excision mechanism may be not fully functional. This deletion/expansion process is still very active and both its occurrence at a rather short-time scale (as observed between Erwe and Erwo) and its susceptibility to environmental changes could participate to explain the diversity of genotypes of *E. ruminantium* encountered in the field and the limited efficacy of vaccines.

The sole identification of the presence of *E. ruminantium* is therefore clearly insufficient for effective control and prevention of heartwater and differential diagnosis at the strain level must be considered. Owing to the expected evolution of isolated populations,[37] the major mutations differentiating Erga from Erwe/Erwo are most likely to be strain specific and represent thus candidates for the development of diagnostic tools. Another specific trait to investigate further is the presence of regions of accumulated differences or RAD in *E. ruminantium*. Phenotypic strain differences like pathogenesis or host range were often related to large insertion–deletion events or to large regions accumulating mutations.[44–47] However, the regions identified in the genome of *E. ruminantium* are instead relatively small mutational regions where contiguous CDS were affected by different kinds of mutations or genome rearrangements over time. These regions might be good targets for strain-specific diagnostics and further investigation should be considered to determine whether they exist in other strains. Interestingly, none of the mutations affecting genes of known functions can explain by itself the observed phenotypic differences between the

Gardel and Welgevonden strains. Candidates must therefore be sought among the other "orphan" genes affected by truncations. Transcriptomics should thus be considered to determine which genes are active and if any differential expression occurs between Erga and Erwe/Erwo as a preliminary step toward more extensive individual gene product analysis. Extending this analysis to the genomes of related bacteria will allow for the identification of genes involved in key mechanisms, such as pathogenesis, virulence, host range, or protection and will thus contribute to a better understanding of the biology of the *Rickettsiales*.

ACKNOWLEDGMENTS

The authors are very grateful to Y. Kandassamy (Cirad), I. Chantal (Cirad), and S. Eychenié (Igh-Cnrs) for technical support. The Welgevonden strain was kindly provided by Dr. Durr Bezuidenhout (Onderstepoort Veterinary Institute, South Africa), in 1988, as an exchange for the Gardel strain from Cirad. This work was supported by Cirad-Cnrs grant # 751745/00.

REFERENCES

1. PROVOST, A. & J.D. BEZUIDENHOUT. 1987. The historical background and global importance of heartwater. Onderstepoort J. Vet. Res. **54:** 165–169.
2. MUKHEBI, A.W., T. CHAMBOKO, C.J. O'CALLAGHAN, *et al.* 1999. An assessment of the economic impact of heartwater (*Cowdria ruminantium* infection) and its control in Zimbabwe. Prev. Vet. Med. **39:** 173–189.
3. BARRÉ, N., G. UILENBERG, P.C. MOREL & E. CAMUS. 1987. Danger of introducing heartwater onto the American mainland: potential role of indigenous and exotic *Amblyomma* ticks. Onderstepoort J. Vet. Res. **54:** 406–416.
4. BURRIDGE, M.J.J., L.A. SIMMONS, T.F. PETER & S.M. MAHAN. 2002. Increasing risks of introduction of heartwater onto the American mainland associated with animal movements. Ann. N. Y. Acad. Sci. **969:** 269–274.
5. PEGRAM, R.P., E.F. GERSABECK, D. WILSON & J.W. HANSEN. 2002. Eradication of the tropical bont tick in the Caribbean: is the Caribbean *Amblyomma* Program in a crisis? Ann. N. Y. Acad. Sci. **969:** 297–305.
6. BEZUIDENHOUT, J.D. 1989. Cowdria vaccines. *In* Veterinary Protozoan and Hemoparasite Vaccines. I.G. Wright Ed.: 31–42. CRC Press. Boca Raton.
7. JONGEJAN, F. 1991. Protective immunity to heartwater (*Cowdria ruminantium* infection) is acquired after vaccination with *in vitro*-attenuated *Rickettsiae*. Infect. Immun. **59:** 729–731.
8. COLLINS, N.E., A. PRETORIUS, M. VAN KLEEF, *et al.* 2003a. Development of improved vaccines for heartwater. Ann. N. Y. Acad. Sci. **990:** 474–484.
9. ZWEYGARTH, E., A.I. JOSEMANS, M.F. VAN STRIJP, *et al.* 2005. An attenuated *Ehrlichia ruminantium* (Welgevonden stock) vaccine protects small ruminants against virulent heartwater challenge. Vaccine **23:** 1695–1702.

10. COLLINS, N.E., A. PRETORIUS, M. VAN KLEEF, *et al.* 2003b. Development of improved attenuated and nucleic acid vaccines for heartwater. Dev. Biol. **114:** 121–136.
11. MAHAN, S.M., A.F. BARBET & M.J. BURRIDGE. 2003. Development of improved vaccines for heartwater. Dev. Biol. **114:** 137–145.
12. MARTINEZ, D., J.C. MAILLARD, S. COISNE, *et al.* 1994. Protection of goats against heartwater acquired by immunisation with inactivated elementary bodies of *Cowdria ruminantium*. Vet. Immunol. Immunopathol. **41:** 153–163.
13. MARTINEZ, D., J.M. PEREZ, C. SHEIKBOUDOU, *et al.* 1996. Comparative efficacy of Freund's and Montanide ISA50 adjuvants for the immunisation of goats against heartwater with inactivated *Cowdria ruminantium*. Vet. Parasitol. **67:** 175–184.
14. MONDRY, R., D. MARTINEZ, E. CAMUS, *et al.* 1998. Validation and comparison of three enzyme-linked immunosorbent assays for the detection of antibodies to *Cowdria ruminantium* infection. Ann. N. Y. Acad. Sci. **849:** 262–272.
15. KATZ, J.B., R. DEWALD, J.E. DAWSON, *et al.* 1997. Development and evaluation of a recombinant antigen, monoclonal antibody-based competitive ELISA for heartwater serodiagnosis. J. Vet. Diagn. Invest. **9:** 130–135.
16. VAN VLIET, A.H., B.A. VAN DER ZEIJST, E. CAMUS, *et al.* 1995. Use of a specific immunogenic region on the *Cowdria ruminantium* MAP1 protein in a serological assay. J. Clin. Microbiol. **33:** 2405–2410.
17. JONGEJAN, F., N. DE VRIES, J. NIEUWENHUIJS, *et al.* 1993. The immunodominant 32-kilodalton protein of *Cowdria ruminantium* is conserved within the genus *Ehrlichia*. Rev. Elev. Med. Vet. Trop. **46:** 145–152.
18. SEMU, S.M., T.F. PETER, D. MUKWEDEYA, *et al.* 2001. Antibody responses to MAP 1B and other *Cowdria ruminantium* antigens are down regulated in cattle challenged with tick-transmitted heartwater. Clin. Diagn. Lab. Immunol. **8:** 388–396.
19. PETER, T.F., S.L. DEEM, A.F. BARBET, *et al.* 1995. Development and evaluation of PCR assay for detection of low levels of *Cowdria ruminantium* infection in *Amblyomma* ticks not detected by DNA probe. J. Clin. Microbiol. **33:** 166–172.
20. ALLSOPP, M.T., E.S. VISSER, J.L. DU PLESSIS, *et al.* 1997. Different organisms associated with heartwater as shown by analysis of 16S ribosomal RNA gene sequences. Vet. Parasitol. **71:** 283–300.
21. BEKKER, C.P.J., S. DE VOS, A. TAOUFIK, *et al.* 2002. Simultaneous detection of *Anaplasma* and *Ehrlichia* species in ruminants and detection of *Ehrlichia ruminantium* in *Amblyomma variegatum* ticks by reverse line blot hybridization. Vet. Microbiol. **89:** 223–238.
22. MARTINEZ, D., N. VACHIERY, F. STACHURSKI, *et al.* 2005. Nested PCR for the detection and genotyping of *Ehrlichia ruminantium*. Use in genetic diversity analysis. Ann. N. Y. Acad. Sci. **1026:** 106–113.
23. UILENBERG, G., E. CAMUS & N. BARRÉ. 1985. Some observations on a stock of *Cowdria ruminantium* from Guadeloupe (French West Indies). Rev. Elev. Med. Vet. Pays Trop. **34:** 34–42.
24. DU PLESSIS, J.L. 1985. A method for determining the *Cowdria ruminantium* infection rate of *Amblyomma hebraeum*: effects in mice injected with tick homogenates. Onderstepoort J. Vet. Res. **52:** 55–61.
25. COLLINS, N.E., J. LIEBENBERG, E.P. DE VILLIERS, *et al.* 2005. The genome of the heartwater agent *Ehrlichia ruminantium* contains multiple tandem re-

peats of actively variable number. Proc. Natl. Acad. Sci. USA **102:** 838–843.

26. FRUTOS, R., A. VIARI, C. FERRAZ, *et al.* 2006. Comparative genomic analysis of three strains of *Ehrlichia ruminantium* reveals an active process of genome size plasticity. J. Bacteriol. **188:** 2533–2542.

27. DURAND, P., C. MEDIGUE, A. MORGAT, *et al.* 2003. Integration of data and methods for genome analysis. Curr. Opin. Drug Discov. Dev. **6:** 346–352.

28. ALTSCHUL, S.F., T.L. MADDEN, A.A. SCHAFFER, *et al.* 1997. Gapped BLAST and PSI-BLAST: a new generation of protein database search programs. Nucleic Acids Res. **25:** 3389–3402.

29. ANDERSSON, S.G., A. ZOMORODIPOUR, J.O. ANDERSSON, *et al.* 1998. The genome sequence of *Rickettsia prowazekii* and the origin of mitochondria. Nature **396:** 133–140.

30. OGATA, H., S. AUDIC, P. RENESTO-AUDIFFREN, *et al.* 2001. Mechanisms of evolution in *Rickettsia conorii* and *R. prowazekii*. Science **293:** 2093–2098.

31. TATUSOV, R.L., N.D. FEDOROVA, J.D. JACKSON, *et al.* 2003. The COG database: an updated version includes eukaryotes. BMC Bioinformatics **4:** 41–54.

32. GRIGORIEV, A. 1998. Analyzing genomes with cumulative skew diagrams. Nucleic Acids Res. **26:** 2286–2290.

33. PERRIERE, G. & J. THIOULOUSE. 2002. Use and misuse of correspondence analysis in codon usage studies. Nucleic Acids Res. **30:** 4548–4555.

34. COLE, S.T., K. EIGLMEIER, J. PARKHILL, *et al.* 2001. Massive gene decay in the leprosy bacillus. Nature **409:** 1007–1111.

35. KLASSON, L. & S.G.E. ANDERSSON. 2004. Evolution of minimal-gene-sets in host-dependent bacteria. Trends Microbiol. **12:** 37–43.

36. ROCHA, E.P., A. DANCHIN & A. VIARI. 1999. Universal replication biases in bacteria. Mol. Microbiol. **32:** 11–16.

37. BERG, O.G., & C.G. KURLAND. 2002. Evolution of microbial genomes: sequence acquisition and loss. Mol. Biol. Evol. **19:** 2265–2276.

38. MIRA, A., L. KLASSON & S.G.E. ANDERSSON. 2002. Microbial genome evolution: sources of variability. Curr. Opin. Microbiol. **5:** 506–512.

39. MORAN, N.A. & A. MIRA. 2001. The process of genome shrinkage in the obligate symbiont *Buchnera aphidicola*. Genome Biol. **2:** 0054.1–0054.12.

40. TAMAS, I., L. KLASSON, B. CANBACK, *et al.* 2002. 50 million years of genomic stasis in endosymbiotic bacteria. Science **296:** 2376–2379.

41. BEKKER, C.P.J., M. POSTIGO, A. TAOUFIK, *et al.* 2005. Transcription analysis of the major antigenic protein 1 multigene family of three in vitro cultured *Ehrlichia ruminantium* isolates. J. Bacteriol. **187:** 4782–4791.

42. BZYMEK, M. & S.T. LOVETT. 2001. Instability of repetitive DNA sequences: the role of replication in multiple mechanisms. Proc. Natl. Acad. Sci. USA **98:** 8319–8325.

43. LOVETT, S.T. 2004. Encoded errors: mutations and rearrangements mediated by misalignment at repetitive DNA sequences. Mol. Microbiol. **52:** 1243–1253.

44. BROSH, R., A.S. PYM, S.V. GORDON & S.T. COLE. The evolution of mycobacterial pathogenicity: clues from comparative genomics. Trends Microbiol. **9:** 452–458.

45. FITZGERALD, J.R. & J.M. MUSSER. 2001. Evolutionary genomics of pathogenic bacteria. Trends Microbiol. **9:** 547–553.

46. FITZGERALD, R.J., D.E. STURDEVANT, S.M. MACKIE, *et al.* 2001. Evolutionary genomics of *Staphylococcus aureus*: insight into the origin of methicillin-resistant

strains and the toxic shock syndrome epidemic. Proc. Natl. Acad. Sci. USA **98:** 8821–8826.
47. CARROLL, I.M., A.A. KHAN & N. AHMED. 2004. Revisiting the pestilence of *Helicobacter pylori*: insights into geographical genomics and pathogen evolution. Infect. Genet. Evol. **4:** 81–90.

Emerging Tick-Borne Disease in African Vipers Caused by a *Cowdria*-Like Organism

JOHNATHAN L. KIEL,[a] RODOLFO M. ALARCON,[a] JILL E. PARKER,[a]
JEEVA VIVEKANANDA,[a] YVETTE B. GONZALEZ,[b]
LUCILLE J.V. STRIBLING,[a] AND CARRIE J. ANDREWS[a]

[a]*Air Force Research Laboratory, Brooks City-Base, Texas 78235-5107, USA*

[b]*Northrop Grumman, Inc., San Antonio, Texas 78228, USA*

ABSTRACT: Heartwater is a tick-borne infectious disease caused by the
rickettsial organism *Cowdria ruminantium*, currently *Ehrlichia ruminantium*. It poses an imminent threat to the Western Hemisphere, where it
could cause mortality in cattle and other ruminant livestock in excess of
70%. It has been reported in the Caribbean; and its vector, *Amblyomma
sparsum*, has been found on imported African spurred tortoises (*Geochelone sulcata*) and leopard tortoises (*Geochelone pardalis*) in southern
Florida in the United States, leading to an importation ban on these reptiles. Symptoms have not been previously reported in reptiles. Here, we
report peracute and acute deaths in African vipers imported from Africa
through Florida. Signs included vomiting mucoid fluid, diarrhea, emaciation, convulsions, and death. Postmortem showed few gross lesions. The
most consistent peracute and acute lesions were the pulmonary lesions
and pericarditis with considerable bloody fluid in the pericardial sac (hydropericardium). These lesions strongly resembled the lesions of heartwater and a coccobacillus of less than 1-micron diameter was isolated in
viper cell culture. The outbreak was brought to a halt by tick control and
treatment of all exposed snakes with tetracycline. This isolation, tetracycline sensitivity, clinical signs, preliminary results with polymerase chain
reaction of pCS20 ORF, and the viper preference of the disease may indicate a Cowdria-related attenuated species that has adapted to infect
reptiles or an emerging new form of this group of microbes.

KEYWORDS: Cowdria; Ehrlichia; viper; heartwater

INTRODUCTION

Heartwater is a tick-borne (*Amblyomma variegatum, Amblyomma hebraeum, Amblyomma lepidum, Amblyomma maculatum,* and other *Amblyomma*)

Address for correspondence: Johnathan L. Kiel, AFRL/HEPC, 2486 Gillingham Drive, Brooks City-
Base, TX 78235-5107. Voice: 210-536-3583; fax: 210-536-4716.
e-mail: Johnathan.Kiel@brooks.af.mil

Ann. N.Y. Acad. Sci. 1081: 434–442 (2006). © 2006 New York Academy of Sciences.
doi: 10.1196/annals.1373.062

infectious disease caused by the rickettsial organism formerly classified as the single member of the Genus Cowdria (*Cowdria ruminantium*), but now classified as *Ehrlichia ruminantium*.[1–3] *E. ruminantium* possesses a life cycle that closely resembles that of Chlamydia, with reticular bodies for intracellular reproduction and elementary (dense) bodies for infection of other cells.[2] Heartwater, or Cowdriosis, poses an imminent threat to the Western Hemisphere, where it could cause mortality in cattle and other ruminant livestock in excess of 70%.[4–7] It has been reported in the Caribbean (Islands of Antigua, Guadaloupe, Marie Galante, and perhaps even Cuba).[6–8] Its vector (*Amblyomma sparsum*), positive for Cowdria by pCS20 polymerase chain reaction (PCR) and DNA hybridization,[9] has been found on imported African spurred tortoises (*Geochelone sulcata*) and leopard tortoises (*Geochelone pardalis*) in southern Florida in the United States, leading to an importation and interstate movement ban on these reptiles.[10,11] Here, we report peracute and acute deaths in African vipers imported from Ghana (a major source of heartwater in West Africa),[12] and subsequent lethal secondary infections in cobras and United States' colubrid snakes, in a private collection, which closely resemble heartwater in signs and gross lesions. Culture, isolation, and molecular biology of the associated rickettsia are described.

MATERIALS AND METHODS

Clinical History and Ticks

On July 8, 2002, a juvenile Gaboon viper (*Bitis gabonica*) was presented dead as the first index case. From that time until February 19, 2003, a total of 22 snakes within the private collection showed similar neurological signs, including convulsions, followed by death. These snakes included eastern Gaboon vipers (*Bitis gabonica gabonica*), western Gaboon vipers (*Bitis gabonica rhinoceros*), rhinoceros vipers (*Bitis nasicornis*), a Sri Lankan cobra (*Naja naja polycellata*), a monocellate cobra (*Naja naja kaouthia*), a black-necked cobra (*Naja nigricollis*), and bullsnakes (*Pituophis melanoleucus sayi*). The outbreak only stopped after chemical removal of ticks with the topical pesticide permethrin (Provent-a-mite®, 0.5% permethrin; Pro Products, Mahopac, NY), and oral treatment of exposed snakes with tetracycline for 2 weeks. Other signs noted were swelling of the head and face, diarrhea, blindness, and vomiting of frothy mucoid material. Tissue samples from the lungs and liver were taken for standard sheep blood agar primary culture and isolation and some were retained for tissue culture in viper cells and bovine endothelial cells.

Two tick species were found on the premises (unfortunately collected following treatment with pesticide). These were the specific reptile tick *Aponomma latum*, which has not been associated with heartwater transmission, and *A. maculatum*, which can transmit heartwater, but has not been reported to parasitize reptiles.[4,8]

Cell Lines, Bacterial Strains, and Culture

Russell's Viper snake spleen epithelial cells (ATCC CCL-129) and bovine pulmonary artery vascular endothelium endothelial cells (ATCC CRL-1733) were obtained from the American Type Culture Collection, Rockville, MD. Viper snake spleen epithelial cells were cultured at 30°C with 5% CO_2 in minimal essential medium (MEM eagles ATCC 30-2003) with 10% fetal bovine serum (FBS; Atlanta Biologicals, Norcross, GA), and pen/strep (Sigma-Aldrich, St. Louis, MO). Liver homogenate was prepared from an isolated infected juvenile Gaboon viper snake liver. One hundred micrograms of the liver was homogenized in 500 μL MEM without FBS. Homogenate was transferred into a sterile microcentrifuge tube, an additional 500 μL of MEM was added, and the mixture was centrifuged at 7500 rpm for 15 min. The supernatant was filter sterilized (0.45 μm filter) and stored at −80°. Cell lines were infected with viper liver homogenate at 30°C with 5% CO_2 in MEM media and cytopathology was determined 24 h postexposure. Slide cultures of infected and mock-infected samples were processed for scanning electron microscopy (SEM).

Sterile swab samples were collected from the interior of lungs of one rhino viper and two eastern Gaboon vipers during postmortem examination. These were cultured on sheep blood agar and subcultured on liquid medium for biochemical analysis at Wilford Hall Medical Center, Lackland Air Force Base, Texas.

Microscopy

Upon receipt of cell cultures that still contained medium, the wells were filled with 3% glutaraldehyde, and the contents were fixed for 5 min at room temperature. The tip of a disposable pipette was placed in the very corner of each well and the medium/fixative mixture was slowly removed. Then, the wells were refilled with 3% glutaraldehyde and fixed for 1–2 h. After removing the glutaraldehyde from each well, the plastic wells and silicone gasket attached to the slide were gently peeled away. The slide wells were rinsed with distilled water and dehydrated with a graded series of ethanol. The slide was scored to separate the samples, mounted on aluminum specimen stubs, sputter-coated with a Hummer Sputter Coater (Hayward, CA), and viewed with a Philips XL20 SEM (Hillsboro, OR).

Primer Preparation and Molecular Biology

Three primers for pCS20 DNA were prepared with the following sequences:

AP126 GTAACACAATCTAAACTCGGTAAG[9]
AP127 CAGCCATACCTGACACGTATTCAT[9]
AP128 ACTAGTAGAAATTGCACAATCTAT[9]
AP129 TGATAACTTGGTGCGGGAAATCCTT[9]
pCS20F CTCACCCAAGTGTTCTTTC[10]
pCS20R GGTAACATTATATACAGCCATACCTGACAC

PCR was performed as described by Mahan *et al.*[9] Samples were run on 3% agarose gels in 1× TAE buffer. PCR products were precipitated using equal volume of 5 M ammonium acetate and two volumes of isopropanol. Samples were left at −20°C overnight. Samples were pooled and run on 3% gels. Bands were cut out and extracted from melted agarose by phenol extraction with lithium chloride and precipitation with ethanol. Precipitated DNA was dissolved in 5 μL DNA buffer and 1 μL run on an agarose gel to check size and concentration. Sequencing was performed.

RESULTS

Postmortem Gross Lesions

The postmortem of the juvenile Gaboon viper (index case) on July 8, 2002 revealed cheesy material in the trachea, a hyperemic lung, and kidneys with unusual red mottling. Acute pneumonia was the immediate cause of death. On August 7, 2002, a rhino viper died of pneumonia and shock based on the postmortem examination. On August 31, 2002, three more snakes were posted—a rhino viper adult (*B. nasicornis*), which had caseous mucoid material in the intestines and lung; a male adult eastern Gaboon (*Bitis gabonica gabonica*) viper with mucus in the esophagus, a hemorrhagic lung with caseous mucus, and a mottled liver; and a female adult eastern Gaboon viper with a hemorrhagic lung with fibrous and caseous mucoid material, large fat bodies, and the other organs essentially normal. On November 12, 2002, a Sri Lankan cobra (*Naja naja polycellata*, male) that died sometime in the last 3 days was found. It had lung hemorrhage with muco-purulent exudates, abundant peritoneal fluid, and dark tubules in kidneys delineated with urate crystals. At this time a juvenile Gaboon viper had died and was posted showing the same lung lesions as the other vipers and cobra. On February 19, 2003, a monocellate cobra (*Naja naja kaouthia*) died. At time of death, it was convulsive, had dry gangrene at tip of tail, and showed evidence of blindness. On February 23, 2003 it was posted, the cobra showed frothy deteriorated, bloody spots and necrosis on inner surface of lung, bloody lung and peritoneal fluid, focal white liver lesions throughout liver, enlarged pale heart muscle, blood that failed to clot in major vessels, abundant fat bodies, bloody fluid coming from mouth, and kidneys dark and swollen with a "bunch of grapes" surface.

Culture, Isolation, and Microscopic Results

Material for routine bacterial culture from the rhino and Gaboon vipers (as described above) yielded a nonviable organism on subculture from the rhino and *Proteus retgerri, Klebsiella oxytoca, Flavobacterium* spp., *Streptococcus uberus, Enterococcus casseliflavus,* and *Staphylococcus sciuri* from primary and subcultures from the Gaboon vipers. The standard bacteriology was inconsistent, with the disease syndrome not being attributable to any specific free-living bacterial agent. This observation led to the co-culturing of liver tissue isolated from the last juvenile Gaboon viper to die with viper cells and bovine endothelial cells. FIGURE 1 shows the cytopathic effects (light microscopy) on viper cells following a week of culture and bovine endothelial cells after

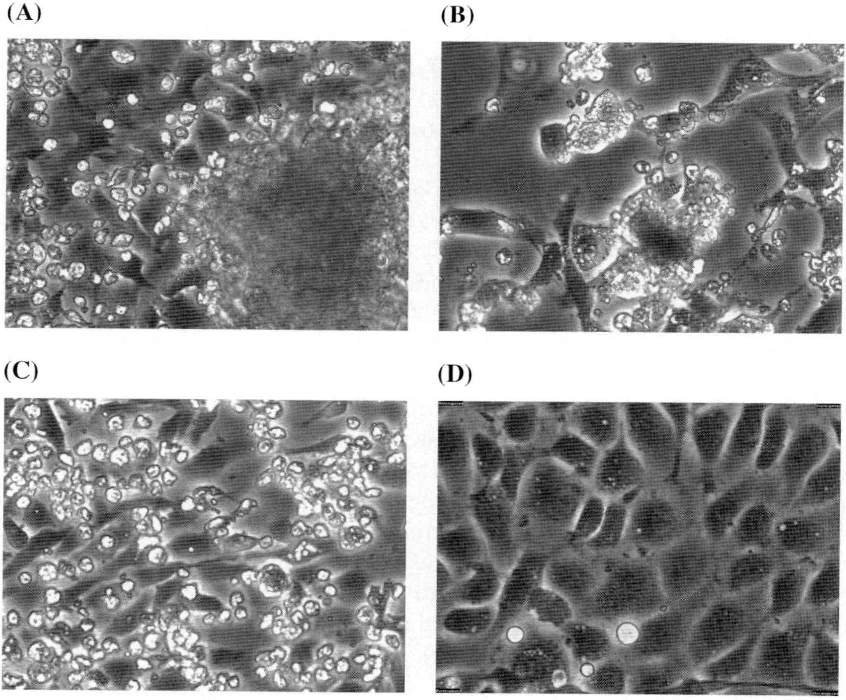

(A)   **(B)**

(C)   **(D)**

FIGURE 1. (**A**) Cytopathic effect (light microscopy) on viper cells following a week of culture with Cowdria-like microbes, and, (**B**), bovine endothelial cells following 24 h of culture with Cowdria-like microbes. Both are compared with their respective controls (**C** and **D**).

(A) (B)

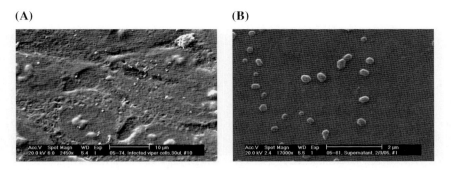

FIGURE 2. (A) SEMs of emerging clusters and individual microbes from the cytoplasm of viper cells. (B) Individual "elementary bodies," or dense bodies, of the microbe isolated from the viper cell cultures (approximately 200 nm in diameter).

24 h of infection with a concentrate from the viper cell culture. FIGURE 2 shows SEMs of emerging clusters and individual microbes from the cytoplasm of the viper cells and displays the individual "elementary bodies," or dense bodies, of the microbe isolated from the viper cell cultures (approximately 200 nm in diameter). FIGURE 3 shows the cellular lesions of the bovine endothelial cell culture at the single cell level.

PCR Results

FIGURE 4 shows PCR results from viper cells and original snake tissues including hepatic tissue from the juvenile Gaboon viper and a bullsnake and heart blood from adult rhino and Gaboon vipers. In many cases, PCR products were produced that matched in both the viper cells and postmortem tissue samples, but the multiple products were significantly different though related to those produced by authentic *E. ruminantium,* according to the literature.[1]

DISCUSSION

On December 21, 1999, the State of Florida Department of Agriculture and Consumer Services, Division of Animal Industry, issued a Florida Fish and Wildlife Conservation Emergency Prohibition against importation of certain African tortoises.[11,12] It banned the importation of African spurred tortoises (*G. sulcata*) and leopard tortoises (*G. pardalis*). The emergency ban was due to the finding that some tortoises were infected with "tropical bont ticks" carrying the rickettsia *E. ruminantium,* causative agent of heartwater. Ticks collected from a Hillsborough County, Florida, reptile facility tested positive for heartwater agent on November 29, 1999. On December 9, 1999, the Florida

(A)   (B)

(C)   (D)

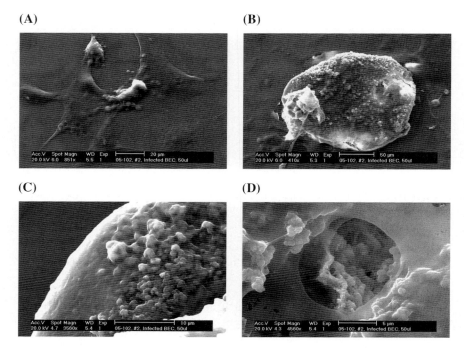

FIGURE 3. (A–D) The cellular lesions of the bovine endothelial cell culture at the single cell level (SEM).

Department of Agriculture and Consumer Services passed an emergency rule restricting the importation into the State of all wildlife without an official Certificate of Veterinary Inspection showing the animals to be free of heartwater and its vectors. The data presented here raises question of whether the rule can be enforced and whether sufficient technology exists to execute the order effectively. Snakes are not routinely examined for the disease or its vectors, in spite of many being imported through Miami, Florida, primarily from a high heartwater incidence area in Africa, Ghana.[13] The snakes reported here showing signs that strongly resemble those of heartwater in ruminants have been reported in the past to carry the vectors of heartwater.[4] The quandary exists, based on the preliminary results described herein, as to whether snakes are reservoirs (carriers) of true heartwater, or of some other disease that closely resembles it or is derived from it (through mutation, attenuation, and adaptation to snakes as hosts and their ectoparasites as vectors), that should be controlled. The successful infection of bovine endothelial cells strongly suggests the first case. What is clear is that the viper disease is highly pathogenic for snakes, crosses over to many species of snakes, and poses a threat to any zoo or private collection into which infected snakes enter. It could also enter native wildlife

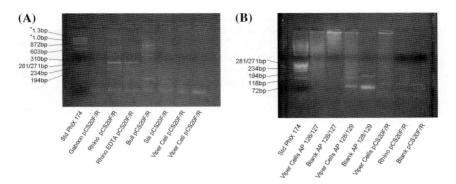

FIGURE 4. (A, B) Electrophoresis gel of PCR products of pCS20 primers interacting with DNA from viper cell cultures and from original snake tissues including hepatic tissue from the juvenile Gaboon viper and a bullsnake, and heart blood from adult rhino viper, Sis = *Sistrurus catenatus edwardsi*, Desert Massasauga rattlesnake, control. *First two bands in panel A are kilobase pairs.

populations of snakes, other reptiles, birds, and mammals. Although control of the tick vectors may be adequate, other blood-feeding arthropods (such as mites) could spread the disease from chronically infected snakes, or this rickettsia may be sufficiently different from *E. ruminantium* to switch to a direct transmission life cycle. At a minimum, the viper disease presents "diagnostic confusion" for the veterinary and regulatory officials who are trying to keep heartwater out of the continental United States. In honor of the discoverer of the disease, acknowledgment of its origin in the snake genus *Bitis*, and its place of origin, Ghana, we recommend, that if it is a new species, it be called *Ehrlichia bishopii v. bitighanae*, or if it proves to be a strain of *E. ruminantium*, that it be called *E. ruminantium v. bishopii*.

ACKNOWLEDGMENTS

We thank Dr. Pete D. Teel of Texas A&M University and Dr. Richard G. Robbins of Walter Reed Army Medical Center for identification of the ticks from the snake collection. This article is dedicated to the memory of Mike Bishop, the amateur herpetologist, who first alerted us to the presence of this viper disease in the United States.

REFERENCES

1. PETER, T.F., S.L. DEEM, A.F. BARBET, *et al.* 1995. Development and evaluation of PCR assay for detection of low levels of *Cowdria ruminantium* infection in *Amblyomma* ticks not detected by DNA probe. J. Clin. Microbiol. **33:** 166–172.

2. WALKER, D.H. & J.S. DUMLER. 1996. Emergence of the Ehrlichioses as human health problems. Emerg. Infect. Dis. **2:** 1–17.
3. DE VILLIERS, E.P., K.A. BRAYTON, E. ZWEYGARTH & B.A. ALLSOP. 2000. Genome size and genetic map of *Cowdria ruminantium*. Microbiology **146:** 2627–2634.
4. BURRIDGE, M.J. 2001. Ticks (Acari: Ixodidae) spread by the international trade in reptiles and their potential roles in dissemination of diseases. Bull. Entomol. Res. **91:** 3–23.
5. UILENBERG, G. 1983. Heartwater (*Cowdria ruminantium* infection): current status. Adv. Vet. Sci. Comp. Med. **27:** 427–480.
6. CAMUS, E., N. BARRE & G. UILENBERG. 1996. Heartwater (Cowdriosis). A Review 2nd ed. Office International des Epizooties. Paris.
7. MONTI, D.J. 2000. Florida not tickled by threat of infestation. J. Am. Vet. Med. Assoc. **216:** 651–655.
8. BURRIDGE, M.J., L.-A. SIMMONS, T.F. PETER & S.M. MAHAN. 2002. Increasing risks of introduction of heartwater onto the American mainland associated with animal movement. Ann. N. Y. Acad. Sci. **969:** 269–274.
9. MAHAN, S.M., S.D. WAGHELA, T.C. MCGUIRE, *et al.* 1992. A cloned DNA probe for *Cowdria ruminantium* hybridizes with eight heartwater strains and detects infected sheep. J. Clin. Microbiol. **30:** 981–986.
10. ALLSOPP, M.T.E.P., H. VAN HEERDEN, H.C. STEYN & B.A. ALLSOPP. 2003. Phylogenetic relationships among *Ehrlichia ruminantium* isolates. Ann. N. Y. Acad. Sci. **990:** 2–7.
11. DEPARTMENT OF AGRICULTURE AND CONSUMER SERVICES, DIVISION OF ANIMAL INDUSTRY. December 9, 1999. Heartwater Disease. 5C-ER-99-1.
12. FLORIDA FISH AND WILDLIFE CONSERVATION COMMISSION. 1999. Emergency prohibition against importation of certain African tortoises. 68A-ER-99-01.
13. KONEY, E.B.M. 1994–1997. Heartwater in Ghana: applying new diagnostic tests in disease epidemiology. **R5971CB:** 95–96.

Identification and Characterization of Merozoite Antigens of a *Theileria* Species Highly Pathogenic for Small Ruminants in China

JOANA MIRANDA,[a] ELISABETE NASCIMENTO,[a] HELDER CRUZ,[a] YIN HONG,[b] ANA COELHO,[a] JABBAR S. AHMED,[c] AND ABEL OLIVA[a]

[a]*Instituto de Biologia Experimental e Tecnologica (IBET)/ Instituto de Tecnologia Quimica e Biologica (ITQB)/ Universidade Nova de Lisboa (UNL), 2781-901 Oeiras, Portugal*

[b]*Lanzhou Veterinary Research Institute (LVRI), Lanzhou, Gansu 730046, People's Republic of China*

[c]*Department of Immunology and Cell Biology, Division of Veterinary Infectiology and Immunology, Research Center Borstel, 23845 Borstel, Germany*

ABSTRACT: A new pathogenic *Theileria* species transmitted by *Haemaphysalis qinghaiensis* was identified in the Northwestern part of China and was shown to be highly pathogenic for small ruminants. The present article aimed at identifying merozoite antigens that might be suitable for developing diagnostic methods and designing a potential vaccine. Absence of other theilerial or babesial infections was confirmed by reverse line blot in all antigen samples used. Extensive Western blot analyses using serum from infected and noninfected animals led to the identification of four potential merozoite immunoreactive proteins at different molecular weights. Further protein characterization using peptide mass mapping by matrix-assisted laser desorption/ionization (MALDI) followed by database searching resulted in two significant hits that identified two proteins of parasite origin, one homologous to a possible MO25-family protein from *Cryptosporidium parvum* and the other with an HSP70 from *Theileria annulata*. Another protein was also identified as a parasite protein but without significant homology. Immunization of rabbits with selected proteins produced antisera that reacted specifically on Western blots with merozoite antigens of the corresponding sizes. This article represents the first identification and characterization of potential antigenic proteins of *Theileria* sp. (China) for veterinary purposes.

KEYWORDS: *Theileria*; merozoites; Western blot; matrix-assisted laser desorption/ionization (MALDI); China

Address for correspondence: Abel Gonzalez Oliva, Biomolecular Diagnostic Laboratory, Av. Republica, Apartado 12, 2780-901 Oeiras, Portugal. Voice: 00351-214469428; fax: 00351-214411161.
e-mail: oliva@itqb.unl.pt

Ann. N.Y. Acad. Sci. 1081: 443–452 (2006). © 2006 New York Academy of Sciences.
doi: 10.1196/annals.1373.063

INTRODUCTION

Theileria organisms are tick-borne protozoan parasites infecting mainly ruminants in tropical and subtropical countries. Although capable of infecting a wide range of vertebrates, theilerial parasites require both vertebrate and nonvertebrate hosts (ticks) to maintain their life cycle. Depending on the *Theileria* species a variety of ticks are responsible for their transmission including *Rhipicephalus*, *Haemaphysalis*, and *Hyalomma*. Theileriosis is still a serious disease because it is responsible for severe economic losses in the livestock industry.[1]

Due to the economic relevance of small ruminants, interest has arisen in sheep-infecting *Theileria* parasites.[2] Recently, a *Theileria* species causing a fatal disease in small ruminants has been identified in the Northwest of China.[3–8] This parasite is transmitted by *Haemaphysalis qinghaiensis* and often occurs in mixed infections with other parasites.[8–10] Depending on the geographic distribution, the rate of morbidity due to the Chinese *Theileria* parasite varies between 19% and 65%, whereas the mortality ranges from 17% to 75%. The highest mortality is observed in lambs and in imported exotic animals. In summary, from 4% to 47% of sheep in the investigated area die due to the infection.[4] The diagnostic techniques for small ruminant piroplasmosis detection are mainly based on the morphological examination of blood smears and clinical symptoms.[11–15] However, these methods require experience in microscopy and are difficult to apply on a large scale for epidemiological studies. Consequently, the development of specific and sensitive diagnostic tools for parasite surveillance, as well as immunoprophylatic means to control and prevent the spread of diseases is crucial. Thus, there is an urgent need for a laboratory diagnostic test combining specificity, sensitivity, and cost effectiveness, such as enzyme-linked immunosorbent assay (ELISA).[16,17] Furthermore, ELISA offers an attractive alternative since reading of the results can be fully automated.

Unlike the leukoproliferative *Theileria* species (e.g., *T. annulata*, *T. lestoquardi*, or *T. parva*), the schizont stage of *Theileria* sp. (China) is very short and until now it could not be cultivated *in vitro*.[18] Additionally, the merozoite stage is the most exposed stage to the host immune system. For this reason the aim of the present article was to identify and characterize merozoite antigens using sera from infected animals. This was achieved by screening lysates of infected erythrocytes as well as purified merozoites in Western blot.

MATERIALS AND METHODS

Antigen and Serum Samples

Experimental infections were conducted in the experimental animal facility of the Lanzhou Veterinary Research Institute, China, using sheep from

Theileria and other protozoa-free areas. Animals were infected by injection of stabilated blood as previously described[19] and were used for the collection of infected erythrocytes (L1, L2, and L3). For the collection of serum samples, sheep were experimentally infected with ticks as described.[7] Negative controls (Ln, Ln3, Ln4) were obtained from sheep held in a *Theileria*-free area (Germany).

Reverse Line Blot

In order to confirm that the biological material used in this study consisted of *Theileria* sp. (China), the samples were analyzed by reverse line blot (RLB) as described previously.[20,21]

Merozoite Antigen Preparation

Merozoite antigenic material was generated by a method previously described[22] with some modifications. In summary, fresh blood from infected sheep was diluted 1:1 (v/v) in Alsever solution (Sigma-Aldrich, St. Louis, MO) and centrifuged at $900g$ for 10 min at $4°C$. The supernatant was discarded; then the pellet was washed three times in Tris–HCl buffer (10 mM Tris–HCl pH 7.4, 150 mM NaCl), and was centrifuged at $500g$ for 10 min at $4°C$. After that, the pellet was diluted 1:5 (v/v) in Tris–HCl, erythrocytes, separated from leukocytes by using a cellulose–powder column, (Whatman cellulose CF11; Millipore, Schwallbach, Germany), and lyzed with α−hemolysin (Sigma) at $37°C$ for 30 min. Merozoite material was generated by a Percoll gradient centrifugation (40% and 60%; Amersham, Munich, Germany) where the merozoite-containing band was localized between the Percoll layers. After collection, merozoites were washed three times at $5000g$ for 10 min at $4°C$, resuspended in Tris–HCl buffer, lyzed by 5 freeze/thaw cycles, and stored at $-70°C$.

Sample Fractionation and Triton X-100 Extraction

Fractionation was performed based on the method of Nagamatsu *et al.*[23] with some modifications. Briefly, 500 μL of erythrocytes obtained from cellulose powder column separation were homogenized in 5 mL of homogenization buffer (10 mM Tris–HCl, pH 7.4, 1 mM EDTA, 250 mM sucrose, 1 mM phenylmethylsulfonyl fluoride, 10 μg/ml leupeptin). Cell debris was removed by centrifugation at $900g$ for 10 min at $4°C$ and the supernatants were collected. The antigen was then ultracentrifuged at $110,000g$ for 75 min at $4°C$. The supernatant fraction (sob) was removed and the membrane-containing pellet was solubilized with solubilization buffer (10 mM Tris–HCl, pH 7.4,

1 mM EDTA, 0.5% Triton X-100, 1 mM phenylmethylsulfonyl fluoride) for 1 h at 4°C. The insoluble material was removed by centrifugation at 14,000g for 10 min at 4°C resulting in a pellet (insoluble fraction, Fi) and a supernatant (soluble fraction, Fs). The insoluble fraction was resuspended in PBS, pH 7.4 and the soluble fraction was concentrated by ultrafiltration using Millipore Centricon ultrafiltration columns with a cutoff molecular weight of 10 kDa. All samples were stored at −70°C.

SDS-PAGE and Western-Blot

Sodium dodecyl sulphate-polyacrylamide gel electrophoresis (SDS-PAGE) was carried out on 8–12% polyacrylamide gels under nonreducing conditions. Proteins were transferred onto PVDF (polyvinylfluoride, Immobilon-P; Millipore) for antigen screening or nitrocellulose membrane (Schleicher & Schuell/Whatman, Dassel, Germany) for immunoblotting with rabbit antisera. For the screening of antigen samples, sheep antisera were diluted to 1:400 in the dilution buffer (3% skim milk powder, 0.05% Tween-20 in TBS) and immunoreactivity was detected by an indirect immunoperoxidase method (donkey anti-goat IgG HRP (Santa Cruz, Santa Cruz, CA) with chemiluminescence detection (WestPico reagent, Pierce, Perbio Science, Bonn, Germany). In addition, fractionated samples were immunoblotted against rabbit antisera, which were raised against the individual protein band (see below). In this case, immunodetection was achieved with goat anti-rabbit alkaline phophatase conjugated antibody (Jackson, West Grove, PA) with BCIP/NBT for chromogenic detection.

MALDI MS Peptide Mapping

Protein SDS-gel bands were excised and polypeptides were subjected to reduction, alkylation, and digestion with modified sequencing-grade trypsin (Promega, VWR International Material de Laboratorio, Lisbon, Portugal) according to Pandey et al.[24] Sample peptides were assayed for peptide mass fingerprint (PMF) in a Voyager-DE STR (Applied Biosystems, Foster City, CA) matrix-assisted laser desorption ionization time-of-flight (MALDI-TOF) mass spectrometer. Peptide crystallization was achieved by using 0.5 L of samples on a plate and adding on top with an equal volume of recrystalized matrix α-cyano-4-hydroxycinnamic acid (CHCA) (10 mg/ml) prepared in acetonitrile (50%, v/v) with trifluoracetic acid (0.1%, v/v). The mixture was allowed to air dry. Monoisotopic peptide masses were used to search for homology and protein identification with Peptide Mass Fingerprint of Mascot (http: //www.matrixscience.com). Searches were done in MSDB database. It was considered a mass accuracy of 50–100 ppm for external calibrations and

Cys carbamidomethylation and Met oxidation as fixed and variable amino acid modifications, respectively. The criteria used to accept the identification were significant homology score achieved in Mascot.[25] Additionally, a minimum of four peptides match, and at least 10% sequence coverage criteria were also considered.

Production of Rabbit Antisera

Three rabbits were immunized in the animal house facility of the Instituto Nacional de Engenharia e Tecnologia Industrial, Portugal, with selected protein bands 2, 5, and 8 (see FIG. 1). The selected gel bands were emulsified and injected four times at 3- to 4-week intervals. Antisera were collected 4 weeks after the last immunization and stored at −20°C.

RESULTS

Antigens Identification

For the identification of parasite antigens, two different types of parasite material were used: (*a*) isolated merozoites of the parasite *Theileria* sp. (China), and (*b*) *Theileria* sp. (China) infected erythrocyte lysated fractions.[26] Noninfected erythrocytes were used as controls. The fractionated erythrocyte lysates and the isolated merozoites were separated by SDS-PAGE under nonreducing conditions.

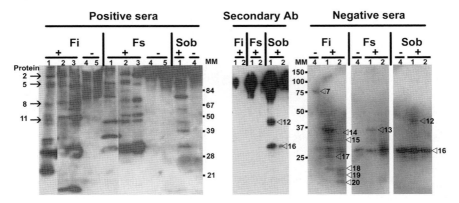

FIGURE 1. Western blots of *Theileria* infected (+; L1 (1), L2 (2), and L3 (3)) and noninfected (−; Ln3 (4) and Ln4 (5)) erythrocyte fractions (Fi, Fs, and Sob) probed with antisera from *Theileria* sp. (China) infected sheep. Protein bands subjected to further analysis are pointed out by arrows (→) and designated with the protein number as mentioned in the text. MM: molecular marker.

The comparative SDS-PAGE analysis of the different fractions revealed different protein band patterns in the higher resolution than unfractionated samples. This allowed the more precise and reproducible detection of several different immunoreactive bands when screened by immunoblotting using different sera of *Theileria* sp. (China) infected sheep. The immunodetection visualized several bands ranging from 11 to 150 kDa (FIG. 1). Despite differences in antibody titers, all the tested sera could recognize the protein bands mentioned above, indicating that these proteins were immunodominant antigens. All negative controls (secondary antibody and serum from noninfected animals) did not specifically react with the material tested (data not shown). The potential antigenic proteins were selected on the basis that they were recognized by all the positive sera tested and not by the negative controls. The serum samples exhibited a similar reaction against purified *Theileria* sp. (China) merozoite antigen samples (FIG. 2 A), resulting in the detection of the same four proteins (proteins 2, 5, 8, and 11). Thus, four potential antigens, with apparent molecular weights of 54 (protein 11), 70 (protein 8), 95 (protein 5), and 119 kDa (protein 2) specific for the merozoite infected erythrocytes fraction, were identified.

Antigen Characterization by Peptide Mass Fingerprint

The results of the peptide mass fingerprint analysis are summarized in TABLE 1. Regarding protein 2, it showed a significant score of 79 to a possible MO25-family protein from *Cryptosporidium parvum,* where protein scores greater than 61 are significant ($P < 0.05$). The spectra results obtained from

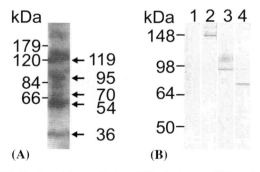

(A)   **(B)**

FIGURE 2. (A) Western blot analysis of *Theileria* sp. (China) isolated merozoites probed with serum from a *Theileria* sp. (China) infected sheep. Corresponding protein bands are indicated on the right. MM: Molecular marker. **(B)** Immunoblot analyses of rabbit antisera produced against proteins from *Theileria* sp. (China), P2, P5, and P8. Rabbit antisera were diluted 1:200 and probed against purified merozoite samples: Lane (1) Rabbit preimmune serum; Lane (2) Rabbit antiserum raised against protein 2; Lane (3) Rabbit antiserum raised against protein 5; Lane (4) Rabbit antiserum raised against protein 8.

TABLE 1. Summary of the peptide mass fingerprint analysis for proteins 2, 5, 8, and 11. Scores greater than 61 are considered significant

Protein	MASCOT score	Coverage (%)	Peptides matched	Highest similarity
2	79	26	14	*C. parvum* possible MO25-family protein (Accession Q7YYL6)
5	39	24	8	Hypothetical *P. chabaudi* protein (Accession Q4XUW9˙PLACH)
8	62	16	8	*T. annulata* 70 kDa heat shock protein (HSP 70.1) (Accession J04653)
11	113	30	11	Actin

protein 5 were quite clear although no significant homologies were found in the database. Protein 8 on the other hand showed some homologies with a HSP70 from *T. annulata*[27] with a significant score when a taxonomic restriction to *Alveolata* species was considered. Finally, protein 11 showed good spectra and was identified as being an actin-like protein.

Specificity of Rabbit Antisera

The rabbit antisera were then characterized for reactivity against the respective proteins and immunoblotting analysis was performed with purified *Theileria* sp. (China) merozoites (FIG. 2 B). Antisera from immunized rabbits, but not preimmune sera, recognized parasite-specific bands that could not be observed in the uninfected erythrocytes fraction. The sizes of detected protein bands corresponded to the appropriate molecular weights of 119, 95, and 70 kDa of proteins used for respective immunization.

DISCUSSION

The present study reports on the identification of antigens of a newly characterized highly pathogenic *Theileria* species of small ruminants in China. As a possible contamination with other *Theileria* or *Babesia* parasites was excluded by RLB, all the potential antigens identified in the present work were of *Theileria* sp. (China) origin. Altogether protein bands with apparent molecular weights of 119 (protein 2), 95 (protein 5), 70 (protein 8), and 54 kDa (protein 11) were identified.

For further antigen identification and characterization, mass spectrometry analysis (peptide mass fingerprint) was performed. Protein 2 had a high homology (with a confidence grade of >95%) to a possible MO25-family protein from *Cryptosporidium parvum* and protein 8 to HSP70 of *T. annulata*. Protein 5 spectra presented no significant homology results, the highest score being obtained with a *Plasmodium chabaudi* conserved hypothetical protein. This finding suggests that protein 5 may be a new nonidentified protein. Protein 11 on the other hand was identified as actin, and was not considered further for diagnostics development due to potential cross reactivity with the highly identical host actin.

Further verification of the parasite origin of the identified antigens was made by using rabbit antisera raised against the respective proteins 2, 5, and 8. These antisera recognized proteins of the respective molecular weights by immunoblots of infected erythrocyte fractions and purified merozoite extracts. These specific rabbit antisera will be employed to screen a *Theileria* sp. (China) merozoite expression library that is under construction to isolate recombinant proteins. The most promising protein will then be used for the establishment of a diagnostic ELISA. In addition, these proteins will be checked for their immunogenic potency and their possible application for perspective candidate vaccine antigens.

ACKNOWLEDGMENTS

We would like to thank Dr. Carlos Novo and Ana Custdio who helped in the immunization experiments. This work was supported in part by the European Union (ICA4-2000-300028) and the Portuguese Foundation for Science and Technology (SFRH/BD/6494/2001).

REFERENCES

1. MEHLHORN, H. & E. SCHEIN. 1984. The piroplasms: life cycle and sexual stages. Adv. Parasitol. **23:** 37–103.
2. FRIEDHOFF, K.T. 1997. Tick-borne diseases of sheep and goats caused by *Babesia*, *Theileria* and *Anaplasma* spp. Parasitologia **39:** 99–109.
3. LUO, J. & H. YIN. 1997. Theilerosis of sheep and goats in China. Trop. Anim. Health Prod. **29:** 8S–10S.
4. SCHNITTGER, L., H. YIN, L. JIANXUN, *et al.* 2000. Ribosomal small-subunit RNA gene sequence analysis of *Theileria lestoquardi* and a *Theileria* species highly pathogenic for small ruminants in China. Parasitol. Res. **86:** 352–358.
5. SCHNITTGER, L., Y. HONG, L. JIANXUN, *et al.* 2000. Phylogenetic analysis by rRNA comparison of the highly pathogenic sheep-infecting parasites *Theileria lestoquardi* and a *Theileria* species identified in China. Ann. N. Y. Acad. Sci. **916:** 271–275.
6. BAI, Q., G. LIU, D. LIU, *et al.* 2002. Isolation and preliminary characterization of a large *Babesia* sp. from sheep and goats in the eastern part of the Gansu Province, China. Parasitol. Res. **88:** S16–S21.
7. YIN, H., J. LUO, G. GUAN, *et al.* 2002. Transmission of an unidentified *Theileria* species to small ruminants by *Haemaphysalis qinghaiensis* ticks collected in the field. Parasitol. Res. **88:** S25–S27.

8. SCHNITTGER, L., H. YIN, J. LUO, *et al.* 2002. Characterization of a polymorphic gene of *T. lestoquardi* and of a recently identified *Theileria* species pathogenic for small ruminants in China. Parasitol. Res. **88:** 553–556.

9. YIN, H., J. LUO, G. GUAN, *et al.* 2002. Experiments on transmission of an unidentified *Theileria* sp. to small ruminants with *Haemaphysalis qinghaiensis* and *Hyalomma anatolicum anatolicum*. Vet. Parasitol. **108:** 21–30.

10. SCHNITTGER, L., H. YIN, M.J. GUBBELS, *et al.* 2003. Phylogeny of sheep and goat *Theileria* and *Babesia* parasites. Parasitol. Res. **91:** 398–406.

11. HOOSHMAND-RAD, P. & N.J. HAWA. 1973. Malignant theilerosis of sheep and goats. Trop. Anim. Health Prod. **5:** 97–102.

12. UILENBERG, G. & B.E. SCHREUDER. 1976. Further studies on *Haematoxenus separatus* (Sporozoa, Theileriidae) of sheep in Tanzania. Rev. Elev. Med. Vet. Pays Trop. **29(2):** 119–126.

13. LEEMANS, I., P. HOOSHMAND-RAD & A. UGGLA. 1997. The indirect fluorescence antibody test based on schizont antigen for study of the sheep parasite *Theileria lestoquardi*. Vet. Parasitol. **69:** 9–18.

14. KIRVAR, E., T. ILHAN, F. KATZER, *et al.* 1998. Detection of *Theileria lestoquardi* (hirci) in ticks, sheep, and goats using polymerase chain reaction. Ann. N. Y. Acad. Sci. **849:** 52–62.

15. AHMED, J., H. YIN, L. SCHNITTGER, *et al.* 2002. Ticks and tick-borne diseases in Asia with special emphasis on China. Parasitol. Res. **88:** S51–S55.

16. SAMUEL, T., R. BOSE & C. SCHELP. 1999. Purification of a 28 kDa *Babesia (Theileria) equi* antigen and a 29 kDa spurius erythrocyte antigen from *in vitro* culture through ion exchange chromatography. Vet. Parasitol. **86:** 63–70.

17. DEMEDTS, P., C. VERMEULEN-VAN OVERMEIR & M. WERY. 1987. Simultaneous detection of *Plasmodium falciparum* crude antigen and red blood cell control antigen in the enzyme-linked immunosorbent assay for malaria. Am. J. Trop. Med. Hyg. **36:** 257–263.

18. YIN, H., G. LIU, J. LUO, *et al.* 2003. Observation on the schizont stage of an unidentified *Theileria* sp. in experimentally infected sheep. Parasitol. Res. **91:** 34–39.

19. YIN, H., G. GUAN, M. MA, *et al.* 2002. *Haemaphysalis qinghaiensis* ticks transmit at least two different *Theileria* species: one is infective to yaks, one is infective to sheep. Vet. Parasitol. **107:** 29–35.

20. SCHNITTGER, L., H. YIN, B. QI, *et al.* 2004. Simultaneous detection and differentiation of *Theileria* and *Babesia* parasites infecting small ruminants by reverse line blotting. Parasitol. Res. **92:** 189–196.

21. GUBBELS, J.M., A.P. DE VOS, M. VAN DER WEIDE, *et al.* 1999. Simultaneous detection of bovine *Theileria* and *Babesia* species by reverse line blot hybridisation. J. Clin. Microbiol. **37:** 1782–1789.

22. HAUSCHILD, S., P. SHAYAN & E. SCHEIN. 1995. Characterization and comparison of merozoite antigens of different *Babesia canis* isolates by serological and immunological investigations. Parasitol. Res. **81:** 638–642.

23. NAGAMATSU, S., J.M. KORNHAUSER, C.F. BURANT, *et al.* 1992. Glucose transporter expression in brain. cDNA sequence of mouse GLUT3, the brain facilitative glucose transporter isoform, and identification of sites of expression by *in situ* hybridization. J. Biol. Chem. **267:** 467–472.

24. PANDEY, A., J.S. ANDERSEN & M. MANN. 2000. Use of mass spectrometry to study signalling pathways. Sci. STKE **37:** 1–12.

25. GONNET, F., G. LEMAITRE, G. WAKSMAN, *et al.* 2003. MALDI/MS peptide mass fingerprinting for proteome analysis: identification of hydrophobic proteins attached to eukaryote keratinocyte cytoplasmic membrane using different matrices in concert. Proteome Sci. **1(1):** 2.
26. MIRANDA, J., B. STUMME, D. BEYER, *et al.* 2004. Identification of antigenic proteins of a *Theileria* species pathogenic for small ruminants in China recognized by antisera of infected animals. Ann. N. Y. Acad. Sci. **1026:** 161–164.
27. SCHNITTGER, L., P. SHAYAN, R. BIERMANN R, *et al.* 2000. Molecular genetic characterization and subcellular localization of *Theileria annulata* mitochondrial heat-shock protein 70. Parasitol. Res. **86:** 444–452.

Purification of Macroschizonts of a Sudanese Isolate of *Theileria lestoquardi* (*T. lestoquardi* [Atbara])

MOHAMMED A. BAKHEIT,[a] ELMAR ENDL,[c] JABBAR S. AHMED,[b] AND ULRIKE SEITZER[b]

[a]*Department of Parasitology, Faculty of Veterinary Medicine, University of Khartoum, 13314 Khartoum North, Sudan*

[b]*Division of Veterinary Infectiology and Immunology, Research Center Borstel, 23845 Borstel, Germany*

[c]*Institute of Molecular Medicine and Experimental Immunology, University of Bonn, 53105 Bonn, Germany*

ABSTRACT: Research on malignant theileriosis is affected by the limited access to biological materials required for studies aiming at controlling the disease through the establishment of diagnostic tools and vaccines. The main aims of this work were to isolate, establish, and characterize a *Theileria lestoquardi*-infected cell culture (line) as a source of biological material and to generate a schizont cDNA library for further studies aiming at the identification of antigenic proteins. The *T. lestoquardi* isolate used originated from a sheep showing typical signs of malignant theileriosis in Atbara town in northern Sudan, and was maintained as an infected cell culture. A high-quality representative schizont cDNA library was established by isolating and purifying the schizonts using a nocodazole/aerolysin protocol followed by Percoll gradient ultracentrifugation. As a parameter to assess the quality of the schizont library, a provisional estimation of the percentage of recombinant phage clones originating from *T. lestoquardi* (Atbara) was undertaken. Ten clones with inserts ranging in size between 600 and 1200 bp were selected randomly, sequenced, and subjected to BLAST similarity searches. As 6 of the 10 sequenced clones showed similarities to *T. parva*, *T. annulata*, and other apicomplexan genes, it was concluded that the majority of the library phage clones originated from the parasite and not from host cell transcripts. The cDNA library will be used for screening of antigenic proteins using sera from infected sheep.

KEYWORDS: schizont; *Theileria*; Sudan; cDNA library

Address for correspondence: Ulrike Seitzer, Division of Veterinary Infectiology and Immunology, Research Center Borstel, Parkallee 22, 23845 Borstel, Germany. Voice: +49-4537-188-413; fax: +49-4537-188-627.

e-mail: useitzer@fz-borstel.de

Ann. N.Y. Acad. Sci. 1081: 453–462 (2006). © 2006 New York Academy of Sciences.
doi: 10.1196/annals.1373.064

INTRODUCTION

Theileria lestoquardi is a pathogen that infects sheep and goats and frequently leads to a fatal disease called malignant theileriosis. The disease is of utmost economic importance, especially in countries where export of sheep and their products is a major component of the national economy. High losses due to malignant theileriosis are recorded in indigenous sheep in Iraq[1] and in Sudan[2] and mortalities in sheep of almost up to 100% in cases of outbreaks have been reported.[3,4] It has been speculated that *T. lestoquardi* and *T. annulata* are the most closely related *Theileria* species and most likely descended from a single direct ancestor. The diversification of *T. lestoquardi* and *T. annulata* from their common ancestor was a relatively recent evolutionary event, which may represent an evolutionary pathway for the establishing of a *Theileria* parasite in sheep (i.e., *T. lestoquardi*), which was independent from the other ovine *Theileria* species, *T. ovis* and *T. separata*.[5] Similar to *T. annulata*, *T. lestoquardi* is transmitted transstadially by *Hyalomma anatolicum anatolicum*. Cross reactions between *T. lestoquardi* and *T. annulata* by the indirect fluorescent antibody test were reported.[6] On the other hand, genetic factors do exist between the two species, which affect their pathogenicity and transmissibility to either the ovine or the bovine host; *T. lestoquardi* does not infect cattle while *T. annulata* can still infect sheep cells.[7,8]

It is of interest to identify and characterize antigenic proteins of *T. lestoquardi* with the aim of controlling the disease through recombinant (or live attenuated) vaccine development and the provision of parasite-specific recombinant protein-based diagnostic tools, such as an enzyme-linked immunosorbent assay (ELISA). The importance of the macroschizont as the most pathogenic stage in *Theileria*'s life cycle has stimulated research targeting at identification and characterization, particularly in genes and proteins expressed by this stage. Due to the scarcity of biological material, isolation and characterization of a *T. lestoquardi*-infected cell culture (line) were required. Highly pure parasite material is affected by the fact that such material isolated from an infected cell line is a mixture of parasite and host nucleic acids and that parasite genes are expressed in a lower number of transcripts.[9] *Theileria*-derived cDNA was found to constitute only 2% of a cDNA library established using mRNA isolated from *T. parva*-infected cells.[10] We report here on the establishment of a *T. lestoquardi* macroschizont cDNA library from schizonts purified from a recently established infected cell line.

MATERIALS AND METHODS

Isolation and Maintenance of T. lestoquardi *(Atbara) Field Isolate*

The *T. lestoquardi* isolate was derived from a naturally infected sheep that was admitted to the governmental veterinary clinic in Atbara town, northern

Sudan in 2001. The animal had shown typical signs of malignant theileriosis as well as schizonts and piroplasms in lymph node biopsy and blood smears, respectively. Lymph node biopsy was collected aseptically and the cells were separated by Ficoll ([Biocoll], Biochrom AG, Berlin, Germany), cultured in RPMI complete medium (RPMI 1640, 2 mg/mL sodium bicarbonate, 2 mM L-glutamine, 100 IU penicillin/mL, 100 μg/mL streptomycin, and 20% heat-inactivated fetal calf serum), and incubated at 37°C in a humidified atmosphere with 5% CO_2. The cell line is referred to as *T. lestoquardi* (Atbara) to note the original source of the infected cells.

Confirmation of the Identity of the Parasite Using Molecular Methods

A multiplex polymerase chain reaction (PCR) was performed to distinguish *T. lestoquardi* (5'-TATGCGAATCGTACTCTG) from *T. ovis* (5'-TGCTCCTTTACGAGTCTT) using a common reverse primer (5'-TGCTGAAGGAGTTAAAAACT) whose sequences were derived from the ssRNA gene and resulted in PCR products of 787 bp and 395 bp, respectively. The second PCR distinguished *T. lestoquardi* from *T. annulata* (using DNA extracted from cells infected with *T. annulata* [Ankara] 288[11]) and was carried out using a *T. lestoquardi*-specific primer set.[12] The 18S rRNA gene was also cloned, sequenced, and confirmed to be *T .lestoquardi* [GenBank AY260185].[13]

Purification of T. lestoquardi *(Atbara) Schizonts*

Macroschizonts were isolated using a modified protocol that was previously published.[14] Host cell tubulin was disrupted by incubation in RPMI complete medium containing 10 μM nocodazole (Sigma, Deisenhofen, Germany) for 18 h. After harvesting, counting, and distribution at 5×10^7 cells in one tube each, pellets were resuspended in 500 μL ice-cold 1 × HEPES buffer (10 mM HEPES, 150 mM NaCl, 20 mM KCl, pH 7.4) containing 1 mM $CaCl_2$ (HEPES-$CaCl_2$). Proaerolysin (Protox Biotech, Victoria BC, Canada) was added to the tubes to a final concentration of 30 μg/mL. The tubes were incubated at 4°C under rotation for 30 min, washed three times in ice-cold HEPES-$CaCl_2$ buffer, resuspended in 1 mL 1× HEPES buffer containing 5 mM EDTA (HEPES-EDTA) and incubated for 15 min at 37°C in a water bath to lyse these cells. One milliliter of cell lysate was added to 3.8 mL lower-phase Percoll (85% in HEPES-EDTA buffer [10 mM HEPES, 1.5 M NaCl, 20 mM KCl, 5 mM EDTA, pH 7.4]) in ultracentrifuge tubes and the volume adjusted to 5 mL with HEPES-EDTA buffer to obtain a lower-phase Percoll concentration of 64.5%. The samples were layered with 7 mL of the upper-phase Percoll (45% in HEPES-EDTA buffer) and were centrifuged at 85,000*g* at 12°C for 30 min. After centrifugation, an upper layer and the small clumps throughout the upper Percoll gradient were removed. The schizont layer (at the junction between the two Percoll gradients) was carefully transferred into new tubes and washed in sterile PBS by centrifugation at 2500g for 5 min at 4°C. Schizont pellets were used for the preparation of cytospins and for the isolation of mRNA. Giemsa staining was performed using Accustain (Giemsa Stain, Sigma) following instructions provided by the manufacturer.

Indirect Immunofluorescence Assay

Cytospin preparations were fixed in 3% paraformaldehyde for 10 min, permeabilized with 0.25% Triton X-100 for 5 min, and blocked in PBS/10% bovine serum albumin (BSA) for 30 min. Mouse anti-tubulin (Sigma) and anti-*T. lestoquardi* sheep serum were applied as primary antibodies. For detection of sheep antibodies, the first secondary antibody (rabbit anti-sheep, Dianova, Hamburg, Germany) was used before applying Alexa 488 conjugated goat anti-rabbit or goat anti-mouse detection antibodies and propidium iodide as a nucleic acid stain (all from Molecular Probes, Leyden, The Netherlands). Specimens were analyzed under a confocal laser scanning microscope (Leica TCS SP, Bensheim, Germany).

Establishment of cDNA Library and Isolation of Clones

Messenger RNA was isolated from purified macroschizonts of *T. lestoquardi* (Atbara). The Micro-Fast Track 2.0 kit (Invitrogen, Paisley, UK) was used for reverse transcription and a SMART cDNA library was established according to the protocol of Clontech® (BD-Biosciences, San Jose, CA). Recombinant phage clones with inserts ranging in size between 600 bp and 1200 bp were isolated and sequenced. The sequences were subjected to BLAST for similarity searches of the nucleic acid and translated proteins against sequences and extended sequence tags (EST) database of the *T. parva* genome database (The Institute for Genomic Research [TIGR] [Rockville, Maryland, http://www.tigr.org/]), the *T. annulata* genome database (The Wellcome Trust Sanger Institute, Hinxton, Cambridge, UK [http://www.sanger.ac.uk/]), and other eukaryotic sequences available at the NCBI, Bethesda, MD (http://www.ncbi.nlm.nih.gov/).

RESULTS

Characterization of the T. lestoquardi (Atbara) Infected Cell Line

Under the light microscope, cells harboring the *T. lestoquardi* (Atbara) schizonts were heterologous in shape and reached up to 20 μM with approximately

(A)   **(B)**   **(C)**

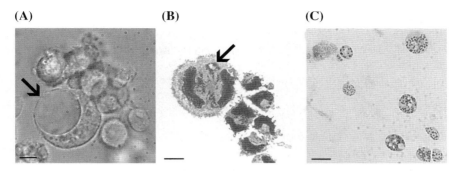

FIGURE 1. *T. lestoquardi* (Atbara)-infected cells and isolated schizonts. (**A**) Nomarski optic image of live cultures (arrow: vacuolated cell). (**B**) Giemsa-stained cytospin prepared from schizont-infected cells (arrow: schizont). (**C**) Demonstration of isolated schizonts in Giemsa-stained cytospin slides. Size bars: 10 μM.

5% of the cells possessing large vacuoles (FIG. 1 A). Sixty times passages did not affect the morphology of the infected cells. Giemsa-stained cytospin preparations also showed heterogeneity in the size of infected cells and the parasitizing schizonts (FIG. 1 B). Infected cells grew only in suspension. Attempts to induce the development of merozoites from *T. lestoquardi* (Atbara) by incubation at temperatures up to 42°C and under 5% carbon dioxide were unsuccessful.

To ensure the absence of contamination with *T. ovis*, which might coexist in sheep in Sudan, a multiplex PCR was performed. An amplified size specific to *T. lestoquardi* (787 bp), using DNA prepared from *T. lestoquardi* (Atbara)-infected cells could be obtained. Neither multiple bands nor a specific band corresponding in size to the one obtained with the genomic DNA template of an isolate of *T. ovis* (395 bp) were observed (FIG. 2 A). A further PCR test differentiated *T. lestoquardi* from *T. annulata*. An amplification of the correct size (785 bp) was demonstrated with the genomic DNA template isolated from *T. lestoquardi* (Atbara)-infected cells, but not with the *T. annulata* (Ankara) 288 genomic DNA template used as a control (FIG. 2 B).

Purification of **T. lestoquardi** *(Atbara) Schizonts*

The effect of nocodazole on the cytoskeleton of the treated cells was examined using immunofluorescence staining for the detection of tubulin. Partial depolymerization of the tubulin network could be seen at concentrations greater than 0.25 μM. The percentage of cells with complete tubulin depolymerization was increased with increasing drug concentration. At ≥ 10 μM, most of the examined cells (~1 × 10⁵ per cytospin) showed complete disruption of the tubulin network (data not shown). Percoll gradient separation of the aerolysin-treated cells resulted in the formation of a layer at the junction be-

(A)   **(B)**

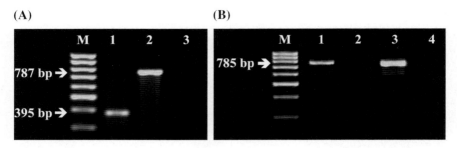

FIGURE 2. PCR verification of *T. lestoquardi* infection. (**A**) Multiplex PCR to distinguish *T. lestoquardi* from *T. ovis*. Lanes: M, DNA molecular weight marker. (1) *T. ovis* control genomic DNA. (2) *T. lestoquardi* (Atbara) genomic DNA. (3) Water control. (**B**) Amplification of genomic DNA of *T. lestoquardi* (Atbara) using *T. lestoquardi* specific primers. Lanes: M, molecular weight marker. (1) *T. lestoquardi* (Atbara) genomic DNA. (2) *T. annulata* (Ankara 288) genomic DNA. (3) *T. lestoquardi* (Fars) genomic DNA control. (4) water control.

tween the upper and the lower Percoll gradients, which contained the isolated schizonts. Cell debris, host cell nuclei, and some intact schizont-containing cells were present in the upper Percoll gradient and tended to form an upper layer just below the rim of the centrifuge tube. Detection of the isolated schizonts using anti-*T. lestoquardi* sheep sera and fluorescence-coupled secondary antibody demonstrated the presence of intact schizont membranes (data not shown). In Giemsa-stained cytospin preparations (FIG. 1 C) only a minor degree (approximately 2%) of contamination with host cell nuclei could be observed.

Random Sequencing Results of the Schizont cDNA Library

TABLE 1 summarizes the results predicted from the highest similarity scores obtained with the BLAST search. Six out of 10 sequenced clones showed

TABLE 1. Sequence analysis of 10 randomly sequenced library clones

Name	GenBank Accession	Similarity[a]
Clone 2	DQ399300	Host protein
Clone 4	DQ399301	*Theileria* gene (conserved ribosomal domains)
Clone 7	DQ399302	*Theileria* putative RAB2 GTPase
Clone 9	DQ399303	Host ribosomal protein
Clone 15	DQ278169	Host protein
Clone 17	DQ399304	Unknown *Theileria* protein
Clone 18	DQ399305	*Theileria* actin
Clone 21	DQ402095/DQ402096	Unknown *Theileria* protein
Clone 22	DQ402094	Conserved gene for elongation factor 1 alpha
Clone 23	DQ862459	*Theileria* gene (lariat-debranching enzyme)

[a]NCBI, TIGR, and Sanger gene banks comparisons. Most probable hits with highest scores are listed.

highest similarities to *T. parva*, *T. annulata*, and other apicomplexan genes, suggesting that they were originating from related organisms, i.e., *T. lestoquardi*. It could, thus, be concluded that the majority of the library phage clones originated from the parasite and not from host cell transcripts.

DISCUSSION

In this study, a new isolate of *T. lestoquardi* originating from northern Sudan was described and was given the name *T. lestoquardi* (Atbara). The isolate constituted a prerequisite for the subsequent steps required to identify, characterize, and test new parasite proteins with the aim of developing diagnostic methods or subunit vaccines to control the disease. As the *T. lestoquardi* (Atbara) isolate was new and originated from a naturally infected sheep, PCR methods were used to verify the nature of this isolate as being *T.lestoquardi*. Thus, using *T. lestoquardi*-specific primers[12] *T. lestoquardi* could be distinguished from *T. annulata,* as has been previously shown to distinguish between *T. lestoquardi* and *T. annulata* in *Hyalomma* vector as well as in sheep and goats.[12,15,16] In the multiplex PCR, the possibility of contamination with *T. ovis* could be excluded. Thus, the results obtained confirmed the nature of the isolate as *T. lestoquardi*.

In the past, the isolation and purification of the *Theileria* schizont stage from infected cells has been attempted by several workers, who applied, in most of the cases, a similar principle used during this study. For example, Sugimoto *et al.*[17] applied a pore-forming toxin in schizont isolation from *T. parva*-infected cells, with a subsequent Percoll ultracentrifugation to separate a schizont layer from a cell nuclei and debris layer. A similar protocol was adopted by Goddeeris *et al.*,[18] who replaced the Percoll gradient with a centrifugation on Nycodenz solution after increasing the buoyant density of the free host cell nuclei by adding 10% metrizamide. In this work, a protocol modified from Baumgartner *et al.*[14] was applied. The strategy of the isolation implied the disruption of the host cell tubulin network, the specific lysis of the host cell, and finally the gradient ultracentrifugation to separate the isolated schizonts from the host cell debris and nuclei.

As host cells microtubules have been shown to be associated with the schizont's surface,[19–21] nocodazole was used to facilitate the release of *T. lestoquardi* (Atbara) schizonts from the host cell cytoskeleton by disruption of the host cell microtubules prior to cell lysis. Since the treatment of the *T. lestoquardi* (Atbara)-infected cells with 10 μM nocodazole for 18 h had no apparent detrimental effects on the viability of cells, while it led to complete disruption of the microtubular network, these conditions were chosen in the schizont isolation trials. The pore-forming toxin, aerolysin, was used to subsequently lyse *T. lestoquardi*-infected, nocodazole-treated cells. Proaerolysin was used during this study without prior trypsin treatment as previously described,[14] since the infected lymphocytes possess sufficient surface enzymes to activate the bound proaerolysine. No lysis was observed during the cell-washing steps at 4°C, possibly due to the retarded activity of surface proteases.

Purified schizonts of *T. lestoquardi* (Atbara) maintained their shape and membrane integrity as examined by the immunostaining and confocal microscopy. However, there was a minor contamination (2%) with intact host cells and nuclei, which could be microscopically detected. The contamination of the schizont layer with host cells, which could not be removed by altering the Percoll gradients, which might be attributed to the heterogeneous cell size of the isolate of *T. lestoquardi* (Atbara) and it was suggested that both schizont-containing host cells and free schizonts had different densities among themselves as well.

As a means of estimating the extent of this contamination with the host cell nucleic material, 10 recombinant λ-phage clones with different insert sizes selected at random from the library were sequenced. BLAST searches were performed with these sequences versus sequences and extended sequence tags of *T. parva*, *T. annulata*, and other eukaryotic sequences available in GenBank. It was concluded that 6 out of 10 clones originated from *T. lestoquardi* (Atbara) and 4 originated from the sheep host. Comparing this to the previous estimation that 10% of the mRNA transcripts isolated from infected lymphocytes were of parasite origin,[9] it can be concluded that the schizont isolation enriched for the parasite transcripts approximately 36 times from the host parasite mixture.

Due to the enrichment of parasite transcripts, the cDNA library should prove to be useful for screening and identification of antigenic proteins using sera from infected sheep. Newly identified *T. lestoquardi*-specific antigenic proteins will in the long term be processed and implemented for the development of diagnostic tools and subunit vaccines.

ACKNOWLEDGMENTS

This work was supported in part by the European Commission within Inco-Dev, project number ICA4-CT-2000-30028. M.A. Bakheit was a doctoral scholarship holder of the German Academic Exchange Services (DAAD). The authors are thankful to the staff of Atbara Veterinary Clinic and the Tick Control Unit (CVRL, Sudan) for the help during the isolation and maintenance of the *T. lestoquardi* cell line.

NOTE ADDED IN PROOF

A further seven clones have been sequenced and analyzed (GenBank DQ278169-DQ278175), six have a high similarity to *T. annulata* and/or *T. parva*.

REFERENCES

1. HOOSHMAND-RAD, P. 1974. Blood protozoan diseases of ruminants. Bull. Off. Int. Epizoot. **81:** 779–792.
2. TAGELDIN, M.H., A.M. ZAKIA, E.G. NAGWA, *et al.* 1992. An outbreak of theileriosis in sheep in Sudan. Trop. Anim. Health Prod. **24:** 15–16.
3. LATIF, A.A., H.M. ABDULLA, S.M. HASSAN, *et al.* 1994. Theileriosis of sheep in the Sudan. *In* Tropical Theileriosis in the Sudan. Proceedings of a Workshop Held at the Sudan Veterinary Association Residence, Khartoum, Sudan, 4–5 May, 1994. A.M. Atelmanan & S.M. Kheir, Eds.: 66–72. Central Veterinary Research Laboratories, Ministry of Science and Technology. Khartoum North, Sudan.
4. ELGHALI, A.A. & A.M. EL HUSSEIN. 1995. Diseases of livestock in Ed-Damer province: a two-years retrospective study. Sud. J. Vet. Sci. Anim. Husb. **34:** 37–45.
5. KATZER, F., S. MCKELLAR, E. KIRVAR, *et al.* 1998. Phylogenetic analysis of *Theileria* and *Babesia equi* in relation to the establishment of parasite populations within novel host species and the development of diagnostic tests. Mol. Biochem. Parasitol. **95:** 33–44.
6. LEEMANS, I., P. HOOSHMAND-RAD & A. UGGLA. 1997. The indirect fluorescent antibody test based on schizont antigen for study of the sheep parasite *Theileria lestoquardi*. Vet. Parasitol. **69:** 9–18.
7. BROWN, C.G.D., T. ILHAN, E. KIRVAR, *et al.* 1998. *Theileria lestoquardi* and *T. annulata* in cattle, sheep and goats: *in vitro* and *in vivo* studies. Ann. N. Y. Acad. Sci. **849:** 44–51.
8. LEEMANS, I., D. BROWN, P. HOOSHMAND-RAD, *et al.* 1999. Infectivity and cross-immunity studies of *Theileria lestoquardi* and *Theileria annulata* in sheep and cattle: I. *In vivo* responses. Vet. Parasitol. **82:** 179–192.
9. GERHARDS, J., A.C. GILL, A.Y.B. EHRFELD, *et al.* 1989. Isolation and characterization of RNA from the intracellular parasite *Theileria parva*. Mol. Biochem. Parasitol. **34:** 15–24.
10. BAYLIS, H.A., B.A. ALLSOPP, R. HALL, *et al.* 1993. Characterisation of a glutamine-and proline-rich protein (QP protein) from *Theileria parva*. Mol. Biochem. Parasitol. **61:** 171–178.
11. SCHEIN, E. 1975. On the life cycle of *Theileria annulata* (Dschunkowsky and Luhs 1904) in the midgut and haemolymph of *Hyalomma anatolicum excavatum* (Koch 1844). Z. Parasitenkd. **47:** 165–167.
12. KIRVAR, E., G. WILKIE, F. KATZER, *et al.* 1998. *Theileria lestoquardi* – maturation and quantification in *Hyalomma anatolicum anatolicum* ticks. Parasitology **117:** 255–263.
13. SCHNITTGER, L., H. YIN, B. QI, *et al.* 2004. Simultaneous detection and differentiation of *Theileria* and *Babesia* parasites infecting small ruminants by reverse line blotting. Parasitol. Res. **92:** 189–196.
14. BAUMGARTNER, M., I. TARDIEUX, H. OHAYON, *et al.* 1999. The use of nocodazole in cell cycle analysis and parasite purification from *Theileria parva*-infected B cells. Microbes Infect. **1:** 1181–1188.
15. KIRVAR, E., T. ILHAN, F. KATZER, *et al.* 1998. Detection of *Theileria lestoquardi* (hirci) in ticks, sheep and goats using the polymerase chain reaction. Ann. N. Y. Acad. Sci. **849:** 52–62.

16. LEEMANS, I., D. BROWN, C. FOSSUM, *et al.* 1999. Infectivity and cross-immunity studies of *Theileria lestoquardi* and *Theileria annulata* in sheep and cattle: II. *In vitro* studies. Vet. Parasitol. **82:** 193–204.
17. SUGIMOTO, C., P.A. CONRAD, S. ITO, *et al.* 1988. Isolation of *Theileria parva* schizonts from infected lymphoblastoid cells. Acta Trop. **45:** 203–216.
18. GODDEERIS, B.M., S. DUNLAP, E.A. INNES, *et al.* 1991. A simple and efficient method for purifying and quantifying schizonts from *Theileria parva*-infected cells. Parasitol. Res. **77:** 482–484.
19. FAWCETT, D., A. MUSOKE & W. VOIGT. 1984. Interaction of sporozoites of *Theileria parva* with bovine lymphocytes *in vitro*. 1. Early events after invasion. Tissue Cell **16:** 873–884.
20. SHAW, M.K. 1999. *Theileria parva*: sporozoite entry into bovine lymphocytes is not dependent on the parasite cytoskeleton. Exp. Parasitol. **92:** 24–31.
21. SHAW, M.K. 2003. Cell invasion by *Theileria* sporozoites. Trends Parasitol. **19:** 2–6.

Identification of Potential Antigenic Proteins of *Theileria lestoquardi*

MOHAMMED BAKHEIT,[a] THOMAS SCHOLZEN,[b]
JABBAR S. AHMED,[b] AND ULRIKE SEITZER[b]

[a] *Department of Parasitology, Faculty of Veterinary Medicine, University of Khartoum, 13314 Khartoum North, Sudan*

[b] *Division of Immunology and Cell Biology, Research Center Borstel, 23845 Borstel, Germany*

ABSTRACT: A PCR strategy was used to identify potential antigenic proteins of *T. lestoquardi* suitable for the development of an ELISA by searching for homologous proteins previously identified in other theilierial parasites to be antigenic.

KEYWORDS: *Theileria lestoquardi*; antigenic protein; ELISA

INTRODUCTION

As with the other pathogenic *Theileria* spp., the diagnosis of *Theileria lestoquardi (T. lestoquardi)* infection is mainly based on the clinical signs and demonstration of the schizont stage in lymph nodes or organ smears, along with the demonstration of piroplasms in blood smears. The availability of an ELISA using an antigenic *T. lestoquardi* recombinant protein would be a useful tool not only for diagnostic purposes but also in epidemiological studies, since it is easy to perform, economic, and amenable to standardization.

METHODS

The strategy used to identifiy potential antigenic proteins of *T. lestoquardi* suitable for the development of an ELISA in this study was to use PCR to search for homologous proteins previously identified in other theilierial parasites.

Address for correspondence: Ulrike Seitzer, Division of Veterinary Infectiology and Immunology, Research Center Borstel, Parkallee 22, 23845 Borstel, Germany. Voice: +49-4537-188413; fax: +49-4537-188627.
e-mail: useitzer@fz-borstel.de

Ann. N.Y. Acad. Sci. 1081: 463–464 (2006). © 2006 New York Academy of Sciences.
doi: 10.1196/annals.1373.065

RESULTS AND DISCUSSION

The cDNA of the homologous gene to the *Theileria annulata* (*T. annulata*) surface protein TaSP[1] [GenBank AJ345067], which was previously found to be present in the genome of *T. lestoquardi*,[2] was cloned from cDNA [GenBank DQ120054] of the *T. lestoquardi* [Atbara] isolate[3] and recombinantly expressed. Western blot experiments revealed a high reactivity of sera from *T. lestoquardi*-infected sheep against this TlSP protein, making it a suitable candidate for ELISA development. Furthermore, the *T. lestoquardi* homolog of the *T. parva* P32 gene[4] [GenBank L47209] could be partially cloned and sequenced [GenBank DQ120059]. Evaluation of the antigenicity of this protein is under examination.

In conclusion, the approach used was successful in identifying potential antigenic proteins in *T. lestoquardi*. The results indicate that the TlSP protein homolog of TaSP, which has been successfully used to establish and validate an ELISA for tropical theileriosis,[5,6] may be a promising candidate for the development of an ELISA for detecting circulating antibodies in *T. lestoquardi*-infected animals.

ACKNOWLEDGMENTS

This work was supported in part by the European Commission (ICA4-CT-2000-30028). M.A. Bakheit was a doctoral scholarship holder of the German Academic Exchange Services (DAAD).

REFERENCES

1. SCHNITTGER, L. *et al*. 2002. Characterization of a polymorphic *Theileria annulata* surface protein (TaSP) closely related to PIM of *Theileria parva*: implications for use in diagnostic tests and subunit vaccines. Mol. Biochem. Parasitol. **120:** 247–256.
2. SCHNITTGER, L. *et al*. 2002. Characterization of a polymorphic gene of *T. lestoquardi* and of a recently identified *Theileria* species pathogenic for small ruminants in China. Parasitol. Res. **88:** 553–556.
3. BAKHEIT, M.A. *et al*. 2006. Purification of macroschizonts of a Sudanese isolate of *Theileria lestoquardi* (*T. lestoquardi* [Atbara]). Ann. N. Y. Acad. Sci. This volume.
4. SKILTON, R.A. *et al*. 2000. A 32 kDa surface antigen of *Theileria parva*: characterization and immunization studies. Parasitology **120:** 553–564.
5. BAKHEIT, M.A. *et al*. 2004. Application of the recombinant *Theileria annulata* surface protein in an indirect ELISA for the diagnosis of tropical theileriosis. Parasitol. Res. **92:** 299–302.
6. SALIH, D.A. *et al*. 2005. Validation of the indirect TaSP enzyme-linked immunosorbent assay for diagnosis of *Theileria annulata* infection in cattle. Parasitol. Res. **97:** 302–308.

The Host Responses in Sheep Artificially Infected with *Theileria* sp. (China)

WU JIAN-SAN, YU JIAN-MIN, WANG ZHI-LIAN, SONG CUI-PING, YUAN JIAN-FONG, YAO BAO-AN

a Animal Quarantine Institute, Ministry of Agriculture, Qingdao 266032, SD, People's Republic of China

b College of Animal Science and Veterinary Medicine, Huazhong Agricultural University, Wuhan, 430070, People's Republic of China

ABSTRACT: Studies on host responses in sheep artificially infected with *Theileria* sp. (China) were discussed and summarized mainly on typical high fever periods, merozoits and schizoon observation, antibody response.

KEYWORDS: Theileriosis; sheep; *Theileria* sp. (China); host; responses

INTRODUCTION

Fatal Theileriosis of sheep and goats in the western part of China has been reported to be due to *Theileria* sp. (China).[1] It was determined that this parasite was most closely related to *T. buffeli/sergenti* and clearly divergent from *T. lestoquardi* and *T. annulata* based on the variation of nucleotide sequences of the small subunit ribosomal RNA(srRNA).[2] The pathogenic mechanism of this Chinese *Theileria* parasite remains to be resolved. For further understanding of this mechanism, studies on host responses have been carried out.

METHODS

Experimental sheep that were 4 to 6 months old were purchased from a *Theileria*-free area in Shandong province. None of the sheep were splenectomized. All were free of tick-borne diseases as determined by clinical and microscopical examination. Adult *Haemaphysalis qinghaiensis* ticks were collected from the pasture in Gannan district, Gansu province, which is an endemic area for ovine theileriosis.[3] Adults female ticks were placed on intact sheep to

Address for correspondence: Wu Jian-San, National Diagnostic Center for Exotic Animal Diseases, China Animal Health and Epidemiology Center (CAHEC), Qingdao, 266032, SD, P.R.China. Voice: +86-532-5631530; fax: 85621552.

e-mail: wujiansan@yahoo.com; wujiansan@epizoo.org

Ann. N.Y. Acad. Sci. 1081: 465–467 (2006). © 2006 New York Academy of Sciences.
doi: 10.1196/annals.1373.066

be fed to engorgement.[4] After infestation with ticks, daily rectal temperatures were taken from experimental sheep. Daily blood smears were prepared and stained, RBC counts were determined and packed cell volume (PCV) was calculated. Needle biopsy of lymph node tissue was done aseptically to determine schizont presence and distribution and for tissue culture attempts.

RESULTS AND DISCUSSION

Clinical responses in sheep typically involved two high fever periods with the highest rectal temperatures ranging from 40.3°C to 41.3°C. Schizonts were observed during the second high fever period and became detectable after 20–23 days. Schizonts existed in a small area in the lymph nodes. The merozoites began increasing 24 h after the appearance of schizonts. Parasitemias ranged from 1% to 39%. Hematology responses indicated a decrease in RBC counts and PCV followed by anemia. Infections resulted in death or recovery with a resultant carrier state.

Antibody response of sheep infected with *Theileria* sp. (China) was measured by IFAT using antigen from *Theileria*-infected erythrocytes produced by cultivation *in vitro*. The kinetics of antibody response indicated that the antibody levels increased on day 10 post infection with peaks at a titer of 5000 (sheep 0110) or 6000 (sheep 0345) on day 40 post infection (sheep 0110) or day 30 (sheep 0345). High antibody levels were sustained for about 2 months then declined gradually until undetectable at 2 months post infection. Sheep infected by tick infestation resulted in higher antibody titers and persisted longer (more than 4 months) in blood than inoculation with merozoites (with a titer of 5000 and persistence of 3 months). Detectable antibody levels occurred after the first high fever, when sporozoites invaded host cells and began the developmental cycle in sheep. The highest antibody levels appear after the second period of high fever when schizonts developed.

ACKNOWLEDGMENTS

This work was financially supported by the Fifth Framework Programme of EU Commission, Project ADDAV, Contract No: ICA4-CT2000-300028.

REFERENCES

1. Luo J. & Y. Hong. 1997. Theileriosis of sheep and goats in China. Trop. Anim. Health Prod. **29:** 8S–10S.
2. Schnittger, L. Y. Hong, L. Jianxun, *et al*. 2000. Phylongenetic analysis by rRNA comparison of the highly pathogenic sheep-infecting parasites *Theileria*

lestoquardi and a Theileria species identified in China. Ann. N. Y. Acad. Sci. **916:** 271–275.

3. SHUZHEN, G., Z. Yuan, G. Wu *et al*. 2002. Epidemiology of ovine theileriosis in Gannan region, Gansu Province, China. Parasitol. Res. **88** (Suppl. 1): S36–S37.

4. YING H, JX LUO, GQ GUAN, *et al*. 2002.Transmission of an unidentified Theileria species to small ruminants by *Haemaphysalis qinghaiensis* ticks collected in the field. Parasitol. Res. **88** (Suppl. 1): S25–S27.

Identification of Homologous Genes of *T. annulata* Proteins in the Genome of *Theileria* sp. (China)

JOANA P.G. MIRANDA,[a] MOHAMMED BAKHEIT,[b] ILKA SCHNEIDER,[b] DANIEL HALLER,[b] JABBAR S. AHMED,[b] HONG YIN,[c] ABEL G. OLIVA,[a] AND ULRIKE SEITZER[b]

[a]*Instituto de Biologia Experimental e Tecnológica (IBET), Apartado 12, P-2781-901 Oeiras, Portugal*

[b]*Research Center Borstel, Parkallee 22, 23845 Borstel, Germany*

[c]*Lanzhou Veterinary Research Institute (LVRI), Xujiaping 11, Lanzhou, Gansu 730046 PR China*

ABSTRACT: Homologues to previously described *Theileria (T.) annulata* genes (*T. annulata* surface protein [TaSP], putative *T. annulata* membrane protein [TaD]) were successfully amplified by polymerase chain reaction (PCR) from *Theileria* sp. (China) merozoite cDNA, with 88% identity to TaD; TcSP partial cDNA, 94% identity to TaSP. Moreover, homologues to a secretory protein of *T. annulata* (TaSE), with a sequence identity of 99% on the cDNA level (TcSE partial cDNA) and to a potential membrane protein of *T. lestoquardi* (Clone-5), with a sequence identity of 100% on the genomic level (Tc Clone-5) but lacking an intron at positions 1894–1928 were identified.

KEYWORDS: *Theileria*; small ruminants; diagnostic tools

INTRODUCTION

Theileria sp. (China) is a newly identified pathogen of small ruminants identified in the northwestern part of China.[1] The development of diagnostic tools for parasite surveillance to control and prevent spread of the disease are needed, thus studies using biochemical techniques were used to identify potential *Theileria* sp. (China) antigenic proteins.[2,3]

Address for correspondence: Ulrike Seitzer, Research Center Borstel, Parkallee 22, 23845 Borstel, Germany. Voice: +49-0-4537-188413; fax: +49-0-4537-188627.
e-mail: useitzer@fz-borstel.de

Ann. N.Y. Acad. Sci. 1081: 468–470 (2006). © 2006 New York Academy of Sciences.
doi: 10.1196/annals.1373.067

METHODS

In this study, polymerase chain reaction (PCR) techniques were employed to identify possible homologous genes of proteins, which have been identified in other *Theileria* species.

RESULTS AND DISCUSSION

Homologs to previously described *Theileria (T.) annulata* genes (*T. annulata* surface protein[4] [TaSP], putative *T. annulata* membrane protein[5] [TaD]) were successfully amplified by PCR from *Theileria* sp. (China) merozoite cDNA and verified by sequencing (TcD [GenBank DQ120056]: 88% identity to TaD; TcSP partial cDNA [GenBank DQ120058] 94% identity to TaSP). Moreover, homologs to a secretory protein of *T. annulata* (TaSE [GenBank AJ512174]) with a sequence identity of 99% on the cDNA level (TcSE partial cDNA [GenBank DQ120057]) and to a potential membrane protein of *T. lestoquardi* (Clone-5 [GenBank DQ004500]) with a sequence identity of 100% on the genomic level (Tc Clone-5 [GenBank DQ120055]) but lacking an intron at positions 1894–1928 were identified.

Preliminary investigations on the humoral immune response to identified proteins demonstrated that no detectable antibody reactivity was present against TaD, TaSE, or Clone-5. The humoral immune response to TcSP was not conclusive and remains to be analyzed using ELISA. Investigations concerning the role of the gene products in the cellular immune response to *Theileria* sp. (China) infection and thus analyzing their applicability for subunit vaccine development are under way.

ACKNOWLEDGMENTS

This work was supported in part by the European Union (ICA4-2000-300028) and the Portuguese Foundation for Science and Technology (SFRH/BD/6494/2001).

REFERENCES

1. SCHNITTGER, L. *et al.* 2000. Phylogenetic analysis by rRNA comparison of the highly pathogenic sheep-infecting parasites *Theileria lestoquardi* and a *Theileria* species identified in China. Ann. N. Y. Acad. Sci. **916:** 271–275.
2. MIRANDA, J. *et al.* 2004. Identification of antigenic proteins of a *Theileria* species pathogenic for small ruminants in China recognized by antisera of infected animals. Ann. N. Y. Acad. Sci. **1026:** 161–164.

3. MIRANDA, J. *et al.* 2005. Identification and characterization of merozoite antigens of a *Theileria* species highly pathogenic for small ruminants in China. Ann. N. Y. Acad. Sci. This volume.
4. SCHNITTGER, L. *et al.* 2002. Characterization of a polymorphic *Theileria annulata* surface protein (TaSP) closely related to PIM of *Theileria parva*: implications for use in diagnostic tests and subunit vaccines. Mol. Biochem. Parasitol. **120:** 247–256.
5. SCHNEIDER, I. *et al.* 2004. Molecular genetic characterization and subcellular localization of a putative *Theileria annulata* membrane protein. Parasitol. Res. **94:** 405–415.

Epidemiology of *Theileria annulata* Infection of Dairy Cattle in the Sudan Using Molecular Techniques

AWADIA M. ALI,[a] MOHAMMED A. BAKHEIT,[a] MAOWIA M. MUKHTAR,[b]
SHAWGI M. HASSAN,[a] JABBAR S. AHMED,[c] AND ULRIKE SEITZER[c]

[a]*Faculty of Veterinary Medicine, University of Khartoum, 13314 Khartoum North, Sudan*

[b]*Institute of Endemic Diseases, University of Khartoum, 11115 Khartoum North, Sudan*

[c]*Research Center Borstel, 23845 Borstel, Germany*

ABSTRACT: This study provides the first epidemiological data regarding *T. annulata* infection of diary cattle in Sudan using a combination of routine microscopic examination and two molecular techniques, PCR and reverse line blot (RLB).

KEYWORDS: *Theileria annulata*; epidemiology; Sudan

INTRODUCTION

In the Sudan tropical theileriosis has been recorded since 1908 and is considered the most important tick-borne disease with substantial economic impact. The epidemiological data of *Theileria annulata* infection by serological surveys showed that the prevalence decreased from 90% in Khartoum State to 13% in the southern parts of the Blue Nile. The aim of this article was to apply molecular techniques to determine the prevalence of *T. annulata* and other hemoparasite infections in the Sudan.

METHODS

Samples (*n* = 162) were analyzed by a combination of routine stained blood smears and two molecular techniques, polymerase chain reaction (PCR)

Address for correspondence: Ulrike Seitzer, Division of Veterinary Infectiology and Immunology, Research Center Borstel, Parkallee 22, 23845 Borstel, Germany. Voice: +49-4537-188-413; fax: +49-4537-188-627.

e-mail: useitzer@fz-borstel.de

Ann. N.Y. Acad. Sci. 1081: 471–472 (2006). © 2006 New York Academy of Sciences.
doi: 10.1196/annals.1373.068

and reverse line blot (RLB). PCR was performed to specifically detect all *Theileria* spp.[1] and *T. annulata*.[2] RLB analysis was designed to detect all *Ehrlichia/Anaplasma*[3] and *Theileria/Babesia*[4] infections, as well as to specifically detect 4 *Anaplasma*, 4 *Ehrlichia*, 6 *Babesia*, and 9 *Theileria* species infecting ruminants.[3–6]

RESULTS AND DISCUSSION

Piroplasms were detected in 16.7% of the animals using stained blood smears, 48.1% animals were positive by PCR, and 65.4% animals were positive by RLB. The agreement between the two molecular tests was 73.4%. The higher positive samples detected by molecular techniques indicate the carrier status of most of the studied animals. RLB allowed the detection of tick-borne parasites that simultaneously infected the animals. Analysis of the field samples also revealed that there may be a new species of *Babesia* and *Ehrlichia/Anaplasma* in the field, which needs to be confirmed by 18 S and 16 S rRNA gene analysis, respectively.

ACKNOWLEDGMENTS

This research was partially supported by the Animal Resources Bank, Sudan, IAEA (NO. SUD04/027), the European Union (ICA4-2000-30028), and the German Academic Exchange Services (A.M. Ali).

REFERENCES

1. ALLSOPP, B.A. *et al*. 1993. Discrimination between six species of *Theileria* using oligonucleotide probes which detect ss rRNA sequences. Parasitology **107:** 157–165.
2. D'OLIVEIRA, C. *et al*. 1995. Detection of *Theileria annulata* in blood samples of carrier cattle by PCR. J. Clin. Microbiol. **13:** 2665–2669.
3. BEKKER, C.P.J. *et al*. 2002. Simultaneous detection of *Anaplasma* and *Ehrlichia* species in ruminants and detection of *Ehrlichia ruminantium* in *Amblyomma variegatum* ticks by reverse line blot hybridization. Vet. Microbiol. **89:** 223–238.
4. GUBBELS, M.J. *et al*. 1999. Simultaneous detection of bovine *Theileria* and *Babesia* species by reverse line blot hybridization. J. Clin. Microbiol. **37:** 1782–1789.
5. OURA, C.A.L. *et al*. 2004. Application of a reverse line blot to the study of haemoparasites in cattle in Uganda. Int. J. Parasitol. **34:** 603–613.
6. SCHOULS, L.M. *et al*. 1999. Detection and identification of *Ehrlichia, Borrelia burgdorferi* and *Bortonella* species in Dutch *Ixodes ricinus* ticks. J. Clin. Microbiol. **37:** 2215–2222.

Investigation of MAP Kinase Activation in *Theileria*-Infected Cell Lines

ULRIKE SEITZER, LEONHARD SCHNITTGER, KATI BOGUSLAWSKI, AND JABBAR S. AHMED

Division of Immunology and Cell Biology, Research Center Borstel, 23845 Borstel, Germany

ABSTRACT: A study on different *Theileria annulata* and *Theileria parva* infected cell lines was performed in order to evaluate the general relevance of the MAP-kinase activation status for *Theileria-* mediated transformation.

KEYWORDS: Theileria; Jun NH2-terminal kinase; extracellular signal-related kinase; P 38

INTRODUCTION

Leukoproliferative *Theileria* are unique intracellular protozoan parasites that transform their host cell to a permanently proliferating phenotype. The molecular signaling involved in this process is complex and poorly understood. Mitogen-activated protein kinases (MAP) function as pivotal components in pathways that control cellular differentiation, proliferation, and apoptosis. It was reported that Jun NH2-terminal kinase (JNK) is constitutively activated in *T. parva*-infected T cells[1] and in *T. annulata*-infected macrophage and B cell lines,[2] whereas the extracellular signal-related kinases (ERK1 and ERK2) and p38 were reported to be silent.[2,3]

METHODS

To evaluate the general relevance of MAP-kinase activation status for *Theileria*-mediated transformation, we performed Western blot analyses to include: (*a*) cell lines established from one animal but infected with *T. annulata* stocks Hissar (TaH2006) or Morocco (TaM2006); (*b*) cell lines established from different animals infected with the same *T. annulata* stock Ankara (TaA288, TaA1272); (*c*) cell lines established from different animals and infected with

Address for correspondence: Jabbar S. Ahmed, Division of Veterinary Infectiology and Immunology, Research Center Borstel, Parkallee 22, 23845 Borstel, Germany. Voice: +49-4537-188-428; fax: +49-4537-188-627.

e-mail: jahmed@fz-borstel.de

Ann. N.Y. Acad. Sci. 1081: 473–475 (2006). © 2006 New York Academy of Sciences.
doi: 10.1196/annals.1373.069

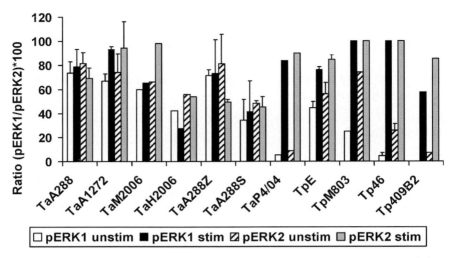

FIGURE 1. Densitometric evaluation of Western blots investigating phosphorylation status of ERK1 and ERK2. Signals obtained for pERK1 and pERK2 without (unstim) and with (stim) stimulation with PMA were set in relation to ERK1 and ERK2 signals. Ta(x): *T. annulata*-infected cell lines; Tp(x): *T. parva*-infected cell lines.

different parasite stocks (TaA288, TaH2006, or TaM2006); (*d*) cell lines established from sheep and goat and infected with *T. annulata* stock Ankara (TaA288S, TaA288Z; (*e*) a *T. annulata*-infected clonal B cell line (TaP4/04); (*f*) a *T. parva*-infected cell line (TpE); and (*g*) *T. parva*-infected clonal B cell (Tp409B2) and T cell (TpM803, Tp46) lines.

RESULTS AND DISCUSSION

As found by others, JNK1 was found to be activated in all cell lines and may thus be regarded as a general concept in cell transformation by *Theileria*. Densitometric evaluation of ERK activation showed that there was a significant difference between *T. annulata*- and *T. parva*-infected cell lines with respect to pERK1 activation without stimulation ($P < 0.05$; FIG. 1). This difference may be due to the fact that these two parasites infect different host cell populations leading to the activation of different signal transduction pathways. The more significant finding was that bulk-infected cell lines showed constitutive ERK1 activation whereas all clonal cell lines showed little to no ERK1 activation ($P < 0.0005$). Thus, investigations of signaling pathways using clonal cell lines may not entirely reflect the complex parasite–host cell interactions involved, resulting in the transformed host cell phenotype.

REFERENCES

1. GALLEY, Y. *et al*. 1997. Jun NH2-terminal kinase is constitutively activated in T cells transformed by the intracellular parasite *Theileria parva*. Proc. Natl. Acad. Sci. USA **94:** 5119–5124.
2. CHAUSSEPIED, M. *et al*. 1998. Upregulation of Jun and Fos family members and permanent JNK activity lead to constitutive AP-1 activation in *Theileria*-transformed leukocytes. Mol. Biochem. Parasitol. **94:** 215–226.
3. BOTTERON, C. & D. DOBBELAERE. 1998. AP-1 and ATF-2 are constitutively activated via the JNK pathway in *Theileria parva*-transformed T-cells. Biochem. Biophys. Res. Commun. **246:** 418–421.

Dermal Mast Cell Counts in F2 Holstein x Gir Crossbred Cattle Artificially Infested with the Tick *Boophilus microplus* (Acari: Ixodidae)

J.R. ENGRACIA FILHO,[a] G.H. BECHARA,[b] AND R.L. TEODORO[c]

[a]*Centro Universitário Barão de Mauá, 14.090-180 Ribeirão Preto, SP, Brazil*

[b]*Faculdade de Ciências Agrárias e Veterinárias-UNESP, 14.884-900 Jaboticabal, SP, Brazil*

[c]*Centro Nacional de Pesquisa de Gado de Leite, Empresa Brasileira de Pesquisa Agropecuária (Embrapa), 36.038-330 Juiz de Fora, MG, Brazil*

ABSTRACT: The role of dermal mast cells (DMC) in the host resistance to ticks has been studied but it is not totally explained yet. Studies have proposed that zebuine cattle breeds, known as highly resistant to ticks, have more DMC than taurine breeds. In the present study, we compared the number of adult female ticks *Boophilus microplus* and the mast cells' countings in the skin of F_2 crossbred Gir × Holstein cattle, before and after tick infestation. F_2 crossbred cattle (n = 148) were divided into seven groups and artificially infested with 1.0×10^4 *B. microplus* larvae and, 21 days afterwards, adult female-fed ticks attached to the skin were counted. Skin biopsies were taken and examined under light microscopy with a square-lined ocular reticulum in a total area of 0.0625 mm^2 in both the superficial and deep dermis. Results demonstrated that infested F_2 crossbred cattle acquired resistance against the cattle-tick *B. microplus* probably associated to an increase in the dermal mast cell number. It is concluded that the tick infestation may lead to an environmental modification in the dermis of parasitized hosts due to the massive migration of mast cells or their local proliferation.

KEYWORDS: dermal mast cells; cattle tick; resistance; crossbred cattle

INTRODUCTION

Host genetic composition determines immune response capabilities and it is well known that both purebred and crossbred cattle of *Bos indicus* genetic

Address for correspondence: G.H. Bechara, Faculdade de Ciências Agrárias e Veterinárias-UNESP, 14.884-900 Jaboticabal, SP, Brazil. Voice: +55-16-32092662; fax: +55-16-32024275.
e-mail: bechara@fcav.unesp.br

Ann. N.Y. Acad. Sci. 1081: 476–478 (2006). © 2006 New York Academy of Sciences.
doi: 10.1196/annals.1373.070

TABLE 1. Mean number of ticks and of DMC per mm^2 from groups of F_2 Gir x Holstein cattle artificially infested with 1.0×10^4 *B. microplus* larvae. Jaboticabal-SP- Brazil, 2004

F_2 Gir x Holstein cattle groups (*n*)	Age (days)	Tick counts	Mast cell number/mm^2	
			BI	AI
1 (22)	418	32.00	28.80	55.71
2 (22)	511	19.91	—	41.31
3 (11)	515	16.09	19.20	91.05
4 (24)	408	18.25	15.27	110.80
5 (20)	788	17.40	71.92	96.16
6 (24)	704	27.25	55.87	108.93
7 (25)	537	27.84	44.54	42.02
Mean (SD)	554.4 (114.8)	22.7 (6.2)	39.27 (22.17)	78.00 (30.74)

composition are more resistant to tick infestation than purebred *Bos taurus*.[1] The role of dermal mast cells (DMC) in the host's resistance to ticks has been studied but it is not totally explained yet. Some studies demonstrated that zebu cattle breeds, known as highly resistant to ticks, have twice the number of DMC than taurine cattle breeds in *Boophilus microplus (B. microplus)*-parasitized skin biopsies.[2,3] This article's objective was to evaluate the DMC counts in F_2 Holstein x Gir crossbred cattle artificially infested with the cattle tick *B. microplus*.

MATERIALS AND METHODS

F_2 crossbred Holstein x Gir cattle (*n* = 148) separated in seven groups were artificially infested with 1.0×10^4 *B. microplus* larvae and, after 21 days, adult female-fed ticks attached to the skin were counted. Before infestation (BI) and 21 days afterward (AI), biopsies of the skin were taken, fixed in formalin 10%, and processed according to routine histotechnology. Sections 5 µM thick were then stained by either hematoxylin-eosin or May-Grünwald and Giemsa for general histopathology and mast cell counting, respectively. DMC of F_2 crossbred cattle were counted under light microscopy with square-lined ocular reticulum and $\times$ 40 objective in both the upper and inner dermis. The comparison of mast cell counting between BI and AI samples collected were accomplished with *F*-test ($P \leq 0.0001$).

RESULTS AND DISCUSSION

Means of age, tick count, and mast cell number from F_2 Gir x Holstein crossbred cattle groups are presented in TABLE 1. The F_2 Gir x Holstein cattle showed high-to-intermediate resistance to cattle tick. All groups displayed a marked increase in the DMC population after tick infestation, excluding group 7, which showed similar values in the mast cell counts performed BI and AI. Statistical analysis of the total means (39.27 BI and 78.0 AI) with F-test showed high significance.

CONCLUSIONS

F_2 crossbred Holstein x Gir cattle was resistant or lightly resistant to *B. microplus* infestation. The artificial infestation with *B. microplus* larvae induced a highly significant rise in the mast cell number in the dermis of F_2 crossbred Holstein x Gir cattle, verified in samples of healthy skin, that is, without any sign of tick attachment. These results suggest that the tick infestation may lead to an environmental change in the skin of parasitized hosts due to the massive migration of mast cells or their local proliferation.

ACKNOWLEDGMENTS

This work was partially supported by the Conselho Nacional de Ciência e Tecnologia-CNPq and facilitated through the Integrated Consortium on Ticks and Tick-borne Diseases (ICTTD-3) supported by the European Union under contract number 510561-INCO.

REFERENCES

1. WIKEL, S.K. 1996. The immunology of host-ectoparasitic arthropod relationships. CAB International. 204–231.
2. MORAES, F.R., J.R.E. MORAES, A.J. COSTA, *et al.* 1992. A comparative study of lesions caused by different parasitic stages of *Boophilus microplus* (Canestrini) in the skins of naturally infested taurine and zebuine hosts. The correlation of tick resistance with mast cell counts in the host's skin. Braz. J. Vet. Res. Anim. Sci. **29:** 378–383.
3. SARTOR, I.F., J.L.H. FACCINI, M.R.G. KUCHEMBUCK & P.R. CURI. 1997. Estudo comparativo da resistência ao carrapato *Boophilus microplus* (Canestrini) (Acari) em bovinos das raças Gir, Holandesa e mestiços $\frac{1}{2}$ Gir-Holandês. Vet. E. Zoot. **9:** 27–47.

Detection of *Hepatozoon canis* in Stray Dogs and Cats in Bangkok, Thailand

SATHAPORN JITTAPALAPONG,[a] OPART RUNGPHISUTTHIPONGSE,[b]
SOICHI MARUYAMA,[c] JOHN J. SCHAEFER,[d] AND ROGER W. STICH[e]

[a]*Department of Parasitology, Faculty of Veterinary Medicine,
Kasetsart University, Bangkok 10900, Thailand*

[b]*PCR MAHALARB Laboratory, Bangkok 24140, Thailand*

[c]*Department of Veterinary Medicine, College of Bioresource Sciences,
Nihon University, Kanagawa 252-8510, Japan*

[d]*Department of Entomology, The Ohio State University, Columbus,
Ohio 43210, USA*

[e]*Department of Veterinary Pathobiology, University of Missouri, Columbia,
Missouri 65211, USA*

ABSTRACT: A rapidly increasing stray animal population in Bangkok
has caused concern regarding transmission of vector-borne and zoonotic
diseases. The purpose of this study was to determine if stray animals in
Bangkok are a potential reservoir of *Hepatozoon*, a genus of tick-borne
parasites that has received little attention in Thailand. Blood samples
were collected from stray companion animals near monasteries in 42
Bangkok metropolitan districts. Both dogs and cats were sampled from
26 districts, dogs alone from 4 districts and cats alone from 12 districts.
Samples were collected from a total of 308 dogs and 300 cats. Light microscopy and an 18 S rRNA gene-based PCR assay were used to test these
samples for evidence of *Hepatozoon* infection. Gamonts were observed in
blood smears for 2.6% of dogs and 0.7% of cats by microscopy. The PCR
assay detected *Hepatozoon* in buffy coats from 11.4% of dogs and 32.3%
of cats tested. The prevalence of infection was the same between male
and female dogs or cats, and PCR-positive dogs and cats were found in
36.6% and 36.8% of the districts surveyed, respectively. There was an
association between the percentages of PCR-positive dogs and cats in
districts where both host species were sampled. Sequences of representative amplicons were closest to those reported for *H. canis*. These results
represent the first molecular confirmation that *H. canis* is indigenous
to Thailand. The unexpectedly high prevalence of *Hepatozoon* among
stray cats indicates that their role in the epizootiology of hepatozoonosis
should be investigated.

Address for correspondence: Dr. Sathaporn Jittapalapong, DUM, Ph.D., Department of Parasitology,
Faculty of Veterinary Medicine, Kasetsart University, Bangkok 10900. Thailand. Voice: 662-942-8438;
fax: 662-942-8438.

e-mail: fvetspj@ku.ac.th

Ann. N.Y. Acad. Sci. 1081: 479–488 (2006). © 2006 New York Academy of Sciences.
doi: 10.1196/annals.1373.071

KEYWORDS: *Hepatozoon canis*; stray dogs and cats; 18 S rRNA gene; PCR; Bangkok; Thailand

INTRODUCTION

Canine hepatozoonosis is caused by the apicomplexan parasites *Hepatozoon canis* and *H. americanum*. Ixodid ticks acquire these protozoa through a vertebrate blood meal that contains gamonts (gamete stages of the parasite), and the parasites are transmitted to vertebrate hosts that ingest infective ticks.[1,2]

There are at least two disease syndromes associated with *Hepatozoon* species known to parasitize canids.[1] One syndrome is caused by *H. americanum*, an agent of canine hepatozoonosis in the Americas that uses the Gulf Coast tick, *Amblyomma maculatum*, as a definitive host. After an infective tick is ingested, *H. americanum* undergoes merogony in skeletal and cardiac muscle of the canine intermediate host, resulting in severe clinical disease that includes exostosis and myositis.[3] Conversely, *H. canis*, an agent of canine hepatozoonosis in both the Old and New Worlds, uses the brown dog tick, *Rhipicephalus sanguineus*, as a definitive host and undergoes merogony primarily in the spleen and liver of the canine host. Canine hepatozoonosis canis is usually mild but can be severe.

Although *Hepatozoon* infections have been found in Asia, including Peninsular Malaysia,[4] Japan,[5] India,[6] Israel,[7] and Sri Lanka,[8] the prevalence of these parasites among companion animals in Thailand is poorly understood. This is mainly because of the difficulty in diagnosing the old world form of the disease, owing in large part to the broad range of nonspecific clinical signs associated with the disease and to the reliance of conventional diagnosis on finding low levels of *Hepatozoon* gamonts in blood smears.

There are several reasons to suspect that *H. canis* is indigenous to Thailand. First, there are reports of microscopic detection of *Hepatozoon* in naturally infected dogs from Thailand.[9,10] Second, *R. sanguineus*, the definitive host of *H. canis*, is considered the most common tick collected from dogs in Thailand,[11] and a survey of canine blood smears suggested that *Hepatozoon* infections were more frequently found in dogs infested with ticks than in dogs without ticks.[9,12] Finally, stray dog and cat populations in Bangkok have increased tremendously during the past decade.[13]

The objective of this article was to determine if *Hepatozoon* is present among stray companion animal populations in Bangkok, Thailand. Thus, blood samples were collected from strays residing near Buddhist monasteries in the Bangkok metropolitan area, and these samples were examined for evidence of *Hepatozoon* infection by light microscopy and with an 18 S rRNA gene (rDNA)-based polymerase chain reaction (PCR) assay.

MATERIALS AND METHODS

Collection of Blood Samples

A cross-sectional study was performed where samples were collected from stray dogs and cats that resided across the Bangkok metropolitan area between October 2002 and September 2003. Animals were sampled from three monasteries of each district. Blood (1 mL) was collected from the saphenous vein of dogs or the jugular vein of cats, into sterile plastic tubes with citrate buffer (EUROTUBO, Bangkok, Thailand). These samples were used to prepare whole blood smears, for microscopical examination with modified Wright–Giemsa stain, then centrifuged at approximately 900 × g before buffy coats were removed and stored at –20°C until needed for DNA isolation.

PCR Assay

For most samples, buffy coats were subjected to proteinase digestion in the presence of sodium dodecyl sulphate (SDS) followed by phenol–chloroform extraction of proteins and ethanol/salt precipitation of DNA as described elsewhere.[14] Some feline samples (approximately 20%) were clotted, and these samples were treated with the UltraClean™ DNA BloodSpin Kit (MO BIO Laboratories, Solana Beach, CA). Each DNA sample was dissolved or eluted into 200 µL of TE buffer (10 mM Tris-Cl, 0.5 mM EDTA, pH 9.0).

An 18 S rDNA-based assay for *Hepatozoon* was performed in 25 µL reactions containing 5 µL of genomic DNA template with primers HepF primer (5′-ATACATGAGCAAAATCTCAAC-3′) and HepR (5′-CTTATTATTCC ATGCTGCAG-3′), and the amplification was performed to generate a 666-bp target amplicon as reported elsewhere.[15–17] These primers were designed to amplify 18 S rDNA of *H. canis, H. americanum,* and *H. catasbianae,* but they are not expected to amplify a 666-bp amplicon from *Plasmodium* or *Babesia* species. Each reaction contained 1× PCR buffer (10 mM Tris-HCl pH 8.8, 50 mM KCl, and 0.1% Triton X-100), 1.6 mM $MgCl_2$, 12.5 pmol of each primer, 0.2 mM of each dNTP, and 0.75 U of Taq DNA polymerase (DyNAzyme: FINNZYMES, Kauklahti, Espoo, Finland). The amplification was performed in a PTC-200 thermal cycler (MJ Research, Inc., Watertown, MA) with an annealing temperature of 53°C. Amplified products (10 µL) were separated on 1.5% agarose gels, stained with ethidium bromide, and visualized using an ultraviolet illuminator.

Representative amplicons were purified with the HiYield Gel/PCR DNA Fragments Extraction kit (Eastern Biotech Real Genomics, Taipe, Taiwan) for automated sequencing. *Hepatozoon* 18 S rDNA sequences were obtained from GenBank for comparison to amplicons generated in this study.[18] The database sequences, with their GenBank accession umbers in parentheses, included 18 S rDNA from *H. canis* (AF176835), *H. americanum* (AF176836), and *H. catesbianae* (AF 176837).

RESULTS

To ensure that results were representative of the entire area, samples were collected from 42 of 50 districts across metropolitan Bangkok between October 2002 and September 2003. Most of the stray dogs sampled were mongrels (including cross-breeds) and cats were native Thai breeds. Blood was collected from totals of 308 dogs from 30 districts and 300 cats from 38 districts. Dogs alone were sampled in 4 districts, cats alone were sampled in 12 districts, and 203 cats and 264 dogs were sampled in the 26 districts where both host species were found.

Gamonts were observed by light microscopy in leukocytes from 8 dogs (2.6%) and 2 (0.7%) cats. An approximately 666-bp amplicon (FIG. 1) was generated from buffy coat DNA of a dog that was confirmed to be infected with *Hepatozoon* by light microscopy. This DNA served as a positive control for PCR assays throughout the study. Similar amplicons were generated from all of the dogs and cats where gamonts were observed by light microscopy. The target amplicon was generated from totals of 35 dogs (11.4%) and 97 cats (32.3%). For districts where both dogs and cats were sampled, 54 cats (26.6%) and 33 dogs (12.5%) tested PCR-positive. There was no apparent difference in prevalence of infection between male and female dogs or cats (TABLE 1). PCR-positive dogs and cats were found in 36.6% and 36.8%, respectively, of the Bangkok districts where they were sampled (TABLE 2).

Interesting differences were observed between the distributions of PCR-positive dogs and cats (FIG. 2). Districts 4, 6, 16, 17, 19, and 21 contained PCR-positive dogs while all cats tested were PCR negative. Districts 22 and 29 contained PCR-positive cats while all dogs tested were PCR negative. Notably, among districts where both dogs and cats were sampled, a moderate correlation between the percentage of PCR-positive dogs and cats from each district was indicated by the Pearson's correlation coefficient ($r = 0.43$), which was statistically significant ($P < 0.05$) according to a two-tailed t-test.[19]

Amplicons generated from 10 naturally exposed dogs and two cats were sequenced to identify the *Hepatozoon* species detected. All of the sequences analyzed were 100% identical to each other and 99% identical to the corresponding 18 S rDNA sequence reported for *H. canis* (AF176835).

DISCUSSION

The results of this study suggest that *H. canis* is indigenous to Bangkok, Thailand. This work represents, to our knowledge, the first demonstration of

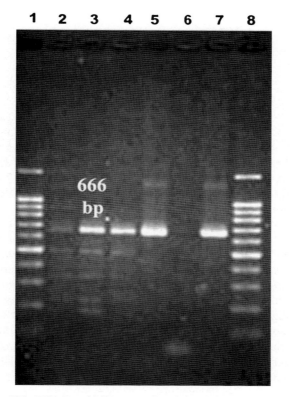

FIGURE 1. 18S rDNA-based PCR assay of peripheral blood from stray dogs. Lanes 1 and 8 contain a 100-bp ladder molecular size standard. Lanes 2–5 represent different stray dogs that tested negative with light microscopy. Lane 6 represents the no-template control and Lane 7 represents the positive control where *Hepatozoon* gamonts were observed with microscopy.

H. canis in stray dogs and cats in Thailand with a PCR technique. Furthermore, to our knowledge this is the first report of feline infections with *Hepatozoon* in Asia.

The results from blood smear examinations were similar to previous studies in Thailand that involved microscopic examination along with clinical signs or post mortem diagnosis.[9,10] One of these earlier reports involved microscopic examination of peripheral blood, liver, spleen, and lymph nodes of anemic dogs from Kasetsart Animal Teaching Hospital.[9] In 1982 a survey for blood parasites indicated that 5.2% of 1892 dogs were infected with *H. canis*, while 1.9% of these infected dogs showed no clinical signs of hepatozoonosis.[10] In our hands, the PCR assay appeared more sensitive than microscopic examination for detection of infection, especially for cats. Moreover, this PCR assay allowed

TABLE 1. *Hepatozoon* infections detected by microscopy and PCR among stray companion animals in Bangkok

Hosts	No. examined	No. positive by microscopy (%)	No. positive by PCR (%)
Stray dogs			
Male	124	2 (1.6)	14 (11.3)
Female	184	6 (3.3)	21 (11.4)
Total	308	8 (2.6)	35 (11.4)
Stray cats			
Male	137	1 (0.7)	42 (30.7)
Female	163	1 (0.6)	55 (33.7)
Total	300	2 (0.7)	97 (32.3)

us to confirm identity of *Hepatozoon* species that were detected. Sequence analysis of amplicons from 10 dogs and 2 cats showed 99% homology to *H. canis*, confirming reports that *H. canis* is present in companion animals in Thailand.

The potential role of stray companion animals as a reservoir or source of pet infections with *H. canis* was not previously reported from Thailand. It is established that *H. canis* can be transmitted between dogs by *R. sanguineus*,[20–22] and there is a high prevalence of *R. sanguineus* reported among stray dogs in Bangkok,[11] suggesting that this tick could vector the parasite between stray dogs and cats as well as pets. Thus, it is not surprising that stray dogs are a possible source of both *R. sanguineus* and *H. canis* parasites of house pets. However, observed differences in geographical distribution of PCR-positive dogs and cats and the high prevalence of *Hepatozoon* infections among cats were both surprising. The former observation could in part be due to difficulty in sampling dogs in certain districts with cultures that are not tolerant of stray dogs.

Several biological explanations could also account for the differences observed between PCR-positive cat and dog populations. First, the PCR assay used for this study might have detected a species other than *H. canis*. This seems unlikely because (*a*) several groups reported utilization of the same assay to identify *H. canis* among naturally infected dogs,[15–17] (*b*) all representative amplicon sequences suggested that *H. canis* was the closest known species, and (*c*) because the correlation between percent PCR-positive dogs and cats of different districts suggested that these different host populations are infected by a common parasite or vector. However, the primers used for this assay also correspond to *H. americanum*, and to our knowledge specificity trials with parasites closely related to *Hepatozoon* were not performed at the time of this report. Therefore, the possibility of reduced specificity is an important caveat for this and other PCR assays based on highly conserved target sequences. Second, dogs and cats could be exposed to *Hepatozoon* at different rates due to different invertebrate vectors of the parasite. Other hematophagous arthropods that parasitize companion animals, including mites, lice, fleas, and

TABLE 2. *Hepatozoon* PCR assay results for stray dogs and cats of Bangkok

District No.[a]	Name	PCR + Hosts ($n =$)	
		Dogs	Cats
1	Phasicharoen	0 (8)	0 (7)
2	Bangkok Yai	0 (7)	0 (6)
3	Phra Nakhon	0 (9)	NA[b]
4	Tailing Chan	3 (13)	0 (6)
5	Bangkok Noi	3 (11)	11(14)
6	Bang Kae	1 (7)	0 (7)
7	Bang Plad	0 (6)	0 (8)
8	Ratchatewi	0 (8)	0 (7)
9	Chatuchak	0 (9)	4 (9)
10	Chom Thong	2 (10)	7 (10)
11	Lak Si	0 (7)	0 (7)
12	Sai Mai	0 (12)	NA
13	Bang Khen	0 (8)	0 (6)
14	Wang Thonglang	0 (7)	NA
15	Pomprap Sattruphai	2 (16)	NA
16	Yannawa	3 (16)	0 (7)
17	Khlong Toei	4 (19)	0 (6)
18	Kannayao	3 (10)	6 (8)
19	Bung Kum	2 (10)	0 (6)
20	Lat Phrao	10 (14)	15 (17)
21	Khlong Samwa	2 (16)	0 (7)
22	Bang Kapi	0 (9)	12 (15)
23	Suan Luang	0 (7)	0 (7)
24	Bang Na	0 (10)	0 (6)
25	Lat Krabang	0 (8)	0 (8)
26	Min Buri	0 (11)	0 (6)
27	Nong Chok	0 (9)	0 (6)
28	Bang Sue	0 (10)	0 (5)
29	Don Muang	0 (10)	5 (7)
30	Dusit	0 (11)	0 (5)
31	Din Daeng	NA	4 (7)
32	Bang Bon	NA	5 (9)
33	Bang Rak	NA	3 (7)
34	Phraya Thai	NA	6 (8)
35	Huai Khwang	NA	7 (10)
36	Thung Kru	NA	0 (7)
37	Bang Khunthian	NA	0 (8)
38	Bang Kholaem	NA	8 (12)
39	Sathon	NA	4 (9)
40	Samphanthawong	NA	0 (8)
41	Nong Khaem	NA	0 (6)
42	Khong San	NA	0 (6)
Total		35 (308)	97 (300)

[a] District numbers correspond to FIGURE 2.
[b] Not applicable: hosts of this species were not sampled in this district.

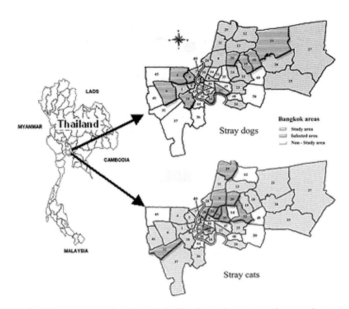

FIGURE 2. Map representing Bangkok districts where stray dogs and cats were tested for *Hepatozoon* infections. Numbers in each district correspond to those in TABLE 2. Districts where each host species was sampled are gray, and districts with PCR-positive hosts are darker. Districts in white are where the respective hosts were not sampled.

mosquitoes, are prevalent among the stray animal population of Bangkok,[11] and potential roles of these ectoparasites as vectors of *Hepatozoon* among cat or dog populations are not reported. Third, exposure rates of cats and dogs to *Hepatozoon* might be different due to differences in host behavior. For example, grooming activity might result in a greater exposure rate of cats due to ingestion of infective arthropods. Also, cats might be less likely to roam between monastery sites, thus the prevalence of cat infections could be more concentrated in areas where the parasite is established. Dogs are thought to roam between districts, especially during mating season, so the prevalence of this parasite among dog populations may be less concentrated as infected hosts leave and uninfected hosts enter an enzootic area. Fourth, there could be differences in host permissiveness, such as innate resistance to *H. canis* infection. Dogs are presumably more commonly parasitized by *H. canis* and possibly more closely adapted to this parasite. Finally, animals that were former pets were less likely to be exposed to *H. canis* at a young age. It is plausible that a larger portion of the Bangkok stray dog population consists of animals that were abandoned at monasteries, while a greater proportion of cats were likely born under feral conditions and exposed to *H. canis* at a potentially more susceptible young age.

In summary, the 18 S rDNA-based PCR assay apparently detected more *Hepatozoon* infections than conventional microscopy, and sequence analysis of representative amplicons suggested that *H. canis* was present in both dogs and cats. A greater than expected prevalence of PCR-positive stray cats suggested that the potential role of these hosts in the epizootiology of hepatozoonosis should be further investigated. Further studies are also warranted to determine the prevalence of *H. canis* among household pets, and to determine if prevalence among pets could be associated with that among stray companion animals. Surveillance of stray companion animals represents an important step toward understanding the role(s) of these populations in the ecology of arthropod-borne diseases in Bangkok, which will be useful for control of vector-borne diseases among animal and human populations in this region.

ACKNOWLEDGMENTS

This study has been partially supported by Faculty of Veterinary Medicine and Kasetsart University Research and Development Institute (KURDI), Thailand. We appreciate the excellent assistance of the 6th year veterinary students, Mrs. Nongnuch Pinyopanuwat and Mr.Wissanuwat Chimnoi.

REFERENCES

1. BANETH, G., J.S. MATHEW, V. SHKAP, *et al*. 2003. Canine hepatozoonosis: two disease syndromes caused by separate *Hepatozoon* spp. Trends Parasitol. **19:** 27–31.
2. EWING, S.A. & R.J. PANCIERA. 2003. American canine hepatozoonosis. Clin. Microbiol. Rev. **16:** 688–697.
3. EWING, S.A., R.J. PANCIERA, J.S. MATHEW, *et al*. 2000. American canine hepatozoonosis. An emerging disease in the New World. Ann. N. Y. Acad. Sci. **916:** 81–92.
4. RAJAMANICKAM, C., E. WIESENHUTTER, F. M. ZIN, *et al*. 1985. The incidence of canine haematozoa in Peninsular Malaysia. Vet. Parasitol. **17:** 151–157.
5. MURATA, T., K. SHIRAMIZU, Y. HARA, *et al*. 1991. First case of *Hepatozoon canis* infection of a dog in Japan. J. Vet. Med. Sci. **53:** 1097–1099.
6. CHRISTOPHERS, S. R. 1906. *Leucocytozoon canis*. Sci. Mem. Off. Med. Sanit. Dep. Gov. India **26:** 1–18.
7. BANETH, G., V. SHKAP, B. Z. PRESENTEY, *et al*. 1996. *Hepatozoon canis*: the prevalence of antibodies and gametocytes in dogs in Israel. Vet. Res. Commun. **20:** 41–46.
8. DISSANAIKE, A.S. 1961. *Hepatozoon canis* infection in dogs in Ceylon. Ceylon Vet. J. **9:** 144–145.
9. PUKKAVESA, C.S., S. DONKAEWBUA & P. NILKUMHANG. 1980. A study of canine hepatozoonosis in Bangkok. Kasetsart Vet. **1:** 31–38.

10. WAJJAWALKU, W. 1982. Survey of canine blood protozoa in Bangkok metropolitan area. Proceedings of the 20th Annual Conference of Kasetsart University, Veterinary Medicine Section, Bangkok, Thailand (Feb 4–5, 1982), 71–72.
11. SANGVARANOND, A., C. SINGHCHAI & W. CHIMNOI. 2000. Ectoparasites (lice, fleas, ticks and ear mites) of stray dogs in Bangkok metropolitan area. Kasetsart Vet. **10:** 1–12.
12. JITTAPALAPONG, S. & S. TIPSAWAKE. 1991. Survey of blood protozoa and blood parasites of pet dogs in Samut Prakan province. Kasetsart J. (Natural Science). **25:** 75–82.
13. JITTAPALAPONG, S., N. PINYOPANUWAT & S. BOONCHOB. 2003. A Guideline of Regulation of Animal Rearing and Maintaining in Public Places. Kasetsart University Publishing. Thailand.
14. BREMER, W. G., J.J. SCHAEFER, E. R. WAGNER, et al. 2005. Transstadial and intrastadial experimental transmission of *Ehrlichia canis* by male *Rhipicephalus sanguineus*. Vet. Parasitol. **131:** 95–105.
15. INOKUMA, H., M. OKUDA, K. OHNO, et al. 2002. Analysis of the 18 S rRNA gene sequence of a *Hepatozoon* detected in two Japanese dogs. Vet. Parasitol. **106:** 265–271.
16. KARAGENC, T. I., S. PASA, G. KIRLI, et al. 2006. A parasitological, molecular and serological survey of *Hepatozoon canis* infection in dogs around the Aegean coast of Turkey. Vet. Parasitol. **135:** 113–119.
17. RUBINI, A.S., K. DOS SANTOS PADUAN, G.G. CAVALCANTE, et al. 2005. Molecular identification and characterization of canine *Hepatozoon* species from Brazil. Parasitol. Res. **97:** 91–93.
18. MATHEW, J.S., R.A. VAN DENBUSSCHE, S.A. EWING, et al. 2000. Phylogenetic relationships of *Hepatozoon* (Apicomplexa: Adeleorina) based on molecular, morphologic, and life-cycle characters. J. Parasitol. **86:** 366–372.
19. SWINSCOW, T.D.V. (revised by M.J. Campbell). 1997. Correlation and regression. Statistics at Square One. Ninth edition. http://bmj.bmjjournals.com/collections/statsbk/11.shtml.
20. INOKUMA, H., S. YAMAMOTO & C. MORITA. 1998. Survey of tick-borne diseases in dogs infested with *Rhipicephalus sanguineus* at a kennel in Okayama Prefecture, Japan. J. Vet. Med. Sci. **60:** 761–763.
21. NORDGREN, R. M. & T. M. CRAIG. 1984. Experimental transmission of the Texas strain of *Hepatozoon canis*. Vet. Parasitol. **16:** 207–214.
22. PANCIERA, R.J., S.A. EWING, J.S. MATHEW, et al. 1999. Canine hepatozoonosis: comparison of lesions and parasites in skeletal muscle of dogs experimentally or naturally infected with *Hepatozoon americanum*. Vet. Parasitol. **82:** 261–272.

Renitelo Cattle Dermatophilosis and PCR–RFLP Analysis of MHC Gene

HANTA RAZAFINDRAIBE,[a] MODESTINE RALINIAINA,[a]
JEAN-CHARLES MAILLARD,[b] AND RAKOTONDRAVAO[a]

[a]FOFIFA-DRZV, B.P. 04 Antananarivo 101, Madagascar

[b]CIRAD-EMVT, Animal Health Program, 34398-Montpellier Cedex 5, France

ABSTRACT: Renitelo breed is a cattle breed created at Kianjasoa station (Madagascar) by a triple crossing Malagasy Zebu × Limousine × Afrikander. This breed besides many valuable advantages, such as rapid growth and drought power, presents a huge disadvantage which is sensitivity to skin disease, dermatophilosis, previously known as streptotrichosis. This disease caused by *Dermatophilus congolensis* is one of the major threats for the population of Renitelo cattle. An allele of MHC gene has been shown to be dramatically associated to hypersensitivity to the disease in other cattle breed. To bring further information to tick borne disease clinical survey, mainly dermatophilosis, we wanted to verify if such allele could be found in this breed. Renitelo cattle included in this study were chosen for the presence of dermatophilosis lesions in more or less severe form (N = 17). These animals were blood sampled and a genetic analysis on the MHC gene *BoLA-DRB3* was performed, by PCR amplification using BOD 31 & BOD 32 primers. Amplified products were analyzed by RFLP using enzymes. Restriction band profiles were characterized according to previously defined patterns. Three cows out of the 17 cattle analyzed for MHC gene presented the hypersensitive allele FDA. Two out of the three hypersensitive cows were pure breed while one was half breed. All the cows presented dermatophilosis lesions at least during rainy season but one of them particularly suffered from severe lesions covering all its body and died of the illness. This study shows that hypersensitivity allele found in other bovine breeds can be found in Renitelo breed. This result seemed to suggest that this characterization could be utilized in breeding program for this breed.

KEYWORDS: dermatophilosis; disease susceptibility; Renitelo cattle; Madagascar; MHC; BoLA-DRB3

INTRODUCTION

Dermatophilosis, formerly known as streptotrichosis, is an exudative skin disease caused by actinomycete, *Dermatophilus congolensis*. It affects mainly

Address for correspondence: Dr. Jean-Charles Maillard, CIRAD-EMVT, Campus de Baillarguet, TA30/G, 34398-Montpellier Cedex S, France. Voice: 33 (4) 67 59 38 35; fax: 33 (4) 67 59 37 24.
e-mail: maillard@cirad.fr

Ann. N.Y. Acad. Sci. 1081: 489–491 (2006). © 2006 New York Academy of Sciences.
doi: 10.1196/annals.1373.072

bovine in tropical area and the presence of *Amblyomma variegatum* tick increases the risk of occurrence of skin lesions.[1] Exotic breeds have been reported to be more sensitive to the disease as compared to indigenous breeds.[2,3] Genetic markers were identified to be associated with sensitivity to the disease in Brahman cattle breed.[4,5] This article outlines association between occurrence of the genetic marker and sensitivity to the disease in Malagasy cattle, the Renitelo cattle breed.

MATERIALS AND METHODS

Kianjasoa station located in the middle west region of Madagascar is the cradle of Renitelo creation. As dermatophilosis is a real threat to Renitelo, cattle reared in extensive mode at the station were followed up. Health monitoring is carried out on a regular basis. Cattle are vaccinated against black leg and anthrax annually. Regular dipping of animals by pour-on or spray of acaricides is made, in order to reduce tick burdens. However, despite acaricide treatment, sporadic cases of dermatophilosis lesions occur among cattle herd. Animals presenting dermatophilosis lesions, mainly during rainy season (from December to April), were blood-sampled for genetic analysis ($n = 17$). Total DNA was extracted from white blood cells, according to the manufacturer's instruction for DNA isolation kit (Puregene®; Gentra Systems Inc., Minneapolis, MN). PCR amplification of exon 2 of MHC class II *BoLA-DRB3* gene was carried out by priming with a couple of primers, BOD31 and BOD32.[4] Amplified PCR product, 304 bp is digested with three different restriction enzymes separately, *Rsa I*, *Mbo I*, and *Hae III*. Restriction fragments are migrated and visualized on 3% agarose gel with size markers. Patterns of bands migration are then compared to the earlier determined patterns.[4]

RESULTS AND DISCUSSION

Among DNA samples of the 17 animals analyzed by PCR–RFLP of exon 2 MHC class II *BoLA-DRB3* gene, three of them presented "FDA*" allele corresponding to susceptibility allele to dermatophilosis.* F, D, and A alleles correspond to a particular restriction pattern obtained after digestion with *Rsa I*, *Mbo I*, and *Hae III* enzymes, respectively.

Cattle showing sensitivity allele were bearing different degrees of Malagasy zebu blood but all of them presented severe form of the disease, as compared to the other ill animals. Moreover, one of them displayed, a few times after sampling, a chronic form of the lesions all over its body and died of the disease.

This study shows that the MHC class II BoLA-DRB3 exon 2 allele, so-called susceptibility allele actually exists among Renitelo cattle breed. Association between this allele and the sensitivity phenotype seemed to be verified although few numbers of samples were included in our analysis. Indeed, we have analyzed animals, which practically every rainy season showed up dermatophilosis lesions, despite regular treatment with acaricides. Some authors mentioned that acaricide treatment becomes inefficient once the disease is settled in the herd.[6] Treatment inefficiency is directly correlated with the exotic blood percentage in the herd.[3]

The fact that one Renito cattle bearing the FDA susceptibility allele has shown severe clinical signs of dermatophilosis, confirms the strong association already described in other cattle breed.[4,5]

Selection based on genetics of animals to breed can be one solution to resolve farmers' problem by reducing the disease occurrence, especially as no vaccine against dermatophilosis is available nowadays. Less sensitivity to the disease may also help farmers in reducing acaricide treatment frequency, which can have double benefit, first in reducing cost treatment and second in environmental preservation by reducing the use of acaricides that are most of the time harmful for environment.

ACKNOWLEDGMENTS

Renitelo cattle maintenance is one of PSDR Project (Composante Recherche Thématique) funded by the World Bank. Laboratory analysis of this work was supported by INCO-DC programme of the European Union under contract n°1C18-CT98-0334 (DG12-SNRD). We are grateful to FAO-AGAH and FSP FORMA Project for supporting H. Razafindraibe's participation to the 8th Biennial Conference of the Society for Tropical Veterinary Medicine.

REFERENCES

1. AMBROSE, N., D. LLOYD & J.C. MAILLARD. 1999. Immune responses to *Dermatophilus congolensis* infections. Parasitol. Today **15:** 295–300.
2. DUMAS, R., P. LHOSTE, N. CHABEUF & J. BLANCOU. 1971. Note sur la sensibilité héréditaire des bovins à la streptothrihose. Rev. Elev. Méd. Vét. Pays Trop. **24:** 349–353.
3. RANAIVOSON, A., R. RANAIVOSON & D. RAMBELOMANANA. 1983. Impact de la dermatophilose sur la production du bétail. Bull. Acad. Malg. t 61/1-2.
4. MAILLARD, J.C., I. CHANTAL, D. BERTHIER, *et al.* 2002. A candidate gene approach and a concrete field application. Ann. N. Y. Acad. Sci. **969:** 92–97.
5. RAZAFINDRAIBE, H., M. RALINIAINA, J.C. MAILLARD & RAKOTONDRAVAO. 2003. Prédisposition du zébu Brahman de Madagascar à résister à la dermatophilose. Proc. Symp. Centenary of Madagascar's Acad. Fasc. XLVIII.
6. RANAIVOSON, A., R. RANAIVOSON & D. RAMBELOMANANA. 1986. Epizootiologie et incidence de la dermatophilose bovine à Madagascar. Rev. Elev. Méd. Vét. Pays Trop. **39:** 279–287.

Polyphasic Taxonomy

GERRIT UILENBERG[a] AND WILL L. GOFF[b]

[a] 'A Surgente,' 20130 Cargèse, France

[b] Animal Disease Research Unit, Agricultural Research Service, United States Department of Agriculture, Pullman, Washington 99164-6630, USA

ABSTRACT: Several organisms from a number of prokaryotic and eukaryotic groups have presented problems for systematists for a long time. Both phenotypic and genotypic methods for sorting out these relationships have been employed. There are limitations with each method when taken alone. Since the purpose of systematics is to determine the correct genealogical relationships among biological organisms, it is necessary to use all available means to arrive at consensus associations, and polyphasic taxonomy, which takes into consideration both methods, is a rational approach. In this short article, we provide a number of examples where polyphasic taxonomy is serving as the means of arriving at the desired consensus.

KEYWORDS: taxonomy; phylogenetics

INTRODUCTION

Taxonomy is important not only for the order which it creates, but for practical reasons related to disease treatment and control when dealing with medically important pathogens. Appropriate classification typically results in clusters of related species or clades with similar characteristics, often sharing similar vector species if they are vector borne, sharing the potential for zoonoses, and being susceptible to similar drug therapies due to related biochemical processes. Molecular phylogeny has become a powerful tool in taxonomy and has taken center stage over the past 20 years. In some cases whole genomes have been sequenced and can be compared, but sequence comparisons are usually based on small parts of the genome (for bacteria 16S rRNA and for eukaryotes 18S rRNA gene sequences are among the first to be chosen). Such sequences are only a tiny part of the whole genome, but nevertheless, there is a dangerous tendency in the last few years to classify organisms solely on such limited comparisons, without taking into account other characteristics, such as life cycle, morphology, habitat, and where applicable, the type of host cell, which

Address for correspondence: Prof. Gerrit Uilenberg, 'A Surgente,' route du Port, 20130 Cargèse (Corse), France. Voice: +33-4-9526-4083; fax: +33-4-9526-4083.

e-mail: uilenber@club-internet.fr

Ann. N.Y. Acad. Sci. 1081: 492–497 (2006). © 2006 New York Academy of Sciences.
doi: 10.1196/annals.1373.073

are determined by the entire genome. However, entire genome sequences are fortunately becoming available for more and more of the prokaryotes, although still exceedingly rare for eukaryotes. Consequently, our knowledge of the taxonomic relationships of many organisms has been greatly increased because of sequence comparisons. It is of course essential to use both approaches in taxonomy; phenotypical characters and sequence comparisons. It is only by using all available approaches that one can hope to arrive at a satisfactory phylogeny and classification of organisms. This is polyphasic taxonomy.

ON RECENT CHANGES IN THE TAXONOMY OF *EPERYTHROZOON* AND *HAEMOBARTONELLA*

These organisms have long been considered as belonging to the order *Rickettsiales*, until it was convincingly shown in 1997 that their closest relatives are the mycoplasms and that they belong to the order *Mycoplasmatales*.[1,2] But this does not necessarily mean that they should be included in the genus *Mycoplasma*, as was proposed.[1] In 2001 and 2002, *Haemobartonella* was merged with *Eperythrozoon* and the inclusion of *Eperythrozoon* spp. in the genus *Mycoplasma* was formally proposed, solely on the basis of 16S rRNA sequence comparisons[3,4] and approved in "Notification Lists" in the International Journal of Systematic and Evolutionary Microbiology (IJSEM). More recently, *Eperythrozoon coccoides* has also been proposed to be included in the genus *Mycoplasma*.[5]

As discussed in a recent paper,[6] this merger is untenable and the genus name *Eperythrozoon* (into which *Haemobartonella* is absorbed) should be conserved as a separate genus of the family *Mycoplasmataceae* for various reasons. First, the percentage of identities between 16S RNA sequences between *Eperythrozoon wenyonii* and one of its closest relatives, *Mycoplasma fastidiosum*, is only some 77%, well below that of micro-organisms belonging to one genus. Second, the habitat of *Eperythrozoon* spp., in circulating blood, is very different from that of classical *Mycoplasma* spp. Finally, there are reasons of priority; the name *Eperythrozoon* was created in 1928, that of *Mycoplasma* a year later, in 1929.

We may add that it is impossible that any species of *Eperythrozoon/ Haemobartonella* and other noncultivable, or at least so far not cultured prokaryotes, such as some of the ehrlichias, described after August 2002, can be recognized as valid, because one of the requirements of the IJSEM and the ICSP (International Committee on Systematics of Prokaryotes) is that authors of new species, new subspecies and new combinations provide evidence that types are deposited in at least two recognized culture collections in two different countries. Obviously, pure bacteriologists have not given much thought to vector-borne prokaryotes; it is true that these were dealt with in the past much more by parasitologists than by bacteriologists.

ON THE TAXONOMY OF *EHRLICHIA PHAGOCYTOPHILA* AND SOME OTHER SPECIES OF THE GENUS

It was shown recently[7] that the genera *Anaplasma, Ehrlichia, Cowdria, Neorickettsia,* and *Wolbachia* are so closely related that they should be grouped in one family, the *Anaplasmataceae.* Within the genus *Ehrlichia* there are various genogroups, and one, consisting of *E. phagocytophila* (including *E. equi* and the agent of human granulocytic ehrlichiosis), *E. bovis,* and *E. platys,* is more closely related to the genus *Anaplasma* than to other genogroups of *Ehrlichia.* It has been proposed to transfer the species of this genogroup to the genus *Anaplasma,* and this transfer was approved in a "Notification List." This transfer is also based on 16S rRNA sequence similarity, a very small part of the genome, and does not take into account the pronounced phenotypical differences existing between these *Ehrlichia* species and classical species of *Anaplasma,* particularly in the type of host cell. Comparing also other gene sequences (still a small part of the whole genome), and the GC content, other authors,[8–10] while confirming the close relationship of the genogroup of *E. phagocytophila* to *Anaplasma,* and the differences with other genogroups of *Ehrlichia,* showed that the genogroup of *E. phagocytophila* is also different from *Anaplasma.* The phylogenic tree constructed from the citrate synthase gene shows more diversity than that constructed from the 16S rRNA gene. The similarity between *A. marginale* and *E. phagocytophila* is only 74.5%, relatively low.[10]

We can only state again that there is much more to taxonomy than the comparison of the sequences of small parts of the genome. Other characters should also be taken into account (polyphasic taxonomy), and phylogenetic trees will also continue to change with more parts of the genomes being compared. There is no justification for rushing into taxonomic changes on thin evidence. It may be necessary to create a new genus name for members of the *E. phagocytophila* genogroup.[6,11]

ON THE TAXONOMY OF *BOOPHILUS*

Recently, it has been proposed to fuse the tick genus *Boophilus* into the genus *Rhipicephalus.*[12,13] Other authors have also shown that *Boophilus* species are very closely related to (classical) species of *Rhipicephalus,* from which they are undoubtedly derived, so closely that from a phylogenetical point they might indeed be considered as belonging to one genus. These conclusions[12,13] are mainly based on molecular studies, but to some extent also on morphological evidence. Nevertheless, the molecular evidence is only based on small parts of the genome, and as said in a recent paper,[6] not even a dissecting microscope is needed to see the obvious morphological differences between them. Without denying the very close relationship between *Boophilus* spp. and *Rhipicephalus* spp., it seems unnecessary to create confusion by synonymizing *Boophilus* and *Rhipicephalus*. Once again, stick to polyphasic taxonomy.

ON THE TAXONOMY OF THE PIROPLASMS (EUKARYOTES)

Reports concerning the life cycle of *"Babesia" equi* in the tick vector, the lack of transovarial transmission, extraerythrocytic schizogony in lymphocytes of equines, and division resulting in four daughter cells within the erythrocyte suggest this parasite is more *Theileria (T.)*-like than *Babesia (B.)*-like.[14,15] However, some of these studies have not yet been confirmed by other investigators, particularly with isolates from other regions, such as the Americas. Things appear to be rather similar for *"Babesia"* microti, where division in the erythrocyte also gives four daughter cells, although beautiful Maltese crosses, such as are observed in *B. (T.) equi* infections, are not so common. Extraerythrocytic schizogony occurs in lymphocytes of the rodent host,[16,17] and the cycle in the vector ticks *Ixodes (I.) scapularis* and *I. ricinus* also resembles more that of *Theileria* than of *Babesia*. Attempts at transovarial transmission with *I. scapularis* and *I. pacificus* failed, but transstadial transmission succeeded with both tick species, as well as with *I. ricinus*.[16,18,19] Based on these reports, *"Babesia"* microti is not a true *Babesia*.

B. equi has been transferred to the genus *Theileria*, on the basis of its life cycle, both in the vertebrate host and in the tick vector.[20-22] This generic change was made before the full development of molecular techniques but molecular phylogeny has, for the most part, supported a change. Parasite surface protein sequence homology between *B. (T.) equi* and *Theileria* spp. has been demonstrated,[23,24] and a number of molecular sequence comparisons, mainly of 18S rRNA gene sequences confirm that the parasite is different from true *Babesia* species.[25,26] However, molecular studies indicate differences with "classical" *Theileria* species too.[26-28] Most of the data suggest that *B. (T.) equi* and *Cytauxzoon felis* are ancestral to the *Theileria*,[27] prompting the suggestion that a new genus name be created.[25] Until confirmation of phenotypic characteristics and life cycle, and/or a new genus name is created, it appears logical to call it *T. equi*.

When comparing 18S rRNA sequences, *B. microti*, like *B. (T.) equi*, is not only different from *Babesia*, but also from the classical *Theileria* species although it appears to be nearer to classical *Theileria* species than to *Babesia*.[29,30] According to some authors it clusters with *B. (T.) equi*,[30] while others place it along with a few other species, including *B. rodhaini* (another parasite that has been extensively used in laboratories for the study of "babesiosis"), in a separate clade.[27] As for *T. equi*, a new genus name, perhaps the same, may have to be created. As long as there is no other genus name, it seems logical to call it *T. microti* (and by the way talk of human theileriosis and not babesiosis, where this species is concerned).

REFERENCES

1. NEIMARK, H. & K.M. KOCAN. 1997. The cell wall-less rickettsia *Eperythrozoon wenyonii* is a *Mycoplasma*. FEMS Microbiol. Lett. **156:** 287–291.

2. RIKIHISHA, Y., M. KAWAHARA, B. WEN, *et al.* 1997. Western immunoblot analysis of *Haemobartonella muris* and comparison of 16S rRNA gene sequences of *H. muris*, *H. felis* and *Eperythrozoon suis*. J. Clin. Microbiol. **35:** 823–829.

3. NEIMARK, H., K.-E. JOHANSSON, Y. RIKIHISA & J.G. TULLY. 2001. Proposal to transfer some members of the genera *Haemobartonella* and *Eperythrozoon* to the genus *Mycoplasma* with descriptions of '*Candidatus* Mycoplasma haemofelis', '*Candidatus* Mycoplasma haemomuris', '*Candidatus* Mycoplasma haemosuis' and '*Candidatus* Mycoplasma wenyonii'. Int. J. Syst. Evol. Microbiol. **51:** 891– 899.

4. NEIMARK, H., K.-E. JOHANSSON, Y. RIKIHISA & J.G. TULLY. 2002. Revision of haemotrophic *Mycoplasma* species names. Int. J. Syst. Evol. Microbiol. **52:** 683.

5. NEIMARK, H., W. PETERS, B.L. ROBINSON & L.B. STEWART. 2005. Phylogenetic analysis and description of *Eperythrozoon coccoides*, proposal to transfer to the genus *Mycoplasma* as *Mycoplasma coccoides* comb. nov. and request for an opinion. Int. J. Syst. Evol. Microbiol. **55:** 1385–1391.

6. UILENBERG, G., F. THIAUCOURT & F. JONGEJAN. 2004. On molecular taxonomy: what is in a name? Exp. Appl. Acarol. **32:** 301–312.

7. DUMLER, J.S., A.F. BARBET, C.P.J. BEKKER, *et al.* 2001. Reorganization of genera in the families *Rickettsiaceae* and *Anaplasmataceae* in the order *Rickettsiales*: unification of some species of *Ehrlichia* with *Anaplasma*, *Cowdria* with *Ehrlichia* and *Ehrlichia* with *Neorickettsia*, descriptions of six new species combinations and designation of *Ehrlichia equi* and 'HGE agent' as subjective synonyms of *Ehrlichia phagocytophila*. Int. J. Syst. Evol. Microbiol. **51:** 2145–2165.

8. INOKUMA, H., P. BROUQUI, M. DRANCOURT & D. RAOULT. 2001. Citrate synthase gene sequence: a new tool for phylogenetic analysis and identification of *Ehrlichia*. J. Clin. Microbiol. **39:** 3031–3039.

9. SHIBATA, S., M. KAWAHARA, Y. RIKIHISA, *et al.* 2000. New *Ehrlichia* species closely related to *Ehrlichia chaffeensis* isolated from *Ixodes ovatus* ticks in Japan. J. Clin. Microbiol. **38:** 1331–1338.

10. TAILLARDAT-BISCH, A.V., D. RAOULT & M. DRANCOURT. 2003. RNA polymerase β-subunit-based phylogeny of *Ehrlichia* spp., *Anaplasma* spp., *Neorickettsia* spp. and *Wolbachia pipientis*. Int. J. Syst. Evol. Microbiol. **53:** 455–458.

11. EUZÉBY, J.P. 2002. *Anaplasma phagocytophilum*. *In* Dictionnaire de Bactériologie Vétérinaire. Available online: http://www.bacterio.cict.fr/bacdico/garde.html and http://www.bacdico.net.

12. BARKER, S.C. & A. MURREL. 2002. Phylogeny, evolution and historical zoogeography of ticks: a review of recent progress. Exp. Appl. Acarol. **28:** 55–68.

13. MURREL, A. & S.C. BARKER. 2003. Synonymy of *Boophilus* Curtice, 1891 with *Rhipicephalus* Koch, 1844 (Acari: Ixodidae). Syst. Parasitol. **56:** 169–172.

14. MOLTMANN, U.G., H. MEHLHORN, E. SCHEIN, *et al.* 1983. Fine structure of *Babesia equi* Laveran, 1901 within lymphocytes and erythrocytes of horses: an in vivo and in vitro study. J. Parasitol. **69:** 111–120.

15. SCHEIN, E., G. REHBEIN, W.P. VOIGT & E. ZWEYGARTH. 1981. *Babesia equi* (Laveran 1901). 1. Development in horses and in lymphocyte culture. Tropenmed. Parasitol. **32:** 223–237.

16. MEHLHORN, H., W. RAETHER, E. SCHEIN, *et al.* 1986. Licht- und elektronen-mikroskopische Untersuchungen zum Entwicklungszyklus and Einfluss von Pentamidin auf die Morphologie der intraerythrocytären Stadien von *Babesia microti.* Dtsch. Tierärztl. Wochenschr. **93:** 400–405.

17. MEHLHORN, H. & E. SCHEIN. 1984. The piroplasms: life cycle and sexual stages. Adv. Parasitol. **23:** 37–103.

18. OLIVEIRA, M.R. & J.P. KREIER. 1979. Transmission of *Babesia microti* using various species of ticks as vectors. J. Parasitol. **65:** 816–817.

19. RUDZINSKA, M., A. SPIELMAN, S. LEWENGRUB, *et al.* 1984. The sequence of developmental events of *Babesia microti* in the gut of *Ixodes dammini.* Protistologica **20:** 649–663.

20. EUZÉBY, J. 1988. Sur la taxonomie des hémosporidies. Cas des piroplasmes. Sci. Vét. Méd. Comp. **90:** 181–200.

21. MEHLHORN, H. & E. SCHEIN. 1998. Redescription of *Babesia equi* Laveran, 1901 as *Theileria equi* Mehlhorn, Schein 1998. Parasitol. Res. **84:** 467–475.

22. UILENBERG, G. 1986. Highlights in recent research on tick-borne diseases of domestic animals. J. Parasitol. **72:** 485–491.

23. KAPPMEYER, L.S., L.E. PERRYMAN & D.P. KNOWLES. 1993. A *Babesia equi* gene encodes a surface protein with homology to *Theileria* species. Mol. Biochem. Parasitol. **62:** 121–124.

24. KNOWLES, D.P., L.S. KAPPMEYER & L.E. PERRYMAN. 1997. Genetic and biochemical analysis of erythrocyte-stage surface antigens belonging to a family of highly conserved proteins of *Babesia equi* and *Theileria* species. Mol. Biochem. Parasitol. **90:** 69–79.

25. ALLSOPP, M.T., T. CAVALIER-SMITH, D.T. DE WAAL & B.A. ALLSOPP. 1994. Phylogeny and evolution of the piroplasms. Parasitology **108:** 147–152.

26. KJEMTRUP, A.M., J. THOMFORD, T. ROBINSON & P.A. CONRAD. 2000. Phylogenetic relationships of human and wildlife piroplasm isolates in the western United States inferred from the 18S nuclear small subunit RNA gene. Parasitology **120:** 487–493.

27. CRIADO-FORNELIO, A., A. MARTINEZ-MARCOS, A. BULING-SARANA & J.C. BARBA-CARRETERO. 2003. Molecular studies on *Babesia, Theileria* and *Hepatozoon* in southern Europe Part II. Phylogenetic analysis and evolutionary history. Vet. Parasitol. **114:** 173–194.

28. NAGORE, D., J. GARCIA-SANMARTIN, A.L. GARCIA-PEREZ, *et al.* 2004. Detection and identification of equine *Theileria* and *Babesia* species by reverse line blotting: epidemiological survey and phylogenetic analysis. Vet. Parasitol. **123:** 41–54.

29. NIJHOF, A.M., B.L. PENZHORN, G. LYNEN, *et al.* 2003. *Babesia bicornis* sp. nov. and *Theileria bicornis* sp. nov.: tick-borne parasites associated with mortality in the black rhinoceros (Diceros bicornis). J. Clin. Microbiol. **41:** 2249–2254.

30. SCHNITTGER, L., H. YIN, M.J. GUBBELS, *et al.* 2003. Phylogeny of sheep and goat *Theileria* and *Babesia* parasites. Parasitol. Res. **91:** 398–406.

Phylogenetic Position of Small-Ruminant Infecting Piroplasms

JABBAR S. AHMED,[a] JIANXUN LUO,[b] LEONHARD SCHNITTGER,[a] ULRIKE SEITZER,[a] FRANS JONGEJAN,[c,d] AND HONG YIN[b]

[a]Research Center Borstel, 23845 Borstel, Germany

[b]Lanzhou Veterinary Research Institute, 730046 Lanzhou, Gansu, China

[c]Division of Parasitology and Tropical Veterinary Medicine, Faculty of Veterinary Medicine, Utrecht University, 3508 TD Utrecht, The Netherlands

[d]Department of Veterinary Tropical Diseases, Faculty of Veterinary Science, University of Pretoria, 0110 Onderstepoort, South Africa

ABSTRACT: *Theileria* and *Babesia* are tick-transmitted protozoa that cause great economical losses in livestock. Recently, interest has risen in sheep-infecting piroplasms and a number of previously unidentified pathogens were described, particularly in China. To address the phylogenetic relationship of *Theileria* and *Babesia* species infecting sheep, the complete sequences of the 18 S small subunit ribosomal RNA genes of a panel of piroplasm isolates, including *T. lestoquardi, T. ovis, T. separata, B. ovis, B. motasi, B. crassa*, and several novel species, were compared. The classification based on the established phylogenetic tree corresponded with traditional systematics and revealed that sheep/goat piroplasm species are of a polyphyletic origin. In addition, these studies revealed the existence of at least two novel sheep/goat piroplasm species, designated *Theileria* sp. (China 1) and *Theileria* sp. (China 2).

KEYWORDS: phylogenetics; piroplasms; *Theileria*; *Babesia*; small ruminants

INTRODUCTION

Theileria and *Babesia* species, the causative agents of theileriosis and babesiosis, respectively, are tick-borne parasitic protozoa and a number of them are highly pathogenic for cattle, sheep, and goats. The economic losses due to theileriosis and babesiosis are enormous in tropical and subtropical areas.[1,2]

Address for correspondence: Jabbar S. Ahmed, Division of Veterinary Infectiology and Immunology, Research Center Borstel, Parkallee 22, 23845 Borstel, Germany. Voice: 49-4537-188-428; fax: 49-4537-188-627.

e-mail: jahmed@fz-borstel.de

Ann. N.Y. Acad. Sci. 1081: 498–504 (2006). © 2006 New York Academy of Sciences.
doi: 10.1196/annals.1373.074

In the past, most attention was given to bovine-infecting piroplasms, whereas ticks and tick-borne diseases of small ruminants received less attention. However, due to the socioeconomic importance of sheep and goats in a number of countries, interest has recently also risen in ovine and caprine piroplasmosis, particularly with respect to infections with *Theileria* ssp.,[3,4] which are transmitted transstadially by a variety of *Hyalomma* ticks. The most prominent *Theileria* species infecting small ruminants is *T. lestoquardi*. In contrast, babesiosis of small ruminants is transmitted by ticks of the genera *Haemaphysalis* and *Rhipicephalus* and the most prominent species are *Babesia ovis* and *B. motasi*.

The classical identification and classification of *Theileria* and *Babesia* species are based on the morphology, host specificity, and mode of transmission by vector ticks. With the advent of molecular methods and, in particular, sequence data analysis, tools are now available for inferring relationships among piroplasms. These tools have been used to define the phylogenetic position of pathogens that were originally classified entirely on the morphological and life history criteria only. The 18 S rRNA genes have been successfully used to assist with the classification of several previously unknown *Theileria* and *Babesia* parasites.[4–11]

Theileria *Species of Small Ruminants*

T. lestoquardi is the most prominent *Theileria* species that causes malignant theileriosis of sheep.[12] *T. lestoquardi* exhibits many similarities to *T. annulata* with respect to serology and morphology[3] and their close phylogenetic relation was confirmed by 18 S rRNA gene comparison.[9]

Recently, a *Theileria* species pathogenic for small ruminants has been identified in the northwestern part of China.[13] This parasite was found to be transmitted by the tick *Haemaphysalis qinhaiensis* and the geographic distribution of the tick is congruent with the distribution of the disease.

Originally, this parasite was reported to be *T. lestoquardi* (formerly *T. hirci*), although a number of properties do not fit the characteristics of *T. lestoquardi*. First, *T. lestoquardi* is transmitted by ticks of the genus *Hyalomma* and not by *Haemaphysalis*.[14] Second, *in vitro* cell culture of *T. lestoquardi* can be established with relative ease,[15] while the macroschizonts of the parasite from China are not amenable to *in vitro* culture thus far.[13] Therefore, we analyzed the 18 S rRNA gene sequence and compared it with that of other *Theileria* and *Babesia* species. The results of these studies clearly demonstrated the affiliation of both parasites (*T. lestoquardi* and the Chinese parasite) to the genus *Theileria*. To further substantiate this finding, we designed primers amplifying DNA of bovine *Theileria* parasites (*T. annulata, T. parva, T. sergenti, T. taurotragi, T. buffeli, T. mutans,* and *T. velifera*)[16] and found that they reacted with the DNA of the Chinese isolate as well as with that of *T. lestoquardi*.

It is noteworthy that these primer pairs did not amplify DNA of *B. bigemina* and *B. bovis.* The established phylogenetic tree of *Theileria* 18 S rRNA genes contains two monophyletic branches: one comprising *T. annulata, T. parva, T. taurotragi,* and *T. lestoquardi,* the latter being closely related to *T. annulata,* while the other branch includes *T. sergenti, T. buffeli,* and the Chinese isolate. Thus the phylogenetic analysis provided evidence that the Chinese *Theileria* species is different from *T. lestoquardi.* It rather seemed to be a distinct *Theileria* species, most closely related to *T. buffeli.* The group of *T. annulata, T. lestoquardi, T. parva,* and *T. taurotragi* represent *Theileria* parasites with a marked intra-leukocytic phase in contrast to the group formed by *T. sergenti* and *T. buffeli.*[9] The Chinese *Theileria* species segregated into the latter group suggesting that it also exhibits a less marked leukocytic phase.[4] This would be in accordance with the observation that the Chinese *Theileria* species like *T. sergenti* and *T. buffeli* are not able to transform cells *in vitro.*

In a further study, the complete 18 S rRNA gene sequences of *Theileria* infecting small ruminants, such as *T. separata, T. ovis,* and *Theileria* sp. (China), were studied by neighbor-joining analysis (summarized in TABLE 1).[17] These analyses revealed that besides the previously described *T.* species (China), another distinct pathogenic *Theileria* parasite occurs in the same region, falling into two separate clusters. Accordingly, these parasites were first designated as *Theileria* sp. (China 1) and *Theileria* sp. (China 2). Both parasites are similar with respect to the vector and host specificity, morphology, and pathogenicity and can at present only be distinguished by molecular approaches. Possibly for these reasons, these two *Theileria* species were not distinguished until molecular classification methods were applied.[18]

Further studies were conducted regarding the phylogenetic relationship between six *Theileria* isolates from China including *Theileria* sp. infective for small ruminants and two isolates of *Theileria* spp. infective for yaks, all transmitted by *H. qinghaiensis,* together with the *T. orientalis/buffeli* group and *T. sinensis.*[18] Two phylogenetic trees were constructed. In the first tree, the *Theileria* sp. infective for yaks was found to be *T. sinensis.* The *Theileria* sp. infective for small ruminants was confirmed to be composed of two separate species of *Theileria* sp. (China). In the second tree, *Theileria* sp. (China 1) was closely related to benign *Theileria* spp., such as *T. buffeli* and *T. sergenti,* while *Theileria sp.* (China 2) was found to be different from the other *Theileria* spp. The results indicated that *H. qinghaiensis* ticks transmit at least three different species of *Theileria,* two of which are infective for sheep and goats, but not yak and one which is infective for yaks and cattle, but not to sheep and goats.

Recently, three further *Theileria* genotypes have been identified, sharing 96.7–97.0% similarity between their 18 S rRNA gene sequences: *T. ovis, Theileria* sp. OT1 (99.6% similarity) with the recently described pathogenic piroplasm *Theileria* sp. (China 1), and *Theileria* sp. OT3. In contrast to the *Theileria* sp. (China 1), the *Theileria* sp. OT1 described in Spain seems to be of relatively low pathogenicity.[19]

TABLE 1. Isolates assigned to piroplasm species by phylogenetic classification

Isolate	Species	Tick vector
T. sp. (Lintan1)	T. sp. (China 1)	*Haemaphysalis qinghaiensis*
T. sp. (Lintan 2)		
T. sp. (Qinghai)		
T. sp. (Madang)		
T. sp. (Ningxian)		
T. sp. (Lintan 3)	T. sp. (China 2)	*Haemaphysalis qinghaiensis*
T. sp. (Zhangjiachuan)		
T. sp. (Longde)		
T. lestoquardi (Lahr)	T. lestoquardi	*Hyalomma a. anatolicum*
T. lestoquardi (Fars)		
T. ovis (Turkey)	T. ovis	*Rhipicephalus evertsi*
T. ovis (Sudan)		
T. sp. G4 (Tanzania)		
T. sp. G6 (Tanzania)		
T. separata (South Africa)	T. separata	*Rhipicephalus evertsi*
B. ovis (Turkey)	B. ovis	*Rhipicephalus bursa*
B. motasi (Ameland)	B. motasi	*Haemaphysalis punctata*
B. motasi (Texel)		
B. crassa (Iran)	B. crassa	Not known
B. sp. (Turkey)		

Based on the available data, the diseases described in sheep and goats occurring in China cannot be attributed to *T. lestoquardi* or *T. ovis* as has previously been published. Until recently, *T. lestoquardi* was considered to be the only pathogenic *Theileria* species for sheep.[12] Our investigations show that apart from *T. lestoquardi*, both *T.* sp. (China 1) and *T.* sp. (China 2) contribute to the spectrum of pathogenic piroplasms in small ruminants. Studies have been initiated to determine if these parasites also occur in other regions.

Other species, such as *T. ovis* from Sudan and Turkey clustered together with isolates of *T.* sp. G4 (Tanzania) and *T.* sp. G6 (Tanzania). The observation that *T. ovis* isolates originating from three entirely different geographic regions cluster together suggests that *T. ovis* does represent a single species.[20,21] Most closely related to *T. ovis* is the sequence of a *Theileria* species isolated from sika deer (*Theileria* sp. CNY1B sika deer [Japan]) and both may have shared a common ancestor. Interestingly, there appears to be another *Theileria* parasite also isolated from sika deer (*T.* sp. CNY2 A sika deer [Japan]) but which clearly represents a different species more closely related to *T.* sp. (China 1) and *T.* sp. CC3 A serow (Japan). Furthermore, the sequence of the ovine piroplasm *T. separata* is most closely related to that of *T.* sp. (sable). If *T. separata* and *T.* sp. (sable) are indeed transmitted by the same tick species, this would provide support for the hypothesis that this parasite was passed on from sable antelope to domestic sheep.[22]

Babesia *Species of Small Ruminants*

Several small ruminant-infecting *Babesia* species have been described. As it is evident from the structure of the generated phylogenetic tree, the genera *Theileria* and *Babesia* have a different evolutionary history: the branch lengths are shortened, and accordingly, the identity among different species is much lower in the branch of *Theileria* than in that of *Babesia* parasites. Under the supposition that the evolutionary rate of 18 S rRNA genes is similar within both groups, this suggests that the genus *Theileria* developed later and has a shorter evolutionary history than *Babesia*.

The most important small ruminant-infecting *Babesia* species is *B. ovis*, which has been reported from Europe, Africa, Asia, and the Far East. In the phylogenetic tree based on 18 S rRNA sequences the closest relation of *B. ovis* (Turkey) appears to be *B. crassa* (93%). Furthermore, *B. motasi* (Ameland) and *B. motasi* (Texel) both isolated from sheep on islands in the north of the Netherlands segregate into the same cluster. *B. crassa* is represented by two geographic variants from Turkey and Iran, which appear to have very similar 18 S rRNA gene sequences.[17]

CONCLUSION

Five different *Theileria* species infecting small ruminants are currently recognized. These are *T. lestoquardi, T. ovis, T. separata, T.* sp. (China 1), and *T.* sp. (China 2). However, one additional species, *T. recondite,* which is considered nonpathogenic and different *from T. ovis* and *T. separata,*[21,23] was not included in this study. Therefore, there may be at least six different *Theileria* species infecting small ruminants.

Three different *Babesia* parasites are currently recognized in sheep and goats. Moreover, one uncharacterized *Babesia* sp. from China was recently reported.[24] This parasite appears to be closely related to *B. motasi*, but (in contrast to *B. motasi),* it is transmitted by *Haemaphysalis longicornis* and is highly pathogenic for sheep as well as for goats.[25]

In conclusion, there are at least ten different *Theileria* and *Babesia* species affecting the health of sheep and goats worldwide. In a manuscript in preparation we propose the following designation for the Chinese parasites: *Theileria* species (China 1) is to be called *T. luwenshuni* and we propose the name *T. uilenbergi* for *Theileria* species (China 2) (Yin *et al.*, in preparation).

ACKNOWLEDGMENTS

This work was supported by the European Commission within the INCO-DEV program, project number ICA4-CT-2000–30028 (ADDAV). We are thankful to the ADDAV consortium members for helpful discussions.

REFERENCES

1. JONGEJAN, F. & G. UILENBERG. 2004. The global importance of ticks. Parasitology **129:** S3–S14.
2. MEHLHORN, H. *et al.* 1994. *Theileria*. In Parasitic Protozoa, Vol. 7. J.P. Kreier, Ed.: 217–304. Academic Press. San Diego.
3. BROWN, C.G.D. *et al.* 1998. *Theileria lestoquardi* and *T. annulata* in cattle, sheep, and goats. *In vitro* and *in vivo* studies. Ann. N. Y. Acad. Sci. 849: 44–51.
4. SCHNITTGER, L. *et al.* 2000. Ribosomal small-subunit RNA gene-sequence analysis of *Theileria lestoquardi* and a *Theileria* species highly pathogenic for small ruminants in China. Parasitol. Res. **86:** 352–358.
5. PERSING, D.H. *et al.* 1995. Infection with a babesia-like organism in northern California. N. Engl. J. Med. **332:** 298–303.
6. QUICK, R.E. *et al.* 1993. Babesiosis in Washington State: a new species of *Babesia*? Ann. Intern. Med. **119:** 284–290.
7. THOMFORD, J.W. *et al.* 1994. Cultivation and phylogenetic characterization of a newly recognized human pathogenic protozoan. J. Infect. Dis. **169:** 1050–1056.
8. HERWALDT, B.L. *et al.* 1997. Transfusion-transmitted babesiosis in Washington State: first reported case caused by a WA1-type parasite. J. Infect. Dis. **175:** 1259–1262.
9. KATZER, F. *et al.* 1998. Phylogenetic analysis of *Theileria* and *Babesia equi* in relation to the establishment of parasite populations within novel host species and the development of diagnostic tests. Mol. Biol. Parasitol. **95:** 33–44.
10. GUBBELS, M.J. *et al.* 2000. Molecular characterisation of the *Theileria buffeli/orientalis* group. Int. J. Parasitol. **30:** 943–952.
11. ALLSOPP, M.T. *et al.* 1994. Phylogeny and evolution of the piroplasms. Parasitology **108:** 147–152.
12. FRIEDHOFF, K.T. 1997. Tick-borne diseases of sheep and goats caused by *Babesia*, *Theileria* or *Anaplasma* spp. Parassitologia **39:** 99–109.
13. LUO, J.X. & H. YIN. 1997. Theileriosis of sheep and goats in China. Trop. Anim. Health Prod. **29:** 8S–10S.
14. HOOSHMAND-RAD, P. & N.Y. HAWA. 1973. Malignant theileriosis of sheep and goats. Trop. Anim. Health Prod. **5:** 97–102.
15. HOOSHMAND-RAD, P. & N.Y. HAWA. 1973. Transmission of *Theileria hirci* in sheep by *Hyalomma anatolicum anatolicum*. Trop. Anim. Health Prod. **5:** 103–109.
16. D'OLIVEIRA, C. *et al.* 1995. Detection of *Theileria annulata* in blood samples of carrier cattle by PCR. J. Clin. Microbiol. **33:** 2665–2669.
17. SCHNITTGER, L. *et al.* 2003. Phylogeny of sheep and goat *Theileria* and *Babesia* parasites. Parasitol. Res. 91: 398–406.
18. YIN, H. *et al.* 2004. Phylogenetic analysis of *Theileria* species transmitted by *Haemaphysalis qinghaiensis*. Parasitol. Res. **92:** 36–42.
19. NAGORE, D. *et al.* 2004. Identification, genetic diversity and prevalence of *Theileria* and *Babesia* species in a sheep population from Northern Spain. Int. J. Parasitol. **34:** 1059–1067.
20. LEEMANS, I., P. HOOSHMAND-RAD & A. UGGLA. 1997. The indirect fluorescent antibody test based on schizont antigen for study of the sheep parasite *Theileria lestoquardi*. Vet. Parasitol. **69:** 9–18.
21. UILENBERG, G. 1981. *Theileria* species of domestic livestock. *In* Advances in the Control of theileriosis. A.D. Irvin, *et al.*, Eds.: 4–37. Martinus Nijhoff. The Hague.

22. THOMAS, S.E., D.E. WILSON & T.E. MASON. 1982. *Babesia*, *Theileria* and *Anaplasma spp.* infecting sable antelope, *Hippotragus niger* (Harris, 1838), in southern Africa. Onderstepoort J. Vet. Res. **49:** 163–166.

23. UILENBERG, G. & M.P. ANDREASSEN. 1974. *Haematoxenus separatus* sp.n. (Sporozoa, Theileriidae) a new blood parasite of domestic sheep in Tanzania. Rev. Elev. Med. Vet. Pays. Trop. **27:** 459–465.

24. ALANI, A.J. & I.V. Herbert. 1988. Morphology and transmission of *Theileria recondita* (Theileriidae: Sporozoa) isolated from *Haemaphysalis punctata* from North Wales. Vet. Parasitol. **28:** 283–291.

25. BAI, Q. *et al.* 2002. Isolation and preliminary characterization of a large *Babesia* sp. from sheep and goats in the eastern part of Gansu Province, China. Parasitol. Res. **88:** S16–S21.

Phylogenetics of *Theileria* Species in Small Ruminants

OLIVIER A.E. SPARAGANO,[a] EVA SPITALSKA,[a,b] MEHDI NAMAVARI,[a,c]
ALESSANDRA TORINA,[d] VINCENZA CANNELLA[d]
AND SANTO CARACAPPA[d]

[a]*Newcastle University, School of Agriculture, Food and Rural Development,
Newcastle upon Tyne, NE1 7RU, United Kingdom*

[b]*Institute of Virology, Slovak Academy of Sciences, Bratislava, 845 05 Slovakia*

[c]*Razi Vaccine and Serum Research Institute, Shiraz Branch, Shiraz, Iran*

[d]*Istituto Zooprofilattico Sperimentale della Sicilia, 90129 Palermo, Italy*

ABSTRACT: Our study is based on the collection of blood and ticks from
sheep in Iran and Italy. Polymerase chain reaction (PCR) testing was performed to target the 18S rRNA gene and RLB was performed using previously published probes. In Italy and Iran 78.7% and 76.0% of the sheep
were PCR positive, which after sequencing and RLB showed that they
were *Theileria ovis* and *Theileria lestoquardi*, respectively. Phylogenetic
analysis was performed using the Clustal W multiple sequence alignment
program and our sequences were compared with more than 50 others already published in the EMBL database. Our *T. lestoquardi* sequences
linked with other *T. lestoquardi* sequences from Iran, Tanzania, and
Sudan and *Theileria annulata* showed the importance of having species-
specific probes between these two species. However, distinctive clades
were found between *T. lestoquardi* ticks and those found in sheep blood.
Italian *T. ovis* seemed to be closer to *Theileria* spp. from Namibia and
Iran than with other *T. ovis* from Spain, Turkey, Tanzania, and Sudan
adding some information to the controversy about this species. However,
some confusion was found on the existing database where the location of
pathogens, years, and species names was inaccurate and when available
sequences were not always appropriately used. This article will discuss
our results and some comparisons with other phylogenetic approaches.

KEYWORDS: Theileriosis; *Theileria ovis*; *Theileria lestoquardi*; sheep;
diagnostic; tick

Address for correspondence: Dr. Olivier A.E. Sparagano, School of Agriculture, Food and Rural
Development, Newcastle University, Agriculture Building, Newcastle upon Tyne NE1 7RU, UK. Voice:
44-191-2225071; fax: 44-191-2226720.
  e-mail: Olivier.sparagano@ncl.ac.uk

Ann. N.Y. Acad. Sci. 1081: 505–508 (2006). © 2006 New York Academy of Sciences.
doi: 10.1196/annals.1373.075

INTRODUCTION

Theileriosis due to *Theileria lestoquardi* is a major problem in small ruminants. However, other less pathogenic species have been described and there is still some confusion within the phylogeny, names, and identification in the Piroplasmida Order. Furthermore, due to the low economic value of small ruminant animals more research has been done on cattle and horses. However, in recent years a few research projects have focused on tick-borne pathogens in small ruminants such as *Anaplasma ovis, Ehrlichia ovina, Theileria lestoquardi*, or *Theileria ovis*. This article will exclusively present data on piroplasmosis in small ruminants.

MATERIALS AND METHODS

Sixty blood samples of sheep blood were collected on the island of Sicily, Italy in the Palermo province in 2000 while 100 samples of sheep blood and 89 tick samples were collected in the Fars region in Iran in 2003.

DNA was extracted from blood and tick samples by using the REDextract N-Amp Blood PCR kit (Sigma, Gillingham, UK) and the QIAamp extraction Tissue kit (Qiagen, Crawley, UK), respectively. Then the DNA was amplified by using two primers previously described for the 18S rRNA gene.[1] Polymerase chain reaction (PCR) mixture and amplification cycles were performed as previously described by Spitalska et al.[2] Previous probes published for *T. lestoquardi* and *T. annulata* unfortunately showed cross-reactivity between the two species and so it was not possible to use this methodology.[3] Therefore, we had to sequence the DNA fragments using an ABI Prism BigDye Terminator Cycle Sequencing Ready Reaction kit, version 1.1. (Applied Biosystems Warrington, UK) and align the sequences and confront our results with existing sequences in the GenBank database.

RESULTS AND DISCUSSION

The PCR results showed 76%, 68.3%, and 52.1% positivity in Iranian sheep blood, female and male ticks, respectively, which is in agreement with similar work in Iran by Razmi et al.[4,5] In Italy PCR positivity was 78.7%. Sequencing analysis showed that *T. ovis* was dominantly present in Sicily, which are the first data published on this island for small ruminants while *T. lestoquardi* was the dominant species in Iran[4] while other colleagues also isolated *Theileria annulata*[6,7] or *Theileria orientalis*.[8] A phylogenetic tree shown in FIGURE 1 is highlighting that *T. ovis* appears to be a single species in agreement with Schnittger et al.[9] while *T. lestoquardi* showed a greater diversity and a very close relationship with *T. annulata* by demonstrating how important these two species should be considered when trying to develop discriminating identification methods. Two clusters were observed between *T. lestoquardi* originating

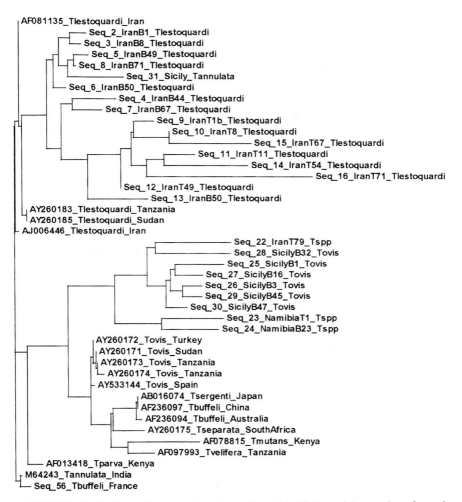

FIGURE 1. Phylogenetic tree of samples collected in Sicily and Iran and confronted with existing GenBank 18S rRNA gene sequences.

from ticks and the same species isolated from sheep blood. A few problems occurred during the comparison with the GenBank data as sequences are sometimes labeled 18S incorrectly when in fact they are related to the 5.5S rRNA gene or because the geographic origin of the species is not clearly stated and therefore we cannot compare effectively the sequences from the same country. It is also unlikely that on the GenBank database we will know if DNA samples have been passed between colleagues and could explain a pattern in the results because they in fact originate from the same source.

ACKNOWLEDGMENTS

This work has been partly financed by a NATO/Royal Society fellowship for Dr. Spitalska, an Iranian visiting fellowship for Dr. Namavari, and grants from the Italian Ministry for Research.

REFERENCES

1. BEKKER, C.P.J., S. DE VOS, A. TAOUFIK, *et al.* 2002. Simultaneous detection of *Anaplasma* and *Ehrlichia* species in ruminants and detection of *Ehrlichia ruminantium* in *Amblyomma variegatum* ticks by reverse line blot hybridization. Vet. Microbiol. **89:** 221–236.
2. SPITALSKA, E., M.M. NAMAVARI, M.H. HOSSEINI, *et al.* 2004a. Molecular surveillance of tick-borne diseases in Iranian ruminants. Small Ruminant Res. **57:** 245–248.
3. SPITALSKA, E., A. TORINA, E.-M. CANNELLA, *et al.* 2004b. Discrimination between *Theileria lestoquardi* and *Theileria annulata* in their vectors and hosts by RFLP based on the 18S rRNA gene. Parasitol. Res. **94:** 28–30.
4. RAZMI, G.R., M. HOSSEINI & M.R. ASLANI. 2003a. Identification of tick vectors of ovine theileriosis in an endemic region of Iran. Vet. Parasitol. **116:** 1–6.
5. RAZMI, G.R., E. EBRAHIMZADEH & M.R. ASLANI. 2003b. A study about tick vectors of bovine theileriosis in an endemic region of Iran. J. Vet Med. B. Infect. Dis. Vet. Publ. Health **50:** 309–310.
6. HASHEMI-FESHARKI, R. 1998. Recent development in control of *Theileria annulata* in Iran. Parasitology **5:** 193–196.
7. HASHEMI-FESHARKI, R. 1988. Control of *Theileria annulata* in Iran. Parasitol. Today **4:** 36–40.
8. UILENBERG, G. & R. HASHEMI-FESHARKI. 1984. *Theileria orientalis* in Iran. Vet. Quart. **6:** 1–4.
9. SCHNITTGER, L., H. YIN, M.J. GUBBELS, *et al.* 2003. Phylogeny of sheep and goat Theileria and Babesia parasites. Parasitol. Res. **91:** 398–406.

Molecular Sequence Evidence for the Reclassification of Some *Babesia* Species

MARIA T. E. P. ALLSOPP[a] AND BASIL A. ALLSOPP[b]

[a] *Onderstepoort Veterinary Institute, Private Bag X5, Onderstepoort 0110, South Africa*

[b] *Department of Veterinary Tropical Diseases, Faculty of Veterinary Science, University of Pretoria, Private Bag X04, Onderstepoort 0110, South Africa*

ABSTRACT: Taxonomic characterization of organisms in the genera *Theileria* and *Babesia* was originally based on observations of morphology and certain general phenotypic characteristics, which enabled many parasites to be unequivocally assigned to a particular genus. However, application of molecular genetic techniques, such as the polymerase chain reaction (PCR) for gene amplification, and DNA sequencing, have revealed gross inconsistencies in the assignation of some parasite genetic variants, particularly those of the *B. gibsoni* and *B. microti* complexes, to the genus *Babesia*. These variants cannot be assigned, on the basis of sequence information and phylogenetic analysis, to either of the genera *Theileria* and *Babesia*. The gene for which most sequence information is available for phylogenetic analysis is the small subunit ribosomal RNA (srRNA) gene. This gene allows clear distinction of the genera *Theileria* and *Babesia* (*sensu stricto*) and reveals that many "*Babesia*" variants are phylogenetically distinct from both genera. This distinction is confirmed, for some of the variants, by β-tubulin sequence data, suggesting that the organisms should be renamed and reclassified.

KEYWORDS: *Theileria*; *Babesia*; small subunit ribosomal RNA gene phylogeny

HISTORICAL PERSPECTIVE

Members of the genera *Babesia* and *Theileria* are tick-borne blood parasites of vertebrates. They are eukaryotes and belong to the phylum Apicomplexa, all members of which are parasitic. Both genera have the potential for worldwide distribution wherever their tick vectors can survive. Microscopic examination of stained blood smears from infected mammalian hosts shows that some *Babesia* and *Theileria* species have a characteristic pear-like appearance in

Address for correspondence: Dr. Maria T.E.P. Allsopp, P.O. Box 13041, Onderstepoort 0110, South Africa. Voice: +27-0-82-484-0890; fax: +27-0-12-529-8312.
e-mail: maria.allsopp@worldonline.co.za

Ann. N.Y. Acad. Sci. 1081: 509–517 (2006). © 2006 New York Academy of Sciences.
doi: 10.1196/annals.1373.076

erythrocytes. This observation led to the widespread use of the name "piroplasm" (Latin, pirum = pear) to describe members of both genera.

The first description of a piroplasm was published in 1888 by Babes,[1] a Roumanian investigator, who identified an organism in the blood of sick cattle as *Haematococcus bovis*, which was renamed *Babesia bovis* by Starcovici in 1893.[2] This was followed shortly afterward by the discovery of another similar cattle parasite, *Pyrosoma bigeminum*, later renamed *Piroplasma bigeminum*, the causative organism of Texas fever.[2–4]

Organisms belonging to the genus now known as *Theileria* were recognized somewhat later. *Theileria parva* was first described by Koch in 1898[5] and the closely related parasite, which causes "tropical piroplasmosis" (*Theileria annulata*) was described in 1904 by Dschunkowsky and Luhs.[6] The causative agent of "tropical piroplasmosis" was observed by these investigators to be present in animals also infected with *Piroplasma bigeminum*, apparently the first reference to mixed piroplasm infections.

THE PARASITES AND LIVESTOCK DISEASES

From the end of the 19th century it was recognized that many intraerythrocytic organisms caused diseases in livestock. The earliest to be characterized were then known as *Babesia bovis* and *Piroplasma bigeminum*, which were responsible, respectively, for the cattle diseases, redwater fever and Texas fever. This was followed shortly afterward by the discovery that ticks were responsible for the spread of *Piroplasma bigeminum* between cattle.[7,8] Another similar parasite, *Babesia ovis,* caused a disease of sheep.[2] The role of *Theileria* parasites as cattle pathogens became very widely known in the early years of the 20th century with the identification of *Piroplasma parvum* (now *T. parva*) as the causative organism of the devastating outbreak of East Coast fever ("Rhodesian tick fever"[9]), which swept through Rhodesia and South Africa between 1902 and 1910. In 1906 Theiler reported details of another cattle parasite that appeared to cause only a mild febrile reaction and which he named *Piroplasma mutans*.[10]

Another disease complex, "biliary fever" in horses, was believed by Koch[11] to be caused by two pathogenic organisms, now known as *Babesia caballi* and *Theileria equi*. Nuttall and Strickland made a clear distinction between the intraerythrocytic forms of both organisms in their detailed observations.[12,13]

THE TOOLS AVAILABLE TO THE INVESTIGATORS

For nearly 70 years, the only tool available to veterinarians, pathologists, and parasitologists for the study of piroplasms was the microscope. The most obvious phenotypic characteristics of the parasites, such as their morphology and the blood cells they infected were recorded in detail. The pathogenicity of the parasites, the lesions they caused in the affected animals, the vector identity, and mode of transmission were also established. This accumulation of new information and the identification of new parasites necessitated periodic revisions of the classification of the organisms. In one such revision, Donatien and Lestoquard[14] stressed the importance of basing a classification on all the information available: morphology, pathological effects, and "biological character." The extension of electron microscopy techniques to the study of piroplasms and related parasites added an extra tool that revealed a wealth of ultrastructural details. For the first time, it was possible to determine the internal structure and morphological changes occurring during all life cycle stages of many of the piroplasms and to confirm their relationship with other parasites, such as *Plasmodium* and the coccidias.[15] Details of fine structure and elucidation of life cycles of the piroplasms have shown that some of the parasites belong unequivocally to the family Theileriidae while others belong to the Babesiidae. There remains, however, a group of piroplasms of "uncertain systematic position"[16] that show some features characteristic of the babesias and other features characteristic of the theilerias. Included among these parasites are *T. equi, Cytauxzoon felis, B. microti*, the newly characterized feline piroplasms[17] and some parasites currently classified as *B. gibsoni.*

RIBOSOMAL RNA GENES AND PHYLOGENETIC RELATIONSHIPS

The most obvious place to seek clarification of problems caused by phenotypic uncertainties is at the level of the gene and 18 S gene sequences from the bulk of the phylogenetic information available for the genera *Theileria* and *Babesia*. The ribosomal RNA genes are under tight structural and functional constraint, substitution rates are low and there is no evidence of lateral gene transfer across lineages. The 28 S (large subunit) gene is long and insufficiently informative to be of general phylogenetic use, while the 5.8 S gene is too short, but the 18 S (small subunit ribosomal RNA) gene has several features that have led it to being widely used for the assignation of organisms to a particular genus. The 18 S gene has both conserved and variable regions, the former allowing unequivocal sequence alignment and the latter providing phylogenetic discrimination. The conserved sequences close to both 5' and 3' ends of the 18 S gene have the practical advantage of allowing the design of primers for polymerase chain reaction (PCR) amplification of near full-length genes in the presence of mammalian DNA.[18] Alignments may then be made of full-length genes, although some workers truncate alignments to eliminate regions where alignments are equivocal or difficult.

PHENOTYPIC CHARACTERIZATION OF *THEILERIA* AND *BABESIA* SPECIES

The most comprehensive survey of phenotypical characteristics of organisms in the genera *Theileria* and *Babesia* is that of Mehlhorn and Schein.[16] In their conclusions, they point out a number of significant differences between members of the two genera, based mainly on life cycle stages. Characteristics unique to the *Babesia* spp. (*sensu stricto*), namely transovarial transmission in the tick vector and division only in erythrocytes of the vertebrate hosts, are not shared either by the theilerias or by the dubiously classified babesias for which life cycle details are known.[19] Only transstadial transmission occurs with *Theileria* spp. and *Theileria* reproduce mainly in lymphocytes, characteristics also shared by *T. equi* (formerly *B. equi*).[20] The effects of chemotherapy in infected vertebrate hosts also differ according to the drugs used and the genus of the infecting parasite.

GENOTYPIC DIVERSITY AT THE GENUS AND SPECIES LEVEL

There are many papers describing *Theileria* and *Babesia* 18 S sequence variants and these genes remain the most useful for distinguishing genus differences. In general, however, it is not possible to use the 18 S gene to decide whether variants represent new species or subspecies.[21] There is relatively little information on the use of other molecules for species/subspecies determination. One study using ribosomal internal transcribed spacer (ITS) sequences has shown that *T. parva* isolates causing the different disease syndromes East Coast Fever and Corridor Disease could and should receive the status of subspecies.[22] Although these variants are both *T. parva* at the genus level, and there is evidence for ongoing genetic recombination between them, there are also indications that they are evolving different host preferences and pathogenicities.[22] *Beta*-tubulin gene sequences have also been used for *Theileria* and *Babesia* species delineation.[23] Several parasite outer membrane protein gene sequences are available (e.g., Tams1, mMPSA),[24,25] but these genes are likely to be under intense selection pressure so they will be evolving at a more rapid rate than core function genes. Such genes will therefore not give reliable phylogenetic information at the species level.

Phylogenetic trees inferred by comparison of a wide range of full-length and truncated 18 S Apicomplexan sequences clearly indicate that many organisms currently classified as *Babesia* are in fact only remotely related to the genus *Babesia* (*sensu stricto*).[17,26] Many of the organisms have been characterized from field isolates only, on the basis of 18 S sequences, and in many cases the vectors are unknown. If it is possible to demonstrate transovarial transmission of the organism, and the 18 S sequences fall into the same clade as *Babesia* (*sensu stricto*), then an organism is unequivocally a *Babesia*. However, many of the organisms for which new 18 S sequences are available have been assigned to the genus *Babesia* simply because no schizonts have been observed in lymphocytes. Piroplasm size, at one time used as a major phenotypic determinant of genus status, is now known to be unreliable for this purpose.

Of particular interest are the organisms currently classified as *B. gibsoni* and *B. microti*. The 18 S sequences obtained from organisms classified as *B. gibsoni* on the basis of host specificity and piroplasm size fall into two widely differing groups: the Asian *B. gibsoni* sequences fall definitively into the *Babesia* (*sensu stricto*) clade,[18] while the North American organisms classified as *B. gibsoni*[18] belong in a group of organisms described as "piroplasms of uncertain phylogenetic position."[16] This description may also be used to cover *B. rodhaini*, the recently characterized piroplasms from felines,[17] and a number of human and cervid piroplasms.[27] These organisms do not form part of either the *Babesia* or *Theileria* phylogenetic groupings. Rather, on the basis of a maximum likelihood inferred tree (FIG. 1) generated using PHYML,[28] *B. microti*, *B. rodhaini,* and the piroplasms from felines constitute a separate group (group C, FIG.1) derived from a common ancestor that preceded the divergence of the *Theileria/Babesia* clades. The human and cervid organisms fall within a clade more closely related to both theilerias and babesias, and included in this clade is an organism currently classified as *B. gibsoni* (group B, FIG.1). Similar tree topologies are described in a paper describing the new piroplasm species detected in felines,[17] in which both neighborjoining (NJ) and maximum likelihood (DNAML) algorithms were applied to 18 S sequence alignments. The algorithm used did not cause any changes in the major groupings, although minor differences were seen if truncated, as against full-length, sequence alignments were used. The conclusion to be drawn is that two new genera should be created to accommodate the two distinct groups, that is, the human and cervid organisms (group B, FIG.1), and *B. microti*, *B. rodhaini,* and the new piroplasms from felines (group C, FIG.1).

The phylogenetic positions of 5 other species remain equivocal, these are *T. equi*, *C. felis*, 2 rhinoceros piroplasms classified as *T. bicornis* and *B. bicornis,*[29] and *T. youngi* from a northern Californian dusky-footed woodrat (*Neotoma fuscipes*) (GenBank reference AF245279). The positions of these organisms in 18 S tree topologies, using both full-length and truncated sequences, vary according to the algorithm used. Distance algorithms tend to place these organisms as a subgroup within the *Theileria* clade, and our most recent phylogram (FIG.1) supports this topology except in the case of *T. equi* (group A, FIG.1). The low bootstrap values on the branches for all 5 species, however, make it impossible to decide whether they should all be reclassified as theilerias or assigned to a new grouping. In contrast, earlier maximum likelihood trees suggested that they evolved from a common ancestor that preceded the *Theileria/Babesia* divergence.[21]

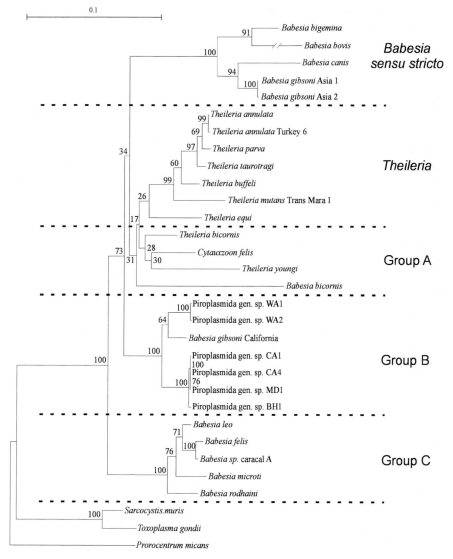

FIGURE 1. Small subunit ribosomal RNA gene "PHYML" phylogenetic tree of *Theileria* and *Babesia* species. Organisms included in the phylogeny, together with their GenBank accession numbers are listed in TABLE 1. *Sarcocystis muris, Prorocentrum micans,* and *Toxoplasma gondii* were used as outgroups to root the tree. Scale bar represents 10 nucleotide changes per 100 nucleotide positions. Figures at nodes represent bootstrap support for branching order over 100 replicates.

TABLE 1. GenBank Accession numbers of organisms included in the phylogeny

Accession number	Organism identity
AF078815	*Theileria mutans* Trans Mara 1
AF158700	Piroplasmida gen. sp. WA1
AF158701	Piroplasmida gen. sp. WA2
AF158702	*Babesia gibsoni* California
AF158703	Piroplasmida gen. sp. CA1
AF158705	Piroplasmida gen. sp. CA4
AF158706	Piroplasmida gen. sp. MD1
AF158708	Piroplasmida gen. sp. BH1
AF175300	*Babesia gibsoni* Asia 1
AF175301	*Babesia gibsoni* Asia 2
AF244911	*Babesia leo*
AF244912	*Babesia felis*
AF244913	*Babesia* sp. caracal A
AF245279	*Theileria youngi*
AF419313	*Babesia bicornis*
AF499604	*Theileria bicornis*
AY508470	*Theileria annulata* Turkey 6
M64243	*Theileria annulata*
L02366	*Theileria parva*
L19077	*Babesia bovis*
L19079	*Babesia canis*
L19080	*Cytauxzoon felis*
L19082	*Theileria taurotragi*
M87565	*Babesia rodhaini*
U09833	*Babesia microti*
X59604	*Babesia bigemina*
Z15105	*Theileria equi*
Z15106	*Theileria buffeli* Marula
M64244	*Sarcocystis muris*
M14649	*Prorocentrum micans*
X68523	*Toxoplasma gondii*

Phenotypic evidence for placing *T. equi* in a separate genus from both *Theileria* and *Babesia* can be deduced from the Mehlhorn and Schein (1984) review of life cycles and sexual stages of piroplasms.[16] These authors acknowledge that there is unlikely to be transovarial transmission of *T. equi*, since there is no reproduction of kinetes in oocytes; in this respect the organism differs from the genus *Babesia* (*sensu stricto*). However, while the fine structure of the erythrocytic stages of *T. equi* is similar to those of *Babesia* spp., the former also possess a micropore, normally only a feature of *Theileria* erythrocytic stages. In contrast, *T. equi* gametes appear more typical of babesias.

In their proposal for reclassification of *B. equi* as *T. equi*, Mehlhorn & Schein[20] cite the susceptibility of the organism to a combined therapy with Imidocarb and Parvaquone as one of the factors supporting the genus change from *B. equi* to *T. equi*. However, while *T. parva* and *T. annulata* are highly susceptible to Parvaquone treatment alone,[30,31] with no parasite recrudescence, Parvaquone treatment alone is ineffective against *T. equi*, and parasites reappear in treated horses even after combined therapy.[20] This situation, with a difference in phenotype and the instability of the tree topology, suggests that *T. equi* could possibly be assigned to a genus other than *Theileria*. The situation in respect of *C. felis*, *T. youngi*, *T. bicornis*, and *B. bicornis* is equally uncertain, with low bootstrap values on the branches to each of these organisms in FIGURE 1. For these parasites phenotypic information is very sparse, but there is little phylogenetic support for including them within the genus *Theileria*, and none at all for including them within the genus *Babesia* (*sensu stricto*), so these organisms may also be assigned to a different genus, or genera, when more information becomes available.

REFERENCES

1. BABES, V. 1888. Sur l'hémoglobinurie bactérienne du boeuf. Comp. Rendues de l'Académ. Sci. **102:** 692–694. Cited in Starcovici, 1893.
2. STARCOVICI, C. 1893. Bemerkungen über den durch Babes entdeckten Blutparasiten und die durch denselben hervorgebrachten Krankheiten, die seuchenhafte Hämoglobinurie des Rindes (Babes), das Texasfieber (Th. Smith) und der Carceag der Schafe (Babes). Central. Bakteriol. Parasiten. **14:** 1–8.
3. SMITH, T. 1889. Investigation into the nature of Texas fever. Medical News. Cited in Starcovici, 1893 Centralblatt für Bakteriologie und Parasitenkunde **14:** 1–8.
4. PATTON, W.H. 1895. The name of the southern or splenic cattle-fever parasite. Amer. Natural. **29:** 498 *et seq.* Cited in Wenyon, C. M. (1926) Protozoology: A manual for Medical men, Veterinarians and Zoologists (2 vols.) **2**. London: Ballière, Tindall & Cox.
5. NORVAL, R. I.A., B. D. PERRY & A.S. YOUNG. 1992. The Epidemiology of Theileriosis in Africa. Academic Press. London.
6. DSCHUNKOWSKY, E. & J. LUHS. 1904. Die piroplasmen der rinder. Central. Bakteriolo. Parasiten. Infektion. **35:** 486–492.
7. SMITH, T. & F.L. KILBORNE. 1893. Investigations into the nature, causation and prevention of Texas or Southern cattle fever. U. S. Depart. Ag. Bureau of Anim. Indus. Bulletin no.1.
8. DU TOIT, P.J. 1918. Zur systematik der piroplasmen. Arvhiv Protist. **39:** 84–104.
9. THEILER, A. 1903. The Rhodesian tick fever. Transvaal Ag. J. **1:** 93–110.
10. THEILER, A. 1906. Piroplasma mutans (N. spec.) of South African cattle. J. Compar. Patholo. Therap. **19:** 292–300.
11. KOCH, R. 1905. Vorläufiger Mitteilungen über die Ergebnisse einer Forschungsreise nach Ostafrika. Deutsche Med. Wochen. **31:** 1865 *et seq.*
12. NUTTALL, G.H.F. & C. STRICKLAND. 1910. Die parasiten der Pferdpiroplasmose resp. der 'Biliary Fever'. Cent. Bakteriolo. Parasiten. Infektion. **56:** 524–525.
13. NUTTALL, G.H.F. & C. STRICKLAND. 1912. On the occurrence of two species of parasites in equine 'Piroplasmosis' or 'Biliary fever'. Parasitology **5:** 65–96.
14. DONATIEN, A. & F. LESTOQUARD. 1930. De la classification des piroplasmes des animaux domestiques. Rec. Méd. Vétérinaire Exotique. **3:** 5–20.

15. LEVINE, N. D. 1971. Taxonomy of the piroplasms. Trans. Amer. Microscop. Soc. **90**: 2–33.

16. MELHORN, H. & E. SCHEIN. 1984. The piroplasms: life-cycle and sexual stages. *In* Advances in Parasitology. J. R. Baker & R. Muller, Eds.: **23**: 37–103. Academic Press. London.

17. PENZHORN, B.L., A. M. KJEMTRUP, L. M. LOPEZ-REBOLLAR & P.A. CONRAD. 2001. *Babesia leo* N. Sp. from lions in the Kruger National Park, South Africa, and its relation to other small piroplasms. J. Parasitol. **87**: 681–685.

18. ZAHLER, M., H. RINDER, E. ZWEYGARTH, *et al.* 2000. '*Babesia gibsoni*' of dogs from North America and Asia belong to different species. Parasitology **120**: 365–369.

19. LEVINE, N. D. 1985. Veterinary Protozoology. Ames: Iowa State University Press.

20. MEHLHORN, H. & E. SCHEIN.1988. Redescription of *Babesia equi* Laveran, 1901 as *Theileria equi* Mehlhorn, Schein 1998. Parasitol. Res. **84**: 467–475.

21. CHAE, J-S., B.A. ALLSOPP, S. D. WAGHELA, *et al.* 1999. A study of the systematics of *Theileria* spp. based upon small-subunit ribosomal RNA sequences. Parasitol. Res. **85**: 877–883.

22. COLLINS, N. E. & B.A. ALLSOPP. 1999. *Theileria parva* ribosomal internal transcribed spacer sequences exhibit extensive polymorphism and mosaic evolution: application to the characterization of parasites from cattle and buffalo. Parasitology **118**: 541–551.

23. CACCIO, S., C. CAMMA, M. ONUMA & C. SEVERINI. 2000. The ß-tubulin gene of *Babesia* and *Theileria* parasites is an informative marker for species discrimination. Int. J. Parasitol. **30**: 1181–1185.

24. KIRVAR, E., T. ILHAN, F. KATZER, *et al.* 2000. Detection of *Theileria annulata* in cattle and vector ticks by PCR using the Tams1 gene sequences. Parasitology **120**: 245–254.

25. KATZER, F., S. MCKELLAR, E. KIRVAR & B. SHIELS. 1998. Phylogenetic analysis of *Theileria* and *Babesia equi* in relation to the establishment of parasite populations within novel host species and the development of diagnostic tests. Mol. Biochem. Parasitol. **95**: 33–44.

26. DANTRAKOOL, A., P. SOMBOON, T. HASHIMOTO & A. SAITO-ITO. 2004. Identification of a new type of *Babesia* species in wild rats (*Bandicoota indica*) in Chiang Mai province, Thailand. J. Clin. Microbiol. **42**: 850–854.

27. KJEMTRUP, A. M., J. THOMFORD, T. ROBINSON & P.A. CONRAD. 2000. Phylogenetic relationships of human and wildlife piroplasm isolates in the western United States inferred from the 18 S nuclear small subunit RNA gene. Parasitology **120**: 487–493.

28. GUINDON, S. & O. GASCUEL. 2003. A simple, fast and accurate algorithm to estimate large phylogenies by maximum likelihood. Syst. Biol. **52**: 696–704.

29. NIJHOF, A. M., B.L. PENZHORN, G. LYNEN, *et al.* 2003. *Babesia bicornis* sp. nov. and *Theileria bicornis* sp. nov.: tick-borne parasites associated with mortality in the black rhinoceros (*Diceros bicornis*). J. Clin. Microbiol. **41**: 2249–2254.

30. MORGAN, D.W.T. & N. MCHARDY. 1982. Comparison of the antitheilerial effect of Wellcome 993 C and halofuginone. Res. Vet. Sci. **32**: 84–88.

31. GILL, B.S., A. BHATTACHARYULU, A. SINGH & D. KAUR. 1984. Chemotherapy of bovine tropical theileriosis: *Theileria annulata* infection. Res. Vet. Sci. **37**: 247–248.

Phylogenetic and Biologic Evidence That *Babesia divergens* Is Not Endemic in the United States

PATRICIA J. HOLMAN

Department of Veterinary Pathobiology, College of Veterinary Medicine and Biomedical Sciences, Texas A&M University, College Station, Texas, 77843 USA

ABSTRACT: The causative agent of human babesiosis in a Kentucky case, which was first identified as *Babesia divergens*, is identical to a parasite of eastern cottontail rabbits on Nantucket Island, Massachusetts based on piroplasm size, morphology, and ribosomal RNA sequence analysis. Studies showing differential infectivity for cattle, host erythrocyte specificity *in vitro*, parasite size and morphology *in vitro*, and ribosomal RNA sequences clearly demonstrate that the parasite from the rabbit (conspecific with the human Kentucky agent) is not the same organism as *B. divergens*.

KEYWORDS: *B. divergens*; human babesiosis; small subunit ribosomal RNA gene; intervening transcribed spacer; eastern cottontail rabbit

BABESIA DIVERGENS IN CATTLE AND HUMANS

Babesia divergens is a bloodborne tick-transmitted protozoan parasite that is the common causative agent of bovine babesiosis in Europe. Reduced milk production and poor weight gain are often associated with the infection, but more severe clinical signs such as hemoglobinuria, anemia, icterus, and diarrhea may occur.[1,2] *B. divergens* is the primary cause of human babesiosis in Europe, with approximately 30 cases reported spanning from Eastern Europe to Italy and Great Britain.[1–3] Human babesiosis due to *B. divergens* most often occurs in rural areas occupied by cattle and corresponds to the seasonal activity of the vector tick, *Ixodes ricinus* (May–September). In addition to location and time of year, predisposing risk factors include splenectomy. The high fatality rate in patients with *B. divergens*-babesiosis is directly associated with prior splenectomy. *Babesia divergens* infection in European patients resulted in fatality rates of 42% and 5% in asplenic and spleen-intact individuals,

Address for correspondence: Patricia J. Holman, Ph.D., Department of Veterinary Pathobiology, College of Veterinary Medicine and Biomedical Sciences, Texas A&M University, College Station, TX 77843. Voice: 979-845–4202; fax: 979-862-2344.
e-mail: pholman@cvm.tamu.edu

Ann. N.Y. Acad. Sci. 1081: 518–525 (2006). © 2006 New York Academy of Sciences.
doi: 10.1196/annals.1373.077

respectively.[2] Parasite-induced hemolytic anemia results in a broad range of symptoms, including fever, fatigue, chills, hemoglobinuria, thrombocytopenia, and hepatomegaly.[4]

Morphologically, *B. divergens* is a small parasite (1.5 × 0.4 μm) most commonly identified as paired merozoites that diverge widely from each other along the margin of the bovine erythrocyte (accolé form), but may also occur as a signet ring or single piriform parasites.[1] Transmission electron microscopy (TEM) reveals a close association with the erythrocyte membrane, resulting in the cell membrane protruding to conform with the parasite shape.[2] In human erythrocytes, the pairs are seen in central or subcentral portions of the cell, with no protrusions of the host cell evident by TEM.[2]

Neither *B. divergens* nor its tick vector, *I. ricinus*, is indigenous to the United States, but two cases of acute human babesiosis in Missouri and Kentucky were attributed to parasites that share similar pathology and morphology to *B. divergens.*[5,6] In the Kentucky case, the patient was a 56-year-old recreational hunter.[5] History included splenectomy 8 years previously and a trip to the Caribbean 9 months previously. Four weeks previous to presentation, he had hunted white-tailed deer and cottontail rabbits, which he dressed in the field. He did not recall being bitten by ticks.

The patient had been treated for 2 weeks with amoxycillin for headaches, but without improvement.[5] At presentation in the emergency room, symptoms included fever, chills, and hemoglobinuria. The clinician immediately ordered doxycycline therapy and blood work, including stained blood films that revealed the presence of numerous intraerythrocytic parasites (FIG. 1 A). Among the parasite forms were paired piriforms in the accolé position characteristic of *B. divergens* in bovine erythrocytes (FIG. 1 A, B). The parasites were clearly distinct from *Babesia microti* (FIG. 1 C), the primary cause of human babesiosis in the United States. Several months later, methanol-fixed unstained blood films were submitted to Texas A&M University for molecular analysis. DNA was successfully extracted from the blood films and the small subunit ribosomal RNA (SSU rRNA) gene was sequenced. Sequence analysis

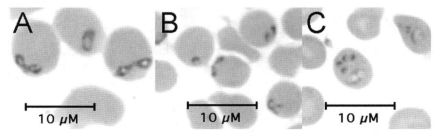

FIGURE 1. Intraerythrocytic forms of **(A)** the KY causative agent of human babesiosis, **(B)** *B. divergens* in bovine erythrocytes, and **(C)** *B. microti* in mouse erythrocytes.

of the SSU rRNA gene showed three base differences, or 99.8% identity, between the human Kentucky (KY) and the Purnell *B. divergens* isolates. Beattie and others reasoned that as this was lesser deviation than was seen among the *B. divergens* SSU rRNA genes listed in the databases at that time (TABLE 1), that the organism was, indeed, *B.divergens*. As a result, based on pathology, morphology, and molecular characterization, the causative agent of human babesiosis in the Kentucky case was thought to be *B. divergens*.[5]

THE RABBIT CONNECTION

A description of *B. divergens* in eastern cottontail rabbits (*Sylvilagus floridanus*) on Nantucket Island, Massachusetts appeared to match the agent identified in the Kentucky case (KY) (FIG. 1 D).[7] Recent reports provide evidence that *B. divergens* is enzootic in this rabbit population with prevalence rates ranging from 11% to 23% over a 5-year period.[7,8] *Ixodes dentatus* ticks are likely responsible for transmission, with 4.6% retaining infection through the molt from the larval to the nymphal stage.[8] The SSU rRNA gene sequence of the cottontail rabbit parasite is identical to that of KY.[8,9]

The fact that the Kentucky patient had hunted and dressed cottontail rabbits prior to the onset of acute babesiosis led to speculation that eastern cottontail rabbits might be the reservoir of infection. The geographic range of the eastern cottontail extends from Canada to South America, including the central United States. Working on the hypothesis that the human parasite found in KY and the rabbit parasite found on Nantucket Island were one and the same, a collaborative effort was undertaken to establish the cottontail rabbit parasite in culture to facilitate further studies.[9]

During 2002–2004, blood samples collected from free-ranging eastern cottontail rabbits live-trapped under a scientific collecting permit issued by the Massachusetts Division of Fisheries and Wildlife were supplied by Drs. Heidi Goethert and Sam R. Telford, III (Division of Infectious Diseases, Department of Biomedical Sciences, Tufts University School of Veterinary Medicine, North Grafton, MA).[9] Giemsa-stained blood smears were examined and the samples were tested for the presence of *Babesia* spp. by a previously described polymerase chain reaction (PCR)[8] prior to shipment to Texas A&M University, College Station, Texas.

TABLE 1. SSU rRNA gene sequence comparisons used to define the agent of human babesiosis in Kentucky as *B. divergens*. GenBank accession numbers are listed

	2002 *Babesia divergens* SSU rRNA gene sequences		
	Purnell U16730	Mackenstedt U07885	Drumaness Z48751
Purnell U16730	1724/1724 (100%)	1665/1672 (99.6%)	1699/1727 (98.4%)
KY agent AY887131	1721/1724 (99.8%)	1662/1672 (99.4%)	1697/1727 (98.3%)

During 2002–2003, 104 samples were collected, of which 12 samples were positive for the parasite.[9] None of the samples collected in 2004 were infected. Of the 12 positive samples, two resulted in continuous parasite cultures designated NR774 and NR831. The conditions that resulted in continuous cultures included human donor erythrocytes and HL-1 medium with 20% human serum and supplements.[9]

COMPARATIVE STUDIES

Ribosomal rRNA Intervening Transcribed Spacer 1 and 2

The SSU rRNA gene produces a functionally conserved product, and therefore has been the gold standard in genetic analysis for Apicomplexan species.[10–12] Within the SSU rRNA gene, there are variable regions that may contain nucleotide sequences that are species-specific. The slight sequence variation that exists between the KY and *B. divergens* genes may not, however, allow for definitive discrimination between the two.[5] What was considered acceptable intra-species variation at that time has been negated by recent re-sequencing of the same three isolates for which SSU rRNA gene sequences were available (GenBank accession nos. U16730, U07885, and Z48751).[13] The same sequence was reported from all three bovine isolates of *B. divergens* (GenBank accession no. AY046576), which is identical to the original sequence for the Purnell isolate SSU rRNA gene (U16730).[12,13] Based on these data, a species assignment of *B. divergens* cannot be made for the KY agent.

Other less highly conserved genetic regions have been investigated for their usefulness in distinguishing among closely related organisms and delineating species within a genus.[14] The rRNA intervening transcribed spacers (ITS1 and ITS2) are nontranslated genetic regions, separated by the smaller 5.8S rRNA gene, which lie between the highly conserved SSU rRNA (5′) and LSU (large subunit) rRNA (3′) genes in most eukaryotic organisms. ITS1 and ITS2 gene region sequence comparisons have reinforced the subspecies separation of *Babesia canis* into *Babesia canis canis, Babesia canis rossi,* and *Babesia canis vogeli* previously based on pathogenicity, vector specificity, and geography.[15,16]

The ITS1–5.8S–ITS2 gene regions amplified from genomic DNA extracted from infected blood from the eastern cottontail rabbit and the KY isolate (described above) and from cultured *B. divergens* (Purnell) were analyzed (TABLE 2).[9,12,17,18] The rabbit parasite and KY ITS1 and the ITS2 regions were identical in length, 449 and 257 base pairs, respectively. The *B. divergens* ITS1 and ITS2 regions were both shorter, at 446 and 246 base pairs, respectively. The ITS1 and ITS2 regions were identical in sequence between the rabbit parasite and KY, but shared only 94% and 90% identity with *B. divergens*, respectively (TABLE 2).

TABLE 2. Summary of differences and similarities among *Babesia divergens*, the Nantucket Island eastern cottontail rabbit parasite, and the causative agent of human babesiosis in the Kentucky case

	Babesia divergens	NR774/831	Kentucky agent
Parasite size in			
Human RBC	3.2 ×1.0 μM[a]	4.3 × 2.0 μM	4.1 × 1.9 μM (blood)
Bovine RBC	2.2 × 0.8 μM[a]	N/A	N/A
CT RBC	N/A	4.2 × 2.0 μM	N/A
Position of pairs in			
Human RBC	Subcentral	Accolé	Accolé
Bovine RBC	Accolé	N/A	N/A
CT RBC	N/A	Accolé	N/A
In Vitro growth in			
Human RBC	Yes[b]	Yes[b]	N/A
Bovine RBC	Yes	No	N/A
CT RBC	No	Yes	N/A
In Vivo infectivity			
Human	Yes	Yes	Yes
Cattle	Yes	No	N/A
SSU rRNA Gene			
B. divergens% identity	100	99.8	99.8
NR% identity	99.8	100	100
KY% identity	99.8	100	100
ITS rRNA			
ITS1 length in BP	446	449	449
ITS2 length in BP	246	257	257
ITS1+ITS2 length in BP	692	706	706
ITS1 *B. divergens*%	100	94	94
ITS1 KY% identity	94	100	100
ITS2 *B. divergens*%	100	90	90
ITS2 KY% identity	90	100	100

[a]Significantly different from NR774/831 and KY agent measurements ($P \leq 0.05$), Student's *t*-test.
[b]No significant difference in growth ($P \geq 0.05$), Student's *t*-test.
N/A = not available; CT = eastern cottontail rabbit.

Infectivity for Cattle

Once cultures of the parasite from the Nantucket Island eastern cottontail rabbits were established, cultured parasites were available for host specificity studies. Inasmuch as *B. divergens* is a pathogen of cattle, in collaboration with scientists at the USDA and Washington State University, Pullman WA (Drs. W.L. Goff and D.P. Knowles, Animal Disease Research Unit, Agricultural Research Service, United States Department of Agriculture and Dr. A. J. Allen, Department of Clinical Medicine and Surgery, College of Veterinary Medicine, Washington State University, Pullman, WA), an experiment was undertaken to compare infectivity of the rabbit parasite for cattle.[19]

Doses of 1×10^5 infected erythrocytes of sixth passage NR831 rabbit parasite culture and eighth passage *B. divergens* culture were inoculated intravenously into Holstein-Friesian calves. Two splenectomized and three spleen-intact animals each received NR831 (experimental group) and one splenectomized and one spleen-intact animal received *B. divergens* Purnell (control group). The calves were monitored by clinical signs, Giemsa-stained blood films, *Babesia* spp.-specific PCR, and blood culture. On day 59 postinoculation the animals were challenged IV with 1×10^5 erythrocytes infected with *B. divergens* Purnell.

The experimental calves that received NR831 did not exhibit clinical signs of infection post and remained negative for all assays. The control calves that received *B. divergens* developed clinical infections and became positive by all assays. Upon challenge inoculation with *B. divergens*, the NR831 experimental calves were fully susceptible to infection.

Host Erythrocyte Specificity In Vitro

This *in vitro* study compared the host erythrocyte specificity of cultured parasites (NR774) from the Nantucket Island eastern cottontail rabbits and *B. divergens* for bovine, cottontail rabbit, and human erythrocytes, based on the known mammalian hosts for each.[17,20] NR774 is a culture-adapted rabbit isolate of the parasite that caused human babesiosis in KY (see molecular comparisons above) and *B. divergens* is a zoonotic parasite of cattle and humans. Although *B. divergens* is also known to infect gerbils,[1] culture with gerbil erythrocytes was not attempted due to the difficulty in obtaining sufficient erythrocytes to complete the study. HL-1 medium with 20% adult bovine serum was used for the bovine erythrocyte cultures; HL-1 medium with 20% human serum was used for both human and cottontail rabbit erythrocyte cultures (it was not possible to obtain cottontail rabbit serum and domestic rabbit serum did not support the parasite).[17,20]

In vitro growth of NR774 was supported in human and cottontail rabbit erythrocytes, but not in bovine (TABLE 2). *B. divergens' in vitro* growth was supported in human and bovine erythrocytes, but not in cottontail rabbit (TABLE 2). Interestingly, there was no significant difference in growth between NR774 and *B. divergens* when cultured in human erythrocytes.

CONCLUSION

The causative agent of the acute human babesiosis case in Kentucky was first thought to be *B. divergens* based on disease pathology, parasite morphology, and small subunit ribosomal RNA gene analysis.[5] However, two facts argued against this:

1. *Babesia divergens* is not indigenous to the United States and there are no reports of cattle infected in the area (or anywhere else in the United States), and

2. *Ixodes ricinus,* the vector tick for *B. divergens,* is not indigenous to the United States.

This series of experiments supports the conspecificity of the eastern cottontail rabbit parasite and the causative agent of the acute human babesiosis case in Kentucky based on infectivity of both for human erythrocytes, position and size of the piroplasms in human erythrocytes, and 100% shared identity between SSU rRNA genes and rRNA regions. Cultures of the eastern cottontail rabbit parasite facilitated further comparisons between this zoonotic agent and *B. divergens.*

This series of studies clearly shows that the KY agent is, in fact, distinct from *B. divergens* as evidenced by the position and size disparity of piroplasms in human erythrocytes, the inability to infect cattle, differential specificity for cottontail rabbit and bovine erythrocytes *in vitro*, and by differences in SSU rRNA gene and rRNA ITS sequences.

ACKNOWLEDGMENTS

The author appreciates the invaluable contributions of each collaborator, Drs. Jim Beattie, Heidi Goethert, Sam R. Telford, III, Will L. Goff, Andrew J. Allen, and Donald P. Knowles, and expresses sincere thanks to all. Many thanks are due the students who were involved in aspects of this project: Angela Spencer, Kylie Bendele, and Lorien Schoelkopf. This study was supported by NIAID NIH RO3 AI054799-01, Texas Agricultural Experiment Station Project 8973, and USDA-ARS-ADRU-CRIS no. 5348-32000-020-00D.

REFERENCES

1. LEVINE, N.D. 1985. Veterinary Protozoology. The Iowa State University Press. Ames, Iowa.
2. GORENFLOT, A., K. MOUBRI & B. CARCY. 1998. Human babesiosis. Ann. Trop. Med. Parasitol. **92:** 489–501.
3. PICCALUGA, P.P., G. POLETTI, G. MARTINELLI, *et al.* 2004. Babesia infection in Italy. Lancet **4:** 212.
4. HOMER, M.J., I. AUGUILAR-DELFIN, S.R. TELFORD, *et al.* 2000. Babesiosis. Clin. Microbiol. Rev. **13:** 451–469.
5. BEATTIE, J.F., M.L. MICHELSON & P.J. HOLMAN. 2002. Acute babesiosis caused by *Babesia divergens* in a resident in Kentucky. N. Engl. J. Med. **347:** 697–698.
6. HERWALDT, B.L., D.H. PERSING, E.A. PRECIGOUT, *et al.* 1996. A fatal case of babesiosis in Missouri: identification of another piroplasm that infects humans. Ann. Intern. Med. **124:** 643–650.
7. GOETHERT, H.K. & S.R. TELFORD III. 2000. Enzootic transmission of *Babesia divergens* among cottontail rabbits on Nantucket Island [abstract]. Am. J. Trop. Med. Hyg. **62**(Suppl):185.

8. GOETHERT, H.K. & S.R. TELFORD III. 2003. Enzootic transmission of *Babesia divergens* among cottontail rabbits on Nantucket Island, Massachusetts. Am. J. Trop. Med. Hyg. **69:** 455–460.
9. HOLMAN, P.J., A.M. SPENCER, R.E. DROLESKEY, *et al.* 2005. *In vitro* cultivation of a zoonotic *Babesia* sp. isolated from eastern cottontail rabbits (*Sylvilagus floridanus*) on Nantucket Island, Massachusetts. J. Clin. Microbiol. **43:** 3995–4001.
10. PRICHARD, R. & A. TAIT. 2001. The role of molecular biology in veterinary parasitology. Vet. Parasitol. **98:** 169–194.
11. ALLSOPP, M.T.E.P., T. CAVALIER-SMITH, D.T. DEWAAL & B.A. ALLSOPP. 1994. Phylogeny and evolution of the piroplasms. Parasitology **108:** 147–152.
12. HOLMAN, P.J., J. MADELEY, T.M. CRAIG, *et al.* 2000. Antigenic, phenotypic and molecular characterization confirms *Babesia odocoilei* isolated from three cervids. J. Wildl. Dis. **36:** 518–530.
13. HERWALDT, B.L., S. CACCIO, F. GHERLINZONI, *et al.* 2003. Molecular characterization of a non-*Babesia divergens* organism causing zoonotic babesiosis in Europe. Emerg. Infect. Dis. **9:** 942–948.
14. BERZUNZA-CRUZ, M., N. CABRERA, M. CRIPPA-ROSSI, *et al.* 2002. Polymorphism analysis of the internal transcribed spacer and small subunit of ribosomal RNA genes of *Leishmania mexicana*. Parasitol. Res. **88:** 918–925.
15. UILENBERG, G., F.F.J. FRANSSEN, N.M. PERIÉ & A.A. SPANJER. 1989. Three groups of *Babesia canis* distinguished and a proposal for nomenclature. Vet. Quart. **11:** 33–40.
16. ZAHLER, M., E. SCHEIN, H. RINDER & R. GOTHE. 1998. Characteristic genotypes discriminate between *Babesia canis* isolates of differing vector specificity and pathogenicity to dogs. Parasitol. Res. **84:** 544–548.
17. SPENCER, A.M. 2005. Molecular and *in vitro* characterization of a *Babesia divergens*-like agent from eastern cottontail rabbits (*Sylvilagus floridanus*) on Nantucket Island. M.S. thesis, Texas A&M University, College Station.
18. PURNELL, R.E., D.W. BROCKLESBY, D.J. HENDRY, & E.R. YOUNG. 1976. Separation and recombination of *Babesia divergens* and *Ehrlichia phagocytophila* from a field case of redwater from Erie. Vet. Rec. **99:** 415–417.
19. HOLMAN, P.J., A.M. SPENCER, S.R. TELFORD III, *et al.* 2005. Comparative infectivity of *Babesia divergens* and a zoonotic *Babesia divergens*-like parasite in cattle. Am. J. Trop. Med. Hyg. **73:** 865–870.
20. SPENCER, A., H.K. GOETHERT, S.R. TELFORD III & P.J. HOLMAN. 2006. *In vitro* host erythrocyte specificity and differential morphology of *Babesia divergens* and a zoonotic *Babesia* sp. from eastern cottontail rabbits (*Sylvilagus floridanus*). J. Parasitol. **2:** 333–340.

An Internet Portal Dedicated to Pig Production and Wild Suids in the Tropics

PigTrop Web Site http://pigtrop.cirad.fr

VINCENT PORPHYRE,[a] CYRICCE GOURMENT,[b] THIERRY ERWIN,[b] AND CHRISTINE NOUAILLE[b]

[a]CIRAD, EMVT Department, Animal Production Unit, PRISE Consortium, Hanoi, Vietnam

[b]CIRAD, DIC, Montpellier F-34398, France

ABSTRACT: Considering that a wide access to updated and relevant data is a key point for livestock development and research improvement in tropics, The PigTrop web site (http://pigtrop.cirad.fr) is dedicated to pig production and pork commodity chains in developing countries. It mainly addresses stakeholders involved in the pig commodity chain, but also researchers, students, or development agencies with an interest in tropical pig breeding. It is run by the French Agricultural Research Centre for International Development (CIRAD).

KEYWORDS: website; pig production; wild suids & peccaries; tropics; research network

INTRODUCTION

This French–English World Wide Web initiative is aiming to gather several institutions within an tropical pig e-network in order to gather relevant data and scientific references to southern researchers, students, NGOs, development agencies, and farmers, support a sustainable development of pig production in Southern countries, and improve international visibility of efforts of North–South research.

METHODS

It announces new publications, special issues, past and upcoming events; as an information database, it gathers research issues, results, current projects,

Address for correspondence: Vincent Porphyre, CIRAD, UPR Systèmes d'élevage, Campus International de Baillarguet, TA 30/A, Montpellier F-34398, France. Voice: +33 4 67 59 38 37; fax: +33 4 67 59 38 25.

e-mail: vincent.porphyre@cirad.fr

Ann. N.Y. Acad. Sci. 1081: 526–527 (2006). © 2006 New York Academy of Sciences.
doi: 10.1196/annals.1373.078

abstract database, and projects presentation. It also gives an overview of publications on pig production in tropical areas, and full text articles and online documents (training material, reports) are available for download.

RESULTS

After the 12 first months, 65,000 visitors have consulted our pages; more than 1000 subscribers in dozens of countries have received the regular updates, and numerous contributions have been published from European and Southern research institutes and universities, journals and e-networks, and development agencies. The scientific pages promote the research results about various disciplines applied to swine; detailed sections address issues on animal health (i.e., disease surveillance, epidemiology, diagnostic and vaccines); animal nutrition (i.e., alternative raw materials and byproducts, nutritional requirements under tropical conditions, economical feeding strategies); genetics and biodiversity (i.e., resistance genes, adaptation to hot climate, local breeds and wild hogs conservation); environment and natural resources protection (i.e., animal wastes management, alternative treatment technologies); socio-economy in pig production sector (i.e., producers organization, market relationships); quality and food safety; and animal husbandry and sustainable practices (i.e., tropical pig production systems, technical and economic performances, productivity and reproduction improvement).

CONCLUSION

This World Wide Web information system is the sole web site meant for pig production in tropics. It provides relevant information for focused beneficiaries in this field. Considering the large and interested feedback from institutions and individuals, it would be the base of a more formal network as a major tool to define research programs and development policies, disseminate results, and improve the visibility of actions in Southern countries.

REFERENCE

For more details: http://pigtrop.cirad.fr/en/

Local Epidemiosurveillance in Swine Diseases in Northern Vietnam

Description and Preliminary Results

VINCENT PORPHYRE,[a] NGUYEN NGOC SON,[b] HA MINH TUAN,[c] STERENN GENEWE,[a] AND CELINE HENRY[a]

[a]CIRAD, EMVT Department, PRISE Consortium in Vietnam, Hanoi, Vietnam

[b]District Veterinary Station, Hoai Duc District, Ha Tay Province, Vietnam

[c]National Institute of Animal Husbandry, PRISE Consortium in Vietnam, Hanoi, Vietnam

ABSTRACT: The REMAPORC is an epidemiosurveillance network in swine diseases and an organizational model for local veterinary services in one district of Northern Vietnam. A strong concern was done on quality of the sanitary information chain from field and feedback to local agents. Based on 4,000 declarations provided by veterinarians and animal health workers involved, preliminary results highlighted the major incidence of porcine respiratory disease complex; digestive affections in piglets, and reproductive disorders in newly raised exotic sows have been also noticed.

KEYWORDS: epidemiosurveillance; swine diseases; veterinary network; Vietnam

INTRODUCTION

The REMAPORC (French acronym for epidemiosurveillance network in swine diseases) is an 18-month-old network and an organizational model located in a district 25 km west from Hanoi (Vietnam). It has initially focused on longitudinal passive monitoring of clinical signs associated with swine enzootic diseases and disorders. This organization was active during 2005 in the early warning program against Avian Flu outbreaks (http://pigtrop.cirad.fr/fr/lemonde/asie_VN_EpidSurv.htm).

Address for correspondence: Vincent Porphyre, CIRAD, UPR Systèmes d'élevage, Campus International de Baillarguet, TA 30/A, Montpellier F-34398, France: Voice: +33 4 67 59 38 37; fax: +33 4 67 59 38 25.

e-mail: vincent.porphyre@cirad.fr

Ann. N.Y. Acad. Sci. 1081: 528–530 (2006). © 2006 New York Academy of Sciences.
doi: 10.1196/annals.1373.079

METHODS

During a preliminary phase, 30 paravets and technicians in veterinary medicine, 1 veterinary district station, 1 research assistant, and 5 veterinary students were involved in monthly reporting of their onfarm syndromic observations through a participatively designed form. A relational database system was designed to manage field information and to ensure an easy and controlled entry. Official reports and epidemiological analysis were performed with reliable data on observed disorders. A monthly newsletter was a major tool in allowing an informative feedback to members.[1] Surveillance targeted various infectious diseases and disorders in swine. Early warning was focused on Foot-and-Mouth disease and Classical Swine Fever.

RESULTS

Preliminary epidemiological analysis based on 4000 declarations highlighted the major incidence of porcine respiratory disease complex (50% of total reported cases). Additional concerns have implied digestive affections in piglets (30% of total reported cases), and reproductive disorders in newly raised exotic sows (10% of total reported cases).

DISCUSSION

Positive key points that were aimed at maintaining and consolidating members' motivation was the monthly training and discussion sessions, clear contractual relationships with veterinary stations at the district level, reasonable incentives, and informative feedback through a monthly newsletter. Even without the use of laboratory analysis to confirm clinical signs, the field data on multifactorial syndromes have constituted original results in Vietnam and can be used to design baseline studies to define specific epidemiological parameters relating to pathogens of economic importance to farmers. Future developments should involve the testing of rapid alert procedures for reporting disease outbreaks,[2] support of specific training programs, creation of rapid and friendly use queries to facilitate data reporting to the provincial veterinary service level, epidemiological assessments regarding spatial disease distribution, defining a more effective means to involve farmers and local extension services, and to promote a better link between field activities and laboratory units.[3]

CONCLUSION

The experience in REMAPORC network has introduced a relevant relationship between the various veterinary professionals at the local level. It would also contribute to a better disease-reporting management scheme for animal disease containment policies, improve capacities of local people involved in animal health, and contribute to the ongoing early warning national veterinary initiatives.

ACKNOWLEDGMENT

We would like to thank the French Embassy in Vietnam RS for its financial support during the year 2005.

REFERENCES

1. CARDINALE, E. 2000. Le réseau sénégalais d'epidémiosurveillance aviaire (RESESAV): présentation et premiers résultats. epidémiologie et santé animale. **37:** 105–116.
2. D'ANDLAU, G., E. CARDINALE, P. GAUTIER & V. PORPHYRE. 2004. "Avian Influenza" support mission to Vietnam: diagnosis and short-term & long-term proposals. Agence Française de Développement. Expert report. From 23/02 to 12/03/2004. **1:** 80 pages.
3. HENDRIKX, P.B.F., J. DOMENECH, M. OUAGAL & A. IDRISS. 1997. Enjeux et contraintes à la mise en place d'un réseau d'épidémiosurveillance national en Afrique: exemple du REPIMAT au Tchad. Epidémiologie et Santé animale **32:** 1–3.

A Study of Edema Disease in Pigs in Vietnam with Particular Reference to the Use of Autovaccine for the Prevention of Disease

CU HUU PHU, N.N. NGUYEN, N.T. DO, X.H. NGUYEN, X.T. AU, T.H. VAN, N.Q. VU AND T.H. DAO

Department of Bacteriology, National Institute of Veterinary Research, Dong da, 84 Hanoi, Vietnam

ABSTRACT: Edema disease caused by *Escherichia coli* is one of the most common diseases in postweaning piglets throughout Vietnam. Verotoxigenic *E. coli* (VTEC) was isolated from 197 of 261 samples (75.5%). All isolates were confirmed by basic biochemical tests and carbohydrate fermentation characteristics. Of these, 70.1% of isolates are hemolytic, 45% isolates belonged to serotypes O149:K91, possessed the VT2e gene, and was the most predominant VTEC pathotype associated with edema disease in pigs. Serogroup O139 accounted for 30% of the isolates, followed by serogroup O138 and O141 (25%). In addition to VT2e gene, the ST (72.7%) and LT (52.7%) genes were also recognized. A total of 10 representative isolates were subjected to toxigenicity testing by intraperitoneal injection in mice and experimental infection in pigs. It was shown that 100% of the mice were killed 17–24 h post injection (p.i.). All pigs experimentally infected with challenge strains and developed typical symptoms of edema disease 36–72 h p.i. A multivalent killed whole-cells vaccine containing aluminum hydroxide was prepared from 5 VTEC strains. The vaccine was 100% safe when administered by the intramuscular route into the pigs. A field trial for over 100,000 pigs (21–90 days old) showed that vaccinated pigs were protected against edema disease at a level of 90% compared to 100% of pigs from unvaccinated groups.

KEYWORDS: edema disease; *E. coli*; Verotoxigenic *E. coli*; serotype

INTRODUCTION

Edema disease caused by verotoxigenic *E. coli* (VTEC) is one of the most common diseases in pre- and postweaning pigs in Vietnam.[1] The disease has

Address for correspondence: Dr. Cu Huu Phu, Department of Bacteriology, 86 Truong Chinh Road, Dong da, 84 Hanoi, Vietnam. Voice: 84-4-8693923; fax: 84-4-8694082.
e-mail: cuhuuphu@netnam.org.vn

Ann. N.Y. Acad. Sci. 1081: 531–533 (2006). © 2006 New York Academy of Sciences.
doi: 10.1196/annals.1373.080

been a major cause of economic loss to the swine industry over the last 10 years. A study to identify the causative agent of disease is needed.

OBJECTIVE

The objective of this study was to examine the virulence factors of bacterial agents, and develop and try an autovaccine to prevent the disease.

MATERIALS AND METHODS

Samples of heart blood, lymph nodes, and intestines ($n = 261$) were taken from pigs (21–90 days old) with clinical signs of edema disease.

Polymerase chain reaction was used for the detection of virulence genes (STa, STb, VT2e, F18).

The conventional method for the preparation of aluminum hydroxide killed whole-cells vaccine was used.

Validated tests for safety, purity, sterility, and potency of vaccine were used.

RESULTS AND DISCUSSION

An epidemiological study undertaken in Vietnam indicated that VTEC was isolated from 197 of 261 samples (75.5%) taken from pigs with the signs of swollen eyelids, ears, nose, and lips. The identity of *E. coli* isolates was confirmed by basic biochemical tests (IMViC) and carbohydrate fermentation characteristics. The result of serotyping is shown in FIGURE 1. Also, distribution of virulence genes of collected VTEC isolates is presented in FIGURE 2.

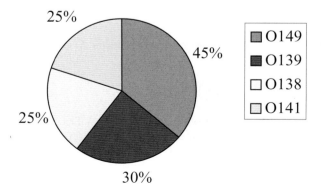

FIGURE 1. O serogroup of collected VTEC isolates.

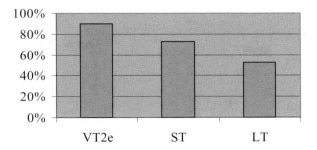

FIGURE 2. The distribution of virulence genes among VTEC collected isolates.

A multivalent killed whole-cell vaccine containing aluminum hydroxide as an adjuvant was prepared from five VTEC strains. The vaccine was 100% safe when administered by the intramuscular route to the pigs. Also, a field trial for over 100,000 pigs aged from 3 to 8 weeks show that vaccinated pigs were protected against edema disease at a level of 90% compared to 100% of pigs from unvaccinated groups.

REFERENCE

1. NGUYEN, N. N., C. H. PHU, N.T. Do *et al.* Edema disease in pigs in Binh Dinh and Ha Tay. The use of an autovaccine to control the disease. Veterinary Scientific Congress of NIVR. 7/2002.

Preliminary Analysis of Tetracycline Residues in Marketed Pork in Hanoi, Vietnam

DUONG VAN NHIEM,[a] PETER PAULSEN,[b]
WITAYA SURIYASATHAPORN,[c] FRANS J.M. SMULDERS,[b]
MOSES N. KYULE,[d] MAXIMILIAN P.O. BAUMANN,[d]
KARL H. ZESSIN,[d] AND PHAM HONG NGAN[a]

[a] Hanoi Agricultural University, Hanoi, Vietnam

[b] University of Veterinary Medicine, A 1210 Vienna, Austria

[c] Chiang Mai University, Chiang Mai 50202, Thailand

[d] Freie Universitaet Berlin, FB Veterinaermedizin, Luisenstr, 56 , D-10177 Berlin,
Germany

ABSTRACT: A cross-sectional survey was designed to investigate the proportion of tetracycline residues in marketed pork in suburb and urban
districts in Hanoi. A total of 290 raw muscle samples were randomly
collected from open markets in these districts. The samples were quali-
tatively screened for tetracycline residues using the agar inhibition test,
and *Bacillus cereus* (ATCC 11778) as the reference strain. The inconclusive samples were then analyzed using high-performance liquid chromatography (HPLC). The positive samples from either test were defined
as positive results. Overall, 5.5% of all collected samples were positive
for tetracycline residues. The proportion of positive samples from shops
in suburb districts was significantly ($P < 0.05$) different from those collected from shops in urban districts. So, the factor of region was identified
as a risk factor of tetracycline residue proportion in raw pork with an
odds ratio (OR) of 4.03 (95% CI = 1.12, 14.45). For the other factors,
such as season, type of shop, type of abattoir, origin of meat, etc., the
difference in proportion of positive samples within each factor was substantial but not statistically significant. These factors were identified as
nonrisk factors. Such a high proportion may pose a potential hazard to
public health, particularly since they might induce drug resistance of
pathogenic micro-organisms.

KEYWORDS: tetracycline; residue; pork; Hanoi

Address for correspondence: Mr. Duong Van Nhiem, Lecturer, Faculty of Animal Science and Veterinary Medicine, Hanoi Agricultural University, GIALAM–HANOI–VIETNAM. Voice: +84-4-8768-270;
fax: +84-4-8276-653.
e-mail: dvnhiem@yahoo.com or dvnhiem@hn.vnn.vn

Ann. N.Y. Acad. Sci. 1081: 534–542 (2006). © 2006 New York Academy of Sciences.
doi: 10.1196/annals.1373.081

INTRODUCTION

Imprudent use of antibiotics in animal production has become a matter of worldwide concern.[1] Recently, a study[2] revealed that, in Vietnam, the application of antibiotics to sick animals by farmers without any veterinary prescription and supervision and laboratory diagnosis is not infrequent. This is facilitated by significant deficiencies in the registration of the numerous antibiotic-containing veterinary medical products (>3000). A substantial proportion of these pharmaceuticals contains tetracyclines (257 of more than 3000[2]).

Thus, antibiotic residues constitute a problem for meat production, as this is one of the major sectors of agricultural production besides paddy rice farming, accounting for 22.3% production value or 5.4% GDP in Vietnam.[3] Pork is the staple product of livestock production in Vietnam. According to statistic data collected by the Ministry of Agriculture and Rural Development (MARD), annual pork production in 2003 reached 1.8 million tons, accounting for 77% total meat production in the country.[4] A great majority of pork production is domestically consumed, and the rest is exported. Hanoi, the capital city of the country with a population of more than 3 million people and a roughly equal number of tourists and in-official immigrants, daily consumes between 180 and 200 tons of pork.[5]

Despite this large scale of meat consumption, and, thus, potential exposure to antibiotic residues, there is only one study on antibiotic residues in environmental samples of aquaculture[6] and one dealing with incurred (suspicious) pork,[7] and, up to now, no information about antibiotic residues in meat retailed to the consumers.

To obtain data for an assessment of the meat-borne exposure of consumers to antibiotic residues, we studied residues of a common antibiotic (tetracyclines) in the most relevant meat type (pork) sold in the markets in the capital of Vietnam (Hanoi). Based on epidemiological considerations, the role of a number of variables was studied, to identify potential risk factors for the presence of antibiotic residues.

MATERIALS AND METHODS

Study Site

Hanoi, the capital city, is located in the Red River Delta in North Vietnam, comprises 14 districts (5 suburbs and 9 urban districts). Climatically, Hanoi falls in the subtropical zone, influenced by tropical humid monsoon. There are four distinct seasons, namely, spring (February–April), summer (May–July), autumn (August–October), and winter (November–January). It can also be divided into two: rainy (May–September) and dry (October–April) seasons. The average temperature in summer is 29.2°C, in winter 17.2°C, and for the whole year 23.2°C. There are about 114 rainy days a year with a mean rainfall of 1800 mm/year.[8]

The study was conducted in the 5 suburb districts, namely Gia Lam, Soc Son, Dong Anh, Tu Liem, and Thanh Tri and the 9 urban districts Cau Giay, Long Bien, Hoang Mai, Tay Ho,Thanh Xuan, Hai Ba Trung, Ba Dinh, Hoan Kiem, and Dong Da of Hanoi. Permanent regular markets in all above districts were selected as sampling sites; meat shops in the markets were defined as study units. This means that 290 different shops were tested.

Sampling

The sampling was conducted in two seasons, early winter and early spring. Meat shops were randomly selected from each market. From each shop, one muscle sample of approximately 300 to 400 g was collected, wrapped in a polyethylene bag, and put in a cool box with dry ice. Samples were then transported to the laboratories and stored in freezers at a temperature no higher than $-18°C$ until analysis. There were altogether 290 samples collected. Number and distribution of samples are shown in TABLE 1. Relevant information, such as location of the market, origin of meat, type of abattoir, product(s) offered on the same shop, and shop owner's profile, was also obtained simultaneously at the time of sampling.

Methods for Analysis

Microbiological Inhibition Test

All samples were analyzed by using the microbiological inhibition test with *Bacillus cereus* (ATCC 11778) as the reference strain, oxytetracycline discs

TABLE 1. Study site and distribution of samples

| No. | Districts | Sampling time | | Total |
		Winter	Spring	
1	Gia Lam	25	20	45
2	Soc Son	13	16	29
3	Dong Anh	16	17	33
4	Tu Liem	16	12	28
5	Thanh Tri	7	13	20
6	Cau Giay	8	10	18
7	Long Bien	11	16	27
8	Hoang Mai	9	11	20
9	Tay Ho	5	6	11
10	Thanh Xuan	12	10	22
11	Hai Ba Trung	4	5	9
12	Ba Dinh	1	4	5
13	Hoan Kiem	5	8	13
14	Dong Da	5	5	10
	Total	137	153	290

(Mast Diagnostics 0.5 μg/disc [Most Group Ltd., Merseyside, UK]) as control, on agar test pH 6 (Merck [MSD Sharp & Dohme, Haar, Germany]).[9,10] The sterile bottles of medium were melted and sterilized in an autoclave at 121°C for 15 min; subsequently placed in a waterbath at 55°C and left for at least 30 min until they reached the temperature of the waterbath. The media were added with the appropriate volumes of inoculums (*Bacillus cereus* spore suspension), gently mixed and poured into 90 mm-diameter sterile plastic plates on a leveling platform with 5 mL/plate. Muscle samples were removed from the freezer and placed at room temperature for up to 20 min. An 8 mm-diameter cylindrical core from each sample was cut using a stainless cork borer. The core was subsequently cut into slices of 2 mm thickness using a sterile scalpel blade. Two slices from each sample were placed opposite each other on a plate using forceps; a positive control disc was placed in the center of plate. Plates were incubated at 30°C for approximately 18 h. Plates were read against a black background with a light from underneath. Zones of inhibition given by the tissue slices and control discs were measured to the nearest mm using a ruler. Positive results were indicated by the complete inhibition of growth around both meat slices in a zone of 12 millimeter diameter or greater (the annular zone not less than 2 mm wide). Negative results were indicated by no inhibition of growth around the meat slices. The inconclusive samples, which showed the annular inhibition zone less than 2 mm wide or incomplete, were then analyzed by the high-performance liquid chromatography (HPLC) briefly described below.

Analysis by HPLC

Samples that were previously considered as inconclusive results were subsequently analyzed by HPLC. These samples underwent three principal stages in the sample preparation (*a*) homogenization and extraction of the sample residues by EDTA/Mc Ilvain buffer; (*b*) precipitation of proteins using trichloroacetic acid and filtration; and, (*c*) cleanup on solid-phase extraction cartridges C_{18}. Tetracyclines are separated on a C_{18} stationary phase and detected by UV absorption at 355 nm. The amount of tetracycline is calculated by interpolation from a calibration curve determined for each of the three compounds: oxytetracycline, tetracycline, and chlortetracycline, taking into account the calculated recovery. The detailed procedures are mentioned in the standard of Agence Française de Sécurité Sanitaire des Aliments (AFSSA) for "determination of tetracycline residues in kidney and muscle by high performance liquid chromatography."[11]

Further Data Processing

A sample that was indicated as a positive result by either above-mentioned methods was defined as positive result in this study. Collected data were

TABLE 2. Two-by-two table of results of each factor. OR = (a/b)/(c/d) = ad/bc

		(+)	(−)	Total
Exposure	(+)	a	b	a+b
	(−)	c	d	c+d
		a+c	b+d	a+b+c+d

analyzed using descriptive (percentage, range...) and inferential statistics (Fisher's exact test) at a confidence level of 95% ($\alpha = 0.05$). Odds ratio (OR) was calculated as given in TABLE 2.

RESULTS AND DISCUSSION

General Relevance of Antibiotics in Food Production

Antibiotics are used in animals as in humans for both prevention and treatment of infections. In animal husbandry, they are also mixed in feeds as growth promotors. In addition, antibiotics are used on a large scale in horticulture and agriculture.[12] Antimicrobials represent the largest proportion of pharmaceutical sales both in volume and money value of any drugs used in animal production.[13] It has been estimated that as much as 50% of total antibiotic production (by weight) is used in animals and plants, with 50–80% used in some countries for growth promotion or disease prophylaxis and the rest used for therapeutic purposes.[14] In the United States alone some 15 million pounds of antibiotics are administered to farm animals annually.[15] Nevertheless, imprudent use of antibiotics has caused adverse consequences to both human and animal health, particularly the increasing presence of antibiotic resistant micro-organisms resulting in difficulties in prevention and treatment of diseases. On the other hand, improper use of antibiotics may cause environmental pollution. For example, a study in aquaculture in Vietnam showed that antibiotic residues were detected in water and mud samples from shrimp ponds in mangrove areas.[6]

Tetracyclines

Tetracyclines are broad-spectrum antibiotics that show activity against Gram-positive and Gram-negative bacteria, including anerobes.[16] They represent one of the five most commonly used groups of antimicrobials in food animals.[17] Despite early warnings about increasing resistances of microorganisms to tetracyclines and the banning of tetracyclines as growth promotors, more than 65% of the antibiotics prescribed for veterinary therapeutic use within the European Community (2294 of 3494 tons) are tetracyclines.[18] In the United States, tetracyclines are the most commonly used antibiotics, approved for use in a variety of animal species (disease treatment and prevention; growth promotion), plants, and humans. Maximum residue levels have been allocated for various tissues, and a number of chemical and microbiological detection methods[10] have been developed for monitoring these residues.

Detection of Tetracycline Residues in Pork Marketed in Hanoi

Results in TABLE 3 show that tetracycline antibiotic residue was detected in 16 out of total 290 analyzed samples or 5.52%. The maximum residue limit of 100 μg/kg muscle, however, was exceeded in two samples (167.4 and 192.3 μg/kg) only. This implies that there might be a much higher proportion of residues of antibiotics in general because the frequency of utilization of tetracycline group accounts for 7.95% total utilization of antibiotics in pig and chicken production[7] and tetracyclines are present in >10% of the antibiotic pharmaceuticals on the market in Vietnam.[2]

To date, no similar study on the prevalence of tetracycline residues in pork in the country does exist. However, a study in the southern province of Binh Duong[7] reports proportion of tetracycline residues in incurred (suspicious) pork samples with oxytetracycline detected in 7 (14.6%) and chlortetracycline in 6 (12.5%) out of 48 samples.

Socioeconomic Factors Associated with the Presence of Tetracycline Residues in Hanoi

The statistical analysis (TABLE 3) demonstrated that most differences, except the one between urban and suburban markets, are not statistically significant or there are no associations between the antibiotic residue proportions and the corresponding factors, respectively. In other words, these factors are identified not as risk factors of getting a higher antibiotic residue proportion at a confidence level of 95% ($\alpha = 0.05$).

The difference in the antibiotic residue proportion between the two areas—urban and suburban, at which the selected markets are located, is statistically significant. This implies that there is an association between the geographical region and the antibiotic residue proportion at a confidence level of 95% ($\alpha = 0.05 > P$ value $= 0.018414$). An OR of 4.03 in this study indicates that raw pork offered on the suburban markets is about four times more likely in being contaminated by antibiotics at detectable levels than those sold in the urban markets.

A possible explanation could be based on the socioeconomic conditions of the two areas. The living standard is usually lower in the suburban area when compared to the urban area; consumers' awareness of food hygiene and safety is poorer and a less strict inspection of slaughter and trade of animals and

TABLE 3. Proportions of tetracycline-positive muscle samples and analysis of potential risk factors

Variables	No. of samples (n)	No. of positive samples	% Positive samples	95% Confidence interval	Fisher's exact test P value (α = 0.05)	Odd ratio (95% CI)
Season						
Early winter	137	6	4.38	[1.79, 9.70]	0.294514	1.53 [0.54, 4.12]
Early spring	153	10	6.54	[3.36, 12.01]		
Region						
Urban	135	3	2.22	[0.58, 6.86]	0.018414	4.03 [1.12, 14.45]
Suburban	155	13	8.39	[4.72, 14.21]		
Type of shop						
Pork only	159	7	4.40	[1.94, 9.21]	0.254633	1.6 [0.58, 4.42]
Pork and other(s)	131	9	6.87	[3.39, 13.01]		
Type of abattoir						
Municipal	45	1	2.22	[0.13, 14.41]	0.257001	2.87 [0.37, 22.39]
Household	245	15	6.22	[3.59, 10.10]		
Origin of meat						
Hanoi	238	14	5.88	[3.38, 9.88]	0.427928	1.56 [0.34, 7.09]
Other provinces	52	2	3.85	[0.67, 14.33]		
Daily offered amount						
Up to 100 kg	252	12	4.76	[2.60, 8.38]	0.142307	2.35 [0.72, 7.71]
>100 kg	38	4	10.53	[3.43, 25.74]		
Residence of owner						
Urban	111	3	2.70	[0.70, 8.28]	0.078638	2.82 [0.78, 10.13]
Nonurban	179	13	7.26	[4.08, 12.36]		
Education attainment of owner						
Primary	125	9	7.20	[3.55, 13.61]	0.201916	1.75 [0.63, 4.84]
Secondary	165	7	4.24	[1.87, 8.89]		
Total	290	16	5.52	[3.29, 8.98]		

animal products is assumed. So, the shop owners tend to buy cheaper meat and live animals including sick or even dead animals that very likely underwent antibiotic treatment. This leads to a potentially higher proportion of antibiotic residue in meat sold in this area.

The present study demonstrates that criteria for food safety may strongly be influenced by social factors, even within one city. It is, therefore, essential to include such factors, when designing further studies to assess the overall exposure of consumers in Vietnam to food-borne antibiotic residues.

REFERENCES

1. TEUBER, M. 2004. Veterinary use and antibiotic resistance. *In* Food Safety and Veterinary Public Health. Vol. 2: safety Assurance During Food Processing. F.J.M. Smulders & J.D. Collins, Eds.: 229–241. Wageningen Academic. Wageningen, NL.

2. BOISSEAU, J. 2002. Registration of veterinary drugs containing antimicrobials. Report of the project Strengthening of Veterinary Services in Vietnam (SVSV) ALA/96/20.

3. FAO. 2004. Review of the livestock sector in the Mekong countries. Livestock sector report. http://www.fao.org/ag/againfo/resources/en/publications/sector_reports/lsr_mekong.pdf, accessed 16th September 2004.

4. MẠNH, M.T. & N.M. TOÀN. 2003. Vì sao lọn Việt Nam có súc cạnh tranh thấp. http://www.vista.gov.vn/Anphamdientu/tapchitrongnuoc/hdkh/2003/so10/17.htm, accessed 28th August 2004.

5. LIÊN, K. 2004. Hà Nội vẫn khan hiếm thịt sạch. http://www.vneconomy.com.vn/vie/index.php?param=article&catid=0999&id=040706154906. Accessed 24th July 2004. Báo điện tử - Thời báo Kinh tế Việt Nam (Vietnam Economy) updated 06/07/2004.

6. TUAN, X.L. & Y. MUNEKAGE. 2004. Residues of selected antibiotics in water and mud from shrimp ponds in mangrove areas in Viet Nam. Marine Poll. Bull. **49:** 922–929.

7. THUẬN, D.T., N.N. TUÂN, V.T.T. AN, *et al.* 2003. Initial survey on antibiotics utilization in farms and its residue in pork and chickens raised in Binh Duong province. Khoa Học Kỹ Thuật Thú Y (Veterinary Science and Technique). **10:** 50–58.

8. VIETNAMTOURISM. 2005. Vietnam country and people: Climate. http://www.vietnamtourism. com/e_pages/country/overview.asp, accessed 17th June 2005.

9. SOP RES 31 V.8. 2002. The detection of residues of anti-bacterial substances in animal tissues (six plate method). Veterinary Sciences Division, Stoney Road, Stormont, BELFAST BT4 3SD.

10. MYLLYNIEMI, A.L., L. NUOTIO, E. LINDFORS, *et al.* 2001. A microbiological six-plate method for the identification of certain antibiotic groups in incurred kidney and muscle samples. Analyst **126:** 641–646.

11. AGENCE FRANÇAISE DESÉCURITÉ SANITAIRE DES ALIMENTS (AFSSA) MV/ITC/P06/25.AN – VERSION 2. "Determination of tetracycline residues in kidney and muscle by high performance liquid chromatography".

12. COMMITTEE FOR VETERINARY MEDICINAL PRODUCTS (CVMP). 1999. Antibiotic resistance in the European Union associated with therapeutic use of veterinary medicines: report and qualitative risk assessment by the CVMP (Report by the CVMP for the European Medicines Evaluation Agency (EMEA)). EMEA. London.
13. MILLER, D.J.S. 1993. Present state and trends in the use of veterinary drugs. Proceedings of the EuroResidue II conference. Veldhoven, the Netherlands. 3–5 May.
14. WHO. 2001. Antibiotic Resistance: synthesis of recommendations by expert policy groups. Alliance for the Prudent Use of Antibiotics. WHO/CDS/DRS/2001.10.
15. WALTER, J.V. 2005. Dietary research: why no animal products. http://www.amazingdiscoveries.org/amazingdiet/modern_animal_husbandry.htm, accessed 13th June 2005.
16. GOODMAN, G.A., L.S. GOODMAN, T.W. RALL & F. MURAD, Eds. 1985. The Pharmacological Basis of Therapeutics, 7th ed. MacMillan. New York.
17. MITCHELL, J., M.W. GRIFFITHS, S.A. McEWEN, et al. 1998. Antimicrobial drug residues in milk and meat: causes, concerns, prevalence, regulations, tests, and test performance. J. Food Protect. 61: 742–756.
18. KÜHNE, M., S. WEGMANN, A. KOBE & R. FRIES. 2000. Tetracycline residues in bones of slaughtered animals. Food Control. 11: 175–180.

Antimicrobial Resistance Phenotypes of ETEC Isolates from Piglets with Diarrhea in North Vietnam

N.T. DO,[a] H.P. CU,[a] N.N. NGUYEN,[a] X.H. NGUYEN,[a] X.T. AU,[a] T.H. VAN,[a] N.Q. VU AND D.J. TROTT[b]

[a]*Department of Bacteriology, National Institute of Veterinary Research, Dong da, 84 Hanoi, Vietnam*

[b]*School of Veterinary Science, The University of Queensland, QLD 4072 Australia*

ABSTRACT: Both disk diffusion and broth micro-dilution assays were employed to determine the level of resistance in Enterotoxigenic *Escherichia coli* (ETEC) isolates ($n = 170$) obtained from preweaning piglet colibacillosis from the two different pig production systems (commercial piggeries and small holder farmers) in Vietnam. Overall, tetracycline, streptomycin, amoxicillin, trimethoprim/sulfamethoxazole, and chloramphenicol showed markedly higher rates of resistance. Both apramycin and ceftiofur are active against all ETEC isolates. These antimicrobials could be recommended as the drugs of choice for the treatment of *E. coli* infections in young pigs in North Vietnam. Resistance to third-generation cephalosporin (ceftiofur, ceftazidime, and cefoxitin) was not observed in Vietnamese ETEC isolates. Multiple resistances to greater than three antimicrobials were widely distributed ($\sim$ 79.4%).

KEYWORDS: pigs; *Escherichia coli* (*E. coli*); colibacillosis; antimicrobial resistance

INTRODUCTION AND OBJECTIVES

Colibacillosis caused by enterotoxigenic *Escherichia coli* (ETEC) is one of the most important diseases of pre- and postweaning pigs.[1] In Vietnam, there exists the potential for antimicrobials to be abused for the control of diarrhea prevailing among piglets. However, a survey has never been conducted to determine the trends in drug resistance in Vietnamese ETEC isolates. The objective of this article was to determine the antimicrobial resistance profiles of ETEC isolates obtained from preweaning piglets with diarrhea to different antimicrobials.

Address for correspondence: Dr. Ngoc Thuy Do, Department of Bacteriology, 86 Truong Chinh Road, Dong da, 84 Hanoi, Vietnam. Voice: 84-4-8693923; fax: 84-4-8694082.
e-mail: dongocthuy73@yahoo.com

Ann. N.Y. Acad. Sci. 1081: 543–545 (2006). © 2006 New York Academy of Sciences.
doi: 10.1196/annals.1373.082

MATERIALS AND METHODS

ETEC isolates ($n = 126$) were obtained from preweaning piglets with diarrhea in North Vietnam. Samples were added to antimicrobial disks (16 types) and Muller–Hilton agar from Oxoid.

Disk diffusion antimicrobial susceptibility testing was performed and interpreted according to National Committee for Clinical Laboratory Standards (NCCLS) guidelines.[2]

RESULTS AND DISCUSSION

Antimicrobial resistance in the isolates definitely appeared to be directly associated with the frequent usage of a particular antimicrobial in pig populations. As expected, the majority of isolates (>65%) showed a high level of individual antimicrobial resistance, as evidenced by high minimum inhibitory concentration (MICs) to antimicrobials commonly used in the treatment of enteric disease in pigs in Vietnam, including tetracycline, streptomycin, amoxicillin, and trimethoprim/sulfamethoxazole (Fig. 1).

There are several important features associated with antimicrobial resistance in Vietnamese ETEC isolates. First, despite the absence of selective pressure associated with current usage, resistance to chloramphenicol was

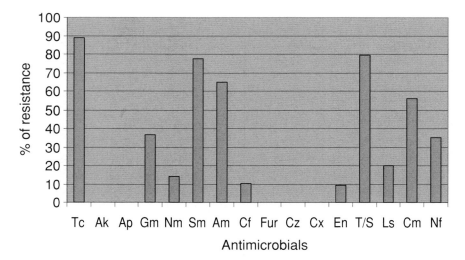

FIGURE 1. Antimicrobial resistance among ETEC isolates obtained from North Vietnam. Tc = tetracycline; Ak = amikacin; Ap = apramycin; Gm = gentamycin; Nm = neomycin; Sm = streptomycin; Am = amoxicillin; Cf = cephalothin; Fur = ceftiofur; Cz = ceftazidime; Cx = cefoxitin; En = enrofloxacin; T/S = trimethoprim/sulfamethoxazole; Ls = lincospectinomycin; Cm = chloramphenicol; Nf = nitrofurantoin.

still observed at a relatively high level ($>45\%$), suggesting the persistence of chloramphenicol-resistant gene(s) among *E. coli* populations. Second, all isolates were highly susceptible to antimicrobials that belonged to the third-generation cephalosporin class, including ceftiofur, ceftazidime, and cefoxitin. In terms of public health impact, this observation is very important as it suggested that the development and selection for extended spectrum β-lactamases (ESBLs) in isolates that could be potentially transferred through the food chain to humans do not occur in Vietnam. Third, multiple resistance to three or more agents was quite prevalent ($\geq 80\%$) among isolates, irrespective of origin. These results are in agreement with a general trend observed in porcine *E. coli* and may suggest a genetic linkage of resistance markers between enterotoxin genes and antimicrobial resistance genes among ETEC isolates, or between resistance genes among non-ETEC isolates.

In conclusion, because of the increasing problem of bacterial resistance, guidelines for the prudent use of antimicrobials, including the implementation of a veterinary antibiotic policy for food-producing animals is of utmost importance to safeguard the efficacy of antibiotic therapy for the future and to minimize public health risks associated with veterinary use in Vietnam.

ACKNOWLEDGMENTS

This work is supported by grants from Australian Centre for International Agricultural Research (ACIAR).

REFERENCES

1. BERTSCHINGER, H.U. & J.M. FAIRBROTHER. 1999. *Escherichia coli* infections. *In* Diseases of Swine. B.E. Straw, S. D'Allaire, W.L. Mengeling & D.J. Taylor, Eds.:431–468. Iowa State University Press. Ames, IA.
2. NCCLS 1999. *Performance Standards for Antimicrobial Disk and Dilution Susceptibility Tests for Bacteria Isolated from Animals; Approved Standard*. The National Committee for Clinical Laboratory Standards. Pennsylvania.

Influence of Different Diets on Growth Performance, Meat Quality, and Disease Resistance in Pig Crossbreeds (PIE × MC-local) and PIE (LW × MC- local)

NGUYEN QUANG LINH, NGUYEN THI BE, AND DINH THI DAO

Hue University of Agriculture and Forestry, 102 Phung Hung St. Hue, Vietnam

ABSTRACT: The present study evaluated the effect of different dietary formulations on the growth rate in pigs and their resistance to infection with hog cholera. Results indicate that growth rates can be enhanced by certain formulations and that there is a correlation between this increased growth rate and increased resistance to infection with hog cholera.

KEYWORDS: growing pigs; diets; growth; antibody titers; resistance

INTRODUCTION

Natural resistance to diseases may play an important role in survival and increased production in pigs. Vaccination programs and improved nutritional approaches may result in improved pig health. Variations in dietary composition can affect antibody levels in animals. Studies[1-5] have shown that the addition of fatty acids, vitamins A and C, and Selenium to the diet contribute to increased resistance to disease. It is thought that dietary-based increases in resistance may result in enhanced growth, particularly when pigs are raised under conditions in which disease transmission pressure is high. Dietary fiber content will impact gut microflora[4] versus using beer byproducts and fishmeal at 15% of the diet. The supplementation of probiotics containing *Bacillus (B.) lichbeniformis* and *B. subtilis* can also improve the health status of piglets. The present research aims at improving pig health status using different dietary formulations to increase growth performance and resistance to hog cholera.

METHODS

The study used 24 growing pigs weighing 7.45 ± 0.52 kg. Animals used were crossbred from the following breeds: Large White (LW), Mong Cai local

Address for correspondence: Nguyen Quang Linh, Hue University of Agriculture and Forestry, 102 Phung Hung St., Hue, Vietnam.
e-mail: edmour.blouin@okstate.edu

Ann. N.Y. Acad. Sci. 1081: 546–548 (2006). © 2006 New York Academy of Sciences.
doi: 10.1196/annals.1373.083

TABLE 1. Growth performance of pigs in different growing phases (g/day)

Age	Trials			
	I (n = 5)	II (n = 5)	III (n = 5)	IV (n = 5)
Month 1	369 ± 25.04	348 ± 27.22	389 ± 25.50	372 ± 25.71
Month 2	379 ± 25.00*	415 ± 24.16	402 ± 25.73*	382 ± 24.60
Month 3	425 ± 24.78	470 ± 24.34	456 ± 25.61	435 ± 25.42
Month 4	503 ± 25.13	495 ± 25.10	543 ± 26.11	520 ± 26.07
Average	481± 24.99^{a**}	471 ± 25.20^b	448± 25.24^{c**}	454± 27.4^d

a, b, c, d: the same row with significant differences, $P < 0.05$; *$P < 0.05$; **$P < 0.01$.

TABLE 2. The blocking (%) of antibody resistance to hog cholera vaccine in pigs

Injection	I (F1D1)	II (F1D2)	III(F2D1)	IV(F2D2)
1	45.38^a	40.32^b	38.48^c	31.2^d
2	49.8*	43.54*	37.86**	34.62**

a, b, c: the same row with significant differences, $P < 0.05$; *$P < 0.05$; **$P < 0.01$.

(MC), and Pietrain, (PIE). Pigs were separated into 4 groups of 6 animals each and fed two diets. Diet 1 (D1) had more dietary composition containing shrimp byproducts and fish meal. Diet 2 (D2) contained soya bean and nut cake meal, 15.5% crude protein, lysine 0.62%, methionin 0.31%, and 11.5 MJME per kg of fresh matter. Pigs were inoculated with hog cholera vaccine at 45 and 65 days of age. Serum samples were collected in two batches and analyzed for antibody titers to swine fever disease.

RESULTS AND DISCUSSION

The results described in TABLE 1 indicate differential growth performance based on differences in weight gains between the two diets and breeds. Pigs of PIE ×MC had higher growth rates than PIE × (LW × MC) (481 ± 45 g/day compared with 448.8 ± 52 g/day) for D1, $P < 0.01$. While pigs of PIE × (LW × MC) were higher than PIE × MC (471 ± 37 g/day compared with 454 ± 49) for D2, the difference was not significant. Meat quality of pigs from formulas (PIE × LW × MC) was better than PIE × MC in both diets. TABLE 2 lists the antibody titers to hog cholera indicating that pigs fed on D1 had higher titers than D2 in the first and second collection, 0.454 of PIE × MC and 0.385 of PIE × (LW × MC) in D1 compared with 0.403 of PIE × MC and 0.312 of PIE × (LW × MC) in first test, 0.498 and 0.379 compared with 0.435 and 0.346, respectively. Results indicate a correlation between growth rate and antibody titer, $R = 0.77$, $P < 0.01$.

REFERENCES

1. BERGERN, L.L. 1997. Zinc: Nutritional and Pharmacological Roles. University of Illinois. USA Ph.D. Thesis.
2. TUREK, J.J., I.A. SCHOENLEIN, B.A. WATKINS & W.G. VAN ALTINE. 1994. Dietary polyunsaturated fatty acids effect on immune cells of porcine lung. J. Leukoc. Biol. **56:** 599–604.
3. TUREK, J.J., I.A. SCHOENLEIN, B.A. WATKINS, *et al.* 1996. Dietary polyunsaturated fatty acids modulate immune responses of pigs to *Mycoplasma Hypopneumonia* infection. J. Nutr. **126:** 1541–1548.
4. NGUYEN, Q.L., H. EVERTS, H.T. HUE & A.C. BAYNEN. 2001. Feeding of spinach or sweet – potato leaves and growth performance of growing pigs kept on small farm in Central Vietnam. Trop. Anim. Health Prod. **26:** 815–822.
5. NGUYEN, Q.L., H. EVERTS & A.C. BEYNEN. 2003. Shrimp by-product feeding and growth performance of growing pigs kept on small holdings in central Vietnam. Aust J. Anim. Sci. **16:** 1025–1029.

Index of Contributors

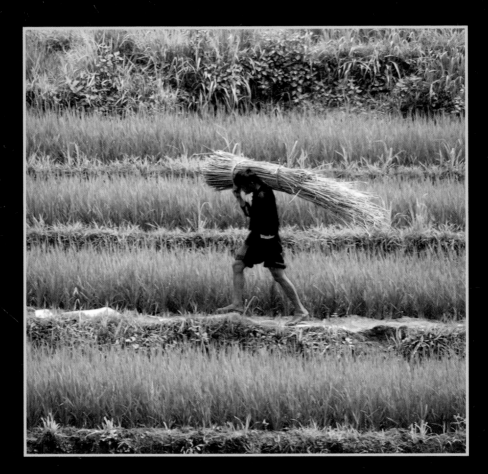

Cover art: Photos by Edmour Blouin
Cover design: Sally Kuzma

ISBN 1-57331-637-7

9 781573 316378